MASSACHUSETTS GENERAL HOSPITAL
Handbook of
General Hospital Psychiatry
Second Edition

MASSACHUSETTS GENERAL HOSPITAL

Handbook of General Hospital Psychiatry

Second Edition

Edited by

THOMAS P. HACKETT, MD

Eben S. Draper Professor of Psychiatry,
Harvard Medical School;
Chief of Psychiatry,
Massachusetts General Hospital,
Boston, Massachusetts

NED H. CASSEM, MD

Associate Professor of Psychiatry,
Harvard Medical School;
Chief, Psychiatric Consultation Service,
Massachusetts General Hospital,
Boston, Massachusetts

PSG PUBLISHING COMPANY, INC.
LITTLETON, MASSACHUSETTS

Library of Congress Cataloging in Publication Data
Main entry under title:

Massachusetts General Hospital handbook of general
  hospital psychiatry.

  Includes bibliographies and index.
  1. Psychiatry—Handbooks, manuals, etc.
I. Hackett, Thomas P. (Thomas Paul), 1928–
II. Cassem, Ned H., 1935–   . III. Massachusetts
General Hospital. IV. Title: Handbook of general
hospital psychiatry. [DNLM: 1. Disease—psychology.
2. Hospitals, General. 3. Mental Disorders.
WM 100 M414]
RC456.M37   1986   616'.001'9   85-28493
ISBN 0-88416-524-8

Published by:
PSG PUBLISHING COMPANY, INC.
545 Great Road
Littleton, Massachusetts 01460

International Standard Book Number: 0-88416-524-8

Library of Congress Catalog Card Number: 85-28493

Last digit is the print number: 9 8 7 6 5 4 3 2

Contributors

William H. Anderson, MD
Chairman, Department of Psychiatry, St. Elizabeth's Hospital;
Lecturer in Psychiatry, Harvard Medical School;
Associate Psychiatrist, Massachusetts General Hospital

Jerrold G. Bernstein, MD
Assistant Clinical Professor, Harvard Medical School;
Assistant Psychiatrist, Massachusetts General Hospital

Carolyn B. Bilodeau, MSN, CS
Independent Consultant and Educator;
Former Psychiatric Clinical Nurse Specialist, Massachusetts General Hospital

Anthony Bouckoms, MD
Assistant Professor of Psychiatry, Harvard Medical School;
Assistant in Psychiatry, Massachusetts General Hospital

Ned H. Cassem, MD
Associate Professor of Psychiatry, Harvard Medical School;
Chief, Psychiatric Consultation Service,
Massachusetts General Hospital

James E. Groves, MD
Assistant Clinical Professor, Harvard Medical School;
Associate Psychiatrist, Massachusetts General Hospital

Thomas P. Hackett, MD
Eben S. Draper Professor of Psychiatry, Harvard Medical School;
Chief of Psychiatry, Massachusetts General Hospital

David B. Herzog, MD
Assistant Professor of Psychiatry, Harvard Medical School;
Assistant Psychiatrist, Massachusetts General Hospital

Michael S. Jellinek, MD
Assistant Professor of Psychiatry, Harvard Medical School;
Associate Psychiatrist, Massachusetts General Hospital

Anastasia Kucharski, MD
Clinical Instructor in Psychiatry, Harvard Medical School;
Clinical Associate in Psychiatry, Massachusetts General Hospital

Theo C. Manschreck, MD
Associate Professor of Psychiatry, Harvard Medical School;
Associate Psychiatrist, Massachusetts General Hospital

George B. Murray, MD
Associate Professor of Psychiatry, Harvard Medical School;
Associate Psychiatrist, Massachusetts General Hospital

Suzanne O. O'Connor, MSN, CS
Nursing Consultant and Educator;
Psychiatric Clinical Nurse Specialist, Massachusetts General Hospital

Mark H. Pollack, MD
Instructor in Psychiatry, Harvard Medical School;
Clinical Fellow in Psychiatry, Massachusetts General Hospital

John A. Renner, Jr, MD
Clinical Instructor in Psychiatry, Harvard Medical School;
Associate Psychiatrist, Massachusetts General Hospital

Jerrold F. Rosenbaum, MD
Assistant Professor of Psychiatry, Harvard Medical School;
Assistant Psychiatrist, Massachusetts General Hospital

Theodore A. Stern, MD
Assistant Professor of Psychiatry, Harvard Medical School;
Assistant Psychiatrist, Massachusetts General Hospital

Thomas D. Stewart, MD
Assistant Professor of Psychiatry, Harvard Medical School;
Director, Consultation/Liaison Service,
Beth Israel Hospital

Owen S. Surman, MD
Assistant Professor of Psychiatry, Harvard Medical School;
Associate Psychiatrist, Massachusetts General Hospital

James M. Vaccarino, JD
Vice President, Johnson and Higgins of Massachusetts, Inc.

Avery D. Weisman, MD
Professor of Psychiatry Emeritus, Harvard Medical School;
Senior Psychiatrist, Massachusetts General Hospital

Charles A. Welch, MD
Instructor in Psychiatry, Harvard Medical School;
Associate Psychiatrist, Massachusetts General Hospital

To Eleanor Mayher Hackett

—T.P.H.

Contents

Preface to the Second Edition

Nearly a decade has gone by since the first edition of this book was published. In the course of that time, consultation psychiatry has contributed to the remedicalization of our specialty and to the burgeoning number of psychiatry services in general hospitals throughout this country. The growth of general hospital psychiatry has become a fact of American hospital life. For example, within the greater Boston area it is hard to find a general hospital that does not contain a psychiatric inpatient service along with outpatient facilities and a consultation service. This is in marked contrast to the health care landscape of the 1960s when it was unusual to find psychiatric facilities in any hospital under 100 beds. A variety of factors account for this proliferation of psychiatric services. Economic incentives are important. Reimbursement policies of insurers are apt to favor psychiatric patients in general hospitals rather than those in psychiatric hospitals. The deinstitutionalization movement has mandated an expansion of alternative psychiatric facilities. In addition, however, is the inescapable fact that psychiatric treatment has become far more effective in the last 15 years than it ever was before and depends much less on long inpatient stays. Psychiatry has emerged from its largely passive psychoanalytic stance of the 1950s and 1960s to become one of the most therapeutically successful clinical specialties in medicine.

The fact that psychiatry has now assumed a role more central to the practice of medicine requires the psychiatrist to insure that his identity as physician is secure. There is no better way to establish medical identity than through consultation psychiatry. Our handbook retains its medical orientation. It is an update of the first edition with a few changes in authorship and two deletions. Chapters on the Private Consultation Service and The Hypnosis and Psychosomatic Clinic have been deleted in the interest of economies of space. The chapter on suicide has been incorporated in the chapter on disruptive patients. All of the psychiatrists who author chapters are members of the Department of Psychiatry at Massachusetts General Hospital (MGH), and most of them are actively involved in the practice of consultation psychiatry. The only exception is James Vaccarino, who was for many years the Director of Legal Affairs at MGH and is now Vice President of the firm Johnson and Higgins, which specializes in medical malpractice.

The practice of consultation psychiatry in the Department of Psychiatry as well as in this hospital enjoys a high priority of support and amenity. We thank what for us must be a benevolent providence for our participation in the life of a hospital that has been a home and a haven to some of the finest clinicians, scientists, and medical leaders in the world.

Thomas P. Hackett, MD
Ned H. Cassem, MD

1

Beginnings: Consultation Psychiatry in a General Hospital

THOMAS P. HACKETT

HISTORY

The history of general hospital psychiatry in the United States is elusive for the student who likes facts and dates neatly packaged. The seeds of consultation psychiatry were sown somewhat haphazardly whenever a medical staff member showed interest in mental disorders, whenever a disturbed patient had a medical problem, or whenever a medical patient had an emotional problem. For those interested in a more detailed account of the development of consultation-liaison psychiatry in the United States, I recommend the work of that doughty and venerable scholar, Z.J. Lipowski. He has provided an encyclopedic guide to the published information on this psychiatric subspecialty, and I commend this sensible and readable review to the student.[1-5]

There has been some controversy over the last few years concerning the use of the term liaison in consultation-liaison (C/L) psychiatry. We believe that using the term liaison is confusing and unnecessary. It is confusing because no other service in the practice of medicine employs the term for its consultation activities. In addition, the meaning it conveys—to teach nonpsychiatrists psychiatric and interpersonal skills —is done as a matter of course during the routine consultation. For quite a while the dual role of the consultant as both clinician and teacher was joined by a hyphen as in consultation-liaison. More recently some writers have emphasized what they consider the greater importance of the liaison component by deleting the word consultation.[6] We prefer to retain the older term and trust that our readers will understand that when we speak of consultation psychiatry, this means that all the necessary liaison activities—teaching the nonpsychiatric caregivers what they need to know about the psychiatric management of the case—will be carried out.

If the course of consultation psychiatry over the last decade is

1

examined, 1975 seems to be the watershed year. Before 1975 scant attention was given to the work of psychiatrists in medicine. Consultation topics were seldom presented at the national meetings of the American Psychiatric Association. Even the American Psychosomatic Society, which has many strong links to consultation work, rarely gave more than a nod of acknowledgement to presentations or panels discussing this aspect of psychiatry. Residency training programs on the whole were no better. In 1966 Mendel surveyed training programs in the United States to determine the extent to which residents were exposed to a training experience in consultation psychiatry.[7] He found that 75% of the 202 programs surveyed offered some training in consultation psychiatry, but most of it was informal and poorly organized. Ten years later Schubert and McKegney found only "a slight increase" in the amount of time devoted to consultation liaison training in residency programs.[8] Today, it is unusual to find a psychiatric residency program which does not include time on a C/L Service. Indeed, C/L training is now mandated by the American Board of Psychiatry and Neurology.

There are a number of reasons for this growth. One was the leadership of Dr James Eaton, former Director of the Psychiatric Education Branch of the National Institute of Mental Health (NIMH). Dr Eaton provided support and encouragement in establishing consultation-liaison programs throughout the country. Another reason for this growth is the burgeoning interest in the primary care specialties, which require skills in psychiatric diagnosis and treatment. The growth of consultation psychiatry has also been stimulated by the attack on psychiatry from an army of self-appointed counselors and psychotherapists, all claiming to possess the same order of skill as the psychiatrist and all demanding recognition by third-party payers. The vigor of competition for patients has caused even those psychiatrists who most avidly sought a career in pure psychotherapy to start closing ranks with their fellow physicians to form a phalanx against the opposition. The medical model has become the guidon around which embattled psychiatrists are attempting to rally. Very little in the training of the psychiatrist is more germane to the medical model than consultation psychiatry. For these reasons of commerce, as well as the natural growth of medicine in psychiatry, consultation work has enjoyed a renaissance.

I trace the origin of organized interest in the mental life of patients at the Massachusetts General Hospital to 1873 when James Jackson Putnam, a young Harvard neurologist, returned from his grand tour of German departments of medicine to practice his specialty. He was awarded a small office under the arch of one of the famous twin flying staircases of the Bulfinch Building. The office was the size of a cupboard and was designed to house electrical equipment. Putnam was given the title of "Electrician." One of his duties was to ensure the proper functioning of various galvanic and faradic devices then used to treat nervous and muscular disorders. It is no coincidence that his office came to be called the "cloaca maxima" by the Professor of Medicine, George Shattuck. This designation stemmed from the fact that patients whose maladies defied diagnosis and treatment—in short, "the crocks"—were referred to young Putnam. With such a beginning it is not difficult for today's consultation psychiatrist to find a familiar anlage in J.J. Putnam. Dr Putnam eventually became a professor of neuropathology and practiced both neurology and psychiatry. He treated medical and surgical patients who developed mental disorders. Dr Putnam's distinguished career, interwoven with the acceptance of Freudian psychology in the United States, is chronicled elsewhere.[9]

In the late 1920s, Dr Howard Means, Chief of Medicine, appointed Boston psychiatrist Robert Herman to study patients who developed mental disturbances in conjunction with endocrine disorders. Dr Herman's studies are hardly remembered today, although he is honored by having a conference room named after him.

In 1934 a Department of Psychiatry took shape when Stanley Cobb was given the Bullard Chair of Neuropathology and granted sufficient money by the Rockefeller Foundation to establish a ward for the study of psychosomatic conditions. Under Dr Cobb's tutelage the department expanded and became known for its eclecticism and for its interest in the mind-brain relationship. A number of European emigrants fleeing Nazi tyranny were welcomed to the department by Dr Cobb. Felix and Helene Deutsch, Edward and Grete Bibring, and Hans Sachs were early arrivals from the Continent. Erich Lindemann came in the mid-1930s and worked with Dr Cobb on a series of projects, the most notable being his study of grief. This came as a result of his work with victims of the 1942 Coconut Grove fire.

When Dr Lindemann became chief of the psychiatric service in 1954, the consultation service had not yet been established. Customarily the resident assigned to night call in the emergency room saw all medical and surgical patients needing psychiatric evaluation. This was regarded as an onerous task, and such calls were often set aside until after supper in the hope that the disturbance might quiet in the intervening hours. Notes in the chart were terse and often impractical. Seldom was there a follow-up. As a result, animosity toward psychiatry grew. To remedy this, Dr Lindemann officially established the Psychiatric Consultation Service under the leadership of Avery Weisman in 1956. As Dr Weisman's resident, I divided my time between doing consultations and learning outpatient psychotherapy. During the first year of the consultation service, 130 consultations were made. In 1958 the number of consultations increased to 370, and we organized an active research program that later became one of the cornerstones of the overall operation.

By 1960 a rotation through the consultation service had become a mandatory part of the MGH residency in psychiatry. Second-year residents were each assigned two wards. Each resident spent 20 to 30 hours a week in the consultation service for a 6-month period. This still holds. Between 1956 and 1960 the service attracted the interest of fellowship students who contributed postgraduate work on psychosomatic topics. Medical students also began to choose the consultation service as part of their elective in psychiatry during this period. From our work with these fellows and medical students, collaborative research studies were initiated with other services. Examples of these studies are (1) the surgical treatment of intractable pain,[10,11] (2) the compliance of duodenal ulcer patients with their medical regimen,[12] (3) postamputation depression in the elderly patient,[13] (4) emotional maladaptation in the surgical patient,[14–17] and (5) the psychological aspect of acute myocardial infarction.[18,19]

By 1970 we had a complement of ten staff members doing almost full-time consultation work (nine of these supported by research grants; the tenth, by hospital salary), six residents, and a chief resident who was assigned full-time to the service. Growth has continued.

We now offer a fellowship program in psychosomatic medicine that has added three fellows and one full-time faculty member to our roster. A private psychiatric consultation service has been established. A somatic therapy unit has been added to evaluate and treat patients for refractory depression and chronic pain syndromes. A consultant is now assigned on a part-time basis to the renal dialysis unit, to the rehabilitation service, and to the medical and surgical intensive care units. There is also an active consultation service in the child psychiatry division. An outpatient psychosomatic clinic continues to function not only as a follow-up facility but as a place where hypnosis, behavioral therapy, and biofeedback are done. The cardiac rehabilitation unit contains an active psychiatric presence in the form of two staff members who carry out psychiatric evaluations, test for type A behavior, and conduct group therapy to modify this behavior pattern. Each month several medical students rotate through the consultation service. Second- and third-year psychiatric residents from other programs also come to us for training in consultation work. Our research has continued to focus on clinical problems. There are active programs investigating the treatment of chronic pain, delirium, dementia, the emotional problems associated with myocardial infarction and cancer, and a variety of other clinical projects. Since there is no basic science facility available to us, our work has been largely devoted to clinical studies, which we encourage our fellows and residents to participate in.

PATIENT CARE, TEACHING, AND RESEARCH

The three functions provided by any consultation service are patient care, teaching, and research. Each of these will be considered separately here.

Patient Care

Approaching a patient in a consultation capacity is different from meeting a patient in the context of outpatient psychotherapy. The consultation patient has not necessarily asked to see a psychiatrist and may, in fact, actively resist the interview. The proper introduction of the consultant to the patient by the referring physician is crucial. If the introduction is made in a relaxed, natural way, particularly if the consultee can make it appear routine, there is seldom much resistance. If, on the other hand, the consultee is uneasy or embarrassed to have his patient seen by a psychiatrist, there is a possibility of discord in the initial contact. The consultation psychiatrist should take every opportunity to let physicians requesting consultation know how important the initial introduction is. Young house officers experience the most difficulty in requesting psychiatric consultations. Those from medical schools where psychiatry is taught well and thoroughly readily use the consultation service with minimal uncertainty or embarrassment. Others, less fortunate in their training, require time to familiarize themselves with our specialty and need our patience and goodwill along the way. By the time these young physicians finish their residency training and join the staff, they have usually assimilated enough diplomacy to make a psychiatric referral without distress to patient or consultant. They have seen first-hand that the psychiatrist can provide effective care without offense to the patient. As the internist and surgeon employ the skills of the psychiatrist they recognize the limitations of our specialty as well as its many uses. Not only do they learn the problems with which the consultant can help, but they also learn the individual consultant's areas of expertise. They also learn to match a specific psychiatrist's style with the patient's temperament or problem.

There has been a growing acceptance in some hospitals of the role of psychiatry in general medicine. At Massachusetts General Hospital approximately 8% to 10% of all general hospital admissions are seen by a psychiatric consultant. This is a high percentage when compared with the national average, but it is not unique. On certain of our services, such as cardiac surgery, with its high incidence of postcardiotomy delirium, the percentage is as high as 40%. The statistics vary from month to month, depending on the energy and interest of the individual consultant and depending on the medical or surgical attending physicians who serve as visits to the wards. (A visit is a staff physician who is assigned to supervise a ward.) A visit who scorns psychiatric intervention is not likely to encourage house officers to call in a consultant. The *MGH News*, a monthly publication for our hospital, in an article on the consultation service, described some typical reasons for psychiatric consultation. Some of these were chronic pain, depression secondary to an illness, and fear of impending surgery. This article clearly enunciates that the psychiatrist does not only deal with the mentally ill, but most commonly handles a variety of problems which occur in conjunction with medical illness. Not a small number of consultees have quoted this article to the patients they refer for consultation to assure them they are not being singled out or regarded as "mental."

Interviewing. Each consultation psychiatrist has a personal style. In the hope that it may be helpful to the novice consultant, I have given a brief description here of my personal approach to the consultation interview.

Generally the first visit is by way of introduction. It takes 15 minutes to peruse the chart, particularly if the patient has been hospitalized for any length of time; another five to ten minutes to contact the nurse; and another few minutes to speak with a family member, if one is present. As a consequence, the initial visit may be in the nature of a sortie during which contact is established—hopefully contact that will dispel whatever alien image the patient may have of a psychiatrist.

I do my best to be friendly when I meet a patient for the first time—not effusive, but decidedly amiable and interested. I want to learn something about this individual in a short time, and to do so I need his help. A frozen professional manner is not apt to elicit anything but hostile reserve. I seldom explain why I have come. My assumption is that has already been discussed by the referring physician. If the patient appears confused, I try to explain my presence, but when there is uncertainty and suspicion about who requested the consultation and why, I often defer further contact until the referring physician can explain the consultation request to the patient.

I usually begin the interview by asking for a brief medical history of the present illness. This assures the patient of my interest in the medical aspects of his condition, underscores my professional identity, and allows me the chance to note how the patient's psychology has unfolded in response to the progression of symptoms. Does he include his emotional reactions to the events he describes? If so, are they appropriate? Is there evidence that his response is influenced by family problems? What limitations or opportunities has his illness elicited? Soon the roles of people and events coincident with the illness begin to take shape. I spend the rest of my time asking questions relevant to the central issues of the apparent problem. If we unearth sensitive material about which the patient appears reluctant to talk, I seldom press the issue. Instead, I will return later in the day or the following day, giving the patient time to question his physician again about my coming. To gain the patient's trust, I make a specific appointment for the second interview. By keeping the appointment, I show the patient through token behavior that I keep my promises. To further encourage trust, I am usually willing to answer most personal questions. I want the patient to know something of me.

I never take notes during the first interview and seldom in subsequent contacts unless the events of the case are complicated. Writing while talking is fine for some, but it does not fit my style. Quite consistent with my style, however, is taking a patient's pulse, listening to his chest, or examining a superficial lesion if it is called for. If I suspect that a medical diagnosis has been overlooked, I will conduct the necessary noninvasive examination.

Depending on the specific information of the case, the initial interview may last anywhere from 15 minutes to 1 1/2 hours. I make it a point to do at least one follow-up visit while the patient is in the hospital. If this cannot be done, I often attempt to contact him by telephone to find out how he is. In any case, I discuss with the patient how often I intend to see him. If I come to believe that he will need psychiatric outpatient treatment, I will refer him to someone else if I am unable to do the task myself. I always explain the reason for this referral. It is my practice to inform patients of any shift in medication, change in plans for surgery, or indeed any alteration in care that stems from my visit. I will give them my opinions, explaining that their physicians will decide how to act on my recommendations.

The consultation environment is unpredictable. The consultant may arrive on the scene only to find visitors present. A nurse or technician may come along to draw blood or record a vital function at an inopportune moment during the conversation. Finding a quiet and private spot is difficult. It requires flexibility and an understanding of hospital life. It is always best to alert the ward charge nurse that a consultant is on the way in order to advise visitors that their stay may be interrupted. A friendly nurse who knows something of the consultant's needs can be helpful in finding a corner where the patient and consultant can meet without interruption. Whenever possible I take the patient to an examining room or a vacant office. If the interview must be conducted in the presence of others, I draw the curtain about the bed and begin my questions. If I sense restraint or uneasiness, I will ask if the patient would prefer a private setting. While such requests are rare, the need for a private setting should be honored even if it means moving other patients away for an hour or two. Oddly enough, one can usually maintain the illusion of privacy behind a drawn curtain or screen.

As a matter of courtesy I sit down when interviewing or visiting patients. Long accustomed to the ritual of making rounds, many physicians remain standing as a matter of course. Standing, physicians remind me of missiles about to be launched, poised to depart. Even if this is not necessarily true, they look the part. Patients sense this, and it limits conversation. In addition, when standing, the physician necessarily looks down on the patient. This disparity in height is apt to encourage the attribution of arrogance. Looking down at a patient who is prone emphasizes the dependency of the position. Sitting at the bedside equalizes station. Sitting with a patient need not take longer than standing with him.

Write-Up.   There are two types of write-up. One is for the medical record; the second is for the central or research file record (discussed in the section on research). The write-up for the patient's chart should be brief and simply written. It should contain a diagnosis and practical suggestions. Rarely is it necessary to cover more than one page of chart paper. Negative findings need not be listed. Confidential information should never be included. If the reason for the consultation request has not been put into the chart by the consultee, it should be stated by the consultant if it can be done without embarrassing the patient. A brief statement of the problems should be made and the pertinent findings listed. A brief differential diagnosis and working diagnosis should be outlined followed by a list of recommendations in numerical order. Some consultants possess a fine literary style. This is commendable. An observation that identifies any unique aspect of the case is apt to enhance the consultation. A sense of humor is always valuable if it is kept in mind that the record can become part of a public document in court.

Conversation with the physician who referred the patient is more than politeness. Only a limited amount can be expressed in a note, however complete it may be. Always there are nuances of feeling and sometimes historical data as well that cannot be committed to the chart. Any exchange by telephone or in person is not only good public relations, but sound medical practice. The language used by the consultant must be compatible with the referring physician's psychiatric vocabulary.

The charge nurse on the floor is a crucial figure to consult in any evaluation of a patient. The nurse will know as much about him as anyone on the floor and perhaps more about his personality and the family interactions than will his physician. The way in which the patient or his family relates to nurses may be informative. Nurses' opinions, when pertinent, should be included in evaluations, and data should be shared with them. If the patient happens to be especially troublesome, a brief visit with all of the nurses at the change of shift, to ensure maximum attendance, is sometimes helpful. If there is a nurse-clinician who has been involved in the patient's case, she should be included in the consultant's plan for treatment.

Teaching

Most consultation psychiatrists believe that teaching psychiatry to medical and surgical house officers cannot be done on a formal basis. When teaching is formalized in weekly lectures or discussion groups, attendance invariably lags. Twenty years ago Erich Lindemann, in an attempt to educate medical house officers about the emotional problems of their patients, enlisted the help of several psychiatric luminaries from the Boston area. A series of biweekly lectures was announced, at which Edward and Grete Bibring, Felix and Helene Deutsch, Stanley Cobb, and Carl Binger, among others, were to share their knowledge and skills. In the beginning, approximately one fifth of the medical house officers attended. Attendance steadily dwindled in subsequent sessions until finally the psychiatry residents had to be forced to attend in order to infuse the lecturers with enough spirit to continue. I believe that if Sigmund Freud could have been resurrected and persuaded to hold luncheon meetings every other week for the medical staff, his reception would have been no more enthusiastic.

Teaching is best done at the bedside on a case-by-case basis. The exceptional house officer who wants more instruction should be given it. Whenever teaching is attempted, the chief of the service involved should be approached to ensure support. Without it the most modest teaching attempt is likely to falter. The chiefs of all services should be made aware that the psychiatric consultant is willing and available to teach.

Good teaching begins with providing information in a good consultation. It can develop further in conversations between consultant and consultee. Discussion with nurses and house officers is desirable and should occur naturally. That should be the initial goal of informed consultation teaching. More formal teaching should generally be avoided, lest the reward be disappointment and unintended rebuff.

We make ourselves available to nursing students and graduate nurses, and offer continuing programs of education as requested. The same is true for social workers and, to a limited extent, for occupational therapists and physiotherapists.

Teaching medical students is a major part of the pedagogic responsibility of the consultation service. Between two and four medical students are assigned to us on an elective basis each month. Each is assigned to a resident on the consultation service with whom they see cases. In addition, they are mentored by the chief of the consultation service who often will see cases with them, particularly in the evening. In addition, we provide them with formal teaching two hours a week and individual supervision for one hour a week. They are encouraged to behave as resident physicians and to carry out their clinical duties responsibly and diligently.

The teaching of psychiatric residents rotating through the consultation service is a more complicated topic. As a general outline, each resident is supervised individually for one to two hours each week. In teaching we have walk rounds five days a week with Dr Cassem, Chief of the Consultation Service. In walk rounds each case seen is reviewed and new cases are examined and interviewed by Dr Cassem. Once a week during walk rounds, I interview a patient in depth and lead a discussion. A weekly psychosomatic conference is held in which a resident presents a topic he has researched. The ensuing discussion is led by a local or visiting expert. The consultation fellows have their own walk rounds with Drs George Murray and Ned Cassem. Each new group of residents is given a set of lecture demonstrations on hypnosis and a course in the fundamentals of consultation psychiatry. Each second-year class receives a series of lectures on the history of psychosomatic medicine and a view of current work in the field.

Research

Research activity by the consultation service is important in building bridges between medical specialties. When physicians from other services are involved in research planning and when there is dual authorship of published accounts, friendships are firmly bonded and differences fade. The general hospital population provides such a cornucopia of research material that a consultation service would be lax or unresponsive not to take advantage of it.

Small research projects are the cornerstone of larger ones. Research need not be funded through federal or state agencies. Projects can be done as "arbeits" and assigned as such to medical students during their month on the service. They can also be suggested to fellows for more extensive development over the course of the year. What begins as an arbeit with results and conclusions to be presented at psychiatric grand rounds can, over a period of a year, develop into full-fledged publication. This in turn might be the starting point for a larger investigation.

A filing system should be designed to keep potential research materials readily accessible. Recently, a system of computer-based records in consultation services has been described. Dr James Strain and his associates have devised this system, and it is now in use in a number of consultation-liaison services throughout the country.[20]

Since the seed of research in consultation psychiatry is the contact between patient and consultant, the recording of this contact is central. In addition to the notes in the patient chart, the consultation psychiatrist should make what we call a context recording for each consultation encounter with patient, family, or hospital staff. This is a technique Dr Avery D. Weisman and I developed while working with dying patients. A context recording is a freely associated dictation on everything that comes to mind about the patient and the interview. It is dictated with no attempt at order in an effort to get every fact, incidental as well as obviously pertinent, into the record. No attempt is made at style, literacy, or organization. It is simply a way of putting on paper all that can be remembered. This method is especially valuable when unusual cases turn up that may have future research value or use as a vignette to illustrate an article. It is designed to be a reservoir of facts for future research.

Activity and lively thinking are the lifeblood of research. In order to keep the circulation flowing, research conferences must be held weekly or monthly to discuss current work and to plan new projects. It seems congruent with consultation psychiatry to emphasize a clinical orientation toward research rather than a laboratory approach, but one does not preclude the other.

Once the direction of the consultation team has been pointed toward research and publication, the results usually fall into line. One of the distressing roadblocks en route to publication is the poor writing skill of many physicians. One or two resource people who can serve as editors and teachers can be of great help. For a number of years we have held a weekly writing seminar in which members submit manuscripts which are reviewed by the seminar group and two senior faculty members. Both of the latter have proven track records for publication and an interest in developing the writing skills of their younger colleagues. Sometimes it is advantageous to hire a professional editor. All efforts seem worth the candle once the printed page is in the author's hand. When a service begins to develop a shelf of publications authored by various members of the team, a pride of accomplishment unfolds, compounding the excitement of the research and stimulating renewed academic effort.

REFERENCES

1. Lipowski ZJ: Psychosomatic medicine: Past and present. Part I—Historical background. Part II—Current state. Part III—Current research. *Can J Psychiatry* 1986; 31:2–21.
2. Lipowski ZJ: Review of consultation psychiatry and psychosomatic medicine. I: General principles. *Psychosom Med* 1967; 29:153–171.
3. Lipowski ZJ: Review of consultation psychiatry and psychosomatic medicine. II: Clinical aspects. *Psychosom Med* 1967; 29:201–224.
4. Lipowski ZJ: Review of consultation psychiatry and psychosomatic medicine. III: Theoretical issues. *Psychosom Med* 1968; 30:395–421.
5. Lipowski ZJ: Consultation-liaison psychiatry: an overview. *Am J Psychiatry* 1974; 131:623–630.
6. Strain JJ, Grossman S: *Psychological Care of the Medically Ill: A Primer in Liaison Psychiatry.* New York, Appleton-Century-Crofts, 1975.
7. Mendel WM: Psychiatric consultation education—1966. *Am J Psychiatry* 1966; 123:150–155.
8. Schubert DSP, McKegney FP: Psychiatric consultation education—1976. *Arch Gen Psychiatry* 1976; 33:1271–1273.
9. Hale NG: *Freud and the Americans.* New York, Oxford University Press, 1971.
10. White JC, Sweet WH, Hackett TP: Radiofrequency leukotomy for the relief of pain. *Arch Neurol* 1960; 2:317–330.
11. Mark VH, Hackett TP: Surgical aspects of thalamotomy in the human. *Trans Am Neurol Assoc* 1959; 92–94.
12. Hernandez M, Hackett TP: The problem of nonadherence to therapy in the management of duodenal ulcer recurrences. *Am J Dig Dis* 1962; 7:1047–1060.
13. Caplan LM, Hackett TP: Prelude to death: emotional effects of lower limb amputation in the aged. *N Engl J Med* 1963; 269:1166–1171.
14. Weisman AD, Hackett TP: Psychosis after eye surgery: establishment of a specific doctor-patient relation and the prevention and treatment of "black patch delirium." *N Engl J Med* 1958; 258:1284–1289.
15. Weisman AD, Hackett TP: Predilection to death: death and dying as a psychiatric problem. *Psychosom Med* 1961; 23:232–257.
16. Hackett TP, Weisman AD: Psychiatric management of operative syndromes I: The therapeutic consultation and the effect of noninterpretive intervention. *Psychosom Med* 1960; 22:267–282.

17. Hackett TP, Weisman AD: Psychiatric management of operative syndromes II: Psychodynamic factors in formulation and management. *Psychosom Med* 1960; 22:356–372.
18. Olin HS, Hackett TP: The denial of chest pain in thirty-two patients with acute myocardial infarction. *JAMA* 1964; 190:977–981.
19. Cassem NH, Hackett TP: Psychiatric consultation in a coronary care unit. *Ann Intern Med* 1971; 75:9–14.
20. Taintor Z, Spikes J, Gise LH, et al: Recording psychiatric consultation: A preliminary report. *Gen Hosp Psychiatry* 1979; 1:139–149.

2
Alcoholism: Acute and Chronic States

THOMAS P. HACKETT

From cases of simple intoxication, when the diagnosis can be made on the basis of breath odor and slurred speech, to the more complicated mental status of withdrawal states, alcohol is responsible for more psychiatric syndromes in general hospitals than any other substance consumed. Even when problem drinking is not in the immediate picture, a past history of alcoholism or heavy social drinking predisposes the patient to postoperative delirium and seems to lower his threshold for other types of delirium as well (see chapters 5, 6). Heavy drinkers have a higher than usual incidence of delirium in conjunction with fever, head trauma, and massive burns. This may be related to the neuropathologic changes in the brain that have been reported to occur in heavy drinkers and alcoholics.

DRUNKENNESS

Inebriation, by far the most prevalent toxic manifestation of drinking, is rarely discussed in the literature of consultation psychiatry. Of the conditions that come to the attention of the psychiatrist in the emergency room or overnight ward of a general hospital, few are potentially more threatening, disruptive, and dangerous. Standard medical textbooks offer little help in handling this problem even though it is the most common drug intoxication found in the United States and has been linked with all manner of violent crimes and assaults. Few sights are more frightening than that of a young and powerful man drunk, mindlessly angry, yet in full possession of his motor coordination and muscular power. Loud, truculent, and unreasonable, such an individual poses a genuine menace to those about him. What are the principles of management in such a case?

Management

For handling these individuals a regimen has been developed at Massachusetts General Hospital (MGH) that has proved effective in

14

most cases. The first principle is to alert the hospital police or security force before starting an interview with a boisterous drunk. While police intervention is seldom required, it is reassuring to have assistance ready if one expects trouble. This is especially true if the patient is armed or has a history of combativeness.

The second principle of our regimen is to suggest that the personal manner of the interviewer be tolerant and nonthreatening. People who possess a skill for disarming the abusive drunk seem to have little or no need to express their authority or toughness even though they may have both qualities in abundance. They can tolerate insults, threats, and oaths because they do not take them personally. Conversely, we have observed that individuals who galvanize the alcoholic person's anger and mobilize his aggression are often autocratic and rigid people whose thin sense of security is easily punctured by invective from the inebriate. The successful interviewer temporarily accepts the drunk as he is; the unsuccessful interviewer instantly attempts to make him civil. The latter effort usually backfires. In approaching the alcoholic person, a handshake of introduction should be extended. Unless the patient is known, he should be addressed by his proper name, for example, "Mr. Smith." For the time being no attempt should be made to change his behavior. Better to listen to a tirade and attempt to make sense of it than to demand that he lower his voice and talk more temperately. This is especially important if you wish to uncover a legitimate grievance or misunderstanding that, if present and correctable, can quickly alleviate the patient's bellicosity.

It is advisable to avoid direct eye contact for more than a few seconds at a time. More than momentary eye contact is often taken as a challenge and becomes the prelude to combat for humans as well as for animals. The interviewer should listen seriously to what the patient has to say and appear puzzled or perplexed rather than angry or amused if the accusation or complaint is absurd. Above all, it is important to avoid any posture of belligerence. A colleague once observed that he patterned his behavior with hostile drunks after the humble-submissive posture assumed by a wolf when bested in battle. Transposed to the human habitus, this physician kept eyes downcast, fists unclenched, and shoulders stooped. Once the patient sees that the interviewer is not going to attack him, his outburst may quiet, his anger slacken.

The third principle is to offer food. Some of the more antagonistic alcoholic individuals have been soothed by the offer of coffee. If the individual is willing to leave the scene with the inducement of coffee, food, and quiet (luring him with the promise of a beer is the last resort), he should be escorted to a lobby or foyer where people are within easy calling distance. Many alcoholic persons are claustrophobic and feel trapped in small rooms. Those with underlying homosexual conflicts, sometimes found in alcoholic persons, might associate the closeness of tiny quarters with the fear of sexual advance. Furthermore, it is discomforting for most physicians to be in an enclosed area with a potentially violent person. The value of offering food, cigarettes, or drink in this case can be justified on empirical evidence only. If the patient will eat, he will lose his fight. The next step is to persuade him to take a sedative and go to bed.

As in handling other conditions of psychotic excitement, it often helps to let the patient know that his behavior is frightening.

> A woman psychiatrist was called to the emergency ward to see a patient who had leaped from the examining table while a scalp laceration was being repaired. He accused the intern of deliberately trying to hurt him and the entire staff of racism. The patient was a large man with a deep, penetrating voice and a menacing manner. The psychiatrist, a tiny attractive woman, asked the others to leave—which they did reluctantly. They heard the patient thunder accusations for 3 to 4 minutes. Then quiet reigned. A shattering scream was expected, but not even a breath could be heard. Five minutes later the psychiatrist emerged and the patient was lying peaceably on the examining table, having consented to an intramuscular injection of a sedative. The psychiatric technique was simple. During a pause for breath in his ranting, she told him she was nearly speechless with fear. She reminded him that she was harmless, that she could do nothing to hurt him, and that she wanted to help him. The tremor in her voice verified her statement. He stared at her for a moment. Then he muttered, "Don't want to scare nobody," and accepted the sedative.

To sedate the intoxicated individual, one must begin with a smaller dose than usual to avoid a deleterious interaction between alcohol and the agent used.[1] Once the individual's tolerance has been established, a specific dose can be safely determined. We favor the use of the benzodiazepines. If parenteral use is required, diazepam (Valium) can be given intramuscularly (IM) or intravenously (IV). Because erratic and slow absorption so often occurs in the IM route, oral or IV use is preferred. The initial dose should be followed by a wait of from one half to one hour before augmenting it. The acutely intoxicated individual does not usually require hospitalization. If there is no risk of withdrawal syndrome, the patient can safely be referred to an alcohol detoxification program. Inpatient detoxification is preferable, especially if the patient is not well known or if this is the first episode of treatment.

PATHOLOGIC INTOXICATION AND ALCOHOLIC PARANOIA
Alcoholic Coma

Alcoholic coma, although rare, is a real medical emergency. It occurs when extraordinary amounts of alcohol are consumed, often in conjunction with another drug. The main goal of treatment is to prevent pulmonary depression and respiratory arrest.

Pathologic Intoxication

The disease state of pathologic intoxication has been described as a condition in which the patient becomes intoxicated on very small amounts of alcohol—as little as 4 oz.[2] There may be subsequent autonomic behavior for which the patient is totally amnesic. This behavior may be violent. If the alcoholic person is known to have a history of pathologic intoxication, he should be sedated heavily and confined until sobriety is assured in order to avoid possible danger to others.

The episode of pathologic intoxication usually ends after prolonged sleep. It may last for only an hour or may last for days. During this time the patient is agitated, impulsive, and often aggressive. Delusions and visual hallucinations may occur. Generally the disorder is marked by hyperactivity, anxiety, or depression. Suicide attempts sometimes occur. It has been postulated that pathologic intoxication is more likely to occur in borderline characters or in epileptic patients—in those individuals who tend toward emotional instability and whose pattern of defense is easily disorganized.

Alcoholic Paranoia

Alcoholic paranoia is somewhat similar to pathologic intoxication. It is a state of disorganization brought about by alcohol and made manifest by strong feelings of jealousy, antagonism, and suspicion. Sometimes the underlying disorder is homosexual in nature; when normal defenses are dissolved by alcohol, homosexual impulses emerge that, in turn, induce paranoid delusions.

The prognosis is poor for patients with pathologic intoxication or alcoholic paranoia.[3] Individuals so afflicted often have a history of violence and aggression with repeated incarcerations. The consultation psychiatrist should be on the watch for emergence of amnesia or the reversal of personality after the alcoholic session has been slept off. Although the premorbid personality of the paranoid alcoholic patient is apt to be somewhat suspicious, it is not nearly as intense or threatening as when under the influence of alcohol.

ALCOHOLIC WITHDRAWAL SYNDROME

"Alcoholic withdrawal syndrome" is now the preferred description rather than the traditional term "delirium tremens" because the latter limits its concern to only one manifestation of the syndrome.[4] However, throughout this discussion the terms will be used interchangeably.

Until open heart surgical procedures spawned new postoperative deliria, delirium tremens was by far the most frequently encountered delirium in a general hospital. Though it was first described in medical literature over 150 years ago and has been frequently observed in general hospitals ever since, delirium tremens is misdiagnosed in an uncomfortably large number of cases.[5] It is missed because physicians tend (or choose) to forget that alcoholism is rampant among people of all possible backgrounds and appearances in the United States. Physicians also fail to suspect the patient who tends, deliberately or unwittingly, to minimize dependence on alcohol and to underestimate the amount consumed. Because 10% of the patients with the full alcoholic withdrawal syndrome and 25% of those patients who have medical or concomitant surgical complications die, it is imperative to be on the alert for this dangerous condition.

Prediction

It is difficult to predict who will develop delirium tremens. Until a few years ago, one could say that delirium tremens rarely developed in patients under the age of 30 years. This is no longer true. Today the condition is not infrequently found in much younger patients. Although regarded as a withdrawal syndrome, there are heavy drinkers who fail to develop delirium after sudden withdrawal of ethanol. Infection, head trauma, and poor nutrition are probably contributing factors toward delirium. History of delirium tremens is an obvious predictor of a repeat episode during an enforced spell of drying out.

> One patient, a 64-year-old wharfinger, entered the hospital with recurrent gout 16 times during a 3-year period. Each time he became tremulous and disoriented during the second night and went on to develop mild visual and vestibular hallucinations that cleared over the next three days. Large ships would issue through the walls or windows and the whole room would rock and sway like a wharf in a storm. The pattern was identical, including his insistence that the only alcohol he ever swallowed was a drop or two from his mouthwash.

Although delirium tremens does not always appear in alcoholic withdrawal, the withdrawal symptoms following the cessation of heavy drinking are predictable. Loss of appetite, irritability, and tremulousness are early features. The appearance of a generalized tremor, fast in frequency and becoming more pronounced when the patient is under stress, is the hallmark of the abstinence syndrome. This tremor may involve the tongue to such an extent that the patient cannot talk. The lower extremities may tremble so that the patient cannot walk. The hands and arms may shake so violently that a drinking glass cannot be held without spilling the contents. The patient will be hypervigilant, have a pronounced startle response, and complain of insomnia. Illusions and hallucinations of a mild variety may appear, producing a sense of vague uneasiness. This picture may persist for as long as 2 weeks and clear without the appearance of a delirium. Grand mal seizures ("rum fits") may occur, usually within the first two days. More than one out of every three patients who suffer seizures develop subsequent delirium tremens.

Diagnosis

If delirium tremens is to occur, it generally does so within 24 to 72 hours after withdrawal. However, there have been reports of cases where the clinical picture of delirium tremens did not appear until seven days after the last drink. The principal features of the state are disorientation (in time or place or person in any combination), tremor hyperactivity, marked wakefulness, fever, increased autonomic arousal, and hallucinations. Hallucinations are generally visual but may be tactile (in which case they are probably associated with a peripheral neuritis), olfactory, or auditory. Vestibular disturbances are common and often hallucinatory. The patient may complain of the floor moving beneath his feet or believe he is on an elevator. The hallucinatory experience is always frightening. Animals, typically snakes, are seen in threatening poses. Mice or lice are felt and seen crawling on the skin. Once the condition manifests itself, delirium tremens usually lasts two to three days. Should it persist for a longer time, one must suspect an underlying disorder, such as infection or subdural hematoma. There are, however, a small number of individuals whose course is characterized by relapses interspersed with intervals of complete lucidity. These patients offer the consultant the most challenging diagnostic opportunities. As a rule of thumb, it is always wise to include delirium tremens in the list of differential diagnostic possibilities whenever delirium appears.

The psychiatric consultant is apt to miss the diagnosis of delirium tremens when the patient's manner, social position, or reputation belie the possibility of alcoholism. For example, the following problem arose after an emergency surgical procedure.

A 54-year-old woman was admitted to the hospital for a cholecystectomy. She was a society matron with all the attendant stereotypical characteristics. She and her surgeon were neighbors. On her third postoperative day (her fifth day without alcohol) the nurses reported that they could not keep her in bed. She got up and walked about her room in a restless, agitated fashion, constantly gazing back over her shoulder as though she feared she was being followed. Soon her peregrinations included other patients' rooms as well as the hospital corridor. She resisted violently every attempt to keep her confined to quarters. The surgeon, when called, described her as "fearful, overactive, stubborn, but polite." While she would not give any reason for her distress, she readily swallowed a 25 mg capsule of chlordiazepoxide hydrochloride (Librium). This produced no change in her behavior after two hours. She talked to herself while she paced but was able to pull herself together and to maintain a shaky semblance of poise when approached by others. Although her physician opposed psychiatric consultation, the nurses prevailed because they feared she might inadvertently hurt herself. When a house officer suggested the possibility of a "small stroke" because of the patient's long history of hypertension, the physician agreed to request psychiatric advice.

After reviewing the history and noting a bilateral hand tremor while observing the patient, the psychiatrist diagnosed delirium tremens. Although the patient refused to speak with him after he identified himself, the psychiatrist maintained his diagnosis because it was the most likely possibility in the absence of other signs. Her personal physician refused to accept the diagnosis, but did follow the recommended regimen of medication (100 mg of chlordiazepoxide each hour) until the patient was able to stay in bed. The medication was then reduced to a maintenance level and supplemented by 50 mg of thiamine daily. Round-the-clock special nurses were also employed. The patient awoke the following morning her normal self. It is characteristic for delirium tremens to terminate suddenly, often after a night of sound sleep.

The patient subsequently admitted drinking four to seven very dry martinis a day, each about 4 oz. She had been doing so for the last 30 years and had gone through all of her maternity confinements without having had delirium tremens. Age may have made the difference. She refused to accept the diagnosis of delirium tremens. However, she was so frightened by her experience that she agreed to enter psychotherapy.

The consultant is also frequently misled when delirium is intermittent and the patient is examined during a lucid stage. Exemplifying this situation is the following case:

A 52-year-old architect was admitted for hematemesis. The patient readily admitted heavy alcohol intake, but had no difficulty in the hospital until the fourth day. He then began to gaze fixedly at a point on the ceiling and to talk in low, menacing tones to an imaginary companion. He sweated, trembled, and thrashed about so wildly that he had to be restrained in bed. He readily described auditory hallucinations of a persecutory nature. These became alarmingly vivid in the evening. The following morning a psychiatrist was called to see him and found him to be fully oriented, lucid, perfectly capable of discussing his hallucinatory experiences of the previous evening, and willing to accept the diagnosis of delirium tremens. However, he pointed out that he had never had delirium tremens before, although he had been a heavy drinker for many years. The psychiatrist noted a probable episode of delirium tremens, but observed that the patient was now lucid and ready for further diagnostic procedures. Restraints were removed.

A few hours later the patient leaped out of bed, ran through the ward, upset tables, and screamed that someone was chasing him. Once again he was forcibly restrained, placed in bed, given 8 mL of paraldehyde orally and 50 mg of chlorpromazine IM. When the psychiatrist returned a few hours later, the patient's mental status was entirely normal and he could recall the violent episode. He was, in fact, so clear-thinking and his mentation so intact that the psychiatrist once again suggested that restraints be removed. Within 20 minutes the patient sprang out of bed, left the ward, and almost left the hospital. After this second unexpected episode the consultant sent him to a mental hospital where he remained for the next 2 weeks with intermittent episodes of delirium.

Although this is a highly atypical course for delirium tremens, it does occur. Consultants should be wary of relinquishing restraints or discontinuing private nurses until the patient has been lucid for 24 hours.

Differential Diagnosis

The differential diagnosis must include the many types of deliria found in a general hospital (see chapter 6). These include postoperative and postconcussive deliria as well as metabolic disorders. Two examples of the latter are: (1) impending hepatic coma and (2) acute pancreatitis. The patient with impending hepatic coma may well be disoriented and confused, but manifests decreased activity rather than agitation. Usually there are no visual hallucinations. Speech is slow and monotonous and the face masklike. Hyperphagia rather than anorexia will exist in impending hepatic coma. Physical signs such as jaundice, hepatomegaly, and fetor hepaticus from elevation of blood ammonia help determine this diagnosis.

There is a delirium that sometimes occurs in acute pancreatitis. In this condition, however, there is generally severe abdominal pain with an elevated serum amylase.

Prognosis

The prognosis for delirium tremens is reasonably good. Death, if it occurs, results from acute heart failure, an infection (chiefly pneumonia), or injuries sustained during the restless period. In a small proportion of patients the delirium may merge into Korsakoff's psychosis, in which case the patient may not regain full mentation. This is more apt to happen with closely spaced episodes of delirium tremens in the elderly.

Treatment

As in the treatment of any delirium the prime concern must be surveillance. The patient must be watched at all times so that he cannot harm himself or others. The necessity for round-the-clock nursing care cannot be overemphasized. Although not necessarily suicidal, delirious patients take terrible unpremeditated risks. Falling from windows, slipping down stairs, and walking through glass doors are common examples of unintended lethal behavior. Restraint should be used only for short periods. It is a point of law that when four-point restraint is used, the patient must be closely observed and relief must be provided every hour. Usually physical restraint can be avoided by using an agent such as chlordiazepoxide 50 to 100 mg given orally every hour until the patient is quiet and 50 mg every six hours thereafter. Haloperidol (Haldol), 10 to 20 mg given orally four times daily, is often used when the patient does not respond to chlordiazepoxide. This is the case when the alcoholism is associated with a psychosis or borderline condition.

Since the B vitamins are known to help prevent peripheral neuropathy and the Wernicke-Korsakoff syndrome, their use is vital. Thiamine, 50 mg, should be given IV immediately and 50 mg should be given IM each day until a normal diet is resumed. A smaller amount of thiamine may be added to infusions for IV use. Since there is frequently a magnesium deficiency, which has been reported to reduce seizure threshold, magnesium sulfate may be given.[6] A high-carbohydrate soft diet should be given containing from 3000 to 4000 calories a day with supplemental vitamins. Phenytoin (Dilantin) may be used in patients with a history of withdrawal seizures. A loading dose of phenytoin must be given (1 g in 50 cc 5% D/W IV over one to four hours). Parenteral diazepam has also been widely used to control seizures.

ALCOHOLIC HALLUCINATIONS
Diagnosis

One of the most bizarre of the alcoholic psychoses is alcoholic hallucinosis. The individual with this condition has vivid auditory illusions and hallucinations occurring in an otherwise clear sensorium.

These hallucinations soon become accusatory and threatening. The individual reacts with fear but is fully oriented and realizes that the voices are hallucinations. However, as the accusations persist, the patient develops ideas of persecution. Although hallucinosis is more apt to occur in the setting of alcohol withdrawal, it is by no means uncommon in individuals who continue to drink. Some authors believe that hallucinosis is programmed by a disturbance of the auditory pathways. Tinnitus is found in many patients who report hallucinosis. Curiously, when tinnitus is one-sided, the hallucinatory experience usually occurs only on that side. Olfactory hallucinations may occur with alcoholic hallucinosis, but visual hallucinations seldom occur. Alcoholic hallucinosis is much less common than delirium tremens.

The clinical picture is one in which auditory hallucinations occur in the absence of tremor, disorientation, and agitation. Usually the male patient hears voices accusing him of homosexual practices and threatening retaliation. It has been reported that in women the hallucinotic voices may vent accusations of promiscuity. Soon after the voices begin, a frightening systematized delusional system develops that may incite the patient to call the police or to arm himself. Then the patient is particularly dangerous. He is capable of acting with an otherwise clear mind. Suicide is a distinct danger in this condition and may occur, as in delirium, without appreciable warning. My first patient with alcoholic hallucinosis came to the hospital on a quiet Sunday morning during my internship.

> A 27-year-old merchant seaman had begun listening to a local disc jockey while at a bar the previous evening. His attention was suddenly caught when he heard his name announced as a third prize winner. He had won 14 sheep, five head of cattle, and a strawberry farm in Kansas. A taxi driver who had listened to him for three hours and had driven him to innumerable radio stations finally insisted on taking him to a hospital. Since this was the early 1950s, the era of the colossal give-aways, the story sounded plausible, especially since the patient told it in a straightforward and reasonable manner. The cab driver was asked if he had heard the announcement on the car radio. He exclaimed, "Oh, no! Not you too! They all believe him instead of me. Ask him what else the voices said." When asked, the seaman grudgingly admitted that the disc jockey, along with announcing his name as a winner, had accused him of homosexual acts. As he spoke he became serious and threatening. He clearly believed these voices to be real. However, he readily agreed to enter the hospital. He seemed certain that the truth of his statement would be quickly discovered if he were hospitalized. A week later he no longer heard voices and had substantially minimized the experience, just as he forgot that alcohol had caused it.

Paranoid schizophrenia is the condition that is apt to be confused with alcoholic hallucinosis. The differential diagnosis is apt to be difficult. The dominance of the auditory component of the disorder and a history of alcoholism can aid in determining this condition.

Treatment

There is no specific treatment for alcoholic hallucinosis. Generally it clears within 30 days, but it may last another month. There are reported instances in which the hallucinosis continued for years. If the individual continues to drink, recurrences are the rule.

The most important aspect of treatment is to determine whether the patient should be in a protected environment. Behavior destructive to self or to others is common enough to require commitment to a mental hospital. Sedation can be given as needed using chlordiazepoxide or chlorpromazine hydrochloride. Since the patients generally feel quite normal after the disappearance of auditory hallucinations, they often insist on being discharged as soon as the voices desist. As in delirium tremens, the course can be intermittent and the patient should be kept in a hospital until a week has passed without hallucinations. He should also be vigorously warned against drinking since the hallucinotic experience is apt to return if drinking is not forsaken.

WERNICKE-KORSAKOFF SYNDROME

Victor et al,[7] in their classic monograph *The Wernicke-Korsakoff Syndrome*, state that "Wernicke's encephalopathy and Korsakoff's syndrome in the alcoholic, nutritionally deprived patient may be regarded as two facets of the same disease. These patients evidence specific central nervous system pathology with resultant profound mental changes."[7] In all of the cases reported by Victor et al, alcoholism was a serious problem and was almost invariably accompanied by malnutrition. Malnutrition is thought to be the causal factor, particularly the absence of thiamine. In addition, there may well be the toxic effect of alcohol itself.

Korsakoff's Psychosis

Korsakoff's psychosis, also referred to as confabulatory psychosis, is characterized by impaired memory in an otherwise alert and responsive individual. This condition is slow to start and only gradually does the memory impairment progress. It may be the end stage of a much longer, gradual process. Hallucinations and delusions are rarely encountered. Curiously, confabulation, long regarded as the hallmark of Korsakoff's psychosis, was exhibited in only a limited number of cases in the large series collected and studied by Victor et al. Most of these patients have no insight into the nature of their illness and a limited understanding of the extent of their memory loss.

The memory deficit is bipartite. The retrograde component is the inability to recall the past and the anterograde component is the lack of capacity for the retention of new information. In the acute stage of Korsakoff's psychosis the memory gap is blatant—the patient cannot recall simple items such as the examiner's first name, the day, or the time, even though he is given this information several times. As memory improves, usually within weeks to months, simple problems can be solved, limited always by the patient's span of recall.

The fact that Korsakoff's psychosis patients tend to improve with time is often forgotten, and too gloomy a prognosis surrounds the condition. In the series of Victor et al, 21% of patients recovered more or less completely, 26% showed no recovery, and the rest recovered partially. During the acute stage there is, however, no way of predicting who will improve and who will not.

The specific anatomical structures pertaining to memory that are affected in Korsakoff's psychosis are the medial dorsal nucleus of the thalamus and the hippocampal formations.

Wernicke's Encephalopathy

Wernicke's encephalopathy appears suddenly and is characterized by ophthalmoplegia and ataxia followed by mental disturbance. The ocular disturbance, which is necessary for the diagnosis, consists of paresis or paralysis of the external recti, nystagmus, and disturbance of conjugate gaze. The patient is apt to be somnolent, confused, and slow to reply. He frequently falls asleep in midsentence. The mental impairment is described by Victor et al as a global confusional state, consisting of disorientation, unresponsiveness, and derangement of perception and memory.[7] Exhaustion, apathy, dehydration, and profound lethargy are also part of the picture. Once treatment with thiamine is started for Wernicke's encephalopathy, improvement is often evident in the ocular palsies within hours. In almost all cases recovery from ocular muscle paralysis is complete within several days or weeks. In the cases reported by Victor et al, about one third recovered from global confusional state within six days of treatment, another third within 1 month, and the remainder within 2 months.[7] The global confusional state is almost always reversible—in marked contrast to the memory impairment of Korsakoff's psychosis.

Treatment

Recommended treatment for both Korsakoff's pyschosis and Wernicke's encephalopathy is identical. Victor et al consider treatment to be a medical emergency.[7] The prompt use of vitamins, particularly thiamine, prevents advancement of the disease and reverses at least a portion of lesions where permanent damage has not yet been done. Ocular palsy is notably sensitive to thiamine. Such administration is, therefore, an important diagnostic aid as well as an essential therapeutic measure. In patients who show only ocular and ataxic signs, the prompt administration of thiamine is crucial in preventing the development of an irreversible and incapacitating amnesic psychosis. In general, the treatment recommended is 50 mg of thiamine given IV immediately and 50 mg IM each day until normal diet is resumed. Parenteral feedings and the administration of B-complex vitamins become necessary if the patient cannot eat. If rapid heart rate, feeble heart sounds, pulmonary edema, or other signs of myocardial weakness appear, digitalization should be started. Since these patients operate with impaired mental function, nursing personnel should be alerted to the patients' possible tendency to wander, to be forgetful, and to become obstreperously psychotic. If the last should occur, benzodiazepines can be given.

MEMORY AND ALCOHOL

The newer investigative methods such as computerized cranial tomography (CT scan) and neuropsychological testing have demonstrated cognitive impairments in individuals who are either alcoholics or heavy drinkers which largely escaped notice until the advent of these modern techniques. Short-term memory, performance on complex memory tasks, visual motor coordination, visual spatial performance, abstract reasoning, and psychomotor dexterity are the areas most seriously damaged. Intelligence scores do not change, and there is sparing of verbal skills and long-term memory. As a consequence of this sparing, it is possible for individuals to appear quite intact unless they are subjected to neuropsychological tests. Abnormalities on CT scan have been reported in 50% or more of chronic alcoholic subjects. These abnormalities can occur in subjects where there is neither clinical nor neuropsychological test evidence of cognitive defects. According to Wells, "It appears that chronic alcoholism can produce defects in neuropsychological functioning or in anatomic structures (or both), but that the two deficits are not necessarily related to each other."[8] These defects, particularly memory disturbances, can be reversed, at least in part, with abstinence. It is thought that the anatomical changes (CT scan abnormalities) may be due in part to brain shrinkage and to brain atrophy. Well says, "The clinical and basic science studies make it clear that alcohol itself is a powerful neurotoxin whose long-term use in excessive amounts causes demonstrable changes in brain function and structure." Wells proposes the label "subacute alcoholic encephalopathy."[8]

REFERRAL AFTER HOSPITALIZATION

The disposition of individuals with an acute or chronic alcohol syndrome is complicated. The principal problem encountered in all therapeutic modalities is the problem of motivation. Most alcoholic patients in the general hospital with problems secondary to drinking have great difficulty admitting their addiction to alcohol. While they may pay lip service to the advice of their physician to seek outside help, they rarely have the tenacity to seek a therapeutic group or an individual counselor. It has been MGH practice to tell each alcoholic patient about the types of treatment programs available in the community. Contact with Alcoholics Anonymous is encouraged because of its success record with this population. Once the community resources have been identified and their differences described, the patient is encouraged to contact the one with the most appeal to him. To ensure the patient's full cooperation, as well as to establish the fact that a recommendation was made, a responsible family member is also informed. It is MGH policy to insist that the patient make the first contact with the treating agency, at which time our name can be used as a referral. When we are contacted by the potential therapist, we furnish a summary of the hospital record and our recommendations. About one in five such patients actually makes contact with a treating agency. With the establishment of a hospital alcohol unit that has personnel available to interview all individuals with alcohol-related problems as noted by the consultation service, the number of self-motivated referrals has increased by 20%. Whether or not this increase implies a record of more enduring sobriety remains to be seen. What may be said, however, is that studies from the National Institute of Alcohol Abuse and Alcoholism (NIAAA) show that 70% of patients who enroll in therapeutic programs improve. This improvement is true with all modalities of treatment.

REFERENCES

1. Hayes SL, et al: Ethanol and oral diazepam absorption. *N Engl J Med* 1977; 296:186–187.

2. Thompson GN (ed): *Alcoholism.* Springfield, Ill: Charles C Thomas Publisher, 1956.

3. Chafetz ME: Alcoholism and alcoholic psychoses, in Freedman AM, Kaplan HI, Sadock BJ (eds): *Comprehensive Textbook of Psychiatry.* Baltimore, Williams & Wilkins Co, 1975, section 23.3.

4. Woodruff RA, Goodwin DW, Guze SB: *Psychiatric Diagnoses.* New York, Oxford University Press, 1974.

5. Cutshall BJ: The Saunders-Sutton syndrome: An analysis of delirium tremens. *QJ Stud Alcohol* 1965; 26:423–448.

6. Jaffe JH, Ciraulo D: Drugs used in the treatment of alcoholism, in Mendelson JH, Mello NK (eds): *The Diagnosis and Treatment of Alcoholism,* ed 2. New York, McGraw-Hill, 1985.

7. Victor M, Adams RD, Collins GH: *The Wernicke-Korsakoff Syndrome.* Philadelphia, FA Davis Co, 1971.

8. Wells C: Chronic brain disease: An update on alcoholism, Parkinson's disease and dementia. *Hosp Community Psychiatry* 1982; 33:111–126.

3
Drug Addiction

JOHN A. RENNER, Jr.

BARBITURATES
Abuse

In addition to the patients who attempt suicide with a barbiturate overdose, we are now seeing an entirely different group of individuals who use barbiturates as a social or recreational drug in the same manner that others use alcohol. The increased nonmedical use of barbiturates and such other sedative-hypnotics as methaqualone, glutethimide, and the benzodiazepines, has produced new clinical problems.

The person intoxicated by barbiturates presents many of the same diagnostic problems associated with alcohol intoxication. Slurred speech, unsteady gait, and sustained vertical or horizontal nystagmus or both occurring in the absence of the odor of alcohol on the breath suggest the diagnosis. Unfortunately, drug abusers frequently combine alcohol with other sedative hypnotic drugs. The clinician may be misled by the odor of alcohol. The diagnosis of mixed alcohol-barbiturate intoxication will be missed unless a careful history is taken and blood and urine samples are analyzed for toxic drugs. The behavioral effects of barbiturate intoxication can vary widely, even in the same person, and may change significantly depending on the surroundings and the expectations of the user. Individuals using barbiturates primarily to control anxiety or stress may appear sleepy or mildly confused as a result of an overdose. In young adults seeking to get "high," a similar dose may produce excitement, loud boisterous behavior, and loss of inhibitions. The aggressive and even violent behavior commonly associated with alcohol intoxication may follow. The prescribed regimen for managing the angry alcoholic individual can also be used for the barbiturate abuser (see chapter 2).

Accidental life-threatening barbiturate overdoses are a common occurrence in individuals who are addicted to barbiturates. As tolerance to barbiturates develops, there is not a concomitant increase in the lethal dose level, as occurs in opiate addiction. As the barbiturate addict gradually increases the dosage to maintain the desired level of intoxication, the margin between the lethal dose and the intoxicating dose becomes smaller. Although the opiate addict may be able to double the regular dose and still avoid fatal respiratory depression, as little as a 10% to 25% increase over the usual daily dosage may be fatal to the barbiturate addict. Thus, a barbiturate overdose should always be considered as potentially life-threatening, especially for drug abusers. Different signs and symptoms may be observed, depending on the drug or combination of drugs used, the amount of time since ingestion, and the presence of such complicating medical conditions as pneumonia, hepatitis, diabetes, heart disease, renal failure, or head injury. At first the patient appears lethargic or semicomatose. The pulse rate is slow but other vital functions are normal. As the level of intoxication increases, the patient becomes unresponsive to even painful stimuli, reflexes disappear, and there is a gradual depression of the rate of respiration and eventually, cardiovascular collapse. Pupil size is not changed by barbiturate intoxication, but secondary anoxia may cause fixed, dilated pupils. In persons who have adequate respiratory function, pinpoint pupils usually indicate an opiate overdose or the combined ingestion of barbiturates and opiates. Such patients should be observed carefully for increased lethargy and progressive respiratory depression. Appropriate measures for treating overdoses should be instituted as necessary. Patients may walk into an emergency room and later lapse into a coma; they should never be left unattended until all signs of intoxication have cleared.

Because there is no cross-tolerance between narcotics and barbiturates, special problems are presented by methadone maintenance patients who continue to abuse barbiturates, or other sedative-hypnotics. If a barbiturate overdose is suspected, the methadone patient should be given a narcotic antagonist to counteract any respiratory depression caused by methadone. We recommend naloxone hydrochloride, 0.4 mg given intramuscularly (IM) or intravenously (IV), because it is a pure narcotic antagonist and has no respiratory depressant effect even in large doses. If the respiratory depression does not improve after treatment with naloxone, the patient should be treated for a pure barbiturate overdose.

Withdrawal

The barbiturate withdrawal syndrome can present a wide variety of symptoms including anxiety, insomnia, hyperreflexia, diaphoresis, nausea, vomiting, and sometimes delirium and convulsions. As a general rule, individuals who ingest 600 to 800 mg/d of secobarbital for more than 45 days will develop physiologic addiction and show symptoms after withdrawal. Minor withdrawal symptoms usually begin within 24 to 36 hours after the last dose. Pulse and respiration rates are usually elevated, pupil size is normal, and there may be postural hypotension. Fever may develop and dangerous hyperpyrexia can occur in severe cases. Major withdrawal symptoms such as convulsions and delirium indicate addiction to large doses (900 mg or more of secobarbital).

Grand mal convulsions, if they occur, are usually seen between the third and seventh day, though there have been cases reported of convulsions occurring as late as 14 days after the completion of a medically controlled detoxification. Because of the danger of convulsions, barbiturate withdrawal should be carried out only on an inpatient basis. Withdrawal convulsions are thought to be related to a rapid drop in the blood barbiturate level. Treatment should therefore be carefully controlled so that barbiturates are withdrawn gradually with minimal fluctuation in the blood barbiturate level. Theoretically, this should decrease the danger of convulsions. Treatment with phenytoin will not prevent convulsions due to barbiturate withdrawal though it will control convulsions due to epilepsy.

Delirium occurs less frequently than convulsions but rarely appears unless preceded by convulsions. It usually begins between the fourth and sixth days and is characterized by both visual and auditory hallucinations, delusions, and fluctuating levels of consciousness. The presence of confusion, hyperreflexia, and fever help distinguish this syndrome from schizophrenia and other nontoxic psychoses.

Treatment for Withdrawal

Several techniques are available for managing barbiturate withdrawal. The basic idea is to withdraw the addicting agent slowly to avoid the danger of convulsions. First, the daily dosage that produces mild toxicity must be established. Since barbiturate addicts tend to underestimate their drug use, it is dangerous to accept the patient's history as completely accurate. Treatment should begin with an oral test dose of 200 mg pentobarbital, a short-acting barbiturate. If no physical changes occur after one hour, the patient's habit probably exceeds 1200 mg pentobarbital/d. If the patient shows only nystagmus and no other signs of intoxication, the habit is probably about 800 mg/d. Evidence of slurred speech and intoxication, but not sleep, suggests a habit of 400 to 600 mg/d. The patient can then be started on the estimated daily requirement divided into four equal doses administered orally every six hours. Should signs of withdrawal appear, the estimated daily dosage can be increased by 25% following an additional dose of 200 mg pentobarbital given IM.

After a daily dose that produces only mild toxicity has been established, the pentobarbital dosage can be decreased each day by 10% of the established daily dosage. An alternative method is to switch the patient from pentobarbital to an equivalent dose of the longer-acting phenobarbital (30 mg phenobarbital equals 100 mg pentobarbital or secobarbital) once the daily dose is established and then withdraw the phenobarbital 30 mg/d. At Massachusetts General Hospital (MGH) we recommend this latter method since the use of a long-acting barbiturate produces fewer variations in the blood barbiturate level and should produce a smoother withdrawal.

Inpatient Management and Referral

Barbiturate addicts can present a variety of psychological management problems. Effective treatment requires a thorough evaluation of the patients' psychiatric problems and the development of long-term treatment plans prior to discharge. Treatment for withdrawal or overdose presents an opportunity for effective intervention in the addict's self-destructive life style. Drug abuse patients have a reputation for deceit, manipulation, and hostility. They frequently sign out against medical advice. It is rarely acknowledged that these problems are usually caused by inadequate attention to the patient's psychological problems. Most of these difficulties can be eliminated by effective medical and psychiatric management. The patient's lack of cooperation and frequent demands for additional drugs are often due to anxiety and to the all-too-real fear of withdrawal seizures. This anxiety will be greatly relieved if the physician thoroughly explains the withdrawal procedure and assures the patient that the staff knows how to handle withdrawal and that convulsions will be avoided if the patient cooperates with a schedule of medically supervised withdrawal.

We sometimes fail to realize that the patient's tough, demanding behavior is a defense against a strong sense of personal inadequacy and a fear of rejection. Addicts have been conditioned to expect rejection and hostility from medical personnel. The trust and cooperation necessary for successful treatment cannot be established unless physicians show by their behavior that they are both genuinely concerned about the patient and medically competent to treat withdrawal. Physicians can expect an initial period of defensive hostility and "testing" behavior and should not take this behavior personally. Patients need to be reassured that their physician is concerned about them.

If the patient manifests signs of a serious character disorder and has a history of severe drug abuse, the setting of firm limits is necessary to ensure successful detoxification. Visitors must be limited to those individuals of known reliability. This may mean excluding spouses and other relatives. Family counseling should be started during hospitalization and should focus on the family's role in helping the patient develop a successful long-term treatment program.

Hospital passes should not be granted until detoxification is completed; however, passes with staff members as escorts should be used as much as possible. An active program of recreational and physical therapy is necessary to keep young, easily bored patients occupied.

The story of a man, aged 21 years, who was hospitalized after having a grand mal seizure illustrates several of the problems that may occur.

> The son of an eminent attorney, the patient described several years of episodic barbiturate and alcohol use and admitted to 3 months of daily barbiturate use after dismissal from college for failing grades. Three days before the patient's seizure, his father discovered that the young man had been ingesting secobarbital tablets taken from the medicine cabinet. The patient agreed to stop using barbiturates but did not realize that he was addicted. After admission to the hospital the young man became a serious management problem. He demanded additional medication and refused to obey hospital regulations. Twice he left the floor without permission and on one occasion he returned obviously "high." A discussion with his physician became an angry shouting match. The patient denied any extra drug use and insisted that he be permitted to leave the ward. He threatened to file a lawsuit for violation of his civil rights. In consultation the patient was hostile and provocative. He denied having any psychiatric problems and suggested that his physician was trying to have him committed to a mental hospital. The patient's hostility disappeared after the psychiatrist indicated that he had no interest in committing him but was concerned that his arguments with his physician and the nurses were interfering with his medical treatment. Once reassured that the psychiatrist did not think he was crazy, he admitted his fear of having more seizures. He did not know what to expect during detoxification and was too frightened to admit his fears to his physician. He finally admitted that he was meeting friends in the hospital cafeteria and they were giving him extra drugs. A meeting was then arranged between the patient and his physician. The physician explained the detoxification procedure in detail including possible causes of seizures and the need for diagnostic tests. The patient was relieved to hear this information and readily agreed to appropriate limitations on visitors and hospital passes. The remainder of his hospitalization passed without incident and he agreed to continue seeing the psychiatrist after his discharge.

In some situations patient management is easier if the patient does not know the exact dosage schedule for withdrawal. A placebo may be given for three or four days following the final dose. This procedure should be used only if the patient agrees to it in advance. It works best with anxious, insecure patients who are able nonetheless to trust their physician, but is clearly contraindicated if the patient is paranoid or incapable of trusting the physician.

Since treatment for detoxification or for an overdose rarely cures an addict, referrals for long-term outpatient or residential care should be made early in the treatment process. Ideally the patient should meet the future therapist prior to discharge. Alcoholics Anonymous or Narcotics Anonymous are useful adjuncts to any outpatient treatment program. If transferring to a halfway house or residential program, the patient should move there directly from the hospital. Addicts are not likely to execute plans for follow-up care without strong encouragement and support.

NARCOTICS

Because of the growing problem of narcotics abuse, the secondary treatment of addiction is becoming commonplace on medical and surgical units. Proper management of such patients necessitates knowledge of Food and Drug Administration regulations, appropriate techniques for using methadone, and community treatment resources.

The classic signs of opiate withdrawal are easily recognized and usually begin eight to 12 hours after the last dose. The patient generally admits the need for drugs and will show sweating, yawning, lacrimation, tremor, rhinorrhea, marked irritability, dilated pupils, and increased respiratory rate. More severe withdrawal signs occur 48 to 72 hours after the last dose and include tachycardia, hypertension, nausea and vomiting, insomnia, and abdominal cramps. Untreated, the syndrome subsides in five to ten days. Withdrawal symptoms are similar in patients addicted to methadone, but they may not appear until 30 to 48 hours after the last dose, and will abate over 2 to 4 weeks.

Food and Drug Administration regulations define methadone maintenance as any treatment with methadone that extends beyond 21 days. Addicts cannot be maintained unless they show physiologic evidence of current addiction (withdrawal signs) and can document a 1-year history of addiction. They must be withdrawn from methadone within 21 days if their addiction history is less than 1 year. The only exception to this rule is for the addict who is hospitalized for the treatment of a medical, surgical, or obstetrical condition. Under these circumstances, the physician has the option of maintaining the addiction of any addict for the duration of the primary illness. At MGH we strongly recommend that the addiction be maintained until the addict has fully recovered from the presenting illness and that the addict be given the option of drug withdrawal treatment prior to discharge.

Establishing the appropriate dose of methadone for a street addict is a trial-and-error process. Since the quality of street heroin is never certain, the addict's description of the size of the current habit is of minimal value. The safest guide to dosage is to monitor the patient's pulse, respiration, and pupil size. After the presence of withdrawal is documented, a hard-core addict should receive 20 mg methadone orally. Only if the patient is well known as a heavy user should the starting dose be as high as 30 mg. A relatively young patient or a patient who describes a small habit can begin treatment with 10 mg given orally. If vital signs have not stabilized or if withdrawal signs reappear after two hours, an additional 5 or 10 mg can be given orally. It is rare to give more than 40 mg during the first 24 hours.

> One woman aged 17 years, admitted for evaluation of fever of undetermined origin and associated epigastric distress, requested large doses of methadone and claimed to have a heroin habit costing $200 a day. Further history revealed that she and her husband had been addicted for less than 3 months and were both relatively naive heroin users. After she began to show signs of opiate withdrawal, she was given 10 mg methadone orally; an additional 5 mg was given ten hours later when her respirations were noted to again be more than 18 per minute. The following day she remained comfortable after a single dose of 15 mg. Later it was discovered that she had regional enteritis.

The addict should be maintained on a single daily oral dose that keeps him or her comfortable and that keeps respiration and pulse rates within normal range. The dose should be reduced 5 or 10 mg if the patient appears lethargic. If the street addict is to be withdrawn from drugs immediately, his methadone can be reduced 10% to 20% a day. If the drug habit has been maintained in the hospital for 2 or more weeks, or if the patient had been using methadone before admission, detoxification should proceed more slowly. The dose can be reduced 5 mg per day until 20 mg per day is reached. Further dose reduction should occur at the rate of 5 mg every three or four days. Chances for successful withdrawal treatment will be enhanced if the patient is aware of the dose and is able to choose the withdrawal schedule within limits established by the physician. By involving the patient in the treatment process and by using a flexible withdrawal schedule, the physician can keep withdrawal symptoms at a tolerable level. Rigid adherence to a fixed schedule of doses is less likely to achieve success and may lead to premature termination of treatment.

If a patient is already in a methadone maintenance clinic prior to admission to the hospital, the methadone dose should be confirmed by the clinic staff and should not be changed without consultation with the clinic physician responsible for the patient's treatment. Under no circumstances should such a patient be withdrawn from drugs unless there is full agreement among the patient, the hospital physician, and the methadone clinic staff on this course of action. Such detoxification is not likely to be successful, particularly if the patient is under stress from some concurrent medical or surgical condition. Withdrawal from drugs may complicate the management of the primary illness. The option of detoxification should not be considered until the patient has fully recovered from the condition that necessitated hospitalization.

Maintenance patients should be continued on daily oral methadone. If parenteral medication is necessary, methadone can be given in doses of 5 or 10 mg IM every eight hours. This regimen should keep the patient comfortable regardless of the previous oral dose. An alternative method is to give one third of the daily oral dose IM every 12 hours. As soon as oral fluids can be tolerated, the original oral dose should be reinstated.

A common problem is determining the appropriate dosage of an analgesic for patients on methadone maintenance.

> A 28-year-old woman was hospitalized for the treatment of acute renal colic. Four years previous to this she had been hospitalized for similar symptoms that subsided after she passed a kidney stone. During the year prior to her second hospitalization, the patient was in a methadone maintenance program and was receiving 60 mg methadone daily. She was doing well in treatment and for the last 6 months was working regularly as a secretary. A psychiatrist was asked to see the patient because she was threatening to sign out of the hospital. She claimed that she was receiving no effective relief for her pain and that she wished to obtain heroin to treat herself. The nurses described her as constantly complaining, demanding, and attempting to manipulate additional doses of narcotics. A review of her chart revealed that she was receiving doses of 5 mg morphine, approximately half the usual analgesic dose in such situations, with strict orders not to repeat the dose sooner than every four hours because of her history of drug abuse. Her physician had assumed that she would require lower doses of morphine because she was taking methadone. After consultation, the physician accepted the psychiatrist's recommendation that the usual dose of 10 mg morphine be given every two hours as circumstances required because the patient would probably metabolize any narcotic more rapidly than normal. This regimen effectively controlled the patient's pain and she suddenly became more cooperative. There was no recurrence of her "manipulative" behavior or other management problems. Two days later she passed several renal stones; she was

discharged several days later. Her physician had not realized that her "demands and manipulations" were legitimate requests for effective doses of analgesics.

The analgesic effect of methadone is minimal in maintenance patients and, at best, lasts only six to eight hours. If control of pain is required addicts should be given normal doses of other narcotics in addition to their methadone. Because of cross-tolerance, a maintenance patient will metabolize other narcotics more rapidly, and may therefore require more frequent administration of analgesics than nonaddicted patients. Pentazocine is contraindicated for such patients; because of its narcotic antagonist effects, this analgesic will produce withdrawal symptoms in opiate addicts.

Discharge planning should be initiated as quickly after admission as possible. For patients not already in treatment, a week or more may be required to arrange admission to a drug-free residential program or to a methadone maintenance clinic. Since a serious illness usually causes an addict to reexamine his behavior and possibly choose rehabilitation, the physician should emphasize the need for long-term treatment. No addict should be discharged while still on methadone unless he is returning to a maintenance program or specifically refuses detoxification. Even when a physician discharges a patient for disciplinary reasons, medical ethics necessitate that the patient be withdrawn from methadone before discharge. Hospital physicians cannot legally give addicts methadone for administration at home.

MIXED DRUG ADDICTION

Increasing numbers of patients are addicted to a combination of drugs including barbiturates, alcohol, and opiates. Accurate diagnosis is difficult because of confusing, inconsistent physical findings and unreliable histories. Blood and urine tests for drugs are required to confirm the diagnosis. The patient who is addicted to both opiates and barbiturates should be maintained on methadone while the barbiturates or other sedative-hypnotics are withdrawn. Then methadone can be withdrawn in the usual manner.

Behavioral problems should be dealt with as previously described. The firm setting of limits is essential to the success of any effective psychological treatment program. Some patients who overdose or present medical problems secondary to drug abuse such as subacute bacterial endocarditis and hepatitis are not physiologically addicted to any drug despite a history of multiple drug abuse. Their drug abuse behavior is usually associated with severe psychopathology. These patients should receive a thorough psychiatric evaluation and may require long-term residential treatment.

AMPHETAMINES
Abuse

Stricter federal controls on the production and distribution of amphetamines have reduced the number of amphetamine abusers to a few. Routine medical evaluation may uncover the most common type of amphetamine abuse seen in the general hospital. This is the patient who began using amphetamines to control obesity and later became a chronic amphetamine abuser. The patient quickly develops tolerance and may use 100 mg or more a day in an unsuccessful effort to control weight. This amphetamine abuse can be treated by abruptly discontinuing the drug or by gradually tapering the dose, whichever is more acceptable to the patient. In either case, the patient should be shown a more appropriate program for weight control.

A more serious problem is the patient who develops a severe psychological dependence on amphetamines and may present the same symptoms seen in younger "street drug" abusers. Typical complaints associated with amphetamine intoxication include anorexia, insomnia, anxiety, hyperactivity, and rapid speech and thought processes (speeding). Adrenergic hyperactivity, such as hyperreflexia, tachycardia, diaphoresis, and dilated pupils responsive to light may be seen. Fortunately, more severe symptoms such as hyperpyrexia and hypertension are relatively rare. Patients may also manifest stereotyped movements of the mouth, face, or extremities.

The other classic syndrome seen in either acute or chronic amphetamine intoxication is a paranoid psychosis without delirium. While typically seen in young people using methamphetamine hydrochloride IV, it can also occur in individuals using dextroamphetamine or other amphetamines orally on a chronic basis. The paranoid psychosis may occur with or without other manifestations of amphetamine intoxication. The absence of disorientation distinguishes this condition from most other toxic psychoses. This syndrome is clinically indistinguishable from an acute schizophrenic reaction of the paranoid type and the correct diagnosis is often made only in retrospect, based on a history of amphetamine use and a urine test positive for amphetamines.

Treatment

Amphetamines can be withdrawn abruptly. If the intoxication is mild, the patient's agitation should be handled by reassurance alone. The patient should be "talked down" much as one would handle an LSD reaction. If sedation is necessary, benzodiazepines are the drugs of choice. Phenothiazines should be avoided. They increase the patient's agitation because they heighten the patient's sense of dysphoria. However, major tranquilizers must be used in cases of severe hypertension or hyperpyrexia.

Chlorpromazine, 25 to 50 mg IM, or haloperidol, 2.5 to 5.0 mg IM, will reverse these life-threatening conditions. If adrenergic hyperactivity is severe, the patient should be given propranolol hydrochloride, 20 to 40 mg orally or 1 to 2 mg IV; but this medication should not be used if the patient has diabetes, asthma, or organic heart disease.

Most signs of intoxication will clear in two to four days. The major problem then is appropriate psychiatric management of postamphetamine depression. In mild cases this will be manifested by feelings of lethargy with the subsequent temptation to use amphetamines again for "energy." In more serious cases, the patient may become suicidal and will require inpatient psychiatric treatment. The efficacy of antidepressants in such cases has not been adequately documented. Even with support and psychotherapy, most patients will experience symptoms of depression for 3 to 6 months following the cessation of chronic amphetamine abuse.

COCAINE
Abuse

Cocaine has emerged as the most psychologically addicting drug in common use. Even mature individuals with normal psychological profiles are vulnerable to compulsive cocaine use. Users experience an intense sense of euphoria often associated with increased sexual desire and improved sexual functioning. These positive rewards are often followed by a moderate to severe postcocaine depression which provides a strong compulsion for further cocaine use.

The signs and symptoms of acute cocaine intoxication are similar to those described in the section on amphetamine abuse. Snorting may produce rhinitis or sinusitis, and rarely, perforations of the nasal septum. "Freebasing" (inhalation of cocaine alkaloid vapors) may produce bronchitis. Grand mal seizures are another infrequent complication. Patients also describe "snowlights," these are flashes of light usually seen at the periphery of the visual field.

The major problem associated with chronic use is a cocaine-induced psychosis manifested by visual and auditory hallucinations and paranoid delusions often associated with violent behavior. Tactile hallucinations, called "coke bugs," involve the perception that something is crawling under the skin. A cocaine psychosis may be indistinguishable from an amphetamine psychosis, but is usually shorter in duration.

Management

Cocaine abusers will be seen in any medical or surgical setting. The problem is becoming common among affluent young people, but all classes and racial groups are potential users. Occasional cocaine use does not require specific treatment, except in the case of a life-threatening overdose. Most lethal doses will be metabolized within one hour by enzymes in the blood and liver. In the interim, an airway and assisted breathing with oxygen may be necessary. Death can be caused by ventricular fibrillation or cardiac arrest. Cardiac status should therefore be monitored closely. Intravenous diazepam should be used to control convulsions.

Chronic cocaine use produces tolerance and severe psychological dependency; true physiologic dependence has not been demonstrated. Detoxification can be accomplished by the abrupt cessation of all cocaine use. A gradual elimination of the drug is not necessary and is not recommended. After withdrawal from cocaine, the chronic user will experience depression, lethargy, and anxiety. These symptoms will begin to resolve within seven days and specific medical treatment is rarely indicated. The major complication of withdrawal is a severe depression with suicidal ideation. If this occurs, the patient requires psychiatric hospitalization and treatment with tricyclic antidepressants.

All cocaine abusers should be referred for individual counseling; participation in Narcotics Anonymous or Alcoholics Anonymous should be strongly recommended. Once compulsive cocaine use has begun, it is almost impossible for the user to return to a pattern of occasional, controlled use. Such individuals are also likely to develop problems with alcohol and other drugs. For that reason, the goal of treatment should be total abstinence from cocaine and all other drugs.

SUGGESTED READINGS

Bernstein JG: *Handbook of Drug Therapy in Psychiatry.* John Wright–PSG Inc, Littleton, Massachusetts, 1983.

Ellinwood EH (ed): *Current Concepts on Amphetamine Abuse.* US Dept of Health, Education, and Welfare publication No. (HSM) 72-9085, National Institute of Mental Health, 1972.

Fultz JM, Senay EC: Guidelines for the management of hospitalized narcotics addicts. *Ann Intern Med* 1975; 82:815–818.

Green AI, Meyer RE, Shader RI: Heroin and methadone abuse—acute and chronic management, in Shader RI (ed): *Manual of Psychiatric Therapeutics*. Boston, Little Brown & Co, 1975.

Shader RI, Caine ED, Meyer RE: Treatment of dependence on barbiturates and sedative-hypnotics, in Shader RI (ed): *Manual of Psychiatric Therapeutics*. Boston, Little Brown & Co, 1975.

Smith DE: Diagnosis, treatment and aftercare approaches to cocaine abuse. *J Substance Abuse Treat* 1984; 1:5–9.

Smith DE, Wesson DR: Phenobarbital technique for treatment of barbiturate dependence. *Arch Gen Psychiatry* 1971; 24:56–60.

Smith DE, Wesson DR: *Diagnosis and Treatment of Adverse Reactions to Sedative-Hypnotics*. US Dept of Health, Education, and Welfare Publication No. (ADM) 75–144, National Institute on Drug Abuse, 1974.

4

The Pain Patient: Evaluation and Treatment

THOMAS P. HACKETT and ANTHONY BOUCKOMS

THE NATURE OF PAIN

Trying to separate functional from organic factors in long-standing pain is both vexing and unprofitable. Nevertheless, it is a task all too frequently requested of consultation psychiatrists. The physician's preoccupation with ferreting psychological issues out of the pain he cannot cure and his desire to implicate the psyche is well known. Like the ritual washing of hands by the Roman tribune eager to absolve himself of responsibility, the request to separate psyche from soma is often a symbolic write-off. The psychiatric consultant must be prepared for this when asked to evaluate a patient with unexplained pain.

The psychiatric consultant's job is to answer four questions: (1) Is the pain intractable because of nociceptive stimuli? (2) Is the pain problem central, mediated by the CNS, that is, have the spinal cord, brainstem, limbic system, and cortex been recruited as reverberating pain circuits? (3) Is the pain complaint primarily suffering as is seen in depression or delusional pain? (4) Has pain behavior supervened, so that associated disability from the pain is now more disabling than the sensory pain itself?

Nociceptive pain is due to activation of A, δ-, or C sensory fibers by stimulation of specialized peripheral pain receptors (nociceptors) by thermal, mechanical, or chemical stimuli. Nociceptive stimulation produces sensory or somatic pain which is direct, sharp, and stimulus-related. Central pain, which is synonymous with deafferentation and neuropathic pain, is burning, exquisitely sensitive pain, characterized by delayed onset after initial injury, spontaneous paroxysmal exacerbations, nonanatomical distribution, trigger zones, and a change in sensory threshold, for example, anesthesia, allodynia, hyperalgesia, or hyperesthesia.

42

Emotional conditions can unquestionably produce pain—a pain that hurts just as much as the pain from a tumor or a gunshot wound. It is equally certain that the severity of the pain resulting from either the wound or tumor can increase or decrease as a function of the patient's apprehensiveness. The most important lesson to remember about pain is that it hurts, whatever its cause. With the exception of five specific conditions which will be described later, pain is rarely generated and maintained by psychological forces alone. It is nevertheless important to weigh the psychological forces bearing on pain. This chapter is designed to give the consultant a basis for evaluating the psychological components of pain. In particular it will attempt to describe the limits of the psychiatric assessment of pain and to offer a framework for consultation when the request is to "rule out the functional."

Long-standing pain is difficult to assess largely because of the limits of our model for pain. Most of what we learn about pain in medical school is based on the concept of acute pain. The patient in acute pain moans, writhes, sweats, begs for help, and gives every appearance of being in great distress. Those in the vicinity of someone in acute pain feel an urgency to help. When pain persists over days and weeks, the individual adapts to it often without realizing that he does so. This adaptation means that the pain becomes bearable without seeming to change in intensity. How this happens is not fully known. The sensation may become intermittent or the sufferer more capable of using distraction. Whatever the reason, the patient learns to accommodate the pain so that he can appear in society without making those around him uncomfortable. The patient becomes able to sit in the physician's examining room complaining of agonizing pain while giving little or no evidence of being in agony. It is ironic that the capacity to adapt to severe pain is often the patient's undoing. It causes the examiner to doubt the patient's veracity as a reporter. The sufferer now finds himself in the position of having to prove that he is in pain. He feels himself on trial. The physician who begins to doubt that the patient is in pain should remember Wilder Penfield's maxim: Believe that pain exists when the patient says so unless the patient is a known malingerer. Generally physicians who have had pain syndromes themselves are in a much better position to assess and to treat long-standing pain in others.

It is helpful in the evaluation of pain to remember some simple definitions. Mersky and Spear state that pain should be defined operationally. "Commonly this implies a disagreeable sensation and tissue damage; and if not, it implies a response by the patient with terms corresponding to those used when there is tissue damage."[1] Ryle, with wry succinctness, says that "pain is a sensation of a special sort which we ordinarily dislike having."[2] The definition we favor comes from the British writer Peter Fleming:

> If you come to think about it, physical pain has many singularities. Of all human experience, it is, as long as it lasts, the most absorbing; and it is the only human experience which, when it comes to an end, automatically confers a real if not perhaps a very high kind of happiness. It is also the only experience this side of death which is by its nature solitary. But the oddest thing about it is that despite its intensity, and despite its unequalled power over mind and body, when it is over, you cannot remember it at all.[3]

Pain can be divided into two components—the original and the reactive. The original component has also been called the primary, organic, or "tissue" component. It is the felt sensation. The reactive component, known also as the processing or secondary component, is the psychological response to the felt sensation. This subdivision is far too simple because it implies that both components must be present and yet distinct in the experience of pain. We know this is not true; for example, pain can be experienced centrally. However, for the sake of this chapter's thesis, the two-part model is appropriate. One could speculate, using this model, that if Van Cliburn or Michael DeBakey had a door slammed on his hand, the pain might be more severe than if the same accident happened to a psychiatrist. The fingers of the pianist or surgeon are his source of livelihood, self-esteem, and pride; as such the reactive component would be considerable. By biting his tongue severely, a psychiatrist might similarly muster a large reactive component in the ensuing pain. The International Association for the Study of Pain has recognized the critical importance of both sensory and emotional components of pain. This recognition has lead to the following definition: "Pain is an unpleasant sensory and emotional experience associated with actual or potential tissue damage, or described in terms of such damage."[4]

Our main focus will be on the reactive or psychological component of pain, not only because it falls naturally to us as psychiatrists, but because it can be altered by distraction, reduced by suggestion, or augmented by fear. Although there is some relationship between the primary sensation and the secondary component, it is by no means direct and linear. We cannot say that the larger the amount of tissue damaged, the greater the psychological effect. Other factors intervene.

PATHOLOGIC VERSUS EXPERIMENTAL PAIN

There are two general types of pain—pathologic and experimental. Familiarity with the difference between experimental and pathologic pain is important to the understanding of the reactive component of pain. Pathologic pain is pain associated with injury, as with laceration, myocardial infarction, or renal calculus. Experimental pain is produced in the laboratory by a variety of means ranging from electrical shock to compression of the Achilles tendon. One would think that both sensations might be equally uncomfortable given a strong enough stimulus. However, the curious nature of pain is such that these experiences are quite different. The difference depends entirely on the reactive or psychological component of pain. An experimental subject experiencing laboratory pain knows that he can bring his discomfort to a halt by crying out. He knows the dimensions of his pain—that it signals no imminent catastrophe, no distant incapacity.

Pathologic pain, in dramatic contrast, is by nature an alerting mechanism heralding the presence of danger. The difference between experimental and pathologic pain is nowhere better demonstrated than in their dramatically different responses to morphine. Massive wounds sustained in accidents or in battle can be made painless by small doses of morphine. In contrast, individuals in severe experimental pain would be no more apt to respond to 15 mg of morphine sulfate than to parenteral sterile saline. Morphine appears to exert its effect not on the primary component of pain but on the reactive. We are indebted to Henry Beecher[5] for illuminating research on this subject.

Another example of the importance of the psychological nature of the painful experience also comes from Beecher. In his study of soldiers shot down at Anzio, all of them seriously wounded yet mentally clear, two thirds did not want morphine. In fact most of them denied any pain. The wound meant relief from combat, an honorable reprieve from mortal peril. In a civilian population suffering far less tissue trauma as the result of abdominal surgery (cholecystecomy) Beecher found that four out of five wanted medication to relieve their pain. The soldier, thankful to have escaped alive from the battlefield, regarded his wound with a feeling akin to pleasure. The civilian, following major surgery, regarded the incident as both disruptive and depressing. Beecher assumed from this that "there is no simple, direct relationship between the wound per se and the pain experience. The pain is in very large part determined by other factors and of great importance here is the significance of the wound." This background will give the reader some idea of the practical importance of psychological factors in the experience of pain. The lesson is that neither the presence nor absence of organic pathology offers much in the way of a guide to the measurement of pain suffered.

Pathologic pain invokes two key elements of the body's response to pain: the psychological stress of the unknown significance of the pain and the biological effects of stress analgesia. The typical delay of minutes to hours between tissue damage and the sensation of pathologic pain illustrates the critical effects of psychological expectancy and the body's biological adaptation to an acute stress. Stress analgesia involves complicated monoamine and opiate mechanisms which are extremely effective in the immediate control of pain and the shock of acute stress. The individual is back in control, albeit briefly, of his environment. When the pain is more protracted, the adaptive mechanism of stress analgesia fails. The biological dynamic of this mechanism is unknown, but may provide an answer to how pain actually becomes an ongoing part of illness.[6]

PERIPHERAL VERSUS CENTRAL PAIN

A major factor that confuses the assessment of pain is the confounding relationship between primary peripheral sensory pain and the central perception of pain. Pain is not conveyed directly from the peripheral injury to the cortex. Most afferent pain information is conveyed diffusely through the brainstem reticular activating system, thalamus, and limbic system. This central component of pain begins right in the dorsal horn of the spinal cord and appears to involve every level of the nervous system up to the cortex. In this way pain can be perceived even without an obvious nociceptive stimulus. Memory can elicit pain. Neuropathic or deafferentation pain is the prototype of central pain as compared to sensory or somatic pain.[7]

Central changes may be associated with 50% of chronic pain states. The evidence for this comes from neurosurgeons who have shown that interruption of the specific pain pathways often does not eliminate the suffering of pain. Limited peripheral nerve damage may result in changes in the receptive fields and recruitment of neurons at multiple levels in the nervous system from the dorsal horn to the brainstem to the thalamus and cortex.[8] For example, stimulation of the anterolateral columns of the spinal cord in patients with deafferentation pain can produce contralateral burning sensations, findings not seen in patients with nociceptive pain. Electrical stimulation of the cerebral cortex is reported to elicit pain in patients with clinical pain of neuropathic origin, whereas stimulation of somatatopically adjacent cortical regions not associated with the site of clinical pain produces only localized parathesias. The centralization of pain through mechanisms like these shows that somatic therapies that are directed only at the peripheral nerve or the spinal segments initially involved in producing the pain syndrome may be ineffective.[9]

PAIN MEASUREMENT

Face to face with an individual in chronic pain, the physician with customary skepticism generally takes steps to convince himself of the presence of authentic pain. However, because the complaint of pain is entirely subjective, the search for a truly objective assessment is a futile effort. It is a myth that an instrument exists by which the presence of pain can be verified. However, while acknowledging the subjective nature of the complaint, objective measurements of the patient's subjective response are possible.

Three sensitive and reliable clinical instruments for pain measurement are:

1. *A pain drawing.* Have the patient draw the anatomical distribution of the pain as he feels it in his body. The subsequent drawing gives a good idea of the anatomy of the problem along with the psychology of the patient and his level of knowledge.

2. *A visual analog scale.* A 100-mm-long visual analog scale with a 0 marking no pain and 10 marking severe pain is readily understood by most patients and is very sensitive to change. The patient can mark this scale once a day or even every hour during therapeutic trials.

3. *Categorical rating scales.* Categorical rating scales using three or five categories of severity of pain are not only simple but very relevant to the patient's perception of his overall problem. These categories are as follows: 0 = no pain, 1 = mild, 2 = discomforting, 3 = distressing, 4 = horrible, and 5 = excruciating pain. The subjective nature of the pain is acknowledged as the outcome variable.

PAIN AND THE PLACEBO

In a further effort to elucidate the nature of pain, the physician may move to the use of placebos. In the entire field of medicine few phenomena are as misunderstood as is the placebo trial. Despite an abundance of excellent research on the topic, most of which has been published in widely read journals and textbooks, people still regard the placebo test as a means of separating functional from organic pain. To compound this error, many of those who conduct placebo trials do so in such an unscientific fashion that they lose whatever useful information might have been gained.

To begin with, it is known that approximately 33% of a population in pain will obtain relief from an inert substance just as if they were given an analgesic.[5] Evans and Hoyle in 1933 used sodium bicarbonate to treat individuals suffering from angina pectoris. In 38% of their subjects they found this agent to be as effective as nitroglycerin.[10] Similar studies have been conducted in various parts of the world and the placebo response is found in about one third of whatever population is tested.

The placebo response is a normal aspect of personality and cannot be linked with any type of psychopathology. The mechanism for the placebo response is probably the endorphin pain-inhibiting system, but it is influenced both by psychological and neurologic factors. It is a complex response which can affect not only pain but other symptoms such as nausea, fatigue, and anxiety as well. Patients with depression, somatoform disorder, or other varieties of emotional disturbance are no more apt to be placebo reactors than are so-called normal people. Following surgery, about one patient out of three obtains pain relief from saline or some other inert substance and is therefore considered placebo-positive. Some investigators believe that a much higher proportion of the population could respond to placebos if suggestion were supplied as well. There is reason to believe that this is correct. Whether the pain is from a metastatic malignancy or is part of a major affective disorder, relief will come to the placebo reactor. Consequently, the only thing learned from a placebo trial is whether or not the patient is placebo-positive. The trial is of no assistance in separating psychogenic from organic pain.

The timeworn custom of slipping in a few saline shots for morphine and calling the deception a placebo trial only demonstrates the ignorance of the perpetrator. If a shot of sterile saline is substituted for one out of six injections of meperidine hydrochloride and the patient responds to this fake shot by obtaining relief, the nature of his pain will be questioned. In fact, his relief is based on the conditioned response. In a valid placebo trial, the inert substance must be given to the patient in a randomized manner along with the usual narcotic under double-blind conditions for at least five days. Without this control the placebo trial is useless. Furthermore, one of the chief hazards of placebo use is that the patient feels tricked. If he discovers that placebos have been used (as he generally does), it is natural for him to feel on trial and wrongly accused. Basically, in clinical practice, there is no reason to conduct placebo trials.

PAIN AND THE PSYCHIATRIC CONSULTANT

The psychiatric consultant should be brought into the case early and ought to be introduced as a regular member of the medical team. The referring physician should take care to ensure that the patient does not interpret the need for a psychiatrist as a sign that his veracity is in doubt. It should be explained that a psychiatrist is routinely asked to evaluate all patients with long-standing pain (which indeed should be the case). As a general rule, when the referring physician is comfortable in using the services of a psychiatrist, the patient accepts the examination without protest. It is only when the psychiatrist is called in at the end of a long, frustrating, and unprofitable hospitalization that the patient balks and protests.

Once the psychiatrist has entered the evaluative arena, what can be expected? To the inexperienced psychiatrist such consultation is often a baffling and frustrating task that grows in complexity with each new attempt to find a resolution. There are a few simple things that can be done without getting bogged down in functional-versus-organic speculation. Indentifying the most common psychiatric conditions associated with pain is often sufficient.

The Psychiatric Examination

Although interviewing the patient with a chronic pain syndrome requires no special psychiatric skill, it does demand that the examiner pay close attention to detail and to the patient's style of discourse. We take a detailed history of when and how the pain began and inquire about the various treatments received and the personalities of the physicians involved. Throughout the history, we look for fluctuations in the course of the pain. Under what circumstances did it improve? Under what circumstances was it exacerbated? Was it the medication that helped or some other factor? How long were remissions, and what life events coincided with exacerbations? It is often valuable to go over the same material more than once, particularly when life circumstances intersect the course of pain and alter it for better or worse. We do this not so much to make a dynamic formulation as to gather facts that will make it possible to predict fluctuations in pain that might otherwise seem inexplicable. As one comes to understand how a patient's pain is shaped by his life, it is sometimes possible to modify the pattern in a small way and thereby reduce suffering.

Since many patients have extensive histories of pain and delight in regaling the examiner with their odysseys through clinics, spas, and hospitals, we often ask them to write detailed accounts of their pain from onset to the present time. Included in this we request information on all medications—those that helped and those that did not—complete with side effects and the reasons for discontinuing those that were stopped. In subsequent sessions we explore the patient's mental life from childhood to the present and take into account the family history and ethnic background as well.

FIVE PSYCHIATRIC CONDITIONS THAT MAY PRESENT WITH PAIN
Depression

Major depressive illness as diagnosed by DSM-III,* or Research Diagnostic Criteria (RDC) is found in about 25% of chronic pain patients.[11] However, 60% to 100% of pain patients have symptoms of a depressive disorder. While some of these depressive syndromes are truly secondary to the pain itself (*adjustment disorders with affective symptoms* (309.00), or *psychological factors affecting physical condition* (316.00), some of these patients have major depression which is denied. Denial of affect, particularly anger, is a significant problem in 44% of chronic pain patients.[12] How does one diagnose an affective disorder when denial of affect is the primary response of the patient being examined? The following tactics are particularly useful in ferreting out the true affective disorders in this group.

1. Ask indirect questions about the affective state through the use of vegetative symptoms. How many times does the person wake from sleep at night? How long does it take to resleep? Do they have early-morning awakening? When was the last time they really enjoyed themselves? Does food taste the same? Do they enjoy eating? Has weight been lost? What do they do that's pleasurable on a given day? Do they have any sexual desire left? What do they do with their anger? Does the pain ever bring them to tears? Would they rather be dead than in their present state? In this way one can pick up the presence of important vegetative signs of depression. (See chapter 12.)

2. Evaluate the person's limbic, that is, real uncensored, response to emotion. Look for denial of strong emotion, particularly anger or depression. Denial, displacement, or suppression of emotions often indicates psychopathology. For example, can they laugh at a joke at their own expense? Can they acknowledge some anger at themselves and others? Do they answer affective questions with affective responses, or is it all avoidance and denial?

3. The Minnesota Multiphasic Personality Inventory (MMPI) with assessment of the subtle scales, the psychosomatic V, and discrepencies

---

* *Diagnostic and Statistical Manual of Mental Disorders*, ed 3. Washington, American Psychiatric Association, 1980.

within the test can be very helpful in picking out covert depression from personality disorder and outright faking.[13]

Somatoform Disorders

The somatoform disorders comprise a group of disorders in which painful physical complaints and irrational anxiety about physical illness are the predominant clinical feature. These concerns exist in the absence of organic findings or known physiologic mechanisms. The following four groups constitute the somatoform disorders: (1) somatization disorder (300.81) (Briquet's syndrome), (2) psychogenic pain disorder (307.80), (3) hypochondriasis (300.70), and (4) conversion hysteria (300.11).

Somatization disorder.   A useful screening device for this disorder is the mnemonic: Somatization Disorder Besets Ladies And Vexes Physicians. These initials stand for Shortness of breath, Dysmenorrhea, Burning genitals, Lump in the throat, Amnesia, Vomiting, and Pain in the extremities. The presence of at least three of the seven screening criteria carries an 80% likelihood of making an accurate diagnosis of somatization disorder.[14] An exact DSM-III diagnosis requires at least 14 symptoms for women and 12 for men. The person must have been treated for these symptoms over the course of a lifetime characterized by sickness beginning before age 30 years. While the strictness of these criteria makes a firm diagnosis quite rare, formes frustes of somatoform illness are plentiful, exhibiting pain in the head, neck, back, and extremities as well as missing work for ill-defined reasons. Like classic hysterics and sociopaths, these patients are the genetic inheritors of alcoholic and sociopathic parents.

Psychogenic pain disorder.   This is a long-standing, severe, nonanatomical pain wherein psychological factors are judged to be etiologic, and it is not due to another mental disorder. It is a useful diagnostic category when: (1) there is a temporal relationship between an environmental stimulus that is apparently related to a psychological conflict and the occurrence of pain; and (2) the pain provides some major secondary gain for the patient.

Hypochondriasis.   This is the unrealistic belief in the presence of a serious disease despite a normal physical examination and medical reassurance. This belief interferes with the individual's social and work life.

Conversion disorders.   Conversion disorders are not diagnosed when symptoms are limited to pain. Diagnosis requires a loss or alteration in physical functioning suggesting a physical disorder; psychological factors are judged to be etiologic. The symptoms are involuntary, and no pathophysiologic mechanism can be invoked.

Psychosis

Schizophrenia, organic psychoses, and dementias can all present with the symptom of pain. The pain will be delusional in nature, often bizarre in both distribution and quality, and usually one part of a mosaic of symptoms which together form the picture of psychosis. Rarely will pain be the only symptom. It is also rare to have pain as the presenting symptom of schizophrenia. In each of the few cases we have seen, the pain was linked to a delusion of persecution.

Pathologic pain does, of course, occur in patients with psychosis, dementia, or hypochondriasis. When this happens, how does one detect it? The denial of pain or its significance is common in schizophrenic patients. This accounts for the unusually large number of silent myocardial infarctions, perforated duodenal ulcers, and ruptured appendices found in mental hospitals. In our experience, when pain is part of a delusional system or represents a fixed idea of the hypochondriac or the demented patient, the sufferer is not eager to have the discomfort removed. In fact, the patient may balk at the suggestion of cure. The physician dealing with psychotic patients must be always vigilant for limps, grimaces, splinting of extremities, and other external indicators of pain.

Compensation Neurosis

Compensation neurosis (under DSM-III this would be called psychological factors affecting physical condition [316.00]) applies to an individual with work-related chronic pain when the amount of distress seems unduly amplified in terms of the discernible pathology or when it persists long past the time most physicians, insurance adjustors, and union stewards think it should. In almost every case the patient has filed a claim for financial compensation. Some psychiatrists consider the term a fiction derived for the convenience of management to pejoratively label unwanted claimants. When the pain is feigned, the individual is called a malingerer. The pain of an individual with compensation neurosis is not feigned. It may seem out of proportion to the injury. It may tax professional mettle not to suspect that the patient is pretending, but it is important to keep in mind that the hurt is real.

Typically, the patient with compensation neurosis is a blue-collar worker who has overworked to compensate for an underlying need to be taken care of. He is a hyperattainer who holds down more than one job and provides abundantly for his family. He considers himself to be a loyal employee and union member, a patriot, a churchgoer, and a family man. He then sustains an industrial accident. The injury may be trivial or major. Whatever the extent, he develops an incapacitating pain that prevents him from resuming the role of provider. He joins the ranks of the dependent. Because he has a history of hard work and accomplishment and because he genuinely enjoyed his active life and takes no conscious relish in being on the dole, he assumes his new role with a sense of entitlement. When he fails to be rehabilitated in the generous allotment of time provided by management, he incurs their emnity. Next he exhausts the patience of his union and soon thereafter, in a domino effect, the patience of his wife, his children, and his friends. He is left with an attorney to bolster him. His pain symbolizes the sum of the frustrations he has endured and becomes a badge of the long hours he has toiled, of the vacations he has postponed, and of the sacrifices he has vainly made for others. Receiving compensation has become the only reward for his suffering. The issue of pain has been transformed into an issue of pride. It has become not only a question of hurt, but of hurt feelings.

In this age of litigation, a lawyer often appears on the scene not far behind the surgeon. As a consequence, nearly every case involves the possibility of some form of compensation. As costs escalate, so lawyers proliferate. Compensation neurosis can be suspected in any case where the pain patient is represented by more than one attorney.

Therapy is often impossible until the legal issues are settled. A transient euphoria usually develops if the case closes favorably. Invariably this is followed by a depression. An exploration of the depression often reveals a long history of dissatisfaction with some aspects of life—marriage, work, or something else of major importance. Antidepressants and psychotherapy can help.

Malingering

The malingerer (V65.20) is a pretender. In order to obtain an end—money, privilege, or the avoidance of an unpleasant duty—the malingerer fakes a complaint. He will seldom undergo painful laboratory procedures for diagnostic reasons. This separates the malingerer from the person with Münchausen's syndrome. (See chapter 14.) More often than not the correlation between the symptom and the goal will be uncomplicated and linear. Malingered pain is more apt to be found in federal, state, and municipal hospitals. Of all the conditions described so far, it is the only pain that is not felt.

The malingerer is not so much treated as discovered. Every specialty has its array of covert techniques to reveal the faker. The MMPI can be used to help make this diagnosis. High, obvious and low, subtle scores; high F scale scores (faking); and extreme changes on repeat testing may indicate malingering, but are not diagnostic alone.

The most practical means of diagnosing the malingerer is to rule out organic pathology through the usual examinations and tests and also to find, through a careful scrutiny of background (particularly old service records), evidence of similar behavior in the past. Like lying, malingering tends to be a character trait used in times of stress from early adolescence through senium. Once revealed, psychotherapy can be offered, but we suspect that the results would be negligible.

CHRONIC PAIN SYNDROMES CHARACTERIZED BY PAIN BEHAVIOR

When each of the five foregoing conditions has been ruled out, the physician often still has a patient suffering from a variety of emotional problems that may contribute to or even cause pain. It is the unusual chronic pain syndrome that does not contain a combination of both psychological and physical components, and it is important to be able to give the referring physician some idea of the relative significance of each to the patient's pain. The concept of *pain behavior* is a valuable aid in understanding this psychology.

Pain behavior is all behavior generated by an individual to reflect the presence of nociception.[15] These behaviors may have begun in response to sensory pain or suffering, but now occur totally because of their environmental reinforcement. For example, the person with inguinal pain who continues to limp after good analgesia has been provided by a nerve block has abnormal learned pain behavior. The recognition of this condition may be made easier by evaluating the patient on the Madison scale. MADISON is an acronym composed of the first initial of seven characteristics that, in our opinion, correlate with the psychogenicity of pain. For those interested in quantification, each characteristic can be rated on a 0 to 4 scale. The higher the total score, the greater the importance of psychological factors.

M   *Multiplicity.* This means the pain is either in more than one place or is of more than one variety. It also means that when one pain disappears through a therapeutic effort, another will replace it.

A   *Authenticity.* Patients who seem more interested in convincing you that their pain is genuine than they are in receiving a cure for it, fall into this category. They want to be believed. We have found this to be especially true for the pain that masks a depression.

D *Denial.* As mentioned earlier, chronic pain patients often deny the presence of emotional problems. This denial can be highlighted when they give an exaggerated account of marital or family harmony. They paint a rosy picture of domestic bliss even in the face of impending divorce. Should they admit the occasional presence of anxiety or depression, it is with the proviso that these affects never influence the intensity of their pain. Pathologic pain is a fluctuating state. It is highly sensitive to the influence of fear, anger, sadness, and tranquillity. When a pain is reported to be unresponsive to these emotions, one should question its nature.

I *Interpersonal relationships.* During the course of an interview the individual may grimace or spontaneously complain of pain when some-one's name is mentioned—someone who has something to do directly, indirectly, or symbolically with the patient. Similarly, if that person should walk into the room during the interview, the patient will give evidence of being in immediate distress such as pressing the nurse call button. Yet, when the patient's attention is drawn to this relationship, the connection will be discounted.

S *Singularity.* This applies to pain that makes the patient unique. The following statements demonstrate singularity: "I am sure you've never encountered a pain like this in your large practice, Doctor." "I have never heard of a pain like this nor has any other physician who has treated me." It is a singular and unusual pain, one that puts the patient into a special category.

O *"Only you."* This is perhaps the most pernicious factor in the Madison Scale in terms of the future of the physician-patient relationship. It reads, "Only you can help me, Doctor." When the patient, soon after meeting you, presents you with a white charger complete with lance and banner bearing the cross of St. George, you should immediately imagine the scores of other physicians who stand behind you in serried ranks with horses crippled, lances bent, and pennons torn.

N *Nothing helps* or *No change.* This means that the pain does not change from hour to hour, day to day, or year to year. If anything, it only gets worse. Nothing helps, including drugs. This defies all that is known about the nature of pathologic pain. Distraction, suggestion, chemical inter-ference, barometric pressure, circadian influences, and political upheaval fail to alter the patient's perception of the discomfort. When asked, "Since drugs don't help, why do you take so many medications?" the answer will be something like, "What else is there to do? If I don't take them I will be worse off." When reminded of the statement that, "nothing helps," the answer is, "Something is better than nothing," or some equally meaning-less cliché. All pathologic pain changes for better or worse during a 24-hour period. Distraction plays a role as does mood. Appropriate pain medication invariably helps. In the absence of some relief, either spontaneous or drug-induced, the consultant should consider another type of distress—more psychological than physical.

These are no more than clues to guide the practitioner in the search for factors that may help in the recognition of underlying psychological issues. When the Madison Score is above 15, some form of psychiatric intervention should be considered.

Understanding and treating pain behavior problems is often more difficult than recognizing them. Several pain clinicians have approached this problem and written about it from slightly different perspectives. Sternbach has described patients' "pain games," emphasizing the secondary gain resulting from them.[16] Blumer and Heilbronn have written about the pain-prone disorder, a syndrome of pain behavior and affective symptoms which they state is part of masked affective pathology.[17] Eric Berne has written about consulting room games, a variety of interpersonal transactions described in terms of parent-child conflict.[18] Bouckoms and Litman have written descriptive analyses of archetypal clinical interviews which underline the patient's narcissistic use of the physician, and describe four common elements that characterize the chronic pain patient's relationship with his doctor: (1) muted anger, (2) demands which are inconsistent with usual good practice, (3) covert depression, and (4) long-standing unrequited wishes for dependency and nurturance.[19]

GENERAL PRINCIPLES OF THERAPY

There are a few general principles which should be followed in the management of chronic pain syndromes. The patient should not have his pain called psychological. The physician should assure the patient that there is no question about the degree of suffering involved. Although psychological factors may play a role—more important in some, less in others—this by no means diminishes either the quality or quantity of pain the patient endures. To this end the physician should be willing to discuss the pain and to take active measures in suggesting remedies that might be helpful.

If warranted, we suggest simple remedies in addition to medication. The application of poultices, unguents, rubifacients, astringent lotions, splints, and hot packs can provide variety to the treatment plan. Massages, rubdowns, hydrotherapy, and physiotherapy all have their place in our therapeutic armamentarium. While these manipulations may seem excessive, some have intrinsic value in soothing the pain, and all share equally in the task of providing tangible evidence of the physician's active interest.

An important principle of management is to assure the patient that treatment will continue even if there is no immediate improvement. One of the fears expressed by many patients in chronic pain is of abandonment—that if they do not improve, the physician will see them no more or will refer them to someone else.

While not requiring a cure, it is important for the physician to be hopeful that the condition will remit or that some method will be discovered to reduce discomfort. The physician should guard against being affected by the patient's sense of discouragement. Great patience is required of the physician who treats the pain patient. Don Lipsitt has described the so-called "crock clinics" that are dumping grounds for chronic pain patients.[20] These are clinics where individuals are free to return for unlimited periods with no expectation of improvement. The symptom, whether pain or another problem, is a "ticket" to establish contact with a physician. As long as the relationship is maintained, the patient seldom decompensates and rarely goes on to find more complex and dangerous treatments. The crock clinic is not a bad model to follow in treating the chronic pain patient. In the long run it is probably quite cost-effective.

An abiding principle in the treatment of chronic pain is to avoid surgery. Very few surgical procedures on the CNS are definitive in the cure or control of pain, and most carry with them a tax that is sometimes worse than the pain. Not only is pain surgery to be approached skeptically, but any type of surgery for the chronic pain patient should be regarded with great care before advising the patient to proceed. In particular, central pain is notoriously refractory to surgery that interrupts afferent pain pathways. This pain is often made worse by procedures such as neurectomies, rhizotomies, and cordotomies.

TALKING AND LISTENING

A strategy to evaluate the feelings and behavior observed in the pain patient is just as necessary as the strategy for evaluating physical aspects of the pain. The skill required is not only a matter of diagnosing the five major psychiatric illnesses that can present with pain. These patients often have a maladaptive style of interaction that requires a different kind of interpretive skill. The physician must be able to relate to the long-suffering pain patient who shows poor judgment of surgical risk, denies anger, and rapidly alternates between idealizing and denigrating his medical caretaker. The fluctuations of both mood and cooperation frequently encountered in the clinical interview are symptomatic of the patient's damaged self-esteem—of his injured narcissism. Chronic pain patients invariably feel damaged not only in the body part afflicted with discomfort, but in self-image and spirit as well, which is what we mean by narcissistic injury. The techniques for interviewing the narcissistically injured pain patient are designed to establish a diagnostic working relationship that will allow an accurate medical history to be elicited, avoid mistrust between physician and patient, and be conducive to the development of an effective treatment plan.

The interviewer should allow the patient to tell his own story. An initial degree of catharsis may be helpful to decrease the patient's anxiety and give the physician a sense of the patient's character. The physician must actively facilitate an alliance with the patient while still maintaining neutrality and avoiding misplaced sympathy. Underlying feelings of fear, anger, resentment, and mistrust are sometimes best uncovered by asking how others view the situation. This will sometimes bare unpleasant affects without incursive questions from the physician. Labeling overt and covert roles assigned by the patient to the physician is an important early intervention. Specifically this means that the physician should point out when the patient is attributing unrealistic curative powers or appears to believe that the physician is indifferent to his suffering. The longer one waits to confront these fantasies, the less effective any intervention will be.

Expression of affect should be encouraged. The physician should help the patient express the feelings he is having but does not want to acknowledge. The physician's assertive pursuit of the patient's true feelings will avoid giving the appearance of unqualified support to feelings that need expression. Too much support not only bypasses psychological problems, but may actually increase conflicted feelings over withholding, control, dependence, and frail self-esteem. The physician's kindness should not be allowed to become a problem for the patient.

Optimal care of intractable pain patients requires the ability to process neurologic and psychiatric data while simultaneously delineating and responding to the phrase-by-phrase manifestations of suffering and pain behavior. In essence, being able to get patients to talk about what they are angry at is just as important as discussing their insomnia or disc herniation. Progress occurs with these needy, angry patients only when there is a clear processing and separation of the reality-based facts of the case from unrealistic expectations. In that way, every clarification of an unrealistic idea can be an introduction to a more realistic alternative. The overall goal is to improve the patient's self-awareness and capacity for insight.

MEDICATION

Judicious and effective use of medicine in chronic pain patients rests on the concise evaluation of the four main components of the pain complaint: nociceptive pain, central pain, suffering, and pain behavior. In its most simplified form, the medical management of these four states employs, respectively, narcotics, anticonvulsants, antidepressants, and behavioral treatment without drugs. Severe intractable nociceptive pain is commonly found in cancer, chronic pancreatitis, or severe peripheral vascular disease. Peripheral tissue damage is the noxious stimulus. Nonsteroidal anti-inflammatory drugs, aspirin, and nerve blocks are often helpful in the early stages of these illnesses. Narcotics are the most effective medicine for these pains when the severity increases.

Principles of Narcotics Usage

Principles for the use of narcotics should be established early in the course of treatment:

1. Use a drug with good oral potency so that parenteral use can be avoided if possible. Methadone hydrochloride is a good first choice because of its oral potency and relatively slow clearance. Morphine, hydromorphone hydrochloride, and levorphanol tartrate may be useful when a stronger drug is required.

2. Avoid pro re nata (prn) or erratic dosing. A steady state of narcotic blood level will require approximately four half-lives to achieve consistency. Dosing prn will make any steady relief impossible. It will also set the patient up for drug-respondent conditioning and hence behavior problems.

3. Avoid meperidine hydrochloride in difficult cases because of its short duration of action (two to four hours) and because its principal metabolite, normeperidine, can cause excitement in patients with malignancy or renal impairment.[1]

4. Check the potency of the drug, its half-life, and absorption by different routes to make sure that the dosage schedule is consistent with these parameters.

The psychiatrist may be asked to see the pain patient because these very principles have not worked. The following is an expanded checklist for review of such a problem case:

1. Are narcotics the drugs of choice in this case? Unduly long clinical trials and ongoing patient suffering may be avoided in the problematic case by giving the patient 10 mg of morphine IV as a single test dose. This is a diagnostic procedure designed to determine if narcotics will relieve the pain. In about 50% of intractable pain patients narcotics do not have any significant analgesic effect. In a minority it is the anxiolytic effect rather than the analgesic effect which is helpful. This information may allow the physician to select another more appropriate drug rather than using a narcotic for anxiolysis.

2. Has the drug been given in adequate dosage and frequency? This requires knowledge of the potency and half-life of the drug as can be

found in a standard text such as Goodman and Gilman.[22] Common problems in this area include the switch from parenteral to oral use without any adjustment for dosage, or the administration of the drug at longer intervals than its half-life.

3. Has the method of administration and type of narcotic been optimized? The commonest problem in severe pain is the three- to eightfold variability of IM absorption. This can be decreased by using narcotics that are hydrophilic rather than lipophilic. Hydrophilic narcotics are morphine and hydromorphone. Fentanyl citrate, methadone, and meperidine are more lipophilic. When more lipophilic agents, (eg, methadone) are used IM, then injections into the deltoid rather than the gluteus muscle are preferable. For reasons that are unclear, this site of injection produces more consistent absorption and higher blood levels and hence more consistent pain relief.

4. The age of the patient is an important factor in the efficacy of the drug. Duration of effect may increase with age up to twofold and hence so does the analgesic effect in a 70-year-old *v* a 20-year-old.[23]

5. There can be problems with mixed agonists-antagonists. Pentazocine and butorphanol are commonly used narcotics because of their mixed antagonist-agonist properties. However, not only are they weaker than the standard narcotics, but if combined with them during a period of transition, the patient may develop withdrawal symptoms, an acute confusional state, or even psychosis. Older people are particularly susceptible to this. Avoidance of mixing drugs with the properties of various agonist-antagonist agents will obviate this problem.

6. The risk of narcotic addiction in medically treated patients is approximately 0.3%.[24] Even in high-risk populations who have been known to have had drug problems, the incidence of addiction is 20%. Therefore, considering the patient as an addict on the basis of difficulties with managing narcotics should be done cautiously and only with hard evidence. Acute sympathetic symptoms from drug withdrawal or tolerance are much more likely to be the problem than addiction per se. Rather than addiction, unrecognized depression is the most frequent immediate source of the excessive need for narcotics.

Narcotic Adjuvants

Pain may be refractory despite the most judicious application of traditional antinociceptive measures such as surgery, nerve blocks, and narcotics. Adjuvants to other analgesics, particularly narcotics, have been used for several decades to help improve pain control. Stimulants, neuroleptics, tricyclic monoaminergic agents, benzodiazepines, anticonvulsants, antihistamines, and prostaglandin inhibitors have their place. There are two indications for narcotic adjuvants: (1) when toxic or pharmacokinetic factors limit further increases in the patient's narcotic dosage, and (2) when pain remains uncontrolled by narcotics in combination with other secondary treatments such as decompression surgery, nerve blocks, or anxiolytic drugs. A narcotic adjuvant is indicated in these situations. For example, a prostaglandin inhibitor (ibuprofen) can be used in metastatic bone pain or clonidine hydrochloride may be added in spinal tolerance to morphine. In general, the choice of adjuvant should be individualized and one should aim for the simplest and most potent combination of drugs. The selection of the adjuvant depends on the symptoms associated with the pain, the character of the pain, and the physician's knowledge of any potential drug interactions.[25] (See Table 4-1.)

The type of pain is as important as its etiology in guiding the choice of an adjuvant. The pain may be characterized as a constant aching somatic pain, as in a fracture, or as a paroxysmal burning deafferentation sensation, as in phantom limb pain. The primary etiology of the pain

Table 4-1. Choosing an Analgesic Adjuvant on the Basis of Target Symptoms

Target Symptoms	Associated Clinical Context	Drug and Dosage
Insomnia	Presence of major depression	Doxepin hydrochloride 50–300 mg/d Trazodone hydrochloride 50–400 gm/d
	Absence of major affective disease	Trazodone 50–200 mg/d
Sedation	Slowed cognition	Dextroamphetamine 5–15 mg/d
Anxiety	Agitation, nausea, delirium	Haloperidol 5–200 mg/d
	Insomnia	Chlorpromazine 10–100 mg/d Doxepin 10–300 mg/d
Nausea	Moderate anxiety, insomnia	Droperidol 5–30 mg/d Haloperidol 2–40 mg/d
	Mild anxiety	Hydroxyzine 100 mg/d
Muscle spasm or myoclonic jerks		Diazepam 5–40 mg/d Clonazepam 1–6 mg/d

Reproduced with permission from Bouckoms.[25]

does not necessarily determine its type or character. For example, the pain of metastatic cancer may be either somatic or neuropathic. The therapeutic importance of recognizing deafferentation pain is not commonly appreciated. This pain is often refractory to narcotics and covers a diverse group of conditions ranging from the pain of rheumatoid arthritis to herpetic neuralgia to atypical facial pain. These patients may respond well to anticonvulsants or tricyclic monoaminergic agents. In general, the more burning deafferentation pains respond best to the tricyclic drugs whereas the more paroxysmal pains respond best to anticonvulsants. However, this is a generalization with many exceptions. In the most difficult ambiguous cases a valuable technique is to use an IV dose of the drug to gain a more rapid and accurate notion of its effectiveness for the long term. Intravenous morphine, lidocaine, and lorazepam can be used in this way to see whether any of these classes of drugs is worth pursuing.

Interactions with adjuvants.   Advantageous and deleterious interactions between narcotics and adjuvants may occur. Neuroleptics such as haloperidol and chlorpromazine bind to opiate receptors, potentially enhancing morphine analgesia. Hydroxyzine (100 mg IM) increases narcotic potency by 50%. Antidepressants enhance analgesia and affect narcotic tolerance.[26] Dextroamphetamine and methylphenidate hydrochloride (Ritalin hydrochloride) are two stimulants that may double the analgesic effect of narcotics. Either class of psychostimulant is also valuable in reducing the sedation that accompanies the use of narcotics.

The use of monoamine oxidase (MAO) inhibitors in combination with meperidine may result in delirium and seizures. Narcotics, chlorpromazine, droperidol, tertiary tricyclics, and MAO inhibitors may all cause postural hypotension. Therefore if a patient is at high risk for hypotension, postural blood pressure changes must be monitored closely. Coffee, tea, and antacid may reduce the absorption of certain neuroleptics and benzodiazepines in the stomach.

Antidepressants for Depression and Pain

Antidepressants have been shown to relieve pain both with or without the relief of depression symptoms. Typical of the optimistic studies are those of Linsey and Wycoff showing 70% to 80% efficacy of four different types of antidepressant in treating chronic pain associated with depression.[27] Blumer and Heilbronn showed a double improvement (60%) in outcome and a halving of the dropout rate (25%) in those pain patients treated with antidepressants.[17] Feinman[28] reviewed the evidence for the efficacy of pain relief with antidepressants when there are associated depressive symptoms. She reviewed the 11 largest and best-designed studies. The antidepressants used ranged from amitriptyline hydrochloride to phenelzine sulfate. The results clearly demonstrated the beneficial role played by antidepressant drugs in the treatment of chronic pain associated with depression.[28] The following guidelines may help the clinician select the proper agent:

1. A trial of antidepressant medication is useful in any intractable pain condition whether or not depression is present.
2. There is no clear evidence for the superiority of any one antidepressant over any other. Amitriptyline and doxepin hydrochloride have been used most often in the clinical studies.
3. Monoamine oxidase inhibitors (MAOIs) may be particularly helpful for the atypical pain associated with atypical depression.
4. Both MAOIs and tricyclics may require a trial of at least 6 weeks for the full benefit to be evident.
5. Low-dosage antidepressants, below the normal therapeutic range for depression, may be helpful in patients with pain and depression. The best results in the largest number of people are obtained, however, when the usual antidepressant dosage of drug is used, that is, 300 mg/d of imipramine hydrochloride or equivalent.
6. Positive results from the drug indicate a maintenance period of from 3 to 6 months.
7. Education of the patient in the rationale for antidepressant treatment is necessary for accurate treatment assessment and compliance.

The mechanism of action of antidepressants is not clear. They may have a primary effect in augmenting the descending inhibitory control of pain mediated by serotonin and norepinephrine. They may potentiate naturally occurring or administered opiates. There may be membrane-stabilizing anesthetic-anticonvulsant effects. They may give pure symptom relief of insomnia or anxiety. Whatever the mechanism, these agents are worth using in the treatment of pain.

TREATMENT OF CENTRAL PAIN STATES

The pain that results from chronic changes in the central somatosensory pathways is called central, deafferentation, or neuropathic pain. The characteristic feature of this type of pain is that it persists without obvious nociceptive stimulus. The seat of this pain in the CNS is the rationale for the use of centrally acting drugs for its treatment. The pain has a number of clinical features: (1) a background of spontaneous burning sensation, (2) paroxysmal jabs that often do not fall within one anatomical region, (3) an elevated sensory threshold with an exaggerated response to a nociceptive stimulus (hyperalgesia), or the perception of a nonnociceptive stimulus as painful (allodynia).

Phenytoin seems particularly effective in treating paroxysmal pain, perhaps because of its membrane effect in reducing the ability of axons to respond to frequent discharge. Trigeminal neuralgia, diabetic neuropathy, and diverse other neuralgias have been the most thoroughly studied. Carbamazepine has also been shown to be useful in these central pain syndromes. It is effective in 80% of trigeminal neuralgia patients within 24 hours of attaining steady state, making it clinically superior to phenytoin. Other types of lancinating pain, such as postherpetic neuralgia, postsympathectomy pain, and posttraumatic pain may also respond to carbamazepine. Unfortunately, long-term efficacy is often limited, and side effects such as dizziness sometimes preclude its use. Clonazepam is the best tolerated anticonvulsant for central pain syndromes. It facilitates both presynaptic and postsynaptic inhibition, increases recurrent inhibition, and decreases the firing rate of normal and epileptic neurons in the brain. In the reports citing clonazepam as a treatment for neuralgia, it appears to be well tolerated and at least as effective as the other anticonvulsants; it may be particularly helpful for allodynia.[29]

EDUCATION

The education we refer to here has to do with the ward personnel, not directly with the patient. For reasons that are unclear, medical people, be they physicians or nurses, view the patient who is in constant need of pain medication with suspicion. Even if the patient is a terminal cancer victim soon to die, medical caretakers still worry about the danger of addiction. Why they do so taxes the imagination, but the fact that they do is easily confirmed by asking the hospitalized pain patient. Marks and Sachar did this and found that 32% of their respondents said they were in severe discomfort; 41% were in moderate discomfort.[30] The authors surveyed the house officers responsible for their care and found that they believed that patients should be pain-free. Why this blatant discrepancy between their beliefs and the facts of their care? Marks and Sachar attributed it to an underestimation of the medication's effective dose, an overestimation of the medication's duration of action, and an exaggerated notion of the danger of addiction. We would add to this the failure in the system of medical education to make doctors sufficiently aware of patients' suffering. Physicians are taught that 50 to 100 mg of meperidine hydrochloride every two to four hours is the proper amount of narcotic to prescribe for severe pain. Rarely are they told to vary the amount depending on the patient's body weight and previous tolerance for the drug. In the list of priorities for the care of patients, patient comfort occupies a place near the bottom.

When the amount of medication a patient requires for the management of pain becomes a cause celebre on the ward, the consultation psychiatrist would be well advised to call a meeting of the house staff, attendants, and nurses, so that all biases and suspicions can be brought into the open. Medical personnel are far more apt to underestimate the amount of narcotic required for a given pain than to overestimate it. In either case, their opinions are usually based more on misinformation or folklore than on fact. Once these are aired and the true issues exposed to reason, the patient usually benefits.

PSYCHODYNAMIC PSYCHOTHERAPY

Psychodynamic psychotherapy when offered as the sole treatment has, in our experience, rarely been successful in alleviating chronic pain. While we have known practitioners who claim success with individuals suffering from low-back syndrome, from migraine, and from other nonspecific painful conditions, their record is far from illustrious. Psychotherapy, however, when used in conjunction with the treatment methods mentioned earlier, might well produce significant benefit, particularly if insight can be given into some of the underlying interpersonal relationships that contribute to pain behavior. An axiom used by those who conduct psychotherapy with chronic pain patients is that providing insight as to why the hurt is there is a great boon to the physician's morale which may, in turn, make the patient feel better for a time. We agree. Rarely does insight alone, no matter how illuminating, relieve pain.

HYPNOSIS

The use of hypnosis in chronic pain syndromes has been discussed at length in the literature. One excellent summary is by Ernest and Josephine Hilgard.[31] Hypnosis depends almost entirely on the patient. Only about one in four subjects is able to achieve a state of concentration of sufficient magnitude for lasting pain control. We have used a system of teaching individuals autohypnosis for the control of pain that is similar to the technique developed by Milton Erickson.[32] It is a method worth looking into, provided the physician knows its limitations and is patient enough and experienced enough in the techniques to give it a full therapeutic trial.

ELECTROCONVULSIVE THERAPY

Electroconvulsive therapy (ECT) has been used by some practitioners, particularly in long-standing pain that is accompanied by depression and is refractory to other forms of treatment. When properly done with judicious case selection, ECT has favorable and long-lasting results. It is the belief of those most skilled in this technique that the mechanisms they are treating in pain patients are those of depression.[33] (See chapter 12.)

SURGERY

There are two types of surgery to be considered. The first type consists of exploratory procedures designed to investigate through direct visualization whether an anatomical structure might be producing the pain in question. The decision to perform this type of procedure will be determined by the medical and psychological circumstances.

The second type of surgery is pain surgery or surgery directed against the central or peripheral nervous system solely for the purpose of removing or easing pain. It need have no connection with the pain's cause and is palliative at best. Rhizotomy, chordotomy, tractotomy, and cingulotomy are some of the procedures used.

Contrary to general belief, in the proper hands a central procedure such as a cingulotomy, performed stereotactically using radiofrequency lesions, does not carry a high psychiatric morbidity.[34] Personality changes, mental dulling, and memory impairment are rare. The benefit provided in the relief of pain is, however, disappointingly short-lived. If pain is reduced, it usually returns within 6 months. As a consequence, the use of such procedures should be limited to pain caused by terminal malignant diseases.

Pain surgery is seldom a desirable alternative. Pain is an elusive sensation with many areas of representation in the nervous system. Melzack believes that chronic pain, in contrast to acute pain, has multiple determinants and that there are no specific pain pathways for this phenomenon.[35] To exemplify this, let us close with the account of an extraordinary case.

> R.C., a 28-year-old mechanic, was thrown from his motorcycle on the way to his wedding. Injury resulted to his brachial plexus, as well as to his left arm, which required an amputation at the shoulder. He developed severe phantom limb pain within 2 weeks of the surgery. Six months later the stump was revised and a neurectomy performed. The pain remained unaltered. The nerve was then severed further into the stump with a similar result. A rhizotomy was then performed that was

unsuccessful, followed by a chordotomy with the same outcome. The patient was then put in individual psychotherapy for a year. There was no improvement. He was then hospitalized and given hypnotherapy, group therapy, and massive doses of phenothiazines and then anti-depressants and anticonvulsants. None of these measures produced improvement. After six sessions of ECT the pain was only intensified. A higher cervical chordotomy was performed without success, and then a mesencephalic tractotomy, again with no relief. He next had both dorsomedial thalamic nuclei ablated using stereotactic electrocautery. During the course of this procedure an electrode slipped and entered his mesencephalon resulting in a 2-week coma. He emerged from this with personality intact, but still with his original pain. Then electrolytic lesions were made bilaterally in the inferior mesial quadrant of the frontal lobe in stages. The pain remained. He then had a left radio frequency amygdalotomy, followed by a left cingulotomy. The pain continued as before. There was no change in his personality as noted by his therapist or his wife. The pain remained for 4 years after the accident, as pristine as it was 2 weeks after the injury. The house in which pain lived had been destroyed, but the sensation, like a stubborn revenant, remained to haunt the patient and his physicians.

Pain continues to be one of man's most important and complicated sensations. In this chapter we have deliberately avoided speculation and have used theory only when it was essential for understanding. Our intention has been to stay close to what is clinically applicable.

REFERENCES

1. Mersky H, Spear FG: *Pain, Psychological and Psychiatric Aspects.* Baltimore, Williams & Wilkins Co, 1967.
2. Ryle G: *Concept of Mind.* London, Hutchinson Publishing Group, 1949.
3. Fleming P: *My Aunt's Rhinoceros and Other Reflections.* New York, Simon & Schuster, Inc, 1958.
4. IASP Subcommittee on Taxonomy: Pain terms: a list with definitions and notes on usage. *Pain* 1979; 6:249–252.
5. Beecher HK: *Measurement of Subjective Responses.* New York, Oxford University Press, 1959.
6. Lewis JW, Terman GW, Shavit Y, et al: Neural neurochemical, and hormonal bases of stress-induced analgesia. *Adv Pain Res Ther* 1986, 6:277–288.
7. Maciewicz R, Bouckoms AJ, Martin JB: Drug therapy of neuropathic pain. *Clin J Pain* 1985; 1:39–45.
8. Wall PD: Alterations in the central nervous system after deafferentation: connectivity control, in Bonica JJ, Lindblom U, Iggo A (eds): *Advances in Pain Research and Therapy.* New York, Raven Press, 1983, vol 5, pp 677–689.
9. Tasker RR, Tsuda T, Hawrylyshyn P: Clinical neurophysiological investigation of deafferentation pain, in Bonica JJ, Lindblom U, Iggo A (eds): *Advances in Pain Research and Therapy.* New York, Raven Press, 1983, vol 5, pp 713–738

10. Evans W, Hoyle C: The comparative value of drugs used in the continuous treatment of angina pectoris. *J Med* 1933; 2:311–338.
11. Reich J, Tupin J, Abramowitz S: Psychiatric diagnosis of chronic pain patients. *Am J Psychiatry* 1983; 140:1495–1498.
12. Antczak-Bouckoms A, Bouckoms AJ: Affective disturbance and denial of problems in dental patients with pain. *Int J Psychosomatics* 1985; 32:9–11.
13. Holmes VF, Rafuls WA, Bouckoms AJ, et al: Covert psychopathology in chronic pain. *Clin J Pain* 1986; 1:6.
14. Ekkehard O, DeSouza C: A screening test for somatization disorder (hysteria). *Am J Psychiatry* 1985; 142:1146–1149.
15. Fordyce WE, Roberts AH, Sternbach RA: The behavioral management of chronic pain: a response to critics. *Pain* 1985; 22:113–125.
16. Sternbach R: *Pain Patients (Traits and Treatments)*. New York, Academic Press, 1974.
17. Blumer D, Heilbronn M: Chronic pain as a variant of depressive disease. The pain-prone disorder. *J Nerv Ment Dis* 1982; 170:381–392.
18. Berne F: *Beyond Games and Scripts*. New York, Grove Press, 1977.
19. Boukoms AJ, Litman RE: Chronic Pain Patients: Clues in the Clinical Interview. *Psychr Med* 1987; In press.
20. Lipsitt DR: Medical and psychological characteristics of "crocks". *J Psychiatry Med* 1970; 1:15–25.
21. Kanko RF, Foley KM, et al: Central nervous system excitatory effects of meperidine in cancer patients. *Ann Neurol* 1983; 13:180–185.
22. Goodman LS, Gilman A (eds): *The Pharmacological Basis of Therapeutics*. New York, Macmillan Publishing Co, 1970.
23. Kaiko RF: Narcotics in the elderly. *Med Clin North Am* 1982; 66:1079.
24. Porter J, Jick H: Addiction rare in patients treated with narcotics. *N Engl J Med* 302:123.
25. Bouckoms AJ: Analgesic adjuvants: The role of psychotropics, anticonvulsants and prostaglandin inhibitors. *Drug Ther* 1981; 6:41–48.
26. Sewall RPE, Spencer PSJ: Interaction of tricyclic antidepressants with opiate receptors. *Biochem Pharmacol* 1980; 29:460–462.
27. Lindsey P, Wyckoff M: The depression-pain syndrome and its response to antidepressants. *Psychosomatics* 1981: 22:571–577.
28. Feinman C: Pain relief by antidepressants: possible modes of action. *Pain* 1985; 23:1–8.
29. Bouckoms AJ, Litman RE: Clonazepam in the treatment of neuralgic pain syndrome. *Psychosomatics* 1985; 26:933–936.
30. Marks RM, Sachar EJ: Undertreatment of medical inpatients with narcotic analgesics. *Ann Intern Med* 1973; 78:178–181.
31. Hilgard ER, Hilgard VR: Hypnosis in the relief of pain, Los Altos, Calif, William Kaufmann, Inc, 1975.
32. Erickson M, in Haley J. (ed): *Advance Techniques of Hypnosis and Therapy*. New York, Grune & Stratton, Inc, 1967.
33. Mandel MR: Electroconvulsive therapy for chronic pain associated with depression. *Am J Psychiatry* 1975; 132:632–636.
34. Bouckoms AJ: Psychosurgery, in Wall PD, Melzack R (eds): *Textbook of Pain*. London, Churchill-Livingstone, 1984, pp 666–678.
35. Melzack R: How acupuncture can block pain, in Weisberg M (ed): *Clinical and Experimental Perspectives*. St Louis, CV Mosby Co, 1975.

5

The Surgical Patient

OWEN S. SURMAN

MEANING OF SURGERY

Several months ago a surgeon colleague presented a letter with a confession of love from a clinic patient who had undergone successful transplant surgery years earlier. The surgeon was advised to send no response and to approach the patient's future visits with customary respect. Beyond the rarity of the incident, the letter was an interesting metaphor for the surgical experience.

Two aspects of surgery speak to the reality and the excess meaning of the experience:

1. Surgery represents a decisive approach to the relief of pain and suffering.
2. Surgery involves a transference relationship with the patient in a role of heightened dependency and expectation.

In most instances surgeon and patient part after the operation with friendliness and mutual respect. Some disappointments are inevitable. With the much publicized advances of medicine come escalating demands on the surgeon's skill and the growing cost of malpractice premiums. As sociologist David Mechanic comments: "Doctors must not only be technically expert but also sensitive to psychosocial stress (their own as well as patients')...".[1] This chapter outlines a pragmatic psychiatric approach to the perioperative stress of surgery.

FEAR OF SURGERY

Some degree of preoperative apprehension is normal. In one study by Janis, patients adapted best who had moderate preoperative anxiety.[2] While there isn't universal agreement on Janis's finding, clinicians should be wary of the patient who appears inappropriately free of concern. Two types of fears are normally encountered in the surgical patient: fear of bodily injury and fear of death, typically fear of not awakening from anesthesia ("narcosis anxiety").[3]

Origins of Excessive Preoperative Anxiety

Past history of trauma. The surgical experience recalls early life stress. Those with a traumatic past are most vulnerable in this respect. For others, the experience of parental separation at a time of childhood surgery, or unpleasant induction-mask exposure may set the stage for abnormal fear of surgery in adulthood.

Identification with others. Abram and Gill described two patients whose emotional adaptation to cancer surgery differed according to expectations based on the cancer experience of relatives.[4] For those with familial disease the experience of forebears is particularly significant.

Expectation of loss vs. gain. Often, surgery is a source of hope and improved identity. Cosmetic procedures and transplantation are examples of this. In other instances, surgery may represent a substantial loss. The burden of mastectomy or colostomy has inspired the formation of successful self-help groups. Of course, there is an implicit gain for the patient whose life is maintained by removal of cancer or whose proximal limb is saved by the amputation of a gangrenous extremity. Critical to emotional outcome is the patient's knowledge and orientation to perioperative events, particularly his realistic appraisal of what can be expected.

Preoperative Psychological Assessment

Individuals with psychopathologic states require identification and specialized medical management. The following are common categories of these states.

Personality disorder. The several types of personality disorder have in common a basic problem with trust typically attested to by a pattern of failed or strained relationships. Problems in medical compliance abound in this setting as does strain in the doctor-patient relationship. Sign-out situations may develop. Costly litigation or, more rarely, personal injury to the caregiver or a colleague may follow from the perceived injustice of a malcontent.[5] Some patients who are unlikely to benefit from surgery may seek an operation or a series of operations in a neurotic attempt to gain love.[6,7] (See chapter 10.)

Affective disorder. The depressed patient may be irritable, agitated, or quietly withdrawn. Postoperative mobilization is a challenge and impaired nutrition undermines the process of surgical repair. Some authors have reported a higher level of postoperative morbidity for depressed patients.[8,9] While this might be expected in primary depression, the type of depression seen in preoperative assessment is sometimes a secondary or reactive depression that varies with the degree of physical disability. The treatment of depression, discussed later in this chapter, is by supportive psychotherapy, psychopharmacologic intervention, and mobilization of social supports. When depression is secondary to surgically correctable physical impairment, successful operative intervention is most often followed by improvement in mood and well-being. (See chapter 12.)

Anxiety disorder. The anxious patient encounters increased suffering and often presents with a demanding nature that may tax the most patient clinician. Monosymptomatic phobias, such as needle phobias, claustrophobia, or pathologic dread of anesthesia are occasionally encountered as are generalized anxiety states and multiple phobias with panic episodes. Often, anxiety may result from misconception about surgery, from anniversary reaction to past trauma, or from the impact of new learning or increased physical impairment on established coping skills. Deniers are especially likely to react anxiously to detailed preoperative information.[10] Treatment of anxiety, discussed later in this chapter, begins with preoperative teaching and formation of a therapeutic alliance. In some instances patients may derive considerable support from contact with others who have successfully completed a similar operative procedure. Those who are unresponsive to these measures or who have chronic anxiety disorders, often benefit from psychotherapy and anxiolytic agents.

Cognitive impairment. This may result from a variety of factors ranging from electrolyte imbalance to mental retardation. The basic issue is impairment of preoperative communication and informed consent, as well as increased risk of postoperative delirium. Impaired cognition on a surgical service is most frequently of metabolic origin. These are often sicker patients with increased risk of postoperative morbidity. Differentiation must be made for the functionally psychotic or demented. Mental retardation is least problematic when stable relationships can be drawn upon in the surgical setting.

Alcoholism. The alcoholic is often both exquisitely sensitive to rejection and also stressed by the perceived obligations of close interpersonal relationships. Pathologic denial increases problems with mutual trust. Anxiety and depression are frequent concomitants of primary alcoholism.[11] Preoperatively it is important to recognize the potential for delirium tremens and the higher risk of postoperative delirium when there is a history of alcoholism. Postoperative delirium may occur in the form of delirium tremens, as a manifestation of alcohol withdrawal; or delirium may occur de novo in an otherwise recovered alcoholic with established sobriety.

INFORMED CONSENT

More than a courtesy, or societally mandated ritual, the consent process is a vital step in the development of the relationship between patient and surgeon or surgical team. In complex procedures the psychiatric consultant may have an opportunity to participate directly. This can be a powerful statement of the team's interest in quality-of-life issues.[12]

Three aspects of the informed consent process can be valuable tools in establishing a good doctor-patient relationship.

1. *Bonding*: Along with a statement of risks and benefits, the consent process is a declaration of clinical goals. A factual, caring presentation marks the beginning of a collaborative bond with established priorities for patient and surgeon. A perfunctory exchange is a harbinger to uncertainty; even technical success may leave in doubt the value of the surgical event.

2. *Teaching*: Patients must be informed of any discomfort associated with the procedure and about the availability of pain medication. The need for intravenous (IV) therapy, indwelling catheters, drains, and endotracheal tubes should be discussed.[13] What is the customary length of the surgery and anticipated recuperative time in hospital and following discharge? What follow-up care is required including medicines, special diet, activity modification, and office visits? An obsessive review complete with pictures of the intraoperative procedure is unnecessary. The patient should know of complications, including psychological difficulties, commonly associated with the procedure. The risk of dying should be addressed in a constructive fashion, emphasizing the positive aspects of surgery. When possible, a visit to specialized areas of postoperative care is beneficial as is opportunity for contact with others who have had similar surgery.

3. *Observing*: The informed consent process allows the surgeon an opportunity for indirect observation of mental status. Preoccupation with excessive detail may be evidence of anxiety or paranoia. Failed comprehension may signal encephalopathy, internal distraction, or deficient intellect. Manner of dress and deportment are a statement of self-worth as well as personal management and socioeconomic status. A despondent, tearful, or lethargic manner signals depression. Attempts by the patient at good-natured evasion of a proper alcohol and drug history may be a clue to pathologic denial. An ingratiating attitude coupled with criticism of former physicians is typical of paranoid individuals, Adjustment problems or evidence of greater psychopathology should be

followed by formal psychiatric consultation and by social service intervention when there is need to mobilize additional perioperative support.

INNOVATIVE SURGERY

The fast pace of medical science has made some former experimental procedures routine. New experiments with the artificial heart and transplantation of multiple organs have aroused the interest of ethicists and health policy planners. Other surgical innovations such as heart and liver transplantation are in transition from experimental to clinical status. The economics of current health care has put a spotlight on quality-of-life aspects for all of these interventions. As a spokesman for this aspect of patient care the psychiatrist has a potentially larger societal role to fill. Exemplary is Willard Gaylin's directorship of The Hastings Center, Hastings-on-Hudson, NY, the medical ethics think-tank. Norman Levy's biannual psychonephrology symposia have multidisciplinary attendance from those with an interest in renal transplantation and dialysis therapy of end-stage renal disease.[14]

Special psychosocial aspects of newer surgical techniques are evident in the following areas:

Resource Allocation

Meaningful long-term survival is increasingly possible following heart transplantation and, to a lesser extent, liver transplantation.[15] One liver transplant recipient at the Massachusetts General Hospital has had the special added benefit of a cure for hemophilia. Despite these successes some have sought to limit availability of these operations because of economic concerns.[16] A limited supply of donor organs (see chapter 19) has proved a natural barrier; and, health care policy planners seek mechanisms for equitable distribution. The healthier the patient, the better the outcome; but those who are sickest and most critically in need have the highest current priority for available organs. Work with the artificial heart raises the possibility of a bridging procedure that would extend the lives of less healthy candidates and expand the list of those awaiting heart transplantation.

Patient Selection

The selection process for emerging surgical technology is based on capacity to benefit from the procedure, degree of present need, and time of initial presentation. Patients with debilitating psychiatric impairment are excluded. The need to prioritize candidacy is a stress for physicians and intensifies with the death of patients who die on the waiting list. Merrikin and Overcast address an important issue in their discussion of the legal limits of the medical selection process. Patients with a specific medical handicap or psychosocial impairment may have differing levels of debilitation. Candidacy for a procedure such as heart transplantation should be individualized, to avoid discrimination.[17]

REDUCTION OF PREOPERATIVE STRESS
Reassurance and Education

Emphasis should be on concerns, common or idiosyncratic, of importance to the individual. Pain is a frequent source of worry. The patient needs to know that pain is normal and that early postoperative mobilization is healthy. Past difficulty with specific analgesic or anesthetic agents is very useful to review along with available alternatives. Patients should be encouraged to request pain medication when it is needed and they should be reassured about fears of addiction. For others, scarring and disfigurement is a source of preoccupation. Such concern may be couched in understatement, for example, "Will I be able to wear a bikini?" Some worry most about sexual function or future capacity to bear children. Patients often voice such issues in a hesitant manner. Those who take pride in active life styles are frequently concerned about return to normal vigor and strength. Loss of privacy is a concern for some. Executives may wish to maintain access to aspects of their work. The elderly may have heard discussion of life support systems and living wills. Dietary considerations, visiting arrangements, and financial issues are meaningful to many, and they may benefit from a preoperative visit with a medical social worker or dietician. Patients with lengthy medical histories, juvenile-onset diabetics, for example, often have firm opinions about their medical needs. In such instances preoperative discussion with nursing is especially beneficial. Where possible it helps a great deal to accommodate to specific needs. But it is equally important to shape expectations and allow patients the opportunity to modify their life styles.

Specialized Intervention

Egbert et al in a classic study showed the advantage of a preoperative visit by the anesthetist over sedation alone.[18] In a later study of patients undergoing abdominal surgery, those who were taught about the normalcy of postoperative pain and encouraged to request needed analgesics had greater postoperative comfort and used far less narcotics than a group receiving no information about pain control.[19]

Supportive preoperative visits by a psychiatrist were shown in two studies to reduce the incidence of delirium following surgery.[20,21] In a third study, preoperative psychiatric support combined with auto-hypnosis training failed to produce a statistically significant reduction in postcardiotomy delirium relative to controls with routine care. However, the setting was one in which all cardiac surgery patients received intensive preoperative preparation from the nursing staff.[13,22] Recent studies on psychological intervention for surgical patients have been reviewed by Mumford et al.[23] While none of these studies were performed blind, patients with psychological intervention averaged less time in hospital than controls.[10]

The use of a psychiatrist preoperatively would be most valuable in procedures where unrealistic fantasies can work to the patient's disadvantage, as in plastic surgery. Whenever a major affective disorder is suspected, or a psychosis, or a history of postoperative psychiatric difficulty, the psychiatrist should be called in.

PERIOPERATIVE MANAGEMENT OF PSYCHIATRIC DISORDERS
Personality Disorder

Once the problem is identified, collaboration among primary physician, psychiatrist, and surgeon is necessary. Consistency is essential. The borderline or marginally adaptive patient should be enlisted in a specific care plan with a minimum of ambiguity. Good communications among caregivers helps with the demanding dependency of such patients and the emotions they may arouse. Paranoid and obsessive individuals manage best when one available member of the team is designated as physician-in-charge. The designated physician is ideally one who can relate to the patient and expend the needed time for repeated questions and detailed review of the care plan. When possible, it is useful to enlist an interested family member who is a reassuring influence. (See chapter 10.)

Depressive disorder. If the patient has a major affective disorder or suffers from a grief reaction, psychiatric help should be requested. (See chapter 12.) Not infrequently, surgery should be postponed and the depression treated. There are exceptions. If a surgically correctable condition is strongly contributory to the mood disorder, there is little benefit in delay. In other instances the surgery may be nonelective or the mood disorder intractable. Appropriate antidepressant medication should be given through the first preoperative day, and resumed postoperatively as soon as the patient can safely take sips by mouth. Some agents, notably imipramine hydrochloride, are available for parenteral administration. In all instances the anesthetist and surgeon should be informed of medication requirements. There has been some controversy about preoperative use of monoamine oxidase inhibitors (MAOIs), but there are reports of safe perioperative administration.[24] If MAOIs are used one should watch for hypotension and avoid contraindicated medications such as demerol. (See chapter 27) A behavioral nursing approach is often beneficial for the depressed patient who is difficult to mobilize postoperatively.

Preoperative depression in the elderly has been discussed by Titchener and Levine, who advocate mobilization of supportive relationships.[25] Depression related to adjustment disorder is often responsive to supportive psychotherapy as illustrated in the following case.

> S.G. a 40-year-old woman with juvenile-onset diabetes mellitus and a 6-year history of successful renal transplantation was admitted to the surgical service for nonunion of a fracture in her left ankle and a secondary infection which had not responded to antibiotic therapy and conservative management. When a below-knee amputation (BKA) was recommended by the infectious disease consultant, the patient was unwilling to proceed. A psychiatric consultation was requested to support her through the hospitalization and to treat her clinical depression.
>
> The patient was able to recount a fear of rejection by her husband's family. She explained that her husband's uncle had been diabetic with multiple complications and that the family was slow to accept her illness. Also, the patient was apprehensive about the impact of her proposed amputation on her 10-year-old daughter.
>
> The consultant began by calling attention to the model of fortitude presented by diabetic patients who were able to persevere in their work or family responsibilites despite multiple complications. Example was given of a young blind diabetic woman who had begun a new business venture while recuperating from a renal transplant. The patient quickly followed with an account of her own volunteer activity in her daughter's Brownie troop.
>
> Next, the patient was enlisted in reviewing the functional limitations of her current condition and the improvement she might expect to experience with a successful BKA. The author commented that diabetics tended to become depressed in the setting of immobilization and infection, both of which were descriptive of the patient's current circumstances and in keeping with her decline in mood. Antidepressant therapy was discussed as a possibility but not implemented. Three days later the author returned to find the patient in improved spirits. She favored the idea of amputation but required her husband's approval. A meeting with the orthopedic surgeon was arranged and the husband proved accepting of the procedure. On the first postoperative day the patient was alert with improved affect. She was encountering moderate

postoperative pain for which ample analgesia was available. She expressed satisfaction with her decision. In keeping with her request to minimize the sedating effect of daytime narcotic use, hypnosis was introduced for the first time as an adjunct for analgesia. The remainder of her postoperative course was uneventful.

Anxiety disorder. Anxiety may be acute in onset and related to fear of surgery, or it may represent a chronic emotional disorder or personality trait. Some patients may not acknowledge distress, or may do so with difficulty because of social custom or personality style. Informing the patient that anxiety about surgery is a common experience may help improve communication. It is best to ask what concerns the patient has rather than to ask if there are concerns. Some patients worry about a specific type of intervention, such as endotracheal tube placement. Many surgical candidates are well-informed but the average patient knows little anatomy. Much can be learned by asking the patient what he thinks the problem is and what understanding he has of the planned intervention.

Prior surgical experience is important. For some, childhood surgical exposure may form the basis for an induction-mask phobia. Others may benefit if assisted in reconstructing earlier traumatic exposure which may relate in anniversary fashion or through other association with the current surgical plan. It is helpful to know how patients have coped with prior surgery and how they deal with other stressful events. At times anxiety is generated by an overly zealous account of the planned procedure. An excessively paternal "leave it to me" approach is insufficient to allow for appropriate expectations.

To reduce anxiety prior to surgery, there should be a sufficient amount of education for the patient to have a judgment about the procedure and an idea of the postoperative course. Minor tranquilizers in the benzo-diazepine class (eg, alprazolam, lorazepam, diazepam) can be used as an adjunct to psychological support. The prescribing physician should be aware of the half-life of these agents and the potential for sedation, particularly in the elderly. Insomnia should be treated with attention to medication to which the patient has been accustomed in the past. Patients with debilitating anxiety that persists, and those who deny anxiety despite evidence to the contrary, should be referred for psychiatric assessment.

Panic disorder. Treatment of panic disorder with agoraphobia is effective with alprazolam, imipramine, or MAOIs. Ideally, MAOIs are best avoided or gradually discontinued 2 weeks before surgery; they can be continued in select situations.[24] Imipramine has a slower onset of response than alprazolam but can be effectively instituted when surgery is elective and is available for parenteral administration. If nonelective surgery is planned, alprazolam is the agent of choice unless there is a specific intolerance. In any case the anesthetist and surgeon must be informed that medication is needed throughout the preoperative and postoperative periods. Sudden cessation following chronic administration of anxiolytics is often associated with rebound anxiety as well as a withdrawal syndrome. When oral medication cannot be administered, a parenterally administered benzodiazepine can be used to provide sedation. Diazepam at 1 mg (= 0.1 mg alprazolam) does not block panic attacks but prevents withdrawal when alprazolam therapy must be interrupted.

Phobic disorder.   Patients with simple phobias are often best treated with standard behavioral therapy when undergoing elective surgery. Alternatively, brief psychotherapy with a combination of supportive and behavioral techniques may be used along with anxiolytic agents.

> A 38-year-old woman (H.D.) approached elective cholecystectomy with an intense fear of death. When 5 years of age the patient had undergone a tonsillectomy. Her mother's subsequent dramatization of the event led the patient to believe she had convulsed from ether. She dreaded that she would succumb to future anesthesia.
>
> On the evening prior to surgery the patient was visited by her surgeon, her neurologist, and a staff anesthesiologist who prescribed lorazepam 2 mg on the night before surgery and, again, with a sip of water on the morning of surgery. A special duty nurse was also provided to remain with the patient through the night. The patient remained unreassured by these supports. She complained of severe anxiety and feared that she would sign out.
>
> The patient was well known to the author, who had treated her for chronic migraine and was familiar with the circumstances of her unhappy marriage to an alcoholic husband. On the day prior to hospital admission an unsuccessful attempt was made to desensitize her phobic anxiety. On the night of admission the history of her childhood surgery was reviewed. Emphasis was placed on the absence of adverse long-term sequelae and the possible benefits of her childhood surgery. Next, attention was directed to her own positive feelings about the hospital, her surgeon, and the anesthesiologist who had approached her in a sensitive and concerned fashion. Questions about potential postoperative complications were candidly discussed, while emphasizing the relative safety of the operating room where extensive medical support would be available. The author next asked the patient to imagine that she was anesthetized and safely undergoing surgery. Once this was accomplished hypnosis was induced, A previously described technique, "postnoxious desensitization,"[26] was then employed to guide her visually through a fantasy of the operative procedure. Beginning with a

theme of successfully completed surgery, she was instructed with hypnosis to visualize a series of images in reverse sequence as follows: awakening in the recovery room with satisfaction upon completing the surgery, safely sleeping in the operating room with the surgery in progress, and thinking ahead toward the surgery with a feeling of improved confidence and reassurance. She was asked to describe the feelings encountered with each image and was encouraged to master each image in turn. Last, a hypnotic suggestion was given that she would be more comfortable through the evening, that she would increase in strength and health with each postoperative day, and that she would employ self-hypnosis at will to further her relaxation. When hypnosis was repeated the patient had a significant reduction of anxiety and proceeded uneventfully with gallbladder surgery.

Hex or predilection to death. Weisman and Hackett[27] give the example of a farmer whose certainty of postoperative fatality presaged his cardiovascular death 3 days after subtotal gastrectomy. These authors called such patients "predilected to death." They are noteworthy for the absence of anxiety or depression. When such a conviction is evident, surgery is best avoided, if possible.[27,28]

Functional psychosis. Psychotic patients often accommodate satisfactorily to the structure of a busy surgical service. Actively suicidal individuals require special duty nurses around the clock as well as standard suicide precautions. Antipsychotic agents should be administered in full dose throughout the pre- and postoperative period. Aliphatic substituted phenothiazines (eg, chlorpromazine, thioridazine) are more likely associated with hypotension than high-potency phenothiazines (eg, trifluoperazine hydrochloride, perphenazine), or haloperidol. (See chapters 26 and 27.) Patients should be managed in a simple direct, relatively concrete manner. Supportive family members or, in select instances, established mental health providers should be mobilized for support. Provocative exploration of sensitive psychodynamics should be scrupulously avoided. On appropriate occasions, arrangements can be made prior to admission to restrict visitors or telephone calls. Wherever possible the patient should be sheltered from toxic interpersonal relations. The patient's competency should be established or appropriate guardianship arranged in consultation with hospital attorneys. (See chapter 29.)

Preoperative encephalopathy. "Organic" CNS disorders should be addressed with an appropriate search for underlying metabolic, infectious, and neurologic causes. An unexpected rise in serum ammonia is sometimes evident in instances where other liver function studies are relatively mildly impaired. Treatment is specific to etiology. Standard orienting techniques should be employed, with clock, calendar, availability of special personal effects, and gentle review of the daily routine. Competency should be established as noted above. Excessive sedation should be carefully avoided. Supportive nursing techniques and reassurance are the principal approach to agitation. Low doses of haloperidol are helpful for persistent agitation and perturbation. Particular caution is necessary in the instance of hepatic dysfunction. Diphenhydramine hydrochloride is a gentle treatment for insomnia. In the elderly, benzodiazepines may be the cause of confusion, but some do benefit from low doses of short-acting agents such as alprazolam, oxazepam, or lorazepam. The best treatment for the behavioral manifestations of encephalopathy on the surgical service is the presence at bedside of a close, level-headed family member.

Postoperative encephalopathy. As in the case of preoperative disturbances in consciousness, supportive care should be coupled with a search for specific etiology. Anesthetic agents or intolerance to specific analgesic agents or their metabolites (normeperidine delirium is an example) (see chapter 6) or intolerance to other drugs should be suspect. In other cases depression of CNS function may be evidence of postoperative cardiopulmonary or infectious complication. Postoperative delirium requires energetic intervention when agitation, mood lability, hallucinations, and delusions pose a threat to medical management. When delirium occurs in the intensive care unit, pharmacologic intervention can include IV morphine, haloperidol, or diazepam. The psychiatric consultant should visit once or more daily and maintain the relationship until the patient's sensorium is clear. Once a frequent complication of cardiovascular surgery, the incidence of postcoronary artery bypass graft and postcardiotomy delirium has declined with improvement in surgical technology.[12,29,30] Among the risk factors for delirium following cardiac surgery are: severity of physical illness, history of substance abuse, history of myocardial infarction, and preoperative organic brain syndrome.[31,32] Steroid-induced psychosis following renal transplantation has become rare (see chapter 19) although a less striking disturbance in consciousness may be associated with methylprednisolone sodium boluses for acute rejection. Another cause of delirium is acute sensory deprivation as in Weisman and Hackett's classic description of their intervention for "black patch delirium" in elderly patients following cataract surgery.[33] Delirium may occur secondary to withdrawal in the active alcoholic or in the recovered alcoholic in the absence of recent alcohol abuse. Complex partial seizures should also be considered in the differential diagnosis.[34]

Alcoholism

The active alcoholic. The one reported drink per night may be from a bottomless glass. Preoperative detoxification is best whenever possible. In the surgical setting prevention of withdrawal is a primary goal. Supplemental nutritional support should be instituted and full doses of chlordiazepoxide begun at four- to six-hour intervals in those patients suspected of being candidates for alcoholic withdrawal. Intravenous alcohol is an alternative. Addictive disorders may provoke an angry response from otherwise caring physicians. Participation of a psychiatric consultant is desirable.

The recovered alcoholic. These patients feel particularly vulnerable. There is typically a history of family discord. And the recovered alcoholic is often apprehensive about a stress-related relapse. Patients who are active in Alcoholics Anonymous are vigilant about the use of medication. If benzodiazepines are thought necessary, pains should be taken to point out the medical indication. Some hospitals such as Massachusetts General Hospital sponsor weekly Alcoholics Anonymous and Alanon meetings. Supportive visits from "safe" companions are usually sufficient to reduce perioperative stress.

The drug-addicted patient. Treatment is similar to that of the alcoholic patient although the two types of disorders have established differences.[10] Barbiturate requirements for patients addicted to depressants is established with a test dose of phenobarbital (see chapter 3). The narcotic addict requiring surgery should not be denarcotized until after the operation. Pain medication is given in addition to what is required for daily maintenance. After surgery, drug withdrawal can be approached in a standard method.[35]

Pain Intolerance

Inadequate analgesia is the most likely factor for the postoperative patient whose complaint is of persisting pain. Tolerance may occur among those receiving frequent daily analgesics over a period of weeks, but addiction is a rare outcome.[36,37] The type of analgesic should be individualized. The oral potency, long half-life, and low abuse potential of methadone are advantageous when a long period of administration is anticipated. Patients who are depressed or anxious and those who have experienced long-term narcotic administration are likely to have increased postoperative analgesic needs. When pain persists in the absence of postoperative complication, it is important to determine if some secondary factor such as depression is operating. An antidepressant added to the analgesic can be highly beneficial, as can other narcotic adjuvants (see chapter 4). Psychiatric consultants should develop familiarity with relaxation techniques and hypnosis or enlist the aid of others who have developed such skills. At Massachusetts General Hospital a relaxation videotape is broadcast on closed circuit television twice daily. Baer and Surman[38] have developed a computerized version which runs on the Apple lle and llc. (See chapters 4, 6, and 18.)

REFERENCES

1. Mechanic D: Physicians and patients in transition. *Hastings Cent Rep* 1985; 15:9–12.
2. Janis IL: *Psychological Stress*. New York, John Wiley & Sons, Inc, 1985.
3. Deutsch H: Some psychoanalytic observations in surgery. *Psychosom Med* 1942; 4:105–115.
4. Abrams HS, Gill BF: Prediction of post-operative, psychiatric complications. *N Engl J Med* 1961; 265:1061.
5. Saxon W: Surgeon slain in hospital, former patient sought. *The New York Times*, Dec 31, 1985, p 1.
6. Meninger KA: Polysurgery and polysurgical addiction. *Psychoanal Q* 1934; 3:173.
7. Abrams HS: Psychological aspects of surgery. *Int Psychiatry Clin* 1967; 4:2.
8. Kimball CP: A predictive study of adjustment to cardiac surgery. *J Thorac Cardiovasc Surg* 1969; 58:891.
9. Tufo HM, Ostfeld AM, Sheteille R: Central nervous system dysfunction following open heart surgery. *JAMA* 1970; 212:1333.
10. Rogers M, Reich P: Psychological intervention with surgical patients: evaluation outcome. *Adv Psychosom Med* 1986; 15:23–50.
11. Schuckit MA: The clinical implications of primary diagnostic groups among alcoholics. *Arch Gen Psychiatry* 1985; 42:1043–1049.
12. Surman OS: The surgical patient, in Hackett TP, Cassem NH (ed): *Massachusetts General Hospital Handbook of General Hospital Psychiatry*. St Louis, CV Mosby Co, 1978, pp 64–92.
13. Surman OS: Psychiatric medicine update, in Manschreck TC (ed): *Massachusetts General Hospital Reviews for Physicians*. New York, Elsevier Biomedical Press, 1981, pp 155–175.
14. Levy NB: *Psychonephrology. 1 Psychological Factors in Hemodialysis and Transplantation*. New York, Plenum Medical Book Co, 1981.
15. Report of the Massachusetts Task Force on organ transplantation. *Law Med Health Care* 1985; 13:8–14.
16. Surman OS: Heart transplantation in Massachusetts and the prince of Denmark, letter. *Law Med Health Care* 1985; 13:189–190.
17. Merrikin KJ, Overcast TD: Patient selection for heart transplantation: When is a discriminating choice discrimination? *J Health Polit Policy Law* 1985; 10:7–32.
18. Egbert LD, Bartlett MK, Tarndorf H, et al: The value of preoperative visits by anesthetists. *JAMA* 1963; 185:553.
19. Egbert LD, Battit GE, Welch CD, et al: Reduction of postoperative pain by

encouragement and instruction of the patient. *N Engl J Med* 1964; 270:825.

20. Lazarus HR, Hagens TH: Prevention of psychosis following open heart surgery. *Am J Psychiatry* 1968; 124:1190.

21. Layne OJ, Yudofsky SC: Postoperative psychosis in cardiotomy patients: The role of organic and psychiatric factors. *N Engl J Med* 1971; 284:518.

22. Surman OS, Hackett TP, Silverman EL, et al: Efficacy of psychotherapy for patients undergoing cardiac surgery. *Arch Gen Psychiatry* 1974; 30:830.

23. Mumford E, Schlesinger HJ, Glass GV: The effects of psychological intervention on recovery from surgery and heart attacks: An analysis of the literature. *Ann J Public Health* 1982; 72:144–151.

24. Gelenberg AJ: MAOIs during surgery and ECT. *Mass Gen Hosp Newsletter Biol Ther Psychiatry* 1985; 8:45–46.

25. Titchener JL, Levine ML: *Surgery as a Human Experience.* New York, Oxford University Press, 1950.

26. Surman OS: Postnoxious desensitization: Some clinical notes on the combined use of hypnosis and systematic desensitization. *Am J Clin Hypn* 1979; 22:54–60.

27. Weisman AD, Hackett TP: Predilection to death. Death and dying as a psychiatric problem. *Psychosom Med* 1961; 23:232–256.

28. Boehnert C: Surgical outcome in "death-mined" patients. *Psychosomatics* 1986; 27:638–642.

29. Breuer AC, Furian AJ, Hanson MR, et al: Complications of coronary artery bypass graft surgery: prospective analysis of 421 patients. *Stroke* 1983; 14:682–687.

30. Aberg T, Ronquist G, Tyden H et al: Adverse effects on the brain in cardiac operations as assessed by biochemical psychometric and radiologic methods. *J Thorac Cardiovasc Surg* 1984; 87:99–105.

31. Dubin WR, Field AL, Gastfriend DR: Postcardiotomy delirium: a critical review. *J Thorac Cardiovasc Surg* 1979; 77:586–599.

32. Heller S, Kornfeld D: Psychiatric aspects of cardiac surgery. *Adv Psychosom Med* 1986; 15:124–139.

33. Weisman AD, Hackett TP: Psychosis after eye surgery: establishment of specific doctor-patient relationship in prevention and treatment of black patch delirium. *N Engl J Med* 1958; 258:1284.

34. Surman OS, Parker SW: Complex partial seizures and psychiatric disturbance in end-stage renal disease. *Psychosomatics* 1981; 22:1077–1080.

35. Jaffe JH: Drug addiction and drug abuse, in Goodman LS, Gilman A (eds): *The Pharmacologic Basics of Therapeutics.* New York, Macmillan Publishing Co, 1970.

36. Hackett TP: Pain and prejudice: why do we doubt that the patient is in pain? *Med Times* 1971; 99:130.

37. Marks RM, Sacha EJ: Undertreatment of medical inpatients with narcotic analgesics. *Ann Intern Med* 1973; 78:173.

38. Baer L, Surman OS: Microcomputer assisted relaxation. *J Percept Motor Skills* 1985; 61:499–502.

6

Confusion, Delirium, and Dementia

GEORGE B. MURRAY

A consultation psychiatrist spends much time in a general hospital diagnosing and treating confusion, delirium, and dementia. This chapter is not intended to be a literature review or an exhaustive study of either delirium or dementia. It is intended primarily as a guide for the consultation psychiatrist in a "what to look for" and a "what to suggest/order" approach. It presupposes some familiarity with confusion, delirium, and dementia.

The consulting psychiatrist is often asked by medical and surgical specialists to determine the mental clarity of a particular problem patient. It is sometimes difficult to assess whether a patient is mildly confused, delirious, demented, or psychotic secondary to a functional or organic disorder. With the increase of longevity and a proportional increase in the elderly hospital population, confusion, delirium, and dementia are more frequently observed. The sphere of dementia in the United States has a prevalence of about 1.3 million cases of which over 50% are of the Alzheimer type. There are an additional 2.8 million patients with mild to moderate impairment.[1] Since the fastest-growing part of the US population is that group over age 85 years we can expect to see increased numbers of dementia patients.

SOME MIDDLE LEVEL THEORY

The term "middle level theory" is used to indicate that what follows is neither, at the start, nonarguable fact level nor is it at the cartesian, clear and distinct, burnished level of universals. What follows lies between these two poles and is an attempt at some heuristic generalities.

Dementia has been defined in many different ways depending on historical context, clinical experience, and the definer's personal interest in dementia. It could be described as the spectrum of mental states resulting from disease of the human cerebral hemispheres. This emphasizes that dementia is not a singular condition but a broad spectrum of dysfunction. Dementia can range from a barely discernible deviation from normal to virtual cerebral death.[2] This is a working definition of dementia and not everyone would agree with it. Engle and Romano[3] maintain that the distinction between delirium and dementia is an arbitrary one, established by convention, with the main discriminating criterion being reversibility *v* irreversibility. However, there is some discussion currently that the idea of irreversibility is no longer necessary for a definition of dementia.[4] Alexander and Geschwind[5] have suggested that the term dementia does not have a sharp boundary and that it refers to a loosely similar group of disabilities in which there is deterioration in one or more behavioral functions that leads to an incapacity for reasonably independent activity. By convention, they say, transient states are often called by other names and one of these is a confusional state.

The definition of delirium presents obvious problems, one of which is confusion with the terminology within the literature. For example, delirium is used interchangeably with acute brain syndrome, acute confusional state, acute brain failure, toxic psychosis, and infectious-exhaustive syndrome, to name a few. Psychiatrist Romano[3] supported by Lipowski,[6] believe that delirium could be described as a reversible global impairment of cognitive processes. The operative words here are "reversible" and "global." Neurologists Adams and Victor[7] try to describe delirium more specifically. They propose delirium as a special type of confusional state characterized by gross disorientation in the presence of alertness and vigilance. This would include disorders of perception and such symptoms as excessive alertness, intense agitation, and frenzied excitement. Their concept uses delirium tremens as its paradigm.

Adams and Victor[7] also distinguish an acute confusional state with three divisions: (1) a delirium, in a narrow sense, that is either hyperkinetic or hypokinetic (so-called quiet delirium), keeping delirium tremens as the prime analogate; (2) a primary mental confusion that may or may not be distinguishable from (3) a beclouded dementia that may be the results of some other disease. The opinion of Engle and Romano[3] and Lipowski,[8] however, is that delirium embraces the whole spectrum of acute confusional states.

In summary, I would suggest that as one approaches the patient clinically, a graded framework be kept in mind, that is, acute confusional states *v* delirium *v* dementia. "Acute confusional state" is a term used to describe the person's afflicted mental status, especially if history or laboratory data are not available on the patient. Chedru and Geschwind[9] have characterized the principle feature of the acute confusional state as reduction of attention. Other symptoms, such as changes in mood and hallucination, are not essential for the diagnosis. Delirium is the term used to describe a more dramatic reversible global impairment of cognitive processes than the more descriptive acute confusional state. The clinician does not know if the impairment is reversible a priori, of course, but one can get a clinical feel from the patient that, at first blush, tends to actuate diagnostic impression more in the delirium or the dementia camp. As a very broad rule of thumb the deliria are thought more often to be due to impairment of general attentional mechanisms (recalling impairment of the reticular activating system and its interaction with cortex) while dementias are usually caused by a deterioration of intellectual capacity secondary to structural "neuron burnout" occurring in a relatively clear consciousness. For the consultation psychiatrist the final judgment remains clinical, depending on theoretical bias, available information, and experience.

CHARACTERISTICS OF DELIRIUM

In 1980 the American Psychiatric Association produced the *Diagnostic and Statistical Manual of Mental Disorders*, third edition (DSM-III).[10] After much effort by many physicians discussing and refining the criteria for diagnosing delirium, and after several drafts, clinical criteria were drawn up for the diagnosis of delirium. In 1985 an attempt to revise the DSM-III, the DSM-III-R, was in effect but there were no changes in the criteria for delirium.

According to the DSM-III the diagnostic criteria for delirium are:

Delirium (DSM-III)

A. Clouding of consciousness (reduced clarity of awareness of environment), as reduced capacity to shift, focus, and sustain attention to environmental stimuli
B. At least two of the following:
   1. Perceptual disturbance; misinterpretations, illusions, or hallucinations
   2. Speech that is at times incoherent
   3. Disturbance or sleep-wakefulness cycle with insomnia or daytime drowsiness
   4. Increased or decreased psychomotor activity
C. Disorientation and memory impairment (if testable)
D. Clinical features that develop over a short period of time (usually hours to days which tend to fluctuate over the course of the day)
E. Evidence from the history, physical examination, or laboratory tests of the specific organic factor judged to be etiologically related to the disturbance

There are usually three general ways in which a delirium presents to the consulting psychiatrist. In the first, the patient has difficulty with memory and is often disoriented, but there is little agitation. The second manner of presentation is where the striking feature is a delusional system, usually paranoid in nature, wherein fear, hyperalertness, and mild agitation are seen. Memory may be impaired but not necessarily. The third general presentation of a delirium is one where psychomotor agitation is full-blown. This type raises staff anxiety on the floor and usually a psychiatric consultation is requested very soon after this psychomotor agitation starts. In this type of presentation, the patient is more apt to have a delusional component, memory impairment, and disorientation. In every delirium or acute confusional state there is reduction in the level of cognition or a clouding of consciousness. This is accompanied by relatively generalized slowing of the electroenceph-alogram (EEG).[3,11]

Delirium secondary to purely psychological cause exists. Internal and external stressors on a patient are inferred to account for a purely psychological delirium. Generally, however, those who see many acute confusional states in all parts of a general hospital feel that the purely psychologically caused delirium is relatively rare and most deliria usually have metabolic determinants. There is some discussion as to whether an "intensive care syndrome" is purely psychological.[12] When anxiety and fear have so escalated that loss of self-identify and self-control are threatened, an acute confusional state can ensue, all other factors ruled out. The most definitive laboratory test to rule out an organic cause is the EEG. If the EEG is abnormal, usually with diffuse slowing, the presumption is that the delirium is not psychological. In our experience those patients seen in an intensive care unit (ICU), labeled with "ICU syndrome" or "ICU psychosis," are usually so labeled by house staff for a delirium whose organic etiology eludes them and who therefore presume that the etiology lies in the "functional" realm.

Important physical signs of delirium are agitation, restlessness, expressions of fear, and demonstration of emotional lability. The patient usually has decreased attention and may have cognitive deficits. Often the patient is slightly, if not frankly, paranoid. He may misinterpret sensory stimuli, that is, have illusions. He may also have frank hallucinations (which have no basis in reality). Often, patients with delirium are hypervigilant, their eyes darting in a scanning motion. On the other hand, a patient may be calmly disoriented, not agitated or hypervigilant. She may even be warm and engaging and may smilingly say that her husband is locked up in the room next door. These latter patients' delusions are well tolerated and cause them a minimum of anxiety. They usually present no behavioral abnormality and are not often seen by a psychiatric consultant since they are no management problem. Some delirious patients who are sleepy, disoriented, hypoactive, and glum-looking, are often labeled "depressed" by the nursing staff; when the psychiatrist sees these patients and points out how disoriented they are this can be an occasion for staff instruction.

Autonomic activation may accompany delirium. One may see signs of tachycardia, hypertension, diaphoresis, dilated pupils, and fever. A delirium from drug withdrawal usually is heralded by autonomic dysfunction. It is important to consider the time in, for example, alcohol withdrawal; if a person was admitted to hospital for acute gastrointestinal (GI) bleeding secondary to alcoholism, sent to surgery immediately where he was anesthetized, and was sedated for three or four days postoperatively, it would not be unusual to see the patient exhibit typical signs of alcohol withdrawal 11 or 12 days "downstream." It is our experience that previous sedation and anesthesia tend to delay alcohol withdrawal symptoms beyond the usual textbook limits for withdrawal. Similarly, with, for example, barbiturate withdrawal, the patient may present with a delirium, even be frankly psychotic in appearance before he shows the more typical signs of physiologic withdrawal such as increased temperature, and tremor. If strongly suspected, it would be important to give the patient a test dose of barbiturate to determine if the symptoms are relieved. Neuroleptic medication may not be the best first approach in these cases since impairment in temperature regulation is a possibility with neuroleptics.

Writing impairment (dysgraphia) is one of the most sensitive indicators of consciousness impairment according to Chedru and Geschwind.[9] In 34 acutely confused patients, they found 33 to have writing impairments. Writing was impaired in its motor, spatial, and linguistic aspects. Motor impairments included letters clumsily drawn, and reduplication of strokes in letters such as "M" and "W"; spatial impairments included inability to align letters properly and orient the letters upward or downward; linguistic errors appeared primarily in spelling. All dysgraphia disappeared when the confusion cleared.

There are three possible outcomes for a delirium: (1) complete recovery, (2) progression to irreversible amnestic syndrome (primary memory loss) or dementia, or (3) progression to irreversible coma and death.[13] A delirium may last anywhere from a minute to months, but on average does not exceed 1 week.

CONSCIOUSNESS

Consciousness is, roughly, that state which allows cognitive processes to occur. This is neither a philosophical nor a neurophysiologic description, both of which are problems for higher level theory.

Cognitive processes include perceiving, thinking, and remembering. The content of cognitive processes is thought to be the result of higher cerebral function and therefore requires the integrity of the hemispheres. Another aspect of consciousness is arousal. Arousal is more general in nature than awareness, and has been likened to the gain control on audio systems. It is thought that the ascending reticular activating system, especially from pons to midbrain and thalamus, is important in this state.[14] Interruption of the reticular activating system can result in unconsciousness. An important key in determining whether delirium or dementia is present is the character of the arousal. The delirious person tends to show high or low levels of arousal over time and unstable variation in the gain or volume of arousal.

What is the substrate or mechanism of delirium? This is, of course, not clearly known. Gross neuropathologic brain cuts do not reveal any pathologic changes of significance in delirium specifically. There are at least three different physical mechanisms that could be suggested. One is in a withdrawal phenomenon such as that seen in withdrawal from ethyl alcohol or barbiturates wherein the withdrawal is thought to trigger a release of inhibitory functions. A second type is that of ingestion of toxins, as might be present in an infectious disease, or as might be the result of a gangrenous limb. A third type of physical mechanism could be destructive lesions such as those found in the brain from the HTLV-III/LAV (AIDS) virus.[15]

Although there are little data at present, our hypothesis is that the basic dysfunction of delirium is a dysfunction in the dopamine and acetylcholine systems of the brain. There is a relatively strong tradition of cognitive dysfunction due to anticholinergic toxicity. Wikler long ago showed the so-called dissociation between behavior and EEG in animals.[16] He showed that, although the EEG shows the classical pervasive slowing of anticholinergic intoxication, in animals there still may be purposeful behavioral patterns. It is not rare to see patients with anticholinergic delirium secondary to tricyclic antidepressants. These patients have disorientation, cognitive dysfunction, and often hallucinations. The EEGs of these patients will reveal diffuse slowing. Blass et al[17] opined that cholinergic dysfunction is the common denominator in metabolic encephalopathies. Studies on primates with scopolamine show they have EEG slowing, purposeful behavior, but cannot learn.[18] On the other hand, it appears that a dysfunction in the dopaminergic system is basically at the root of increased agitation and delusions in the patient. It is postulated that dopamine controls the process of association and learning which, if it is speeded up with too much dopamine, can produce delusions.[19] Similarly, an excess of dopamine can increase the agitation of a patient as is seen in manic and amphetamine-toxic patients. Our experience with intravenous (IV) haloperidol as a dopamine blocker indirectly supports this idea that an excess of dopamine is the culprit in delusions and agitation.[20] In summary, it seems there are two major transmitter system breakdowns involved in delirium—an excess of dopamine and a deficiency of acetylcholine. This may explain why some people have only cognitive difficulty, such as disorientation, with a disordered cholinergic system, whereas other patients in a delirium may be quite agitated with some delusions, but remember everything that went on during that delirious period. It might be said of them that they had a superabundance of dopamine in the system and a relatively regularized cholinergic function.

Are there any specific types of delirium? This depends to a great extent on one's point of view. One may contend that all delirium is the same or that there are different types of deliria, depending on whether one tends to be a "lumper" or "splitter" in using diagnostic categories. Probably the basic agreement would be that most deliria are phenomena due to multiple organic or psychogenic causes. Stressors, internal and external, act on the mind-brain complex to produce delirium. To call a delirium toxic is clinically helpful but not scientifically satisfying. Various deliria have been described in association with internal and external stressors: For example, lesions in limbic structures such as the hippocampus and cingulate gyrus can have an associated agitated delirium[21]; cerebro-vascular disease has elicited deliria[22]; personality dissociation may be manifest as hallucinations, release of primary process material, and agitation. For a helpful and thorough "grocery list" of the causes of delirium, see Aita.[23]

Several clinical features of delirium follow[24]:

1. The onset of delirium can be rapid or slow. There may be mild transient symptoms, disturbed sleep or nightmares.

2. The patients can be aware of the dysfunction and may use the defenses of denial, projection, conversion, or withdrawal to master the feelings this dysfunction may incur. Patients may therefore make it more difficult for the psychiatric examiner by denying to themselves and to the examiner what they are really experiencing.

3. Nocturnal exacerbations may occur, possibly due to a decrease in sensory stimuli. The phenomenon of "sundowning" is common in general hospitals, and is usually found in the more elderly population. Some older people report that soft background music during the night is reassuring to them. Although the causes of sundowning are not known,

there are various theories that it may be connected to decreased sensory input and/or connected with circadian rhythms and/or sleep disorder.

4. There is always some disorientation in delirium. Patients may mistake unfamiliar persons or places for the familiar. They may believe they are in a local hospital and act perfectly reasonable otherwise. They may confuse what should be familiar names. It is important for the physician to do a formal mental status examination of patients, that is, to press the patients for specific answers to questions and not accept general answers.

5. The patient's grasp of the environment may be faulty. His former grasp was the product of complex cognitive processes usually impaired by delirium. For example, patients may know they are in the hospital, but may believe it is primarily for a follow-up GI series for their duodenal ulcer whereas, in fact, they have been admitted for bleeding esophageal varices and knew it at the time of admission.

6. Attention and arousal are key areas. There may be a selective central influence related to the reticular activating system important in serving up sufficient arousal to guarantee attention. It is not fully clear whether selective or global attention impairment can be of diagnostic significance. Mesulam et al[25] have argued that the main deficit in the acute confusional state is in the function of selective attention. Usually there is an inverse correlation between attention and distractibility—as one increases, the other decreases. Attention needs a certain amount of arousal; too little or too much impairs attention.

7. Thinking is an effort for delirious patients. Bizarre thoughts may intrude into the patient's conversation or general thought stream. Delirious patients tend to be more concrete than abstract. Psychotic patients with formal thought disorders can be quite abstract rather than concrete. Delusions may appear but are usually transient. They may change in response to environmental stimuli. They are usually unsystematized and persecutory, in contradistinction to the neatly formed paranoid delusions of the patient who has paranoid schizophrenia or paraphrenia. Because of the jumbled and poorly linked thought processes, the examiner may wonder if a formal thought disorder exists. This can be put to rest, for the most part, because with delirium there is always some clouding of consciousness which is generally not the case with the schizophrenic.

8. The patient with delirium commonly has perceptual impairment or illusions. It may be helpful to consider illusions as a sort of premature and improper labeling of percepts. Visual illusions tend to predominate.

9. Hallucinations have been estimated to vary from 39% to 100% in

delirious patients.[6] They are probably less common in the older person than in the younger person. Visual hallucinations predominate over auditory or sensory hallucinations. Auditory hallucinations are particularly predominant in paranoid schizophrenia and are often cited as the major mode of hallucination in so-called alcoholic hallucinosis. Since the arrival of the "near-death" literature, it is clear that there are out-of-body sensations, which could be listed as kinesthetic hallucinations. Whether, in fact, near-death is an artifact of delirium remains to be seen. Visual hallucinations may take on Lilliputian proportions as, for example, in a patient seen by the author who was toxic from digoxin. The patient was seeing small, 4-in.-tall figures marching up and down on his left leg dressed in British uniforms from our American Revolution.

10. In delirium, short-term memory is impaired. This was alluded to previously as possibly explained by a deficit in acetylcholine. As demonstrated by Hebb, a certain amount of arousal is required in order to remember.[26] The graph of the memory-arousal correlation is like an inverse U; too little arousal gives no memory, a certain amount gives peak memory, and intense arousal decreases memory. In most deliria there is either not enough or too much arousal. Katz et al[27] differentiate global and selective cognitive impairment; global is associated with hypokinetic delirium and selective is associated with hyperkinetic delirium. In their experience, global impairment was due more often to an organic lesion, whereas a selective impairment was due more often to environmental stress.

11. The affects most commonly found in deliria are anxiety, fear, and depression, alone or in combination.

12. Psychomotor behavior may be slowed or agitated. Agitation may take the form of picking at the sheets or some bizarre type of behavior such as trying to find the toilet in the clothes closet.

Differentially, acute confusional states or fully developed deliria may result from meningitis, ictal states, postictal states, drug intoxications, metabolic problems, pulmonary embolism, carcinoma, withdrawal states, fever, pneumonia, congestive heart failure, myocardial infarction, fat emboli syndrome, urinary tract infections, postoperative states, hypothermia, dehydration, lack of sleep, other underlying medical problems, and external environmental stress.

CHARACTERISTICS OF DEMENTIA

Dementia is more easily diagnosed if it is seen longitudinally. When seen once or over a relatively brief time it can be difficult to diagnose. This difficulty is compounded when there is no opportunity to discuss the patient with family members or others who can give some historical background and commentary on how the patient has behaved. Early behavioral characteristics seen in demented persons include:

1. A lack of initiative
2. An increase in irritability over and above former normal behavior
3. Some loss of interest in various areas of their lives
4. Impaired performance

This last characteristic comes to the attention of the family often in the form of the inability of patients to "hold their liquor" as they used to. It is not uncommon for a family member to say that grandpa becomes silly or irascible after only one drink now. Evolution of dementia may be a slow process taking from 3 to 8 years. Some of the late characteristics are:

1. Distractibility
2. Inability to think clearly and intellectual fatigue
3. Lack of perseverance in performance of tasks
4. Defective memory (although this may be an early sign also)
5. Alteration in mood, especially depression, and lack of insight

Since 1976[78] a change in the usual custom of considering Alzheimer's disease as a presenile dementia and senile dementia as a separate entity has been developing. It is now thought that both presenile and senile dementia are similar, and that someone with senile dementia over the age of 65 may be termed as having senile dementia of the Alzheimer type (SDAT).[29] Strictly speaking, Alzheimer's disease is still only certain when the neuropathologic features of it are found either by autopsy or brain biopsy. In 1980 the DSM-III considered the senile and presenile dementias together in their category of Primary Degenerative Dementia. For the diagnosis of any dementia they laid out the following criteria[10]:

Dementia (DSM-III)

A. A loss of intellectual abilities of sufficient severity to interfere with social or occupational functioning
B. Memory impairment
C. At least one of the following:
   1. Impairment of abstract thinking, as manifested by concrete interpretation of proverbs, inability to find similarities and differences between related words, difficulty in defining words and concepts, and other similar tasks
   2. Impaired judgment
   3. Other disturbances of higher cortical function, such as aphasia (disorder of language due to brain dysfunction), apraxia (inability to carry out motor activities despite intact comprehension and motor function),

agnosia (failure to recognize or identify objects despite intact sensory function), "constructional difficulty" (eg, inability to copy three-dimensional figures, assemble blocks, or arrange sticks in specific designs)

4. Personality change (ie, alteration or accentuation of premorbid traits)

D. State of consciousness not clouded (ie, does not meet the criteria for delirium or intoxication, although these may be superimposed)

E. Either (1) or (2):

1. Evidence from the history, physical examination, or laboratory tests, of a specific organic factor that is judged to be etiologically related to the disturbance

2. In the absence of such evidence, an organic factor necessary for the development of the syndrome can be presumed if conditions other than Organic Mental Disorders have been reasonably excluded and if the behavioral change represents cognitive impairment in a variety of areas

A further attempt to ascertain criteria for the clinical diagnosis of Alzheimer's disease was published in 1984 by a work group cosponsored by the National Institute of Neurological and Communication Disorders and Stroke (NINCDS) and Alzheimer's Disease and Related Disorders Association (ADRDA). They established seven categories[30]:

I. The criteria for the clinical diagnosis of PROBABLE Alzheimer's disease include:

Dementia established by clinical examination and documented by the Mini-Mental Test, the Blessed Dementia Scale, or some similar examination, and confirmed by neuropsychological tests

Deficits in two or more areas of cognition

Progressive worsening of memory and other cognitive functions

No disturbance of consciousness

Onset between ages 40 and 90, most often after age 65

Absence of systemic disorders or other brain diseases that in and of themselves could account for the progressive deficits in memory and cognition

II. The diagnosis of PROBABLE Alzheimer's disease is supported by:

Progressive deterioration of specific cognitive functions such as language (aphasia), motor skills (apraxia), and perception (agnosia)

Impaired activities of daily living and altered patterns of behavior

Family history of similar disorders, particularly if confirmed neuropathologically

Laboratory results of:

Normal lumbar puncture as evaluated by standard techniques

Normal pattern of nonspecific changes in EEG, such as increased slow wave activity

Evidence of cerebral atrophy on computed tomography (CT) with progression documented by serial observation

III. Other clinical features consistent with the diagnosis of PROBABLE Alzheimer's disease, after exclusion of causative dementia other than Alzheimer's disease, include:

Plateaus in the course of progression of the illness

Associated symptoms of depression, insomnia, incontinence, delusions, illusions, hallucinations, catastrophic verbal, emotional, or physical outbursts, sexual disorders, and weight loss

Other neurologic abnormalities in some patients, especially with more advanced disease and including motor signs such as increased muscle tone, myoclonus, or gait disorder

Seizures in advanced disease

CT normal for age

IV. Features that make the diagnosis of PROBABLE Alzheimer's disease uncertain or unlikely include:

Sudden, apoplectic onset

Focal neurologic findings such as hemiparesis, sensory loss, visual field defect deficits, and incoordination early in the course of the illness

Seizures or gait disturbances at the onset or very early in the course of the illness

V. Clinical diagnosis of POSSIBLE Alzheimer's disease:

May be made on the basis of the dementia syndrome, in the absence of other neurologic, psychiatric, or systemic disorders sufficient to cause dementia, and in the presence of variations in the onset, in the presentation, or in the clinical course

May be made in the presence of a second systemic or brain disorder sufficient to produce dementia, which is not considered to be *the* cause of the dementia

Should be used in research studies when a single, gradually progressive severe cognitive deficit is identified in the absence of other identifiable cause

VI. Criteria for diagnosis of DEFINITE Alzheimer's disease are:

The clinical criteria for PROBABLE Alzheimer's disease

Histopathologic evidence obtained from a biopsy or autopsy

VII. Classification of Alzheimer's disease for research purposes should specify features that may differentiate subtypes of the disorder, such as:

Familiar occurrence

Onset before age of 65

Presence of trisomy 21

Coexistence of other relevant conditions such as Parkinson's disease

A relatively new and controversial entity in the domain of dementia is subcortical dementia, originally described by Albert et al.[31] It has been seen especially in progressive supranuclear palsy, Huntington's disease, and Parkinson's disease. It is distinguished from cortical dementia by impaired timing and activation. Subcortically demented persons have been described as forgetful, but with a good memory. They do not have aphasia, their cognition is impaired, especially with poor problem solving produced to a great extent by their slowness, forgetfulness, and impaired strategy and planning, all of which is evident in their slow processing time. They often may have an affective disorder, and it is not unusual that treatment-resistant depressions may well have a component of subcortical dementia. Generally, they have a posture and/or gait dysfunction, sometimes being dysarthric, and can have movement disorders such as chorea, tremor, or ataxia. The basis for the distinction between cortical and subcortical dementia is that in the cortical species the cortex is largely involved and the basal ganglia, thalamus, and mesencephalon are largely spared; whereas it is just the opposite in subcortical dementia.

From a clinical point of view there are two basic types of dementia, the treatable and the nontreatable.[32] One of the more important treatable types of dementia is normal pressure hydrocephalus (NPH) in which the triad of (1) ataxia, (2) dementia, and (3) urinary incontinence is seen.[33] Dementia due to NPH can present with symptoms of depression such as apathy, inattentiveness, agitation, and poverty of thought.[34]

There has been increased focus on the so-called entity of pseudo-dementia in recent years.[35] It is known that a clinical depression can affect the cognitive aspect of the patient, and it is thought by some that there is a so-called dementia of depression.[36] A middle-aged or elderly patient who is substantially depressed may be erroneously classified as demented. There is an argument in the field as to whether this concept of pseudodementia is, in fact, helpful or not.[37] When the word "pseudo-dementia" is used alone it usually means the pseudodementia of depression. There are other types of pseudodementia, for example, of hysteria, which are less frequently seen.[38]

It is this author's opinion that the psychiatrist should be able to diagnose the depression from a face-to-face confrontation with the patient who displays in the interview not only cognitive but, more important, limbic features of depression. If one relies primarily on "paper-and-pencil tests" such as the Hamilton Depression Rating Scale[39] to make diagnoses, one can very seriously miss whether a patient has a depression or dementia. Tests such as these are often helpful in assessing severity of depression but they fail to capture limbic phenomenology, crucial in the diagnosis of depression.

One of the quickest ways to a diagnostic clue, in a hospitalized patient, whether a pseudodementia or a real dementia exists, is to give the patient 5 mg of dextroamphetamine at 8 AM and come by and see him about an hour later. The depressed patient, in general, will be more alert, and will exhibit more cognitive sharpness; whereas if the patient is primarily demented, he will be more alert, have increased animation, but, against this background, most often there will be an intensification of his memory and cognitive impairment secondary to a dementia.

Although with deliria structural changes are rarely seen, SDAT, Alzheimer's disease, and Pick's disease do show structural neuro-anatomical correlates. In 1907, Alois Alzheimer demonstrated neurofibrillary tangles and senile plaques (now generally called neuritic plaques)[40] in patients with presenile dementia. There is also some discussion as to whether normal aging, if it goes long enough, shows processes similar to those in Alzheimer's disease.[41] In normal aging the locus ceruleus and the substantia nigra undergo significant neuronal loss.[42] Neuritic plaques are present in the neocortex during aging and may be found in 80% of normal brains. In general, the number of plaques in the neocortex correlates with the patient's mental status. Ignored for many years, there is increasing interest in the ravaging of aging and Alzheimer's disease on limbic system structures.[43] The neurofibrillary tangles of Alzheimer's disease occur in the hippocampus during normal aging and may be found in more than 90% of all human brains by the ninth decade. The highest concentration of neurofibrillary tangles found in SDAT are in the hippocampus and the parahippocampal area, including the amygdala.[44] In fact, a Canadian group has cogently argued that Alzheimer's disease is basically a hippocampal dementia.[45] In SDAT there is also a decrease in the number of dendritic spines. The substantia innominata (which includes Meynert's nucleus basalis, thought to be the reservoir of acetylcholine) is affected in SDAT.[46] An important feature that is especially consoling to the relatives of an Alzheimer's patient is that there is no convincing evidence that psychosocial factors can or have predisposed a patient to SDAT.

Differentially, dementia may result from degenerative causes such as Alzheimer's disease and Huntington's chorea; metabolic causes such as myxedema and Wilson's disease; vitamin deficiencies such as lack of vitamin B_{12}; neoplastic causes such as glioma and metastasis; mechanical causes such as trauma as in dementia pugilistica (punch-drunk syndrome); vascular causes, the most common of which is multi-infarct dementia; toxic causes such as alcohol and the outlawed absinthe; and infectious causes such as general paresis and Creutzfeldt-Jakob disease.

APPROACH TO THE PATIENT

An important point to determine in approaching the patient is whether the consult is urgent or allows some leisure on the part of the consultant. This means the consultant has to know why he is being called—a point not always clear in large teaching hospitals. Is he being called because the patient is such a management problem that he is tying up two or three nurses during each shift? Or is it that the principal physician would like to have some help selecting a sedative for the patient's management? If the consult does not need urgent attention, it is important to check the chart of the patient. This means more than just riffling through the chart. The consultant must look in the chart for various key items. These include:

1. *Previous psychiatric intervention.* One should check for previous psychiatric hospitalizations. If found, what were the diagnoses, hospital course, prognosis, discharge medications, and follow-up? Was there ever any psychiatric evaluation? A history or previous physical examination may mention this. (In teaching hospitals more than one history and physical examination report are usually in the chart—the medical student's usually being the most thorough.)

It is also helpful to keep an eye out for any neurologic information that may be in the chart, for example, previous CT scans, previous EEGs.

Most hospitals have social service units and a case history written by the social worker may be present. Often this is an invaluable aid, especially concerning the patient's relationships with family. The consultant has to judge whether a full reading or quick scan is sufficient.

2. *Vital signs.* One should check for hypotension and possible anoxic changes. Hypertension over long periods can produce small lesions which affect behavior slowly, yielding such symptoms as mood lability, drive reduction, insomnia, and impaired judgment. One has to notice whether there had been a febrile course with the patient, and what his present status is. What was the highest recorded temperature?

3. *Operative procedures and use of anesthesia.* Surgery is traumatic and postoperative confusion is not a rarity.[47] The consultant should check the anesthesiologist's work sheet in the chart, not only to notice blood loss and replacement but, more important, to evaluate the blood pressure readings taken during surgery. It is not infrequent that a systolic blood pressure would dip below 100 mmHg in a difficult surgery. A mild hypoxia may be well tolerated by the young without detectable behavioral consequence. In the elderly, however, a mild hypoxia may produce subtle mental changes and discrete motor changes such as intermittent darting of the tongue to one side. Such subtle changes may go unrecognized in the hospital during the postoperative period.

Surgery itself, or time on the respirator, may induce inappropriate antidiuretic hormone (ADH) secretion and thereby cause a relative hyponatremia that can affect mental status. This hyponatremia need not necessarily be drastically reduced. It is known that sodium concentration of 125 mEq/L effects mental changes.[48] It is entirely possible that the idiosyncratically sensitive brain may show mental changes at sodium concentrations of 130 mEq/L. We have seen three cases of mild hyponatremia, none of the sodiums being less than 128 mEq/L, which resulted in nonconvulsive, complex partial seizure with an attendant confusional state. No treatment was needed other than to correct the electrolyte imbalance.

4. *Nurses' notes.* Speaking to the nurses in charge of the patient gives a more longitudinal window on patient behavior. Since the consultant is usually not present during all three nursing shifts, it is useful to peruse the nurses' notes for possible significant behavioral observations. This is especially important when one is called to see a delirious patient, since, almost invariably, the nurses' notes document disorientation before the attending physician.

5. *Laboratory values.* Psychiatric residents, unless specifically taught to do so, do not often skim "the numbers" on the patients they are asked to see. Unless the resident is shown otherwise, he may have the impression that he is to see the patient using only his "talking skills." One of the functions of a consultant is to come in fresh—not close to or heavily invested in a specific diagnosis. Coming in fresh, the consultant may notice high or low normal laboratory test values and his suggestions may lead to the repetition of a study with positive results.

Scanning the numbers over the hospitalized period gives the consultant an idea of trends in the patient's physiology. The brain is a sensitive organ and can vary in its individual sensitivity to calcium, sodium, or other electrolytes. Therefore, borderline high or low normals may be a key to mildly confusional states or incipient deliria. A nonexhaustive list of laboratory values with a sampling of pathologic states associated with each is given here. The consultant may do well to keep these in mind:

Hemoglobin (Hb): Anemia, dehydration?

White blood cells (WBC): Infection?

Red blood cells (RBC): Anemia?

Mean corpuscular volume (MCV): Vitamin B_{12} deficiency, folate deficiency, history of alcoholism?

Blood urea nitrogen (BUN): Starvation, dehydration, uremia?

Magnesium (Mg): Weakness, depression?

Calcium (Ca): Endocrine disorder, depression?

Sodium (Na): Hyponatremia?

Potassium (K): Weakness, depression?

Liver function tests: Encephalopathy, clue to delirium tremens?

Arterial blood gases (ABG): Respiratory insufficiency, CO_2 narcosis?

Osmolality (serum and urinary): Hyponatremia?

Input and output: If not critical can be checked in a rough way with the nursing staff

Familiarity with the basic elements of brain function in the critically ill can prepare the consultant better for intensive care unit consultation.[49]

6. *Medications.* This topic is vast and could be the subject of a paper in itself. Consultants must know about general hospital medication—those commonly used on medical and surgical services. Medication may be responsible for a decompensated mental state. It is necessary also to understand the pharmacology of the patient's medication in order to make intelligent recommendations for further management of the patient. Table 6-1 is a nonexhaustive list of therapeutic drugs that have either appeared in the literature or that our consultant team have associated with a clinical delirium.

The psychiatric side effects of drugs is another subject in itself and cannot be gone into in depth here. Although the general psychiatric consultant is not necessarily a pharmacologist with grocery lists of side effects at the ready, some clear side effects mentally tucked away will help him to be a more intelligent consultant. Psychiatrists as a group also tend to be rather diffident in urging the discontinuance of a drug if the attending physician is resistant to changing it. This was the case when cimetidine first appeared. After stressful surgery many surgeons place their patients on IV cimetidine. Not surprisingly, there were many confusional states secondary to this. The surgeons were generally resistant to discontinuing the cimetidine until the bulk of clinical evidence showed that it can indeed produce a confusional state. We have seen, on a smaller scale, similar reactions with IV acyclovir. The consultant cannot *prove* that a medication is the culprit in delirium, but a hard reading of the chart and, following, of the temporal course of medication use and the confusional state with its waxings and wanings can often produce serious circumstantial evidence as to what the culprit is.

Meperidine hydrochloride is used in large quantities, especially postsurgery in many hospitals. Kaiko et al[50] have shown that a metabolite of meperidine, normeperidine, can build up with increased dosage and cause "the shakes", myoclonus, anxiety, and, ultimately, seizures. This is not as well known to clinicians as it should be. We have seen several cases thought to be delirium tremens postsurgery which in fact were due to meperidine use. The diagnosis is important since the treatment is to discontinue the meperidine and not to treat with a neuroleptic or benzodiazepine for delirium tremens. Normeperidine toxicity can also present first as pure paranoid state with trembling and myoclonus following it.[51]

Table 6-1. Some Therapeutic Drugs Associated with Clinical Delirium

ACTH	LAsparaginase
Acyclovir	Levodopa
Alprazolam	Lidocaine
Amantadine hydrochloride	Lithium carbonate
Aminoglycosides	Lorazepam
Aminophylline	Meperidine hydrochloride (normeperidine)
Amitriptyline hydrochloride	Methotrexate
Amodiaquine hydrochloride	Methyldopa
Amphetamine	Metrizamide
Amphotericin B	Metronidazole
Atropine	Mexiletine
Baclofen	Naproxen
Barbiturates	Pentazocine
Benztropine mesylate	Phenelzine sulfate
Bromocriptine	Phenylephrine hydrochloride
Captopril	Phenylpropranolamine hydrochloride
Cephalosporins	Phenytoin
Chloramphenicol	Podophyllum resin
Chloroquine	Prednisone
Cimetidine	Procainamide hydrochloride
Clonidine hydrochloride	Procarbazine hydrochloride
Colistin	Propranolol hydrochloride
Cyclosporine	Protriptyline hydrochloride
Cytorabine hydrochloride	Ranitidine
Digitalis	Rifampin
Diisopropamide	Scopolamine
Dipipanone hydrochloride	Sulfonamides
Disulfiram	Sulindac
Ephedrine	Tamoxifen citrate
Ergotamine tartrate	Tetracyclines
Ethambutol hydrochloride	Theophylline
Fluorouracil	Thioridazine
Gentamicin sulfate	Ticarcillin
Methenamine	Trihexylphenidyl hydrochloride
Ibuprofen	Vancomycin hydrochloride
Indomethacin	Vinblastine sulfate
Isoniazid	Vincristine sulfate

Mental Status Examination

A mental status examination should be done on all patients. It may not be possible to do a formal mental status examination, however, in conversation with the patient much clinical information regarding mental status may be garnered. A consultation psychiatrist may not be allowed the time or cooperation to perform a complete psychiatric mental status examination of the type given in an inpatient psychiatric unit. An examination that can easily be repeated allows for better follow-up and assessment of progress or decline.

There are various ways of assessing a patient. Some psychiatrists use a technique called JOMAC, an acronym for the testing of Judgment, Orientation, Memory, Affect, and Consciousness or intellect. In our consultations we find most helpful, and use most often, the "Mini-Mental State" examination of Folstein et al.[52] (An example of this test is shown in Fig. 6-1.) Eleven questions concentrate on the cognitive functions and these can be given in five to ten minutes. The examination can be repeated often and can serve as a numerical key recordable in the chart to show progress or decline. The mini-mental state examination assesses more properly the cognitive aspects of mental status and is not meant to adequately assess the affective state of the patient. Therefore, it behooves the psychiatrist to investigate various affects such as anger, sadness, euphoria, and others that in and of themselves also affect the cognitive state. The psychiatrist must have a precise understanding of the differentiation of delusion from hallucination, dissociation from psychosis, hypomania from joviality.

Differentiating Delirium from Dementia

In differentiating delirium from dementia a key clinical observation is the patient's arousal. The demented person generally, but not always, tends to have about the same degree of arousal as a general state. The patient with delirium usually does not exhibit a constant level of arousal. He may wax or wane. He may be sometimes more, sometimes less aroused. This is a major distinction between delirium and dementia. Attention, obviously, is linked to arousal, but there are different types of attention. A demented person may be sufficiently aroused, but he may be distracted by some persistent thought or sensory input and not attend to the matter at hand. The delirious patient can also be distracted, but it may have a different quality in that the "gain" of his arousal tends to vary, being either turned down or turned up. The delirious patient gives the impression of being oblivious to, or, conversely, jumpy in response to environmental stimuli. The delirious person's arousal and correlative attention tends to vary more than that of the demented person, who generally maintains a constant amount of arousal with a constant amount of attention or inattention.

Familiarization with the various entities that can cause a delirium or confusional state is helpful. The following is a sampling of some of these entities that are frequently missed:

Patient _____
Examiner _____
Date _____

"MINI-MENTAL STATE"*

Maxi-mum score	Score	
		Orientation
5	( )	What is the (year) (season) (date) (day) (month)?
5	( )	Where are we? (state) (country) (town) (hospital) (floor).

Registration

3 ( ) Name 3 objects: 1 second to say each. Then ask the patient all 3 after you have said them. Give 1 point for each correct answer. Then repeat them until he learns all 3. Count trials and record.
Trials _____

Attention and Calculation

5 ( ) Serial 7's. 1 point for each correct. Stop after 5 answers. Alternatively spell "world" backwards.

Recall

3 ( ) Ask for the 3 objects repeated above. Give 1 point for each correct.

Language

9 ( ) Name a pencil, and watch (2 points)
Repeat the following "No ifs, ands or buts." (1 point)
Follow a 3-stage command:
"Take a paper in your right hand, fold it in half, and put it on the floor" (3 points)
Read and obey the following:

Close your eyes (1 point)

Write a sentence (1 point)
Copy design (1 point)
Total score
ASSESS level of consciousness
along a continuum _____

Alert Drowsy Stupor Coma

Figure 6-1. Mini-Mental State Examination (reproduced with permission from Folstein et al[52]).

INSTRUCTIONS FOR ADMINISTRATION OF MINI-MENTAL STATE EXAMINATION

Orientation

(1) Ask for the date. Then ask specifically for parts omitted, e.g., "Can you also tell me what season it is?" One point for each correct.

(2) Ask in turn "Can you tell me the name of this hospital?" (town, country, etc.). One point for each correct.

Registration

Ask the patient if you may test his memory. Then say the names of 3 unrelated objects, clearly and slowly, about one second for each. After you have said all 3, ask him to repeat them. This first repetition determines his score (0–3) but keep saying them until he can repeat all 3, up to 6 trials. If he does not eventually learn all 3, recall cannot be meaningfully tested.

Attention and calculation

Ask the patient to begin with 100 and count backwards by 7. Stop after 5 subtractions (93, 86, 79, 72, 65). Score the total number of correct answers.

If the patient cannot or will not perform this task, ask him to spell the word "world" backwards. The score is the number of letters in correct order. E.g., dlrow = 5, dlorw = 3.

Recall

Ask the patient if he can recall the 3 words you previously asked him to remember. Score 0–3.

Language

Naming: Show the patient a wrist watch and ask him what it is. Repeat for pencil. Score 0–2.

Repetition: Ask the patient to repeat the sentence after you. Allow only one trial. Score 0 or 1.

3-Stage command: Give the patient a piece of plain blank paper and repeat the command. Score 1 point for each part correctly executed.

Reading: On a blank piece of paper print the sentence "Close your eyes", in letters large enough for the patient to see clearly. Ask him to read it and do what it says. Score 1 point only if he actually closes his eyes.

Writing: Give the patient a blank piece of paper and ask him to write a sentence for you. Do not dictate a sentence, it is to be written spontaneously. It must contain a subject and verb and be sensible. Correct grammar and punctuation are not necessary.

Copying: On a clean piece of paper, draw intersecting pentagons, each side about 1 in., and ask him to copy it exactly as it is. All 10 angles must be present and 2 must intersect to score 1 point. Tremor and rotation are ignored.

Estimate the patient's level of sensorium along a continuum, from alert on the left to coma on the right.

1. *Withdrawal from barbiturates.* Occasionally, a few days after admission to a medical or surgical unit, either postoperatively or not, a middle-aged or geriatric patient will show unexpected signs and symptoms, for example, confusion, fever. A detailed review of the medications the patient had been taking prior to hospitalization is often helpful. In several cases we have found that the patient has been taking a barbiturate for sleep for perhaps 12 years, and this need only be, say, 100 mg of secobarbital every night. Upon hospitalization the barbiturate had been abruptly stopped. These patients did not appear as the usual barbiturate addict. A dramatic response is seen in these patients when treated with the addition of a barbiturate and subsequent weaning is begun.[53] This has also occurred with medications such as methaqualone (Quaalude) and ethchlorvynil (Placidyl).

2. *Metrizamide.* Metrizamide (Amipaque) can be the etiologic agent of confusion secondary to seizure.[54] It is important not only to review previous medications of the patient but also to be aware of medications used in special testing procedures.

3. *Hyperviscosity syndrome.* Although the hyperviscosity syndrome is rare, it is not unusual that mental changes accompany it.[55]

4. *Fat emboli syndrome.* A confusional state is probably more common with fat emboli showers than is reported. We have been asked to see several patients thought to be in delirium tremens. Upon reviewing the history and examining the patient, signs consistent with emboli showers were found and a diagnosis of fat emboli syndrome was made which more cogently explained the disordered mental status.[56] It is important to remember that fat emboli are most often seen in fractures of the long bones and will therefore be seen more on orthopedic units.

5. *Complex partial seizures.* One of the least recognized causes of confusion in our collective consultation experience has been nonconvulsive partial seizure.[57] For most physicians, neurologists included, there is a reluctance to make a clinical diagnosis of partial seizure without the presence of some convulsive activity (muscle activity).[58] The EEG is relied upon for the diagnosis. However, in 40% of patients with complex partial seizure there is no "diagnostic" EEG available.[59] Although difficult to prove without implanted electrodes, it is our clinical conviction that there is a much greater incidence of complex partial status epilepticus than is appreciated.[60] Ictal confusion in later life is also not as infrequent as is generally taught.[61] We have found IV lorazepam (2 to 4 mg) to be quite effective in both treatment of the seizure phenomenon and in support of the clinical diagnosis.

If the patient is thought to be demented there are two bedside tests that may be helpful. The first is the simple Set Test of Isaacs and Kennie.[62] This test requires the patient to name ten items in four general categories such as animals, colors, fruits, and towns. One point is given for each different item named. Naming less than 15 out of a possible 40 or more items is consistent with dementia, and a score of 15 to 24 is consistent with possible dementia.

Another test is the Blessed Dementia Scale (Fig. 6-2).[63] This test assesses two items in general: the first is the activities of daily living, and the second is memory per se. The combined score of these two parts gives the Blessed score. Obviously, a score of 0 is the normal non-demented score and it is helpful with an escalating score to see that it correlates with increased dementia. Within certain limits there is also good correlation of the Blessed Dementia Scale with the Mini-Mental State examination.[64]

Much information about delirium and dementia may be gathered in examining the patient by asking him to preform various tasks. Cortical release phenomena can often be noted. The most prominent of the various physical signs associated with dementia are the grasp, glabellar, blink, palmomental, Babinski, and sucking reflexes.[65]

Asking the patient to perform simple commands, such as left hand on right elbow, right hand on left elbow, left hand on left elbow, and observing how the commands are executed may be revealing. If there is undue hesitation or confusion in carrying out such commands, a suspicion of organic disease must be entertained. Testing for reproduction of "kinetic melodies"[66] may give information substantiating a frontal lobe dysfunction. Kinetic melodies is a term coined by Luria to describe the performance of complex movements generalized in time. All good drummers have excellent control of kinetic melody. As a test for frontal lobe function the examiner has only to "play" his left (L) and right (R) fingers on a desk in a pattern such as RRL, LLR and ask the patient to repeat it. One can then progress to a paradiddle, such as RLRR, LRLL. The degree of difficulty experienced in performing these kinetic melodies gives a rough estimate of frontal lobe dysfunction. Any suspicion of hepatic precoma should prompt the examining psychiatrist to test extended arms for asterixis. Asterixis is not specific for hepatic disease and is seen in a variety of metabolic diseases such as chronic pulmonary disease. The important point is that the patient's arms may be extended for as long as 30 seconds before there is a lapse.

If it is not clearly evident whether the patient is delirious or demented, more laboratory tests are indicated. Although the EEG is not usually ordered for this type of differential diagnosis, it may be helpful.[67]

NAME _____

Date _____

NEMCH # _____

BLESSED DEMENTIA SCALE

Changes in Performance of Everyday Activities

1. Inability to perform household tasks   1 ½ 0
2. Inability to cope with small sums of money   1 ½ 0
3. Inability to remember short list of items, e.g. in shopping   1 ½ 0
4. Inability to find way about indoors   1 ½ 0
5. Inability to find way about familiar street   1 ½ 0
6. Inability to interpret surroundings (e.g. to recognize
   whether in hospital or at home, to discriminate between
   patients, doctors, nurses, relatives, hospital staff, etc.)   1 ½ 0
7. Inability to recall recent events (e.g. recent outings, visits
   of relatives or friends to hospital, etc.)   1 ½ 0
8. Tendency to dwell in the past   1 ½ 0

Changes in Habits

9. Eating:
   - Cleanly with proper utensils   0
   - Messily with spoon only   2
   - Simple solids, e.g. biscuits   2
   - Has to be fed   3
10. Dressing:
   - Unaided   0
   - Occasionally misplaced buttons, etc.   1
   - Wrong sequence, commonly forgetting items   2
   - Unable to dress   3
11. Complete sphincter control   0
   - Occasional wet beds   1
   - Frequent wet beds   2
   - Doubly incontinent   3

Changes in Personality, Interests, Drive

No Change   0
12. Increased rigidity   1
13. Increased egocentricity   1
14. Impairment of regard for feelings of others   1
15. Coarsening of affect   1
16. Impairment of emotional control, e.g. increased petulance
    and irritability   1
17. Hilarity in inappropriate situations   1
18. Diminished emotional responsiveness   1
19. Sexual misdemeanor (appearing *de novo* in old age)   1
    Interests retained   0
20. Hobbies relinquished   1
21. Diminished initiative or growing apathy   1
22. Purposeless hyperactivity   1

TOTAL _____

Information-Memory-Concentration Test

Information Test

Name	1
Age	1
Time (hour)	1
Time of day	1
Day of week	1
Date	1
Month	1
Season	1
Year	1
Place—Name	1
Street	1
Town	1
Type of Place (home, hospital, etc)	1
Recognition of persons (cleaner, doctor, nurse, patient, relative; any 2 available)	2

Memory

(1) Personal

Date of Birth	1
Place of Birth	1
School attended	1
Occupation	1
Name of sibs/spouse	1
Name of any town where pt. had worked	1
Name of employers	1

(2) Non-personal

Date of World War I	1
Date of World War II	1
President	1
Vice-President	1

(3) Name and address (5 min. recall)
   Mr. John Brown
   42 West Street

Cambridge, Ma.	5

Concentration

Months of year backwards	2	1	0
Counting 1–20	2	1	0
Counting 20–1	2	1	0

TOTAL DEMENTIA SCALE _____

Figure 6-2. The Blessed Dementia Scale.[63]

A CT scan can demonstrate cortical atrophy and possibly some other masked lesion. If not already ordered, so-called crazy chemistries are very useful. These include BUN, blood ammonia, sugar, magnesium, calcium, and electrolytes. Calcium concentrations above 15 mg/100 mL are frequently coupled with mental disturbance with paranoid trends.[68] It is also helpful, if suspicion is aroused, especially in the emergency room consultation, to obtain blood and urine specimens for toxic screen of substances that patients may have taken and denied having taken. It is usually not standard practice to get nuclear magnetic imaging of the brain or neuropsychological testing while in consultation. It may be necessary, however, since the outcome may determine treatment and/or postdischarge planning.

Table 6-2 lists the possible laboratory evaluations for dementia or delirium. A minimal work-up for delirium will include a complete blood count; and determination of electrolytes, including magnesium and calcium; BUN; creatinine; blood sugar; and liver function tests.

Table 6-2. Laboratory Evaluation of Dementia or Delirium

CBC	Serum B_{12}	Protein electrophoresis
Serology	Serum folate	CSF protein
Electrolytes, including Ca, Mg	Thyroid tests T_4 T_3 uptake Skull x-ray films	Lipid profile Cholesterol
ESR	Chest films	Urine analysis
BUN	EEG	NH_3
Creatinine, serum	CT scan	Nuclear magnetic imaging
Glucose fasting	Oxygen Tension, p_{O_2} Tension, p_{CO_2}	
Osmolality		
Liver function tests SGOT Alkaline phosphatase LDH Bilirubin	ECG Neuropsychological testing	

CBC = complete blood count, LDH = lactic dehydroqenase, T_4 = thyroxine, T_3 = triiodothyronine, CT = computed tomography.

Delirium and dementia usually have organic causes. However, clinical experience leads to the conclusion that some deliria result from so-called functional or nonorganic causes. Hackett et al[69] urge caution in attributing psychiatric difficulties in an ICU to the "intensive care syndrome." Functional delirium can result from a dissociation or other form of hysterical psychogenic process.

A formal thought disorder can generally be distinguished clinically from the cognitive disorder of delirium by two points: (1) A formal thought disorder often gives the examiner an impression of a "secret logic code" linking the loosely associated thought content. (2) There is consistency of the arousal and attention level in formal thought disorder.

Management

Once the diagnosis is made, the next step is treatment and management. In some urgent cases time is not available for comfortable diagnosis and the physician may have to manage the patient on the basis of a quick provisional impression. An example of this is the patient in a postictal confusional state from complex partial seizure who attempts to force his way out of the hospital. Intervention is obviously necessary with this patient before a more studied diagnosis can be made. In general, the diagnosis is known and there are four areas of concern in management.

1. Treatment of the underlying cause when possible
2. Orientation of the patient
3. Human contact with the patient, such as staff interactions, visits by relatives, visits by professionals
4. Medication, whether used for chemical restraint, anxiety reduction, or treatment of the cause of the delirium itself

Of the four elements listed above, the most important for the practicing consultant psychiatrist is the fourth. It is true that orienting the patient with clocks and calendars in the room, having human contact, and so forth, is consoling to the patient and helpful in his management. Nevertheless, all the human contact in the world and the placement of the maximum of orientation devices in the room will not do as much for the patient as correcting either his electrolyte balance, his cholinergic or dopaminergic system dysfunction, or whatever encephalopathogenic cause is at work.

Presuming that the cause of the delirium is rectified or there is no cause discoverable, the psychiatrist has to make a clinical decision whether to medicate the patient or not. The clinical condition of the patient is the guide in this decision. If the patient has mild memory dysfunction and mild paranoia with no agitation and it does not trouble the patient, a decision not to medicate and watch may be in order, being mindful of the quick turns that delirium can take and therefore being ready to quell agitation with medication.[70] The use of restraints may be contraindicated, for example, after thoracic surgery, and in any event are not calming to the patient.

On the other hand, moderate to severe agitation will require medication. Agitation is rarely seen in isolation; there is almost invariably an underlying delirium.[71] Our experience has been that the quickest way to control agitation is the use of IV haloperidol.[20,71-73] Mild agitation usually responds to between 0.5 mg to 2.0 mg of IV haloperidol; moderate agitation to 5.0 mg to 10.0 mg, and severe agitation to 10.0 mg or more. If agitation persists 20 minutes after administration, another dose, doubled, can be given and repeated in 20 minutes if agitation still has not subsided. The dose is doubled up to the control of agitation or the clinician's assessment of effectiveness.[72] Intravenous haloperidol has almost no effect on pulmonary or cardiovascular values.[73]

We have been impressed with the lack of extrapyramidal side effects in high-dose IV haloperidol relative to the oral or intramuscular (IM) route.[74] The reason for this is not clear, but we suspect it is due to the γ-aminobutyric acid–dopaminergic balance since most patients medicated with haloperidol will also have been administered diazepam or lorazepam. Adams et al, who also find scant evidence of extrapyramidal signs in using IV haloperidol, treat their agitated patients with regular IV haloperidol and IV lorazepam.[75]

Oral or IM neuroleptics can also be used if delirium and/or agitation is minor and there is relatively good patient cooperation.

The management of a patient with agitated delirium lies not just in the use of pharmacology. In the broader sense good management of the patient must include interaction with the patient's other caregivers. Accordingly, allying anxiety in staff with appropriate explanations and listening is to be encouraged, as is being available for sudden changes in the patient's condition.

REFERENCES

1. Terry RD, Katzman R: Senile dementia of the Alzheimer type. *Ann Neurol* 1983; 14:497–506.
2. Wells CE: The symptoms and behavioral manifestations of dementia, in Wells CE (ed): *Dementia*. Philadelphia, FA Davis Co, 1971, pp 1–12.
3. Engle GL, Romano J: Delirium, a syndrome of cerebral insufficiency. *J Chronic Dis* 1959; 9:260–277.

4. Mahendra B: Depression and dementia: The multifaceted relationship. *Psychol Med* 1985; 15:227–236.

5. Alexander MP, Geschwind N. Dementia in the elderly, in Albert ML (ed): *Clinical Neurology of Aging.* New York, Oxford University Press, 1984, pp 254–276.

6. Lipowski ZJ: Delirium, clouding of consciousness and confusion. *J Nerv Ment Dis* 1967; 145:227–255.

7. Adams RD, Victor M: Delirium and other acute confusional states, in Thorn GW, et al: *Harrison's Principles of Internal Medicine,* ed 8. New York, McGraw-Hill Book Co, 1977, pp 145–150.

8. Lipowski ZJ: *Delirium: Acute Brain Failure in Man.* Springfield, Ill, Charles C Thomas Publisher, 1980.

9. Chedru F, Geschwind N: Writing disturbances in acute confusional states. *Neuropsychologia* 1972; 10:343–353.

10. American Psychiatric Association: *Diagnostic and Statistical Manual of Mental Disorders* [DSM-III], 3rd ed. Washington, American Psychiatric Association, 1980.

11. Obreck R, Okhomina FOA, Scott DF: Value of EEG in acute confusional states. *J Neurol Neurosurg Psychiatry* 1979; 42:75–77.

12. Holland J, Sgroi SM, Marwit SJ, et al: The ICU syndrome: fact or fancy. *Psychiatr Med* 1973; 4:241–249.

13. Weddington WW: The mortality of delirium: an underappreciated problem? *Psychosomatics* 1982; 23:1232–1235.

14. Plum F, Posner JB: *The Diagnosis of Stupor and Coma,* ed 3. Philadelphia, FA Davis Co, 1980, pp 13–15.

15. Koenig S, Gendelman HE, Orenstein JM, et al: Detection of AIDS virus in macrophages in brain tissue from AIDS patients with encephalopathy. *Science* 1986; 233:1089–1093.

16. Wikler A: Pharmacologic dissociation of behavior and EEG "sleep patterns" in dogs: morphine, N-allylnormorphine, and atropine. *Proc Soc Exp Biol Med* 1952; 79:261–265.

17. Blass JP, Gibson GE, Duffy TE, et al: Cholinergic dysfunction: a common denominator in metabolic encephalopathies, in Pepeu G, Ladinsky H (eds); *Cholinergic Mechanisms.* New York, Plenum Medical Book Co, 1981, pp 921–928.

18. Murray GB, Jasper HH: The role of cholinergic mechanisms in the learning of a tactile discrimination in the monkey, in *Cellular Mechanisms of Conditioning and Behavioral Plasticity.* Seattle, University of Washington Press, 1986, p 44.

19. Miller R: Major psychosis and dopamine: controversial features and some suggestions. *Psychol Med* 1984; 14:779–789.

20. Tesar GE, Murray GB, Cassem NH: Use of high-dose intravenous haloperidol in the treatment of agitated cardiac patients. *J Clin Psychopharmacol* 1985; 5:344–347.

21. Medina JL, Rubino FA, Ross E: Agitated delirium caused by infarctions of the hippocampal formation and fusiform and lingual gyri. *Neurology* 1974; 24:1181–1183.

22. Horenstein S: Effects of cerebrovascular disease on personality and emotionality, in Benton AL (ed): *Behavioral Change in Cerebrovascular Disease.*

New York, Harper & Row Publishers Inc, 1970, pp 171–194.

23. Aita JA: Everyman's psychosis—the delirium. *Nebr Med J* 1968; 53:424–427.

24. Lipowski ZJ: Delirium (acute confusional state), in Frederiks JAM (ed): *Handbook of Clinical Neurology*. New York, Elsevier Biomedical Press, 1985, vol 2, pp 523–559.

25. Mesulam M-M, Waxman SG, Geschwind N, et al: Acute confusional state with right middle cerebral artery infarctions. *J Neurol Neurosurg Psychiatry* 1976; 39:84–89.

26. Hebb DO: Drives and the C.N.S. (conceptual nervous system). *Psychol Rev* 1955; 62:243–254.

27. Katz NM, Agle DP, DePalma RG, et al: Delirium in surgical patients under intensive care. *Arch Surg* 1972; 104:310–313.

28. Katzman R: The prevalence and malignancy of Alzheimer disease. *Arch Neurol* 1976; 33:217–218.

29. Katzman R, Terry RD, Bick KL, (eds): *Alzheimer's Disease: Senile Dementia and Related Disorders. Aging*, vol 7. New York, Raven Press, 1978.

30. McKhann G, Drackman D, Folstein M, et al: Clinical diagnosis of Alzheimer's disease: Report of the NINCDS-ADRDA Work Group. *Neurology* 1984; 34:939–944.

31. Albert ML, Feldman RG, Willis AL: The "subcortical dementia" of progressive supranuclear palsy. *J Neurol Neurosurg Psychiatry* 1974; 37:121–130.

32. Cummings J, Benson DF, LoVerme S Jr: Reversible dementia: illustrative cases, definition, and review. *JAMA* 1980; 243:2434–2439.

33. Black PM: Idiopathic normal-pressure hydrocephalus: results of shunting in 62 patients. *J Neurosurg* 1980; 52:371–377.

34. Rosen H, Swigar ME: Depression and normal pressure hydrocephalus. *J Nerv Ment Dis* 1976; 163:35–40.

35. Wells CE: Pseudodementia. *Am J Psychiatry* 1979; 136:895–900.

36. Folstein MF, McHugh PR: Dementia syndrome of depression. *Alzheimer's Disease: Senile Dementia and Related Disorders. Aging*, vol 7. Katzman R, Terry RD, Bick KL (eds). New York, Raven Press, 1978, pp 87–93.

37. Reifler BV: Arguments for abandoning the term pseudodementia. *J Am Geriatr Soc* 1982; 30:665–668.

38. Lishman WA: *Organic Psychiatry: the Psychological Consequences of Cerebral Disorder*. London, Blackwell, 1978, pp 561–575.

39. Hamilton M: A rating scale for depression. *J Neurol Neurosurg Psychiatry* 1960; 23:56–62.

40. Katzman R: Alzheimer's disease. *N Engl J Med* 1986; 314:964–973.

41. Berg L: Does Alzheimer's disease represent an exaggeration of normal aging? *Arch Neurol* 1985; 42:737–739.

42. Creasey H, Rapaport SI: The aging brain. *Ann Neurol* 1985; 17:2–10.

43. Hooper WW, Vogel FS: The limbic system in Alzheimer disease. *Am J Pathol* 1976; 85:1–20.

44. Herzog AG, Kemper TL: Amygdaloid changes in aging and dementia. *Arch Neurol* 1980; 37:625–629.

45. Ball MJ, Hachinski V, Fox A, et al: A new definition of Alzheimer's disease: a hippocampal dementia. *Lancet* 1985; 1:14–16.

46. Coyle JT, Price DL, De Long MR: Alzheimer's disease: a disorder of cortical cholinergic innervation. *Science* 1983; 219:1184–1190.

47. Dubin WR, Field HL, Gastfriend DR: Postcardiotomy delirium: a critical review. *J Thorac Cardiovasc Surg* 1979; 77:586–594.

48. Arieff AI, Llach F, Massey SG: Neurological manifestations and morbidity of hyponatremia: correlation with brain water and electrolytes. *Medicine* 1976; 55:121–129.

49. Siesjo BK, Carlsson C, Hagerdal M, et al: Brain metabolism in the critically ill. *Crit Care Med* 1976; 4:283–294.

50. Kaiko RF, Foley KM, Grabinski PY, et al: Central nervous system excitatory effects of meperidine in cancer patients. *Ann Neurol* 1983; 13:180–185.

51. Fogarty T, Murray GB. Psychiatric presentation of meperidine toxicity. *J Clin Psychopharmacol* 1987; 7.

52. Folstein MF, Folstein SE, McHugh PR: "Mini-Mental State," a practical method for grading the cognitive state of patients for the clinician. *J Psychiatr Res* 1975; 12:189–198.

53. Wikler A: Diagnosis and treatment of drug dependence of the barbiturate type. *Am J Psychiatry* 1968; 125:758–765.

54. Vollmer ME, Weiss H, Beanland C, et al: Prolonged confusion due to absence status following metrizamide myelography. *Arch Neurol* 1985; 42: 1005–1008.

55. Stern TA, Purcell JJ, Murray GB: Complex partial seizures associated with Waldenström's macroglobulinemia. *Psychosomatics* 1985; 26:890–892.

56. Jacobson DM, Terrence CF, Reinmuth OM: The neurologic manifestations of fat embolism. *Neurology* 1986; 36:847–851.

57. Stern TA, Murray GB: Complex partial seizures presenting as a psychiatric illness. *J Nerv Ment Dis* 1984; 172:625–627.

58. Murray GB: Complex partial seizures, in Manschreck TC (ed): *Psychiatric Update: Massachusetts General Hospital Reviews for Physicians.* New York, Elsevier Biomedical Press, 1981, pp 103–118.

59. Murray GB: Psychiatric disorders secondary to complex partial seizures. *Durg Ther* 1985; 15:145–155.

60. Tomson T, Svanborg E, Wedlund J-A: Nonconvulsive status epilepticus: high incidence of complex partial status. *Epilepsia* 1986; 27:276–285.

61. Ellis JM, Lee SI: Acute prolonged confusion in later life as an ictal state. *Epilepsia* 1978; 19:119–128.

62. Isaacs B, Kennie AT: The Set Test as an aid to the detection of dementia in old people. *Br J Psychiatry* 1973; 123:467–470.

63. Blessed G, Tomlinson BE, Roth M: The association between quantitative measures of dementia and of senile change in the cerebral grey matter of elderly subjects. *Br J Psychiatry* 1968; 114:797–811.

64. Thal LJ, Grundman M, Golden R: Alzheimer's disease: a correlational analysis of the Blessed-Information-Memory-Concentration Test and the Mini-Mental State Exam. *Neurology* 1986; 36:262–264.

65. Paulson GW: The neurological examination in dementia, in Wells CE (ed): *Dementia.* Philadelphia, FA Davis Co, 1971, pp 13–33.

66. Luria AR: Frontal lobe syndromes, in Vincken PJ, Bruyn GW (eds): *Handbook of Clinical Neurology.* New York, John Wiley & Sons, 1969, vol 2, pp 725–757.

67. Rabins PV, Folstein MF: Delirium and dementia: diagnostic criteria and fatality rates. *Br J Psychiatry* 1982; 140:149–153.

68. Sachar EJ: Endocrine factors in depressive illness, in Flach FF, Draghi SC (eds): *The Nature and Treatment of Depression*. New York, John Wiley & Sons, 1975, pp 397–411.

69. Hackett TP, Cassem NH, Wishnie HA: The coronary care unit: an appraisal of its psychological hazards. *N Engl J Med* 1968; 279:1365–1370.

70. Adams F: Neuropsychiatric evaluation and treatment of delirium in the critically ill cancer patient. *Cancer Bull* 1984; 36:156–160.

71. Dudley DL, Rowlett DE, Loebel PJ: Emergency use of intravenous haloperidol. *Gen Hosp Psychiatry* 1979; 1:240–246.

72. Tesar GE, Stern TA: Evaluation and treatment of agitation in the intensive care unit. *J Intensive Care Med* 1986; 1:137–148.

73. Sos J, Cassem NH: Managing postoperative agitation. *Drug Ther* 1980; 10:103–106.

74. Menza MA, Murray GB, Holmes VF, et al: Decreased extrapyramidal symptoms with the use of intravenous haloperidol. *J Clin Psychopharmacol.* In press.

75. Adams F, Fernandez F, Andersson BS: Emergency pharmacotherapy of delirium in the critically ill cancer patient. *Psychosomatics* (suppl) 1986; 27:33–37.

7

Limbic Music

GEORGE B. MURRAY

"Limbic Music" is a strange title for a chapter in a handbook of psychiatry in the general hospital. However, it would appear to be clinically relevant. First of all, it must be stressed that this chapter is primarily heuristic. Some license is taken with philosophical assumptions not adequately substantiated, there are arguable statements, and the anatomy and physiology upon which this structure is based may change, although probably not in a major way, in coming years. Mesulam mentions that the concept of the limbic system has ebbed and welled to fit the preference of individual authors.[1] This is another case of it. It is hoped that the use of limbic music will aid the clinician in assessing the affective component in the patient.

Usually in discussing delirium and dementia, and in reading the literature, attention is paid to the cerebral hemispheres and to the arousal systems. It is rare to find any mention of the limbic system. Several reasons may account for this. First, the limbic system is difficult to reach within the brain; one has to traverse much cortex to get to it. Second, the limbic system is not a neatly discrete structure and some, such as Brodal,[2] would say that it does not exist as a system at all. A third reason, not usually stated, but detectable in casual discussion, is that the limbic system does not subserve "higher function" and as a result has the bias associated with it as mediating man's "lower elements."

First, let us briefly review some aspects of the mind-body arena. Psychobiology is a word coined by Adolph Meyer by which he hoped to compress and unite the concept of mind-brain. When we first heard this word, those of us who had an interest in the mind-brain connection thought that this concept of psychobiology would contain the kernel which would dispel the problems involved with mind-brain. Unfortunately after carefully reading Adolph Meyer's works, we find that kernel is still difficult to come by. In the relatively recent tradition of psychosomatic medicine, a word again tries to compress the two ideas of mind-brain into one word implying a unity therein. As one reads the literature in this area and discusses the term with experts in the field one finds much left to be desired for an understanding of the relationship of mind to brain and vice versa.

An important feature with regard to psychosomatic medicine is that there are no residency training programs in the subject. This fact of no residencies tells us something about psychosomatic medicine in the pragmatic world. It tells us, in William James's words, that "it bakes no bread." It may be quite interesting in itself, but as a collected fund of knowledge it does not allow the physician to *do* much with psychosomatic medical knowledge.

On the other hand there is a certain animosity among psychosomatocists with regard to those who would split man into mind and brain. In traditional philosophical thinking there are two core poles: They are realism and idealism. Those with a more idealistic bent strive for global unity, tend to dislike fractionation and atomization, tend to charge the so-called realists as being those who would disunite, and reduce everything to its smallest biological parts, that is, realists are practitioners of reductionism. The charge goes on to say that in reductionism what one reduces and gets rid of is, in fact, mind. The idealist smiles when the charge is made that the realist has a mindless brain only; however, when the idealist is charged with having a brainless mind as a subject of study, the smile turns to a frown.

The culprit for this great, supposed split between brain and mind is usually thought to be Descartes. His most famous treatise, *Discourse on Method*,[3] outlined his philosophical approach to using methodic doubt in obtaining philosophical proof by the use of reason alone.

One often hears the phrase "Cartesian dualism," and it is presupposed that Descartes, in isolating the mind from the body to study it more specifically, has in fact initiated the great nonunion of mind and brain.[4] It is here submitted that it was primarily Descartes' followers who pragmatically operated on the premises of a split between brain and mind. Since Descartes is often quoted and rarely read, it is not difficult to see why he "takes the rap" for dualism. Descartes operated in no different way than, for example, a cardiac surgeon does today. The cardiac surgeon isolates his interests and bears his intensity upon how he may best make an intervention on the physiologic function of a failing heart, and he does not pay much attention to the gastrointestinal system, endocrine system, and so forth. Similarly, Descartes set his intensity upon looking at the mind and did not, in fact, negate the importance of the body, just as the cardiac surgeon would not negate the importance of the endocrine system and the fact that man lives by all of his physiologic systems as well as mind. Though Descartes' criteria of clarity and distinctness of ideas led him to emphasize a real distinction between mind and body—soul and body to him—he still did not accept the idea that the soul (read: mind) is just lodged in the body. What he does say in his *Replies to Objections* is, "Mind and body are incomplete substances, viewed in relation to the man who is the unity which they form together."[5]

Most psychiatrists in using the term Cartesian dualism use it in a pejorative sense, as if to castigate someone for not being an idealistic upholder of "holism." Most persons interested in psychosomatic medicine have an interest in how the body may influence the mind, how the mind may influence the body, and there have been no "clear and distinct" theories that settle this question to everybody's satisfaction.

It is submitted here that a partial key to the understanding of the mind-brain or mind-body meld is the limbic system. The limbic system can be considered in the Cartesian manner as part mind and part body. Mind consists of many things, intellect, imagination, affect, cognition, and motivation among others. There is no one definition of mind that satisfies everybody's view of it. If the neocortex is more "intellectual," certainly the limbic system is more affectual. In fact, it is often stated that the limbic system is the substratum of emotion in man and animals.

The history of the development of the concept of the limbic system is interesting. Of the many names in the history of its development, four stand out: Broca, Papez, MacLean, and Nauta. Pierre Paul Broca (1824–1880), a French surgeon, founded the Societé d'Anthropologie in Paris in 1859, the year, by the way, of Darwin's *On the Origin of Species by Means of Natural Selection*. In 1861, a patient named Laborgne came under Broca's care. Laborgne had had aphasia for 21 years; all he could say was "tan-tan-tan." After his death a postmortem examination was carried out and Broca found a softened area in the left frontal cortex, now described as Brodmann's area 44, and more popularly known as Broca's area. In the medical sciences Broca is best known for his work in aphasia. M Laborgne's brain is still extant, housed in L'École de Médicine in Paris, as is, interestingly enough, Broca's brain.

Broca is less well known as an author of a remarkable 113-page monograph on the comparative neuroanatomy of mammals. The title of this monograph is *De circonvolutions cerebrals*. Its subtitle is *Le grande lobe limbique*.[6] This work was published in *Revue d'Anthropologie* in 1878, 2 years before Broca's death. The monograph is a fascinating, comparative neuroanatomical study of all of the mammals, containing drawings of what the author called the great limbic lobe (limbic meaning border).

What Broca called the great limbic lobe includes for us today the cingulate gyrus, retrosplenial cortex, and the parahippocampal gyrus (gyrus fornicatus).

Neuroanatomical knowledge progressed with its characterizations of nuclei and connections, but there was no stimulating discussion of the limbic lobe until 1937 when James Papez published his classic paper, "A Proposed Mechanism of Emotion," in the *Archives of Neurology and Psychiatry*.[7] Dr Papez (1883–1958), was a 1911 graduate of the University of Minnesota Medical School; at the time of writing the paper cited he was a neuroanatomist at Cornell University Medical School when it was still in Ithaca, New York State. When he published the paper, it did not create much stir. According to Paul MacLean, Papez wrote this paper because of some ongoing discussion in England on the subject; Papez felt that the discussion did not reflect the tradition of emotion and neuro-anatomical structures already known, and thus he elaborated the idea of the limbic structures subserving the emotions.[8]

From this paper came the popular name of the Papez circuit. This circuit was so called because Papez himself hypothesized that a neuroimpulse could leave the hippocampus via the fornix, travel on up the fornix under the corpus callosum, and traverse the septal area into the mammillary bodies. At the mammillary bodies a synaptic connection would be made to the anterior nucleus of the thalamus and then radiate up onto more primitive cortex, the cingulate gyrus. This impulse would then be captured at the level of the cingulate gyrus, be returned in a neurobundle, the cingulum, and brought down and again entered into the hippocampus. Thus the circuit shown in Figure 7-1.

What Papez postulated was precisely that this circuit was the basis for the feeling of emotions in man. The cingulate gyrus in particular, not a neocortical structure but composed of archicortex and mesocortex, allows the human to "know" that he is having his present feelings.

There was not much stir until 1947 when Paul MacLean ran across Papez's paper in the library at Massachusetts General Hospital. At this time MacLean was a United States Public Health Service Fellow. MacLean, with Stanley Cobb as his mentor, was doing EEG recordings in mesobasal structures of the brain on patients with temporal lobe epilepsy. In effect, when MacLean saw Papez's paper he cried "Eureka." Discussion with Cobb about the significance of the Papez circuit resulted in MacLean's visiting Papez with Cobb's help.

After his discussion with Papez, MacLean wrote a paper entitled "Psychosomatic Disease and the 'Visceral Brain': Recent Developments Bearing on the Papez Theory of Emotion," which appeared in *Psychoso-*

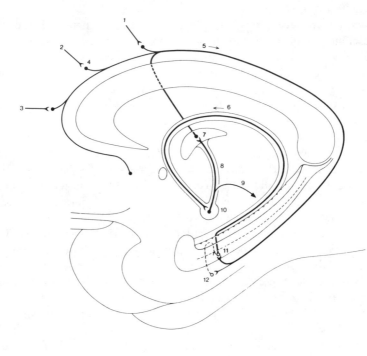

1=Brodmann areas 6, 8; 2=area 9; 3=areas 10, 11; 4=area 24; 5=cingulum; 6=fornix; 7=anterior nucleus of the thalamus; 8=mamillothalamic tract; 9=mamillotegmental tract; 10=mamillary body; 11=subiculum; 12=area 28.

Figure 7-1. The Papez circuit.

matic Medicine in 1949.[9] MacLean used the term visceral brain because he wanted to communicate the notion of "gut feeling." This was a commonly used expression at that time to designate a true or genuinely felt intuition. In those years, for the most part, this area of the brain was called the rhinencephalon or the "nose brain."[8] It turned out that visceral brain did not catch the wind and soar effectively either.

In 1952, after further research, MacLean published another paper entitled "Some Psychiatric Implications of Physiological Studies on the Frontotemporal Portion of the Limbic System (Visceral Brain)."[10] This, then, was the first coining of the words "limbic system." This concept *did* catch the wind and soars today as a concept for those structures that subserve emotion in man.

Walle J.H. Nauta, neuroanatomist at Massachusetts Institute of Technology, has been instrumental both in his own meticulous work, and in influencing his students in careful delineation and expansion of the limbic system. In tracking down frontal lobe connections to the limbic system he has effectively expanded it forward. Connections to the midbrain indicate an expansion of the limbic concept backward or "downstream."[11,12]

More important, the limbic system can serve as an integrating concept for the clinical side of psychiatry and neurology. Various approaches to the study of the limbic system can be taken: morphologic,[13] evolutionary,[14] polymodal,[1] or an overview![15] Perhaps Nauta gives us the most contemporary view—a look at emotions and their anatomy.[16]

Roger Sperry, the Nobel laureate, has shown movies of "split brain" subjects that had had corpus callosotomies for intractable epilepsy. In one film the contents of a slide were flashed into the right cortex of a woman's brain and, of course, she could not speak about it since there was no Broca's area in the right cortex. Every slide flashed into her left cortex only was described adequately in words; in those pictures flashed to her right cortex only, the left brain chattered on in a manner not relevant to the slide shown to the right mute brain. At one point a risqué slide was shown to the right brain and the woman flushed, and showed other aspects of autonomic arousal, for example, rapid respirations, increased systolic blood pressure, increased pulse rate. Not surprisingly, her left brain did not know why. All the left brain said was "Oh my! That's something isn't it!" Even though the left brain did not know what was occurring and the right brain did, the limbic system also "knew" what was going on in order to have the affectual engagement of the autonomic system. It became clear that many things can happen affectually without all of the neocortex being aware of what is "really going on" in the total human person.

The limbic system is involved with motivation, attention, emotion, and memory. It can also be looked at in an "animal" way or a "human" way. In a cavalier fashion, it is often said that the limbic system mediates "the four F's"—fear, food, fight, and fornication. This is a view from the Olympian hill of the cerebral cortex. A more "noble" consideration is that the limbic system mediates gender role, territoriality, and bonding.[17] So, for example, as far as territoriality is concerned, what the limbic system mediates is how one feels about his financial position, his military position, the situation with his family, his rights, "keep off the grass," and other areas that have a spatial or relational component. As far as bonding goes the limbic system mediates strongly how one bonds to one's spouse, family, father, country, flag, religion—in sum, loyalty. If this be true then most of the actions performed daily are already set limbically before man neocortically intellectualizes and these three elements constitute much of the work or, in fact, are *the* subject of the psychiatrist's work.

The neocortex, with Broca's area, is the substrate for the lyrics or the words of what one thinks and feels. The limbic system has no Broca's area, has no words, but is the locus of the music of one's affect. Psychiatric interviewers hear what people verbalize, but often much more important is what one sees, what one feels, and what one hears as the affective music or tune from the person interviewed.

A crude analogy may be helpful in how the neocortex and limbic system may work in the human. If one views a slide of Death Valley he perceives that slide neocortically in the primary visual area pretty much the same as all other humans. However, limbically, one could have at least two different feeling states on seeing the slide. One could have a subtitle or label at the bottom of the slide reading "The sparse grandeur of the West," or at the other end of the spectrum one could label the Death Valley slide as "the devil's fiery hell." The limbic system supplies the affective tone when information is perceived or recalled.

A smile and a laugh are probably as limbically wired as the wagging of a dog's tail. Although the dog does not speak, his affective state is announced by the performance or nonperformance of his tail. One aspect of smiling is that it is the behavioral sign of the recognition and valuing of reality before this reality is formally intellectually known.

At the bedside one can use the so-called Frank Jones story to test acute confusional states. The supposition here is that the neocortex is usually affected in confusional states earlier and more severely than the limbic system. Let us say that the psychiatrist has been called because there is suspicion of a postoperative acute confusional state. One of the things he can do is say to the patient, "Now, sir, how does this strike you? I have a friend, Frank Jones, whose feet are so big he has to put his pants on over his head." If the limbic system is grossly intact the patient will smile or chuckle. There are usually three responses with patients at the bedside. With type 1—the normal response—the patient usually chuckles indicating that he "gits it" and when he's asked, "Can he do it?," he usually says, "Hell no, its goofy. . . . The crotch—he can't go up on both sides," meaning that he also "gets it," that is, he has intellectual insight. A type 2 answer usually indicates that the limbic system is intact, but the neocortex is impaired. When told the Frank Jones pants story he usually smiles and laughs and gives the limbic music that there's something funny to it. However, when asked, "Can he do it," he will usually say something like, "Well, whatever you say, doc," or, "Well, if he tries hard enough." This type 2 patient "gits it" but does not "get it."

The type 3 response indicates that both the limbic system and the neocortex are impaired. When one tells the patient the story about putting the pants on over the head, the patient does not smile, shows no facial quizzicalness, gives no special limbic response at all, and then when one asks, "Can he do it?," the answer usually is something like, "Well, doctor, he must have to have special shoes but sure he can do it." He neither "gits it" nor "gets it." He has limbic and neocortical confusion. With a type 3 response, one has to suspect an underlying dementia.

Quietly confused hospital patients are frequently seen after surgery. They are often not recognized by the treating physician as having an impairment of higher cortical function. The impairment is usually missed because the patient is alert and gets along very well, as it were, "grooving with the vibrations" of the doctor. The patient smiles, says he's doing OK, but if he were pressed as to exactly where he is, or what year it is, he would not know. The point to emphasize here is that the limbic system, even without neocortical clarity, can take us as humans quite far in everyday life, and it is probably that which really gets us through the day. That is, the limbic system and not the higher intellectual activity of the neocortex, save for the primary motor and sensory areas, is where most of man's mental activity occurs. Much resistance to this notion exists, especially from intellectuals, theologians, humanists and others who, perhaps unconsciously, have a bias against the limbic system because it mediates those raw, crude, baser elements of man, that is, the emotions.

Not long ago I was asked to see a patient who was in the Massachusetts Eye and Ear Infirmary for presumed hysterical blindness. She had had an extensive work-up, including visually evoked potentials, and no clinical findings were found to support an organic lesion. Unfortunately, the diagnosis of a conversion disorder is often made without primary data for the diagnosis, but only on secondary, substantive corollary data from the psychosocial realm. This woman had quite a bit of psychosocial perturbation having to do with a violent husband and an appearance in court. In fact, the day she was seen she was to have appeared in court against her husband, but "unfortunately" she was hospitalized.

As I stood before the patient and interviewed her I noticed that she looked away from me. Gradually I moved over in front of her again as I was talking, and noticed that gradually her eyes moved off to the other side, looking away again. I continued to do this, moving in front of her gaze several times, and she always shifted her gaze. I performed the usual test of threatening her eyes with my hand. She did not blink. I then moved over in front of her gaze again and as I continued to speak I put both of my hands on the side of my head, contorted my face, and wiggled my fingers as little children do. (The incongruity of finger wiggling and serious physician's voice should evoke *some* response in the normal patient.) There was a slight smile on her lips and her eyes shifted away again. I repeated this maneuver several times and each time it was apparent that the patient revealed a slight smile which immediately disappeared. Then it was clear: This lady sees. My interpretation of what happened is that the patient perceived in the occipital cortex my funny business with the hands and screwing-up of my face, but heard in her auditory cortex a serious physician's voice. Before she could employ "neocortical squelch," her limbic system assigned a valence[18] to the incongruity of voice and pantomime, thus activating, presumably, the nucleus accumbens[19] and the limbic basoganglion,[20] and evoking a slight smile that appeared just slightly out of her immediate neocortical control.

In conclusion there are several points to be emphasized:

1. The use of the term "limbic system" here is not hard, scientific usage; it partakes of metaphor.

2. The limbic system can be helpful in understanding the so-called rift between mind and body.

3. The stuff of clinical psychiatry is primarily mediated by the limbic system and not by the nonsensory structures of the neocortex.

4. Limbic music is a term that denotes the existential, clinical, "raw feel" emanating from the patient. It is a more true rendering of the patient's clinical state than articulate speech. Limbic music never lies.

REFERENCES

1. Mesulam M-M: Patterns in behavioral neuroanatomy: association areas, the limbic system, and hemispheric specialization, in Mesulam MM (ed): *Principles of Behavioral Neurology.* Philadelphia, FA Davis Co, 1985, pp 1–70.
2. Brodal A: *Neurological Anatomy* (2nd ed). New York, Oxford University

Press, 1969, pp 537–539.

3. Descartes R: *Discourse on Method of Rightly Conducting the Reason and Seeking for Truth in the Sciences*, 1637, in Adam C, Tannery P (trans-eds): *Works of Descartes*, Paris, 13 vols, 1897–1913.

4. Brown TM: Descartes, dualism and psychosomatic medicine, in Bynum WF, Porter R, Shepherd M (eds): *The Anatomy of Madness*. New York, Tavistock, 1982, vol 1, pp 40–62.

5. Descartes R: *Objections and Replies to Objections*, in Adam C, Tannery P. *Works of Descartes*. Paris, vol 7, chap 13, section 2, p 175.

6. Broca P: Des circonvolutions cerebrales: le grand lobe limbique et al scissure limbique dans la série des *mammifères*. *Rev Anthropol* 1878; 1:385–498.

7. Papez JW: A proposed mechanism of emotion. *Arch Neurol Psychiatry* 1937; 38:725–743.

8. MacLean PD: Challenges of the Papez heritage, in Livingston KE, Hornykievicz O (eds): *Limbic Mechanisms*. New York, Plenum, 1976, pp 1–15.

9. MacLean PD: Psychosomatic disease and the "visceral brain": recent developments bearing on the Papez theory of emotion. *Psychosom Med* 1949; 11:338–353.

10. MacLean PD: Some psychiatric implications of physiological studies on frontotemporal portion of limbic system (visceral brain). *EEG Clin Neurophysiol* 1952; 4:407–418.

11. Nauta WJH: Connections of the frontal lobe with the limbic system, in Laitinen LV, Livingston KE (eds): *Surgical Approaches in Psychiatry*. Baltimore, University Park Press, 1973, pp 303–314.

12. Nauta WJH, Domesick VB: Neural associations of the limbic system, in Beckman AL (ed): *The Neural Basis of Behavior*. New York, Spectrum, 1982, pp 175–206.

13. White LE: A morphologic concept of the limbic lobe. *Int Rev Neurobiol* 1965; 8:1–34.

14. MacLean PD: *A Triune Concept of the Brain and Behaviour*. Toronto, University of Toronto, 1973.

15. Swanson LW: The hippocampus and the concept of the limbic system, in Seifert W (ed): *Neurobiology of the Hippocampus*. New York, Academic Press, 1983, pp 3–19.

16. Nauta WJH, Feirtag M: Affect and motivation; the limbic system, in *Fundamental Neuroanatomy*. New York, WH Freeman Co, 1986, pp 120–131.

17. Henry JP, Stephens PM: *Stress, Health, and the Social Environment*. New York, Springer-Verlag, 1977.

18. Gloor P: Role of the human limbic system in perception, memory, and affect. Lessons from temporal lobe epilepsy, in Doane BK, Livingston KF (eds): *The Limbic System: Functional Disorders and Clinical Disorders*. New York, Raven Press, 1986, pp 159–170.

19. Graybiel AM: Input-output anatomy of the basal ganglia, in symposium lecture. *Proc Soc Neurosci*, Toronto, 1976.

20. Mogenson GJ, Jones DL, Yim CY: From motivation to action: functional interface between the limbic system and the motor system. *Prog Neurobiol* 1980; 14:69–97.

8

Functional Somatic Symptoms and Somatoform Disorders

NED H. CASSEM

Although only 26 years old, the young woman has had abdominal pain for 10 years. Multiple contrast radiographic, ultrasonographic, computer tomographic, endoscopic, and colonoscopic studies and three exploratory laparotomies failed to diagnose an organic etiology for the pain. Although active, energetic, and healthy in appearance, she had become progressively incapacitated by the symptom. Admitted to the surgical service, the patient was referred for psychiatric evaluation with questions about diagnosis, prognosis, advisability of proceeding to laparotomy, and, above all, acute and chronic management recommendations.

Called by Lipowski[1] the borderland between medicine and psychiatry, somatization, meaning here complaining about physical symptoms for which there are no discoverable organic abnormalities, presents a fascinating challenge to the consultation psychiatrist. In an excellent review of functional somatic symptoms, Kellner[2] noted that 60% to 80% of the normal population will experience one or more somatic symptoms in any one week of their lives. When a patient approaches a physician with a somatic complaint, no organic cause can be found between 20% and 84% of the time. Commonest among these functional somatic symptoms are chest pain, headache, fatigue, and dizziness. For patients who persist in their search for a medical disease which could be causing their functional symptoms, the dangers of invasive diagnostic procedures, unnecessary surgery, and misdirected therapeutic drug trials can be life-threatening, and the unwarranted costs of these measures further strain limited medical resources.

DIFFERENTIAL DIAGNOSIS OF FUNCTIONAL SOMATIC SYMPTOMS

Asked to evaluate a patient whose somatic symptoms show no causative physical abnormality or seem far out of proportion to any abnormalities found, the psychiatrist should not think first of the somatoform disorders. Of psychiatric disorders, depression will be found

126

Table 8-1. Differential Diagnosis of Functional Somatic Symptoms: Diagnoses Producing Somatoform Complaints

1. Physical disease etiology?
2. Affective disorders
3. Anxiety disorders
4. Substance use disorders
5. Psychotic disorders
6. Organic brain syndromes
7. Voluntary symptom production
    Malingering
    Factitious disorders
8. Somatoform disorders
9. Personality disorders
    Dependent
    Passive-aggressive
    Antisocial
    Borderline
    Narcissistic
    Compulsive
    Histrionic
    Paranoid
    Schizoid
    Schizotypal

far more often when the patient is examined. As with any condition, a systematic differential diagnostic approach is required. Table 8-1 lists the diagnoses most likely to produce somatoform complaints.

The approach to these patients must include the standard thorough history and examination: past and family psychiatric history, psychosocial history, past medical history, current medications, and current laboratory examination results. In fact, the first question in differential diagnosis for the consultant is always: What organic disease, possibly still undiagnosed, could account for these symptoms? When the latter are functional somatic symptoms, the first question remains the same. Reading both the current and the (too often formidable) old chart is an indispensable beginning. One of the main reasons a psychiatrist makes the diagnosis of a physical disease is that something about the patient (personality, behavior, affect, odd cognition) may have effectively distracted the primary physician and/or consultants.

Affective Disorders

First of all, many of the symptoms of major depression *are* somatic (sleep, anhedonia, fatigue, anorexia, true motor agitation or retardation). Moreover, depressed patients have more functional somatic symptoms (aches and pains, dizziness, and the like) than do other patients. There is good evidence that hypochondriacal preoccupations during depressive episodes increase with age. (For further coverage of affective disorder, see chapter 12, Depression.) When major depression is diagnosed, it should be treated. Ordinarily both the affective and functional somatic symptoms will clear with the treatment, although, as shall be discussed, sometimes only the affective episode will remit, leaving functional somatic symptoms still to be dealt with. Depression should be treated first. Depression with somatoform complaints is far more common than a somatoform disorder.

Anxiety Disorders

Symptoms of anxiety intermingle with and pervade functional somatic symptoms. As noted in chapter 9 on anxiety disorders, the symptoms of panic disorder *are* somatic: dyspnea, palpitations, chest pain, choking, dizziness, paresthesias, hot and cold flashes, sweating, faintness, trembling. Anxiety, however, is not nearly as likely as depression to escape the notice of a primary physician—although panic, phobia, and obsessive-compulsive disorder are as commonly undiagnosed as affective disorders. Patients with these three disorders are often recognized as anxious and often placed on benzodiazepines. Since the latter are not the treatment of choice for the disorders, specific treatment will have to be initiated by the consulting psychiatrist. Anxiety is also one of the commonest features of major depression. Important to remember as well is that when present with pain, anxiety can lower pain threshold dramatically, causing some who care for the patient to interpret the marked discrepancy between pain complaints and objective findings as one of the more intractable or malignant forms of somatizing (drug abuse, personality disorder). Because many of these patients cannot distinguish anxiety from pain ("No, I am not frightened; I hurt!"), diagnosis can be delayed and frustrations intensified. Neuroleptics, not benzodiazepines, are the treatment of choice for this anxiety, and a small dose of, for example, haloperidol or fluphenazine (1 mg orally three times a day), may significantly reduce narcotic analgesic requirements.

Substance Use Disorder(s)

Alcohol abuse should always be considered when a patient continues to have multiple, vague somatic symptoms. Whether the patient simply lies to conceal his disorder or fails to make the connection, diagnosis may be elusive. Information from the patient's family may help ("What he calls headache and chest pains, Doctor, I call a hangover."). Because alcoholism systematically disrupts sleep, patients may begin using sedative-hypnotic substances as well. Insomnia, morning cough, extremity pains, dysesthesias, palpitations, headache, gastrointestinal (GI) symptoms, fatigue, bruises—none are strangers to the alcoholic. See chapters 2 and 3 on diagnosis and treatment of substance abuse disorders.

Psychotic Disorders

Patients with psychotic depression may have somatic delusions, such as the conviction that all organs in the abdominal cavity are decomposing. Such patients are much more likely to be mistakenly diagnosed as being schizophrenic than as physically ill. The material in chapter 11 (Psychotic Patients) applies here. When a schizophrenic patient complains of a functional symptom, for example, headache or weakness (not as dramatic as a somatic delusion), his psychosis may be missed. Making such a diagnosis with a thorough psychiatric history and examination is ordinarily no problem. Schizophrenic patients can present with true conversion symptoms, for example, left-sided paresis shortly before discharge from hospital. In such a case the proper diagnosis is a conversion symptom in a schizophrenic patient, not "conversion disorder."

Organic Brain Syndromes

Although it would be reasonable to argue that somatization disorder and hypochondriasis are themselves the result of structural brain abnormalities (as one might say of schizophrenia), the diagnosis of organic brain syndrome here refers to either the dementias or to the psychiatric disorder on axis I produced by a medical disease on axis III, such as stroke-induced depression. Viewed in this way, no organic brain syndrome is known to produce specifically functional somatic symptoms (another way of saying that "somatizing" cannot at this time be localized either to a specific brain structure or site or to a brain system, like a neurotransmitter system). However, patients with organic brain disease do have functional somatic complaints. For the psychiatric consultant careful examination easily detects cognitive dysfunction that may have gone unnoticed prior to the consultation.

Voluntary Symptom Production

Malingering. Of the two types of voluntary symptom production, malingering is simple enough: the patient lies about the symptom's presence or severity. The false or exaggerated symptom may be psychological as well as somatic (eg, flashbacks or nightmares). The main criterion for making this diagnosis is the obvious recognizability of the symptom's goal (always presupposing that no organic abnormality can be found or what is found is far out of proportion to the magnitude of the complaint). Excruciating back pain may be postponing trial or court-martial, the key to disability payments, or the justification for the patient's requests for narcotic analgesics. The consultant should not be cowed by the pejorative connotations of the diagnosis. The latter does not depend on an analysis of the patient's virtue but on the readily understandable nature of the symptom as a means to an end. In fact, one could say that these patients have a *good* reason for lying—in some cases so good that they may almost come to believe their own stories. Whether the patient believes the story is irrelevant to the diagnosis. Malingering could be part of heroic action, as when a prisoner of war feigns illness in order to make an escape attempt.

The American Psychiatric Association's *Diagnostic and Statistical Manual of Mental Disorders*, third edition (DSM-III)[3] actually forces the diagnosis of malingering to be made more frequently, since older labels like "compensation neurosis" have been (fortunately) discarded. More-over, a high suspicion of malingering should be aroused if any combination of the following four factors is present: (1) medicolegal context, for example, the patient is referred by his attorney for examination; (2) marked discrepancy between the claimed distress or disability and the objective findings; (3) lack of cooperation with the diagnostic evaluation and/or prescribed treatment regimen, for example, the patient refuses to take the Minnesota Multiphasic Personality Inventory (MMPI), co-operate with physical therapy, use the transcutaneous nerve stimulator (TENS), accept a trial of nighttime amitriptyline hydrochloride, release permission for obtaining past medical records, and the like; (4) the presence of *antisocial personality disorder*.[3] When the goal is truly obvious (money, work status) there is no point in hiding from the patient that failure to comply with any portion of the evaluation and treatment will almost surely be seen as implying malingering.

Factitious disorders. *Factitious illness* can be quite complicated. Unlike malingering, where the goal obtained has obvious value to the patient, the simulated "disease" of the patient with factitious illness confers no obvious advantage on the patient. The patient who warms his thermometer to 103 °F on the morning of transfer to a nursing home is a malingerer, even though this could be called a "factitious" fever. It is wiser to reserve the term for patients with psychopathology which drives them to sustain their contrivance of illness without apparent self-advantage and often at considerable risk to their health. Patients with factitious illness are commonly liars, and, in fact, exercise remarkable ingenuity in fooling the physicians caring for them. While they do produce the false symptoms voluntarily, their "control" is seldom as complete as that of the malingerer. The woman who takes warfarin sodium, is covered with bruises, and suffers a serious gastric hemorrhage resulting in hospitalization, is driven by pathologic motives. A psychiatrist might say that the sympathy she received from telling her associates that she had leukemia is an obvious advantage. It is also obviously sick. Moreover there is a driven quality to the behavior and the patient may have little or no insight into the reasons for the self-destructive behavior. In one form of factitious disorder, known as pseudologia fantastica, the lies of the patient form the core of the presenting history. It can be difficult to determine whether the lies are delusions or conscious deceptions.[4] The patients suffer from borderline personality disorders.

Ford's review of these disorders is excellent.[5] From the viewpoint of the psychiatric consultant, two aspects of diagnosis can be summarized: the detective aspects and the spectrum of pathology. So inventive are these patients with self-inflicted diseases that an exhaustive list is not possible, but stalwart sleuthing by clinicians in the past leaves us with a few helpful strategies worth listing. Factitious fever is relatively common.[6] Patients warm their thermometers on light bulbs, radiators, by friction or flame, or anything convenient. Some keep a supply of "preset" thermometers hidden in the hospital room, ready for substitution after the nurse leaves the patient alone. To counteract this the nurse may remain with the patient or use an electronic thermometer which registers temperature rapidly. Comparison of a freshly voided urine specimen with simultaneous body temperature is another method.[7]

Room search for pre-set thermometers has been used. Even an electronic thermometer can be outwitted, as by one patient who consistently went to the bathroom prior to having her temperature taken and rinsed her mouth out with hot water. She refused to have a rectal temperature taken.[8] Other patients produce a real fever by infecting themselves, usually by injecting contaminated material into their skin or veins, including sputum, feces, tuberculous and other organisms, foreign bodies, and lighter fluid. A skin biopsy of such a lesion might be helpful, with culture and microscopic analysis.

Skin is commonly attacked as well, producing any number of dermatitides. Excoriations of all kinds occur. One patient in our hospital applied a blowtorch to his own arm, then maintained a nonhealing wound by reinfecting his grafts. Exposure of the factitious nature of the wound is more difficult, especially since these patients usually improve in the hospital, only to return with a markedly worsened condition. Subcutaneous tissue has also been damaged in order to create the appearance of legitimate disease. Air has been injected into the tissues, presenting as an "ulcer" on the forearm, but also raising concern about gas gangrene.[9] Another patient in our hospital presented with creatine phosphokinase (CPK) values which would rise intermittently to 1000 U/L or more. X-ray films diagnosed both factitious disorders. In the first a needle was discovered beneath the skin. In the second an even, circumferential band 1 in. in width of compressed adipose tissue was found. The patient's muscle had been traumatized by tightening a band around her gastrocnemius muscles. Also in her case, careful inspection of the bruises on her legs revealed a distribution limited to the lateral surface of the right and the medial surface of the left—a right-handed distribution.

"Hematologic" disorders have been mentioned and include anemia, usually induced by performing a phlebotomy on oneself, but one patient induced a severe hemorrhage by lacerating her colon with a knitting needle. Blood dyscrasia or leukemia is most commonly simulated by surreptitious self-administration of warfarin or heparin sodium.[10-12] Psychogenic purpura or "autoerythrocyte sensitization" has long been studied by investigators at Case Western Reserve in Cleveland and has been recently reviewed by Ratnoff.[13] Patients also simulate blood in other body products, especially sputum, with a classical history for pulmonary embolus; urine, with a classical history for renal stone; and stool. A self-inflicted cut or abrasion is the commonest source of the blood (it is simple to urinate over a cut finger into the specimen cup). These are exceedingly difficult, if at all possible, to detect. One patient who produced great quantities of blood was discovered by blood analysis, which revealed nonhuman blood.

Of bogus endocrine disorders, hypoglycemia is probably the commonest and is usually produced by insulin injection or oral ingestion of sulfonylureas. Scarlett et al showed that the triad of simultaneous demonstration of low plasma glucose, high immunoreactive insulin, and suppressed C-peptide immunoreactivity is pathognomonic of exogenous insulin administration.[14] Because C-peptide and insulin are secreted from the pancreatic β-cells in equimolar concentrations, the ability to measure C-peptide and produce this diagnostic triad answered prior difficulties of the radioimmunoassay technique posed by the interfering presence of insulin antibodies in insulin-treated diabetics and the difficulty of accepting antibodies, in patients not supposed to be taking insulin, as definite proof of exogenous insulin administration.

When the sulfonylurea ingester presents with a possible diagnosis of insulinoma, either his plasma sulfonylurea can be determined or tolbutamide can be administered. If insulinoma is present plasma insulin will rise. In factitious hypoglycemia it will remain the same or fall. Moreover, the inexplicable cases of "brittle diabetes" may sometimes be the result of self-induced difficulties. Schade et al[8] reported five cases, including self-injection of insulin, watered-down insulin bottles (explaining the "high" insulin requirements), and faked "shortness of breath" after insulin injections which had been erroneously labeled as "allergy" to purified pork insulin. The patient was diagnosed when pulmonary function tests were normal. There is recent evidence to suggest that self-administration of insulin in juvenile diabetics, not for glucose regulation but as a manifestation of psychiatric disorder, may either be more common than realized or is a recourse taken by the patient whose recurrent ketoacidosis has become too closely watched for the patient to secretly cause it any longer.[15]

Ingestion of large amounts of thyroxine simulate thyrotoxicosis, although determinations of thyroxine, triiodothyronine, the ratio of the first to the second, thyroid-stimulating hormone, and serum thyroglobulin are usually sufficient to diagnose excess exogenous ingestion.[16,17]

Another endocrine disease to be simulated was pheochromocytoma, suspected because the elevated urine catecholamines consisted of epinephrine only. It was diagnosed when a room search revealed an empty vial of epinephrine.

Factitious asthma has also been reported, and in these cases pulmonary function tests and arterial blood analysis helped demonstrate that the "wheezing" of the patients was self-induced. In the three patients studied, Downing et al[18] defined blood gas values for an acute asthmatic attack as an oxygen partial pressure less than 80 mmHg and alveolar-arterial oxygen tension difference greater than 25 mmHg. Corresponding pulmonary function values included a one-second forced expiratory volume (FEV_1), the FEV_1 as a percentage of the vital capacity (FEV_1/VC), and the midmaximal expiratory flow rate (MMEFR) as all less than 80% of the predicted values.

Laxative abuse presents with abdominal pain, diarrhea, hypokalemia and acid-base abnormalities, weight loss, vomiting, steatorrhea, and skin pigmentation. It should always be considered when a patient presents with chronic diarrhea of unknown etiology. The most helpful test to confirm laxative use is the demonstration of phenolphthalein in the stool.[19] In the test the stool specimen is alkalinized; when present, phenolphthalein causes the solution to turn pink. An informative case from the published records of our hospital illustrates the differential diagnostic and detective work required to solve the chronic diarrhea and weight loss of a 60-year-old laxative abuser.[20]

Self-induced vomiting can cause several metabolic abnormalities, especially hypokalemia. Workups can be extensive—for example, the patient may be thought to have a renal disease like Bartter's syndrome. This abnormal behavior is most commonly associated with anorexia nervosa and/or bulimia. A clue signalling that the patient induces vomiting is the presence of "bulimia calluses," lesions on the dorsal surface of the hand, caused by abrasion by the teeth in the induction of emesis.[21] Of course, in the eating disorders self-induced vomiting is often combined with laxative and diuretic abuse, leading most commonly to metabolic alkalosis, hypochloremia, and hypokalemia.[22] One survey finds that 13% of adolescents indulge in purging behaviors of this type.[23] The medical complications of anorexia and bulimia can be life-threatening.[24]

A variant, occasionally mistakenly called "postprandial vomiting," is the more rare "rumination syndrome," a repeated, effortless regurgitation of gastric contents into the mouth immediately after a meal. Part of the contents is chewed and reswallowed, and part is spit out. This process may continue for up to four to five hours.[25] The etiology was unclear. In eight of 12 patients the onset of the behavior occurred after an acute illness or event associated with nausea and vomiting. Manometric study showed the motility pattern of this pseudoregurgitation to differ distinctly from that of vomiting.

Factitious renal colic has been mentioned and is one way to obtain narcotic analgesics. Some patients may also present the physician with factitious stones. Stone analysis quickly reveals the nature of the hoax. Yet some of these patients traumatize their urethras as well, inserting the "stone" and then reporting that they heard the sound of it falling into the bedpan or other container. Some have even urinated in the presence of a family member or a nurse, adding authenticity to the appearance of the "stone."

Detective work is an essential feature of most of these evaluations. Consultants here are usually called before the suspicion of factitious disorder is confirmed. It is intellectually stimulating and occasionally the most enjoyable part of the consultation, especially if symptom production can be unambiguously proved. Because a room search can be one of the most successful diagnostic procedures, ethical questions can arise about violation of the patient's privacy. Like Ford and Abernethy we evaluate each case individually and refer the reader to a summary of a conference on this subject.[26] Psychiatrists seldom hesitate to intervene when a patient slices his wrists; self-injection of feces or insulin is no less self-destructive. Room searches are routine for hospitalized suicidal patients.

Factitious disorders can include psychological symptoms as well as the many physical ones described above. The 300.16 designation of DSM-III, *factitious disorder with psychological symptoms*, was apparently used originally to describe those patients formerly called Ganser's syndrome, pseudopsychosis, or pseudodementia. Since factitious bereavement has been reported, in which patients presented with depression and suicidal ideation after fabricated deaths,[27] these cases may best fit in the 300.16 category as well. However, many of the patients described also had histories of factitious physical disorders as well. Ganser's syndrome, helpfully reviewed by Whitlock,[28] has a complex history. This diagnosis is far too nonspecific to be helpful.

There is no substitute for thorough diagnostic evaluation: when dementia is present it is so labeled, and likewise delirium, depression, malingering, factitious disorder, and the like. An almost humorous variant of factitious disorder with psychological symptoms is the patient who presented himself to a hospital emergency room, demanding immediate hospitalization because he suffered from Munchausen syndrome. The unnecessary surgeries he claimed to have undergone were denied by the physicians and hospitals he cited, and the scars covering his abdomen washed off with soap and water.[29]

Finally, one must realize that there exists a form of "proxy" factitious disorder, in which the patient is usually a child and the author of the sham is the child's mother. In one case of "brittle diabetes" the parents had spent more than $80,000 in the year prior to this discovery, including evaluations at three major medical centers in the United States and Canada.[8] The child's mother was injecting heparin into the child's central line. Later the mother injected contaminants, producing recurrent gram-negative sepsis. Reviewing the numerous reports of this variant of child abuse which have appeared since 1977, Ford[5] noted that at least one child had died as a result of this pathologic maternal behavior.

Spectrum of psychopathology in factitious disorder. When confronted by the phenomenon of factitious disorder the consultant is best served by examining each patient individually, with routine careful diagnostic attention devoted to both axis I and II. Generalizations are therefore difficult when considering the entire spectrum. However, inspection of the reported cases will show that the majority of patients are female, under 40 years of age, and have invariably gained medical sophistication from being a nurse, medical technician, or physician; having a physician parent, or having an illness. The milder end of the spectrum includes patients with diagnosis of hypochondriasis and possibly depression. Typical is a 15-year-old boy reported by Reich et al[30] who repeatedly contaminated his urine with feces. At age 2 he had undergone surgery for hypospadias. Convinced that something was genuinely wrong with his bladder which his doctors had thus far failed to discover, he kept contaminating his urine by retrograde injections so that continued medical examinations would reveal an abnormality which could be repaired. When supportively confronted he confessed his action and this seemed to restore him to his senses. After brief psychotherapy his behavior remained normal and he resumed normal peer relationships.

The more severe forms of factitious disorder have extensive axis II pathology. Immature, dependent, passive, masochistic, and histrionic traits are described, but most of the patients with factitious disorder of several years duration are most likely to have borderline personality disorder. In an excellent review of 41 cases of factitious disorder found during a 10-year period, Reich and Gottfried[31] stress the possibility of finding forms milder than the most extreme form of this disorder, Munchausen syndrome (described in detail in chapter 14). Two thirds of the presentations were accounted for by sepsis, nonhealing wounds, fever, and electrolyte disorder. Two thirds of the patients had medical occupations. Self-contamination, surreptitious medication use, and wound exacerbation accounted for the methods used by 29 of the 41 patients. Fourteen room searches led to ten diagnostic discoveries. No patient was found to have had a diagnosis of borderline personality disorder.

Our MGH experience has not found the patients so benign. Despite bland and passive exteriors many of these patients reveal hostility and intense projected self-hatred. Each patient, of course, must be individually evaluated. Because factitious illness tends to generate anger, it is important to consider this as distinct and beware of countertransference feelings which arise in response to the patient.

Treatment of the patient with factitious disorder. All treatment depends on the specific diagnosis. Before any plan can be executed, the question arises as to how best to confront the patient with the evidence or the opinion that the disorder is self-induced. The primary physician may prefer to do this alone or with the consultant present. The option should always be offered. As Reich and Gottfried indicate,[31] these patients, whatever their motives, were seeking medical care and, at least in the beginning, enlisted their physicians as allies rather than as adversaries. One can begin the confrontation with a list of the patient's strengths and long history of suffering. After the current evaluation or room search it is also clear that there is now a serious emotional problem present because of the evidence compiled. There need be no insistence that the patient admit to inflicting the symptoms on herself. At the same time the best stance is the quiet conviction that this is unnecessary because its truth is known by the physician. Since psychiatric treatment is what the patient needs, the physician can, after the patient has been given an opportunity to discuss the situation, stress that the focus remains on what is best for the patient, namely, psychiatric treatment.

If present, the psychiatrist should secure some agreement from the patient while the primary physician is still there, offering to remain to discuss this or to return. The more severe the patient's pathology, the more likely he is to reject offers of help, express indignation at the physicians' lack of trust, and leave the hospital. Any anger in the confronting physician(s) will increase the likelihood of this reaction. At the heart of the confrontation is the concern for self-inflicted wounds, dangerous diagnostic or therapeutic measures, and whatever help the patient needs to replace the destructive with constructive behaviors. Each effort of the patient to provoke an angry encounter about the "accusation" of factitious disease should be quietly countered by a reminder of how reassuring it is that there is no untreatable infection, malignancy, or other life-threatening illness and how important it is to help the patient with the genuine psychiatric difficulty remaining.

Personality Disorders

Although included in the differential diagnostic list of Table 8-1, personality disorders do not "cause" functional somatic symptoms. However, for the patient with axis II disturbance, the somatic symptom is a means to an end. For the *antisocial personality* pain is a means to get narcotics, get out of work, escape trial, and so on. For the dependent personality, functional weakness gains the attention and nurturance of others. For the borderline patient the somatic symptoms are the focus about which the physicians and nurses are engaged in a sadomasochistic struggle, beginning with a helping relationship and ending with the disappointed and outraged patient being accused of wrongdoing and rejected. The "end" for this patient is the emotionally charged (usually hostile) relationship. Somatic symptoms are exaggerated by patients with histrionic personality and may be so intensely fixated upon by compulsive, paranoid, schizotypal, and schizoid personalities as to make these patients take on a hypochondriacal character, reinforcing their symptoms by their personality styles.

The Somatoform Disorders

The five categories of Somatoform disorders in DSM-III are called "somatoform" because the patients complain of physical symptoms suggesting a physical disorder for which there are no demonstrable organic findings or known physiologic mechanisms and a strong presumption that the symptoms are linked to psychological factors or conflict.

Conversion disorder is perhaps the most classic form of somatoform disorder. This disorder involves a loss or change in physical function, suggestive of a physical disorder, in which the causal role of psychological factors is based on the temporal closeness of symptom onset to environmental factors, or the symptom's enabling the patient to escape something noxious, or its enabling him to get some benefit. A patient who developed functional blindness may be found to have seen her husband with another woman on the night before she complained of being unable to see. The conversion symptom is not under voluntary control, although the patient may to some extent alter its severity, as in the patient with a functional gait disturbance or weak arm who, with intense concentration, can demonstrate slightly better control or strength. DSM-III has eliminated pain from the list of symptoms which qualify ("conversion" pain syndromes are now called psychogenic pain disorder), leaving symptoms which mimic neurologic disease (paralysis, aphonia, seizures, gait or coordination disturbances, blindness, tunnel vision, anesthesia), autonomic or endocrine disease, asthma, vomiting, dysphagia, pseudocyesis, and other symptoms.

Reviewing conversion, Ford and Folks recommended that it be treated clinically as a symptom rather than a primary diagnosis.[32] The sex ratio is equal in children presenting with conversion symptoms, while in adults more women are seen than men. Two notable situations in which men have been said to show with conversion symptomatology are industrial accidents and military service—although DSM-III would now cast the majority of them as malingerers. Predisposing factors are important for both diagnosis and treatment. A prior illness is a common source for the symptom. If a viral illness accompanied by vertigo occurs when a patient is under stress, the illness may "rescue" him from the stress and bring attention and support from loved ones. At a later time, when stress recurs, the symptom of vertigo may recur, this time as a conversion symptom. By definition this is beyond the patient's conscious control.

Patients with seizures, especially complex partial seizures (where consciousness is preserved), are repeatedly exposed to a phenomenon which instantaneously removes them from responsibility for what they are doing and may evoke sympathy and help from a loved one. Pseudoseizures commonly coexist with true seizures and can be exceedingly hard to discriminate, particularly when cortical electrodes of the EEG show nothing or nonspecific slowing. Exposure to others with conversion symptoms is a definite factor and can result in a chain reaction or "mass hysteria." Patients with histrionic and passive-dependent personalities are more likely than others to develop conversion symptoms. Finally, extreme psychosocial stress may be the most important of all factors. The presence of this in the history provides stronger and more reliable evidence for the diagnosis of conversion than either escape of responsibility or getting nurturance. Some authors have presented evidence for a predominance of conversion symptoms, when unilateral, on the nondominant side in females.[33,34]

The diagnosis of conversion cannot rest comfortably on the inability to find physical pathology. Caution in making a diagnosis of conversion symptoms is based on the reports of 13% to 30% of those with this diagnosis going on to develop an organic condition which seemed to account for it.[35] For this reason one usually hopes to demonstrate that function is normal in the symptomatic body part. Electromyograms (EMGs), evoked responses of vision and hearing, slit lamp, funduscopic and retinoscopic examinations, pulmonary function tests, and barium swallow are examples of tests in which normal function should be demonstrable. This negative phase is critical, requiring meticulous review by the psychiatrist. Positive evidence includes not only the psychological data but also any demonstration of normal function in the supposedly disabled body part. Detective work begins with close observation of the patient, including times when he is not aware of the observer's presence. In part one is trying to discriminate the malingerer as well. If the patient moves his arm normally when he is unaware of observation and displays a flail arm when watched, he is most likely malingering.

Conversion symptoms are usually sustained, but sometimes only for a certain activity. The patient who cannot lift his leg adequately in walking may be observed to cross it over his good one during conversation. Deviation of the eyes toward the ground no matter which side the semicomatose patient lies on is functional and sometimes demonstrates lack of organic pathology.[36] One may lead the patient with functional blindness around obstacles like chairs; the conversion patient usually avoids them (a malingerer is more likely to bump into them). Carefully watching the "blind" patient's eyes and face while taking a roll of money out of one's wallet, suddenly menacing (careful to avoid creating a draft or noise) or making a face at him is another way to assess intactness of the visual system. Sensory testing on the patient in both prone and supine positions checks consistency. A malingerer is more likely to become hostile and uncooperative during the examination, probably in the hope of shortening it.

Prognosis and treatment. Despite the warnings about the patients who went on to develop organic pathology, the literature supports an optimistic outlook for these patients, at least in the first few years. From 50% to 90% of patients have recovered by the time of discharge from the hospital, with Folks et al recording a 50% rate of complete remission by discharge in a group of patients diagnosed with conversion symptoms in a general hospital.[37]

Suggestion that the conversion symptom will improve is the commonest form of treatment. This ordinarily begins with reassuring news that tests of the involved body system show no damage and therefore recovery is certain. Predicting that recovery will be gradual, with specific suggestions (vague shapes will become visible first; weight-bearing will be possible and then steps with a walker; standing up straight will come before full steadiness of gait; clear liquids can be kept down, then a steadily advanced diet; strength in squeezing a tennis ball will be followed by strength at the wrist and then elbow joints; feeling will return to the toes first; and so on), will usually succeed, provided the diagnosis is conveyed with serene confidence and the suggestions with supportive optimism. Lazare points out that the psychiatrist is also discussing the patient's life stresses, trying to detect painful affects and to assess how the symptom socially communicates between the patient and others.[35] Confrontation is seldom helpful. However, some patients may ask what the psychiatrist thinks caused their condition and others sense a relationship between the stressful psychosocial conditions and the conversion symptomatology.

An approach which has been acceptable to some of these persons has been to say that the body, mysterious in many ways, can be smarter than we are. It may help us out before we realize we need it. When the stress in our lives becomes excessive, especially when our nature is more to overlook it or to grit our teeth and prevail, our body, by its symptoms, may blow the "Time out!" whistle, forcing us to stop, take a rest, and get some help. This approach invites the patient to greater insight. It may not be necessary. Resolution of the stressful situation becomes the target of intervention. Since stresses are social, couple or family therapy may be instrumental in achieving final resolution. Some patients will not improve with suggestion. Since they occupy a nonpsychiatric bed, they must be told, should they maintain they are not well enough to leave the hospital, that their transfer to a psychiatric hospital or unit will then be arranged. Symptoms that have not responded to earlier suggestion may then improve sufficiently to permit discharge. One would have to entertain in this patient the possibility that the more proper diagnosis may be malingering.

Psychogenic pain disorder. For diagnostic purposes the most practical way of clinically conceptualizing this diagnosis is as a conversion disorder in which the symptom is pain. DSM-III criteria for this condition are essentially identical to those for conversion. In this condition, however, it is pain which is the focus because examination shows the symptom distribution to be neuroanatomically inconsistent, without any structural pathology or pathophysiologic mechanism to account for it, or, when there is some related organic pathology, the complaint of pain is grossly in excess of what would be expected from the physical and laboratory findings. Pain is the subject of an entire chapter in this book (chapter 4).

As a complaint pain may be part of the diagnoses listed in Table 8-1. The diagnosis of psychogenic pain disorder should be reserved for that patient who, in a setting of intense psychosocial stress, develops pain. It will persist until the stress is resolved, although, as the diagnostic criteria indicate for this and other conversion symptoms, development of pain tends to partially "solve" the stressful situation or relieve some of the pressure by permitting the sufferer to avoid noxious responsibilities and gain nurturance and attention.

Typical was the man who developed a painful exacerbation of an old back injury the day after his wife attended a birthday party in her honor, given by a neighborhood bachelor, to which the patient had not been invited. Physical, neurologic, and radiologic examinations showed either normal function or no change. No immediate knowledge of this association was in evidence and was gained only when the patient, questioned independently about his relationship with his wife (which he said was "excellent") and specifically asked if she had ever seen another man, produced this anecdote. He readily admitted anger and hurt. It was only when he asked the date of his wife's birthday that the consultant noted it was the day before symptom onset. When asked whether there might be a connection, the patient sincerely said he was sure no relationship existed—even though he could see why the consultant might see a causal relation. An MMPI suggested conversion symptomatology. Projective testing revealed many concerns about dependency and nurturance, including a story of marital infidelity and other references to fear of loss of love.

The spectrum of reactions of these patients is likely to mimic that for conversion, mentioned above. The same therapeutic approach is recommended, with the reassurance that the body parts in question appear to be normal or no worse and the suggestion that the pain will gradually subside. Some patients can accept their manifest need to resolve the stress which has been uncovered (and can be told that it is worth working on even if it is not at all related to the pain). Use of their own productions in the psychological testing can be sometimes presented to them as helpful evidence of the existence of concern in their subconscious or unconscious minds. The "wisdom" of their body in warning them about their stress by means of pain may be helpful as well. The longer the duration of the pain, the less likely that the cause is as uncomplicated as psychogenic pain disorder. Treatment of patients with this disorder usually is limited to individual, marital, or family therapy. If it has continued for a longer time, other treatments for chronic pain patients such as relaxation, TENS, and physical therapy may be needed. Much more clinical and epidemiologic information must be gathered on this new diagnostic category.

Somatization disorder.   Originally identified as hysteria or Briquet's syndrome and now given the DSM-III designation of somatization disorder, this condition has been solidly established as clinically and epidemiologically distinct. The disorder tends to occur in women of low socioeconomic, often nonwhite and rural, status, at a prevalence rate of 0.4% in the general population.[38] Twenty percent of first-degree female relatives suffer the same disorder, while male relatives show increased incidence of alcoholism and sociopathy. Women with this disorder tend to have histories as children of missing, disturbed, or defective parents, marry sociopathic males oftener than chance would predict, and tend to be poor parents themselves.[38-43] Given these unfortunate circumstances and their roughly 75% chance of having one or more additional psychiatric diagnoses (commonest being affective disorder, anxiety disorder, and drug and alcohol abuse[44]), it is no surprise that marital discord is also the rule for those who are married.

DSM-III diagnostic criteria have been simplified from the initial criteria of the Washington University group[45] and now include:

A history of physical symptoms of several years' duration beginning before the age of 30

Complaints of at least 14 symptoms for women and 12 for men from the 37 symptoms listed below

To count a symptom as present the individual must report that the symptom caused him or her to take medicine (other than aspirin), alter his or her life pattern, or see a physician. The symptoms, in the judgment of the clinician, are not adequately explained by physical disorder or physical injury, and are not side effects of medication, drugs, or alcohol. The clinician need not be convinced that the symptom was actually present, for example, that the individual actually vomited through her entire pregnancy; report of the symptom by the individual is sufficient.

Sickly for a good part of life

Conversion symptoms: dysphagia, aphonia, deafness, double vision, blurred vision, blindness, faintings, memory loss, seizures, trouble walking, paralysis or muscle weakness, urinary retention or difficulty urinating

GI symptoms: abdominal pain, nausea, vomiting spells (other than pregnancy), bloating (gassy), intolerance (gets sick) of a variety of foods, diarrhea

Female reproductive: Judged as occurring more frequently or severely than in most women: painful menstruation, menstrual irregularity, excessive bleeding, severe vomiting throughout pregnancy or causing hospitalization during pregnancy

Psychosexual: for the major part of the individual's life after opportunities for sexual activity. sexual indifference, lack of pleasure during intercourse, pain during intercourse

Pain: in back, joints, extremities, genital area (other than during intercourse); pain on urination; other pain (except headaches)

Cardiopulmonary: shortness of breath, palpitations, chest pain, dizziness

Despite initial fear that reducing the number of symptoms from 25 to 14 (or 12) would invalidate the diagnostic evaluation, these newer criteria have been shown to be equally effective in identifying patients with this disorder.[46] Still more recently Othmer and DeSouza[47] have introduced a clever mnemonic for the diagnosis of somatization disorder based on a screening for only seven symptoms, three of which must be present for a preliminary diagnosis of somatization disorder. This is presented in Table 8-2.

The results of Othmer and DeSouza indicated that three symptoms accurately identified 91% of the patients with somatization disorder with a sensitivity of 87% and specificity of 95%. Despite the shorter list of symptoms to verify, the clinical diagnosis remains cumbersome, and

Table 8-2. Seven-Symptom Screen Test for Somatization Disorder

Mnemonic	Symptom	System
Somatization	Shortness of breath	Respiratory
Disorder	Dysmenorrhea	Female reproductive
Besets	Burning in sex organs	Psychosexual
Ladies	Lump in throat	Pseudoneurologic
And	Amnesia	Pseudoneurologic
Vexes	Vomiting	Gastrointestinal
Physicians	Painful extremities	Skeletal muscle

From Othmer and DeSouza.[47]

is almost always impossible without the past records. These tend to be voluminous, scattered among a host of hospitals, lost, or a combination of the three. Notoriously poor historians, these patients will say they cannot remember past admissions or clinic visits, deny a history of a symptom which the chart lists as a chief complaint on a past visit, and, in general, show little motivation or interest in giving a precise history. A clinical pearl from Goodwin and Guze[48] is that menstrual difficulties and sexual indifference are so common in these patients that the diagnosis should be made with caution if the menstrual and sexual histories are normal.

In the absence of the chart, contact with prior treating physicians or family may help in establishing the symptom count. In person, the patient usually presents her complaints in a histrionic fashion ("Why I bled so much—I've never seen so much blood!!—that I passed out on the bed and my family said I was in coma for three days!"), with symptoms so exaggerated that a psychogenic etiology may be suspected from the outset. The other consistent trait these patients possess is a peculiar difficulty communicating. Histories are vague and symptomatic details are extremely elusive or downright inconsistent. Efforts to clarify may be so frustrating that the clinician wonders whether the language spoken, despite the familiar words, is actually English. Emotional distress is openly expressed ("I'm not getting *anywhere*, Doctor! No one can tell me anything! What's happening to me?!!"), but if one tries to identify the emotion, for example, telling the patient she seems very anxious, that emotion is more likely to intensify ("Well, wouldn't anybody be?! It's been a whole month and nobody—nobody, Doctor—knows what's going on with me!!"). This type of response tends to drive the physician back to a cognitive search—onset, duration, radiation, intensifying or relieving factors, etc, only to encounter once again the fogbound and trackless wastes of imprecision, inconsistency, and lapsing memory.

Contemporary medicine's shift from clinical to economic priorities has only heightened attention to somatization disorder. Smith et al[49] have documented that the average patient with this disorder spends an average of seven days per month sick in bed (compared to 0.48 days for the average person), and accrues annually (mostly unnecessary) hospital care expenditures of $2382, physician services of $1721, and total care charges of $4700—charges which are roughly six times, 14 times, and nine times higher, respectively, than those of the average person in the population between the ages of 15 and 64 years. This happens in spite of their remarkably stable clinical course, with a 90% probability of not developing a new medical or psychiatric disorder in the next 6 to 8 years following diagnosis. Quill referred to this disorder as "one of medicine's blind spots."[50]

Clinical and research evidence for the distinctiveness of somatization disorder has increased progressively.[39] In an effort to clarify distinctive verbal patterns of somatization patients, Oxman et al[51] took 500 word samples of free speech from 11 patients and compared them to similar samples from patients with major depression, paranoid disorders, and medical disorders. The distinctive pattern revealed by content analysis was that of a confused, negative self-identity. The authors noted two major factors, the first a sort of unrelenting negativism, "the relentless modification of objects and actions by their negative attitude." The second centered on self-identification patterns which the authors likened to pathologic narcissism in the impoverished interpersonal relations and little empathy, or a bogus empathy manifested as a pseudodependence on others. Yet there appeared to be little of the ambition, exploitativeness, and dependency on admiration and acclaim commonly associated with narcissism.

In a study based on extensive neuropsychological testing of these patients compared to patients with psychotic depression, schizophrenia, and normal controls, Flor-Henry et al[52] demonstrated bifrontal hemispheric impairment of cognitive processes with, globally, greater impairment of the nondominant hemisphere. The nondominant abnormalities were postulated by the authors to be responsible for depression, psychogenic pain, asymmetrical conversion symptoms, and the histrionic pattern, while dominant hemisphere abnormalities were seen to mediate the subtle impairment of verbal communication, peculiar incongruity of affective responsivity, and abnormal sensory motor integration and mobility control.

Treatment of somatization was formulated by Murphy.[53] It is best managed by primary care physicians according to a conservative plan based on (1) providing a consistent other person, (2) preventing unnecessary and/or dangerous procedures, and (3) supportive inquiry into the areas of stress in the patient's life. The last occurs during the physical examination, without inferring to the patient that the real cause for the increase in somatic complaints was increased psychosocial stress (which is what most authors believe). Smith et al at Little Rock[54] codified treatment recommendations in a letter to the primary care physician of each somatization disorder patient, including regularly scheduled appointments (eg, every 4 to 6 weeks); a physical examination performed at each visit to look for true disease; advice to avoid hospitalization, diagnostic procedures, surgery and the use of laboratory assessments, unless clearly indicated; and advice to avoid telling patients "it's all in your head." In a randomized controlled trial these investigators demonstrated that this intervention resulted in a 53% reduction in quarterly health care charges, largely due to decreases in hospitalization.[54] Neither the health of the patients nor their satisfaction with their care was affected by implementation of the advice.

Hypochondriasis. Although continued investigation has brought considerable unity to the concept of somatization disorder, no impression exists or can be well supported that hypochondriasis is a distinct disorder. The phenomenon of being preoccupied with symptoms for which there is no discoverable organic basis is common. Kenyon's early work on this topic remains classic,[55] and Kellner provides an invaluable contemporary review.[2] Following the work of Barsky and others at our own hospital,[56-59] a systematic approach to the description of hypochondriacal symptoms can be outlined and applied to the clinical examination.

DSM-III singles out as the predominant disturbance of hypochondriasis (A) an unrealistic interpretation of physical signs and sensations as abnormal, leading to a preoccupation with the fear or belief of having a serious disease. The diagnostic criteria include: (B) Thorough physical evaluation does not support the diagnosis of any physical disorder that can account for the physical signs or sensations or for the individual's unrealistic interpretation of them. (C) The unrealistic fear or belief of having a disease persists despite medical reassurance and causes impairment in social or occupational functioning. (D) The signs and sensations are not due to any other mental disorder.

Barsky et al[58] have operationalized these four criteria as follows:

A. 1. Somatic symptoms
   2. Disease conviction

      3. Disease fear
      4. Bodily preoccupation
B. 5. Absence of medical disorder that could account for the hypochondriacal symptoms
C. 6. Illness behavior
      7. Disability
D. 8. Absence of major psychiatric disorder of which hypochondriacal symptoms are a feature

It is the three hypochondriacal attitudes, disease conviction, disease fear, and bodily preoccupation, which are the focus of this diagnosis. It is not at all clear whether this is a single diagnostic entity or a continuous spectrum, along which most persons would take a position at least transiently during their lifetimes. But the feature which differentiates the hypochondriac from the somatization disorder patient is that the former has an interpretation for the functional somatic symptom (disease conviction or fear). Moreover, the cognitive style of the hypochondriacal patient tends to be obsessive, whereas that of the somatization patient tends to be histrionic. Compulsive traits are common. The diagnosis is made with equal frequency in males and females. The course of the disorder, in Kenyon's study of primary hypochondriasis, could be phasic, fluctuating, or constant—with most of the latter progressively worsening.[55]

Origins of hypochondriacal attitudes are not understood, but disease in the patient at an early age or disease in the family, overprotective parents, and other conditioning factors have been noted. The first onset of the syndrome may occur in the context of a physical illness (a patient remains preoccupied with functional somatic symptoms after undergoing cardiopulmonary bypass, for example) or after the death of a loved one. Kenyon[55] could find no precipitant in over half of the cases. When a patient has a myocardial infarction, for example, it is normal for bodily preoccupation with the chest area to be heightened in the ensuing 2 to 3 months. Is this hypochondriacal? If it is so designated, it is probably of little clinical significance unless it is abnormally prolonged. Yet one could be hard pressed to define the normal limits of duration. Such a definition is of far less interest to the consultant than the patient who can describe a bodily preoccupation from childhood. In Kellner's review[2] he notes that such patients are more likely to be augmenters and sensitizers than reducers and repressors.

When confronted with a patient who appears to have the triad of symptoms comprising the hypochondriacal attitude, the consultant should systematically search for affective disorder, anxiety disorder, and obsessive-compulsive disorder—and treat them if present. These specific diagnoses are associated with hypochondriasis, and when they are treated the hypochondriasis may either disappear entirely or diminish significantly. In the patients who are "hard-core" hypochondriacs, improvement can occur when these three other psychiatric disorders are treated, but the basic disorder remains. In addition, clinical lore notes on axis II in these patients hostile, obsessive, compulsive, masochistic, and paranoid traits—none of which facilitate the treatment process.[59] Much less is known about this disorder than about somatization.

The prognosis of these patients has been considered poor traditionally. Kenyon, for example, found that of those hospitalized patients with primary hypochondriasis, only 21% were judged recovered or much improved at the time of discharge, and 40% were either unchanged or worse than when they were admitted.[55] On the other hand, Kellner finds reason to be optimistic, especially when the illness was associated with a duration of less than 3 years, there was no personality disorder, and possibly when the patient belonged to a higher social class.[60] Adler commented that "clinical success with such a patient is an achievement that rarely receives the recognition it deserves."[61]

Kellner[60,62] describes psychotherapy for hypochondriasis, delivered in ten sessions over a 5-month period, starting once weekly and then tapering, in which the following are featured. (1) The patient must be persuaded that his disease beliefs are false. (2) Repeated physical examinations, including emergency examinations, are performed to reassure the patient that no physical disease accounts of his symptoms. (3) Education is provided stressing the role of accurate information, selective perception's role in strengthening hypochondriacal attitudes, the need for unlearning certain patterns of response, clarification, and repetition. (4) Acceptance and empathy accompany each encounter. (5) Suggestion is used, for example, relax and you will feel less pain. (6) In some cases patients progressed to insight-oriented, dynamic psychotherapy, such as examination of the similarity of their somatic symptoms to those of a deceased loved one, and its implications for unresolved grief. (7) Those who remain invalids are referred to a pain clinic or a rehabilitation program. (8) All but three of the patients received antianxiety drugs at one time or another during treatment. Of the 36 patients, 23 (64%) recovered or improved during therapy.

Atypical somatoform disorder. DSM-III reserves this category for those particular disorders referred to as the dysmorphophobias, and, in our interpretation, monosymptomatic hypochondriasis. Thomas notes that the former is an overvalued idea and the latter a solitary delusion.[63]

A diagnostic check list for monosymptomatic hypochondriacal psychosis is presented by Munro and Chmara.[64] It is characterized by a single delusional system, distinct from the remainder of the personality.[65-67] The first of the three commonest forms of this disorder consists of delusions of infestation, such as parasites, insects, worms, or foreign bodies under the skin. The skin of such a patient may be severely excoriated. These individuals tend to be in their mid-fifties at onset and about 70% are women. Second is the olfactory reference syndrome, in which the patient is convinced he emits a foul odor or has halitosis when no objective evidence for this exists. This occurs typically in a younger age patient, in the mid-twenties, and males outnumber females in this category. Finally, dysmorphophobia is the belief that one is misshapen and unattractive. The average age of these patients is about 30, with males and females equally represented. A typical male will present himself to a plastic surgeon with the conviction that his nose is too large and/or deformed. The typical female, convinced that her breasts are too large and/or deformed, making her appearance grotesque, will seek a reduction mammoplasty.

Despite the encapsulation of symptoms the lives of these patients are severely disrupted by the illness. Anxiety and paranoia are common. They are usually intensely ashamed, convinced that they are under constant scrutiny. Alcohol abuse is common, especially in younger males. Two patients, one with dysmorphophobia and the other with olfactory reference syndrome, presented at our hospital with symptoms of major depression. After treatment with tricyclic antidepressants, the hypochondriacal delusions of both remitted.[68]

Ordinarily these patients do not respond to antidepressants or neuroleptics, with the exception of pimozide, now the agent of choice.[64] A single morning dose is administered daily, starting with 2 mg and moving up in 2-mg increments every three days or so. Munro states that one seldom needs to exceed a total daily dose of 12 mg.[64] Antiparkinsonian agents can be given if dystonic symptoms are experienced. Complete or partial improvement occurs in about 80% of cases, usually within 2 weeks, although treatment failure should not be accepted before a 6- to 8-week course of the drug. Maintenance therapy is probably the rule. Stress can exacerbate the delusion, but restarting or temporarily increasing the pimozide usually restores equilibrium. These beliefs are strongly entrenched. The patient may be quite difficult to get started on pimozide. It will be refused because it is prescribed by a psychiatrist, because the patient will not accept that a psychotropic drug could correct his physical defect, or, once started on pimozide, may stop taking it without informing his physician. One may never be able to get the patient to accept the delusional nature of the disorder, even after significant improvement. Hard pressed to justify the recommendation of a neuroleptic, one may even tell the patient that these insects or odors are best "cleansed" from within the system, hence the need for a drug. On the other hand, some will more easily accept the notion that the body is more vulnerable to parasitic infestation or odor generation during times of greater stress.

Much remains to be learned about these disorders, and many other symptom approximations exist which are not covered by the three categories mentioned above. Clinical vigilance remains necessary in the care of these patients. One report describes the progression of an olfactory reference syndrome to mania.[69]

When one thinks of "somatizers," the somatoform disorders may be the first diagnostic category to come to mind. In general hospital patients, other psychiatric diagnoses, particularly major affective disorders, the anxiety disorders, and organic mental syndromes, are more likely to be discovered at the end of the history and examination. These require treatment. When the psychiatric disorder remits, the functional somatic symptoms usually subside. The diagnostic tests we find helpful are the MMPI, an excellent screening device for conversion, somatoform, and axis II parameters; the projective tests to help both physician and patient understand conflicts in the patient's life which may not be in the patient's awareness; and full neuropsychological test batteries, which delineate precise areas of cognitive deficiency.

The treatment, as noted, is prescribed according to the diagnosis. When the disorder is somatization disorder or hypochondriasis, treatment guidelines are hard to find and controlled studies rare, except for the excellent demonstration by Smith et al[54] that intervention by the primary physician for somatization disorder significantly reduced costly and potentially harmful interventions without compromising the health or satisfaction of these patients. Kellner[2] has pioneered treatment for those hypochondriacs a bit nearer the healthy end of the disorder spectrum, a program rather similar to those designed to reactivate patients suffering with chronic pain.

REFERENCES

1. Lipowski ZJ: Somatization: A borderland between medicine and psychiatry. *Can Med Assoc J* 1986; 135:609–614.
2. Kellner R: Functional somatic symptoms and hypochondriasis. *Arch Gen Psychiatry* 1986; 42:821–833.

3. *Diagnostic and Statistical Manual of Mental Disorders*, ed 3. Washington, American Psychiatric Association, 1980.

4. Snyder S: Pseudologia fantastica in the borderline patient. *Am J Psychiatry* 1986; 143:1287–1289.

5. Ford CV: *The Somatizing Disorders*. New York, Elsevier, 1983.

6. Aduan RP, Fauci AS, Dale DC, et al: Factitious fever and self-induced infection. *Ann Intern Med* 1979; 90:230–242.

7. Murray HW, Tuazon CU, Guerrero IC, et al: Urinary temperature. A clue to early diagnosis of factitious fever. *N Engl J Med* 1977; 296:23–24.

8. Schade DS, Drumm DA, Eaton RP, et al: Factitious brittle diabetes. *Am J Med* 1985; 78:777–784.

9. Kusumi RK, Plouffe JF: Gas in soft tissues of forearm in an 18-year-old emotionally disturbed diabetic. *JAMA* 1981; 246:679–680.

10. O'Reilly RA, Aggeler PM: Covert anticoagulant ingestion: study of 25 patients and review of world literature. *Medicine* 1976; 55:389–399.

11. Schmaier AH, Carabello J, Day HJ, et al: Factitious heparin administration. *Ann Intern Med* 1981; 95:592–593.

12. Kim HC, Kosmin M: Heparin and factitious purpura, letter. *Ann Intern Med* 1982; 96:377.

13. Ratnoff OD: Psychogenic bleeding, in Ratnoff OD, Forbes CD (eds): *Disorders of Hemostasis*. New York, Grune & Stratton, 1984, chap 19.

14. Scarlett JA, Mako ME, Rubinstein AH, et al: Factitious hypoglycemia. Diagnosis by measurement of serum C-peptide immunoreactivity and insulin-binding antibodies. *N Engl J Med* 1977; 297:1029–1032.

15. Orr DP, Eccles T, Lawlor R, Golden M: Surreptitious insulin administration in adolescents with insulin-dependent diabetes mellitus. *JAMA* 1986; 256:3227–3230.

16. Mariotti S, Martino E, Cupini C, et al: Low serum thyroglobulin as a clue to the diagnosis of thyrotoxicosis factitia. *N Engl J Med* 1982; 307:410–412.

17. Pearce CJ, Himsworth RL: Thyrotoxicosis factitia, letter. *N Engl J Med* 1982; 307:1708–1709.

18. Downing ET, Braman SF, Fox MJ, et al: Factitious asthma. *JAMA* 1982; 248:2878–2882.

19. Devore CD, Ulshen MH, Cross RE: Phenolphthalein laxatives in factitious diarrhea. *Clin Pediatr* 1982; 21:573–574.

20. Falchuk ZM, Butterly LF, Stern TA: A 60-year-old woman with chronic diarrhea and weight loss. *N Engl J Med* 1985; 313:1341–1346.

21. Winn DR, Martin MJ: A physical sign of bulimia, letter. *Mayo Clin Proc* 1984; 59:722.

22. Mitchell JE, Pyle RL, Eckert ED, et al: Electrolyte and other physiological abnormalities in patients with bulimia. *Psychol Med* 1983; 13:273–278.

23. Killen JD, Taylor CB, Telch MJ, et al: Self-induced vomiting and laxative and diuretic use among teenagers. *JAMA* 1986; 255:1477–1449.

24. Brotman AW, Rigotti N, Herzog DB: Medical complications of eating disorders: outpatient evaluation and management. *Compr Psychiatry* 1985; 26:258–272.

25. Amarnath RP, Abell TL, Malagelada JR: The rumination syndrome in adults. *Ann Intern Med* 1986; 105:513–518.

26. Ford CV, Abernethy V: Factitious illness: a multidisciplinary consideration of

ethical issues. *Gen Hosp Psychiatry* 1981; 3:329–336.

27. Phillips MR, Ward NG, Ries RK: Factitious mourning: painless patienthood. *Am J Psychiatry* 1983; 140:420–425.

28. Whitlock FA: The Ganser syndrome and hysterical pseudo-dementia, in Roy A (ed): *Hysteria.* New York, John Wiley & Sons, 1982, pp 185–209.

29. Gurwith M, Langston C: Factitious Munchausen's syndrome, letter. *N Engl J Med* 1980; 302:1483–1484.

30. Reich P, Lazarus JM, Kelly MJ, et al: Factitious feculent urine in an adolescent boy. *JAMA* 1977; 238:420–421.

31. Reich P, Gottfried LA: Factitious disorders in a teaching hospital. *Ann Intern Med* 1983; 99:240–247.

32. Ford CV, Folks DG: Conversion disorders: an overview. *Psychosomatics* 1985; 26:371–383.

33. Galin D, Diamond R, Braff D: Lateralization of conversion symptoms: more frequent on the left. *Am J Psychiatry* 1977; 134:578–580.

34. Stern DB: Handedness and the lateral distribution of conversion reactions. *J Nerv Ment Dis* 1977; 164;122–128.

35. Lazare A: Conversion symptoms. *N Engl J Med* 1981; 305:745–748.

36. Henry JA, Woodruff GHA: A diagnostic sign in states of apparent unconsciousness. *Lancet* 1978; 2:920–921.

37. Folks DG, Ford CV, Regan WM: Conversion symptoms in a general hospital. *Psychosomatics* 1984; 25:285–295.

38. Swartz M, Blazer D, George L, et al: Somatization disorder in a community population. *Am J Psychiatry* 1986; 143:1403–1408.

39. Swartz M, Blazer D, Woodbury M, et al: Somatization disorder in a U.S. southern community: use of a new procedure for analysis of medical classification. *Psychol Med* 1986; 16:595–609.

40. Guze SB: The validity and significance of the clinical diagnosis of hysteria (Briquet's syndrome). *Am J Psychiatry* 1975; 132:138–141.

41. Cloninger CR, Reich T, Guze SB: The multifactorial model of disease transmission: III. Familial relationship between sociopathy and hysteria (Briquet's syndrome). *Br J Psychiatry* 1975; 127:23–32.

42. Coryell W. A blind family history study of Briquet's syndrome. *Arch Gen Psychiatry* 1980; 37:1266–1269.

43. Zoccolillo M, Cloninger CR: Parenteral breakdown associated with somatisation disorder (hysteria). *Br J Psychiatry* 1985; 147:443–446.

44. Liskow B, Othmer E, Penick EC, et al: Is Briquet's syndrome a heterogeneous disorder? *Am J Psychiatry* 1986; 143:626–629.

45. Feighner JP, Robins E, Guze SB, et al: Diagnostic criteria for use in psychiatric research. *Arch Gen Psychiatry* 1972; 26:57–63.

46. DeSouza C, Othmer E: Somatization disorder in Briquet's syndrome. *Arch Gen Psychiatry* 1984; 41:334–336.

47. Othmer E, DeSouza C: A screening test for somatization disorder (hysteria). *Am J Psychiatry* 1985; 142:1146–1149.

48. Goodwin DW, Guze SB: *Psychiatric Diagnosis,* ed 2. New York, Oxford University Press, 1979.

49. Smith Jr GR, Monson RA, Ray DC: Patients with multiple unexplained symptoms. *Arch Intern Med* 1986; 146:69–72.

50. Quill TE: Somatization disorder, one of medicine's blind spots. *JAMA* 1985;

254:3075–3079.
51. Oxman TE, Rosenberg SD, Schnurr PP, et al: Linguistic dimensions of affect and thought in somatization disorder. *Am J Psychiatry* 1985; 142:1150–1155.
52. Flor-Henry P, Fromm-Auch D, Tapper M, et al: A neuropsychological study of the stable syndrome of hysteria. *Biol Psychiatry* 1981; 16:601–626.
53. Murphy GE: The clinical management of hysteria. *JAMA* 1982; 247: 2559–2564.
54. Smith Jr GR, Monson RA, Ray DC: Psychiatric consultation in somatization disorder. *N Engl J Med* 1986; 314:1407–1413.
55. Kenyon FE. Hypochondriasis: a clinical study. *Br J Psychiatry* 1964; 110:478–488.
56. Barsky AJ: Patients who amplify bodily sensations. *Ann Intern Med* 1979; 91:63–70.
57. Barsky AJ, Klerman GL: Overview: hypochondriasis, bodily complaints, and somatic styles. *Am J Psychiatry* 1983; 140:273–283.
58. Barsky AJ, Wyshak G, Klerman GL: Hypochondriasis. *Arch Gen Psychiatry* 1986; 43:493–500.
59. Murray GB: Hypochondriasis, in Manschreck TC (ed): *Psychiatric Medicine Update*. New York, Elsevier, 1979, pp 125–134.
60. Kellner R: Prognosis of treated hypochondriasis. *Acta Psychiatr Scand* 1983; 67:69–79.
61. Adler G: The physician and the hypochondriacal patient. *N Engl J Med* 1981; 304:1393–1396.
62. Kellner R: Psychotherapeutic strategies in hypochondriasis: a clinical study. *Am J Psychother* 1982; 36:146–157.
63. Thomas CS: Dysmorphophobia: a question of definition. *Br J Psychiatry* 1984; 144:513–516.
64. Munro A, Chmara J: Monosymptomatic hypochondriacal psychosis: a diagnostic checklist based on 50 cases of the disorder. *Can J Psychiatry* 1982; 27:374–376.
65. Bishop ER Jr: Monosymptomatic hypochondriasis. *Psychosomatics* 1981; 21:731–747.
66. Goldberg RL, Buongiorno PA, Henkin RI: Delusions of halitosis. *Psychosomatics* 1985; 26:325–331.
67. Andreasen NC, Bardach J: Dysmorphophobia: symptom or disease. *Am J Psychiatry* 1977; 134:673–675.
68. Brotman AW, Jenike MA: Monosymptomatic hypochondriasis treated with tricyclic antidepressants. *Am J Psychiatry* 1984; 141:1608–1609.
69. Davidson M, Mukherjee S: Progression of olfactory reference syndrome to mania: a case report. *Am J Psychiatry* 1982; 139:1623–1624.

9

Anxiety

JERROLD F. ROSENBAUM and MARK H. POLLACK

The clinical challenges in the diagnosis and treatment of anxiety are apparent in the general hospital setting: discerning normal from pathologic anxiety, differentiating medical from psychiatric causes, and choosing effective therapeutic approaches. In addition to knowledge of medical and psychiatric differential diagnosis, the clinician must rely on a variety of strategies and interventions including pharmacologic, psychodynamic, interpersonal, behavioral, and cognitive skills. The ubiquitousness of anxiousness and the nonspecific nature of anxiety symptoms can confound the care of the patient with pathologic anxiety. Pathologic anxious symptoms and behavior may be attributed to other physical causes, or when viewed as "only anxiety," may be prematurely dismissed as insignificant.

Anxiety is indistinguishable from fear, except as to cause. The former is the same distressing experience of dread and foreboding as the latter, except deriving from an unknown internal stimulus, inappropriate to the reality of an external stimulus or concerned with a future stimulus. Anxiety is manifest in the physical, affective, cognitive, and behavioral domains. The possible physical symptoms of anxiety reflect autonomic arousal and include an array of bodily perturbations (see Table 9-1). The anxious state ranges from edginess and unease to terror and panic. Cognitively, the experience is one of worry, apprehension, and thoughts concerned with emotional or bodily danger. Behaviorally, anxiety triggers a multitude of responses concerned with diminishing or avoiding the distress.

The importance of recognizing and attending to the suffering of the anxious patient may not always be apparent given the universality of the experience of anxiety. Anxiousness is expected and normal as a transient response to stress and may be a necessary stimulus to adaptation and coping. Excessive or pathologic anxiety, however, is no more a normal state than the production of excess thyroid hormone.

Pathologic anxiety is distinguished from normative response by four criteria: (1) autonomy, (2) intensity, (3) duration, and (4) behavior.

154

Table 9-1. Physical Signs and Symptoms of Anxiety

Anorexia	Muscle tension
"Butterflies" in stomach	Nausea
Chest pain or tightness	Pallor
Diaphoresis	Palpitations
Diarrhea	Paresthesias
Dizziness	Sexual dysfunction
Dyspnea	Shortness of breath
Dry mouth	Stomach pain
Faintness	Tachycardia
Flushing	Tremulousness
Headache	Urinary frequency
Hyperventilation	Vomiting
Lightheadedness	

Autonomy refers to suffering that to some extent, has a "life of its own," a minimal basis in recognizable environmental stimuli, an apparently "endogenous" component. *Intensity* refers to the level of distress; the severity of symptoms are such that the patient's level of anguish moves the physician to offer relief. The patient's capacity to bear discomfort has been exceeded.

The *duration* of suffering also can define anxiousness as pathologic: symptoms that persist, rather than transient, possibly adaptive responses, indicate disorder, and are a call to evaluation and treatment. Finally, *behavior* is a critical criterion; if anxiety impairs coping, if normal function is disrupted, or if special behavior such as avoidance or withdrawal result, the anxiety is of a pathologic nature.

Stereotyped syndromes of pathologic anxiety are represented in the American Psychiatric Association's *Diagnostic and Statistical Manual of Mental Disorders*, third edition (DSM-III) Anxiety Disorders (Table 9-2). In epidemiologic studies, anxiety disorders were found to be among the most common psychiatric disorders in the general population.[1] This observation would predict that a significant percentage of the general hospital population would also suffer anxiety symptoms. In addition to those patients who suffer anxiety disorder prior to admission to hospital for medical care, medical and surgical settings will also be associated with *onset* of anxiety symptoms as a consequence of hospitalization, medical illness, or its treatment (eg, adjustment disorder with anxious mood and "organic anxiety disorder."[2]).

DESCRIBING ANXIETY

Despite the protean physiologic manifestations of anxiety, the experience of anxiety can be divided into two broad categories: (1) an acute,

Table 9-2. Anxiety Disorders

Panic disorder: Recurrent panic attacks ranging in severity from severe (experienced as terror, "going to die" or "lose control") to mild (only "limited symptom attacks" or rare panic attack). If complicated by fear of places of restricted or embarrassing escape or where help is unavailable, by travel restriction (or need for a companion), or endurance of such situations despite intense anxiety, the diagnosis is panic disorder with (mild, moderate, or severe) agoraphobia.

Phobic disorders
  Simple phobia: Intense fear of and attempt to avoid specific objects or situations (eg, heights)
  Social phobia: Intense anxiety or discomfort in situations of scrutiny by others with typical fear of embarrassment or humiliation (eg, stage fright)
  Agoraphobia (without history of panic disorder)

Generalized anxiety disorder: Six-month history of anxious symptoms, but not panic attacks, with cognitive (worry) and autonomic symptoms

Posttraumatic stress disorder: A syndrome with onset following a traumatic, usually life-threatening, event. The course may resemble panic disorder with the herald attack a real life threat rather than spontaneous panic. Recurrent images of the original event frequently occur

Obsessive-compulsive disorder: Recurrent intrusive unwanted thoughts and images as well as compulsive behaviors such as rituals characterize this disorder. Panic attacks and generalized anxiety also occur

The most common form of anxious suffering in a hospital population, however, is most likely transient situational reactions or adjustment disorders with anxiety.

From *Diagnostic and Statistical Manual of Mental Disorders,* ed 3. Washington, American Psychiatric Association, 1980.

severe, and brief wave of intense anxiety with impressive cognitive, physiologic, and behavioral components, and (2) a lower-grade persistent distress, quantitatively distinct and with some qualitative differences as well. Pharmacologic and epidemiologic observations suggest a clinically relevant distinction between these two states.

In light of phenomenologic similarities, fear and anxiety likely reflect a common underlying neurophysiology. The first category of anxiety resembles acute fear or alarm in response to life-threatening danger: a cognitive state of terror, helplessness, or sense of impending disaster or doom, with autonomic but primarily sympathetic activation, and an urgency to flee or seek safety. The second type of anxiety would correspond to a state of "alert" with heightened sense of vigilance to possible threats with less intense levels of inhibition, physical distress, and behavioral impairment.

The two fear states resemble the clinical syndromes of panic attacks and generalized or anticipatory anxiety. As innate responses for protecting the organism and enhancing survival, panic and vigilance are normal when faced with threatening stimuli. As "anxiety" or psychopathologic symptoms, other factors besides actual physical threat must be implicated as "triggers" or cause. Of several explanatory models proposed, the *biological* model places emphasis on the nervous system, the *psychodynamic* on meanings and memories, and the *behavioral* on learning.

Animal and neuronal receptor studies suggest that there are, indeed, two central systems involved in fear and pathologic anxiety.[3,4] The alarm or panic mechanism is likely to have a critical component involving central noradrenergic mechanisms, with particular importance placed on a small retropontine nucleus, the primary source of the brain's norepinephrine, the *locus ceruleus* (LC). When this key to sympathetic activation is stimulated in monkeys, for example, an acute fear response can be elicited with distress vocalizations, fear behaviors, and flight. Alternatively, destruction of LC leads to abnormal complacency in the face of threat.[5] Biochemical perturbations that increase LC firing similarly elicit anxious responses in animal and man that are blocked by agents that decrease LC firing, some of which are in clinical practice as antipanic agents (eg, tricyclic antidepressants, alprazolam).[6]

A second system appears to involve benzodiazepine receptors with particular emphasis on limbic system structures, especially the septohippocampal areas. An important role of the limbic system is to scan the environment for life-supporting and threatening cues as well as to monitor internal or bodily sensations. Vigilance or its psychopathologic equivalent, generalized anxiety, most probably involves limbic system activity: "limbic alert." Benzodiazepine receptors in high concentration in relevant limbic system structures may play a role in modulating limbic alert, arousal, and behavioral inhibition[7] by increased binding of the inhibitory neurotransmitter γ-*aminobutyric acid* (GABA).[8] As one might expect, there are neuronal connections between the LC and limbic systems. Increased firing rate of LC neurons may serve as a rheostat to generate levels of arousal from vigilance to alarm.

Psychodynamic principles are less concerned with the neurophysiology of anxiety symptoms and more with intrapsychic activation of these mechanisms. While Freud's early writing implied a more physiologic basis for anxiety attacks in terms of undischarged libido, later emphasis was on anxiety as a signal of threat to the ego, signals elicited because of events and situations with similarities (symbolic or actual) to early, developmental experiences which were threatening to the vulnerable child (traumatic anxiety) such as separations, losses, certain constellations of relationships, and symbolic objects or events (eg, snakes, successes). More recent psychodynamic thinking would emphasize object relations and the use of internalized objects to maintain affective stability under stress.

Behavioral formulations of anxiety disorder antecedents focus on learning, wherein anxiety symptoms or avoidant behavior become associated with benign settings or objects due to generalization from earlier traumatic experiences; for example, a child ridiculed by peers because of a mistake during "show and tell" associates embarrassment and shame with speaking before groups and continues thereafter to manifest anticipatory anxiety and avoidance of all public speaking. Self-defeating cognitive "habits" sustain the syndrome with unrealistic catastrophic thinking, "expecting the worst." Misinterpretation of bodily stimuli with exaggerated cognitive and behavioral responses also serve to maintain the behavior.

Phobic disorders, whose sufferers may experience panic, anticipatory anxiety, or no anxiety symptoms at all (depending on the success of avoidance behavior), serve to illustrate the differing models of understanding anxiety. The biological view recognizes the stereotyped nature of phobias. Most of the objects and situations in everyday life that truly threaten us are rarely selected as phobic stimuli; children, who proceed normally through a variety of developmental phobias (strangers, separation, darkness, etc), rarely become phobic of objects and situations that parents attempt to associate with danger (eg, electric outlets, roads); and most phobic stimuli have meaning in the context of biological preparedness and were presumably selected through evolution.[9] Most human phobias are of objects and situations that make sense in the context of enhancing survival before the dawn of civilization: places of restricted escape, groups of strangers, heights, and snakes, for example. Social phobias, for example, fear of scrutiny by others, resemble the intense discomfort elicited in primates introduced into a new colony or in any animal simply being stared at—a glare is a threat. When panic attacks and anticipatory anxiety heighten the general sense of danger and insecurity, a variety of phobias may become manifest as part of the patient's increased concern with security and safety. Genetic factors are presumed to be primary in determining vulnerability to these disorders.

Psychodynamic observations underscore the use of defense mechanisms such as displacement and the contribution of meanings and symbolic representations of phobic objects and situations. Learning theory presumes some real or perceived prior traumatic experience with the object or situation. As with most of human experience, psychopathology rarely can be reduced to one explanatory framework, and clinical observation and research indicate contributing roles for all three models as determinants of behavior and symptoms and as guides to therapeutic strategies.

ANXIETY IN THE MEDICAL SETTING

While some distress from anxiety is expected as a routine consequence of hospitalization, anxiety may also be a significant clinical issue in the treatment of patients in a medical setting. The hospitalized patient encounters a world of both internal and external dangers: assaults on bodily integrity in the form of uncomfortable procedures and forced intimacy with strangers; the atmosphere of illness, pain, and death; and separation from loved ones and familiar surroundings. The patient typically experiences uncertainty about his illness and its implications for his capacity to work and maintain social and family relationships. Just as depression has been described as a "psychobiological final common pathway" of a number of interacting determinants,[10] it is likely that anxiety too represents a multidetermined expression of the variety of psychological, biological, and social factors having impact on the patient.

The anxious patient can be a diagnostic challenge. The presence of anxiety may represent the patient's reaction to the meaning and implications of medical illness or to the medical setting, a manifestation of the physical disorder itself, or the expression of an underlying psychiatric disorder. The distinction between anxiety as symptom and anxiety as syndrome may be difficult to make in the medical setting where there may be overlap between "normal" situational anxiety or "fear," anxiety-like symptoms resulting from a variety of organic disease states and their treatments, and the characteristic presentation of anxiety disorders.

Methodologic obstacles surface in attempts to identify the nature and prevalence of anxiety in medical patients.[11] Studies of anxiety in the medical setting are often difficult to interpret because of a lack of clarity of case definition and assessment measures, heterogeneity of the study populations, absence of appropriate control groups, and the nonspecific and often transitory nature of the anxiety symptoms themselves.

Approximately 60% of patients with psychiatric conditions are treated by primary practitioners; the most common disorders are depression and anxiety.[12,13] In a study of patients presenting to a group of primary care physicians, anxiety was the fifth most common diagnosis overall;

others suggest this may be an underestimate.[14,15] The high rate of prescribing benzodiazepines by primary care physicians reflects the frequency of anxiety in the medical setting.[16] Panic disorder has a reported prevalence of 1% to 2% in the general population,[17] as compared to 6% to 10% of patients in a primary care setting[18] and 10% to 14% of patients in a cardiology practice.[19] The number of patients with anxiety disorders, furthermore, is but a subgroup of those for whom anxiety is a complicating factor in their diagnosis and treatment in hospital.

Considering the likely frequency of "normal" anxiousness in this setting, there must be special circumstances surrounding those patients identified by primary caregivers as deserving psychiatric attention. While some overly anxious patients go unrecognized, those who generate concern must have impressed their caregivers in some way by the autonomy, intensity, duration, or behavior associated with their distress. Several typical scenarios of anxiety in the general hospital can be recognized.

ANXIETY FROM THE FAILURE TO COPE

For most patients the potentially overwhelming stressors of hospitalization are mitigated by a variety of coping mechanisms. The sources of threat and the flood of perceptions signalling potential danger are managed by common strategies: rationalization and self-reassurance ("I've come this far," "the doctors know what they're doing," "safest place in the world"), denial and minimization ("the chest pain is just heartburn," "these machines will protect me"), religious faith, support from family and friends, and other strategies determined by the patient's personality style.

Even for those without pre-illness anxiety disorder, coping strategies may fail, yielding to a sense of fear and vulnerability. A host of factors may be implicated in this failure: personality features with brittleness or tendency to regress in the face of threat (or paradoxically in a setting evoking passivity and offering access to nurturance), the suddenness of onset of threat (acute, life-threatening medical or surgical disease), unavailability of familial or other social support, feelings of aloneness or abandonment, or the unconscious meaning of the particular illness or injury. The patient becomes frightened, trembles, cannot sleep, repeatedly seeks attention and reassurance, registers excessive pain complaints and other physical symptoms, becomes disruptive, unable to manage the fear. For many, especially the young or retarded, catastrophic emotional responses are more readily triggered.

Case: A psychiatric consultation request was received for a 17-year-old high school junior following above-the-knee amputation for osteogenic sarcoma, without evidence of metastasis at the time of surgery. He had returned to school with a prosthesis and had done well. Some months later, a pulmonary metastasis was discovered and he was rehospitalized for surgery and chemotherapy. Although anticipating a favorable outcome at this point, he behaved unlike his prior hospitalization. He raged at caregivers, acted panicky, and withdrew from contact. Consultation sought treatment for his anxiety.

He was a tall, handsome, athletic, narcissistic young man admired by his peers, a "leader" who managed his life with bragadoccio and pseudoindependence. For the first time in his illness he was overwhelmed and frightened. Two critical issues emerged from interview. In the past he had a great deal of support from his peers, but had lately refused their visits. He was embarrassed by hair loss from chemotherapy. Secondly, during this hospitalization, his father, feeling overwhelmed by this turn of events, had decreased the frequency of visits to his son, citing increased work demands.

Two interventions calmed the acute anxiety. First, effort was made to find a well-suited wig; secondly, a psychotherapeutic contact with the father helped him to adequately manage his grief to permit renewed frequency of visits, and thereby relief for his son's separation anxiety.

While the oncologist's request was for an anxiolytic prescription, recognition of the loss of coping ability yielded the appropriate therapy for the acute anxiety.

This case serves to underscore two points: (1) Previously well-adapted individuals can become anxious in the face of serious or life-threatening illness; (2) despite the "appropriateness" of anxiety in the face of serious illness, other factors, potentially remediable, may be involved in triggering anxious symptoms or behavior. In this case troublesome behavior was evident; for others, only more subtle physical symptoms may have occurred.

ANXIETY INTERFERING WITH EVALUATION OR TREATMENT

A request for consultation may be a consequence of anxiety that interferes with a patient's evaluation or treatment: refusal of workup or treatment because of fear of pain or discomfort; catastrophic interpretation of physical symptoms or of the planned workup ("they're looking for cancer") with excessively fearful response; or alternatively the need to minimize or deny a potentially serious condition and its implications limiting cooperation with evaluation.

Case: Examination of a 38-year-old woman revealed a large breast lump. Although initially reluctant, she eventually agreed to a mammogram. In the waiting room, she became increasingly anxious and when her name was called refused to come in for the test. A psychiatric consultation was called to provide management of the patient's anxiety to permit the mammogram.

An attractive woman, she had stopped working as a teacher 12 years earlier after marrying a successful business executive and having the first of her two children. On interview she spoke of a favorite aunt who had died of breast cancer after disfiguring surgeries, and her own fear of a similar lesion. She was plagued by the thought that loss of a breast would cause her husband to lose interest and abandon her. She had not informed her husband of her current medical situation.

Meeting subsequently with both husband and wife, the psychiatrist gave explicit information about the possibility of malignancy and treatment options. The husband's manifest interest, support, and affection were reassuring; following the mammogram a benign lump was removed.

Discovery of the meaning to the patient of the illness and procedure permitted an intervention that sufficiently reduced her anxiety to allow evaluation and treatment. As with any "situational" anxiety, the fear of serious or fatal illness can be managed with education, support, cognitive and behavioral strategies, and at times the short-term use of benzo-diazepines.

Anxiety that occurs in patients with a known and potentially fatal illness is more accurately termed "fear," as there is a known danger. Such fear, however, can adversely affect the course of illness and treatment. Study of survivors of myocardial infarction (MI), for example, indicate 95% evidenced increased tension and anxiety and of one group of post-MI patients discharged from the hospital, 40% did not return to work; in 80%, psychological impairment, including anxiety, was the cause.[20] Worry that activity will cause further heart damage or death interferes with rehabilitation and the return to autonomous functioning. Most effective therapeutic approaches for these patients center on education, group discussion, and support and stress management techniques.[21] Anxious patients with a diagnosed serious or fatal illness require treatment that includes education in addition to possible use of supportive or insight-oriented psychotherapy, cognitive-behavioral techniques, and anxiolytic or antidepressant medications.

Among patients with medical disorders such as gastrointestinal (GI) disorders or allergies, the course and symptoms of illness may be exacerbated by anxiety.[21,22] Anxiety, like other emotional responses, may adversely affect normal physiologic function; asthma symptoms are exacerbated by emotional arousal or stress and the increased symptoms generate further anxiety.[23] Psychological and emotional responses and behavior possibly affect the survival of patients with cancer through effects on the immune system.[24]

MEDICAL ILLNESS MIMICKING ANXIETY DISORDER

Anxiety symptoms may be the principal manifestation of an underlying medical illness.[25] Of patients referred for psychiatric treatment, 5% to 42% have been reported as having underlying medical illness responsible for their distress with depression and anxiety as frequent complaints.[26,27] Twenty-five percent of reported cases of medical illnesses causing anxiety symptoms have been secondary to neurologic problems and 25% to endocrinologic causes, with 12% attributed to circulatory, rheumatoid-collagen vascular disorders, and chronic infection, and 14% to miscellaneous other illnesses.[25] A most common "organic" cause of anxiety may be alcohol and drug use, resulting from either intoxication, or more typically, withdrawal states.[28]

The clinical presentation of anxiety in the medical setting takes many forms: The bewildering array and variable nature of the physical and psychic symptoms reported by anxious patients may lead the physician to overlook symptoms related to another disorder.[29] The relative contribution of situational, psychiatric, and physiologic factors to the presentation of anxiety-like symptoms in a medical patient is often murky. The number of medical illnesses, furthermore, that may generate or exacerbate anxiety symptoms (Table 9-3) obviously renders an exhaustive evaluation for each of them impractical. A thorough yet efficient

Table 9-3. Medical Causes of Anxiety

Endocrine
    Adrenal cortical hyperplasia (Cushing's disease)
    Adrenal cortical insufficiency (Addison's disease)
    Adrenal tumors
    Carcinoid syndrome
    Cushing syndrome
    Diabetes mellitus
    Hyperparathyroidism
    Hyperthyroidism
    Hypoglycemia
    Hypothyroidism
    Insulinoma
    Menopause
    Ovarian dysfunction
    Pancreatic carcinoma
    Pheochromocytoma
    Pituitary disorders

Table 9-3. (cont.)

Premenstrual syndrome
Testicular deficiency
Drug-related
  Intoxication
    Analgesics
    Antibiotics
    Anticholinergics
    Anticonvulsants
    Antidepressants
    Antihistamines
    Antihypertensives
    Anti-inflammatory agents
    Antiparkinsonian agents
    Aspirin
    Caffeine
    Chemotherapy agents
    Cocaine
    Digitalis
    Hallucinogens
    Neuroleptics
    Steroids
    Sympathomimetics
    Thyroid supplements
    Tobacco
  Withdrawal
    Ethanol
    Narcotics
    Sedative-hypnotics
Cardiovascular and circulatory
  Anemia
  Cerebral anoxia
  Cerebral insufficiency
  Congestive heart failure
  Coronary insufficiency
  Dysrhythmias
  Hyperdynamic β-adrenergic state
  Hypovolemia
  Mitral valve prolapse
  Myocardial infarction
  Type A behavior
Respiratory system
  Asthma
  Hyperventilation
  Hypoxia
  Pneumonia
  Pneumothorax
  Pulmonary edema

Pulmonary embolus
Immunologic-collagen vascular
  Anaphylaxsis
  Polyarteritis nodosa
  Rheumatoid arthritis
  Systemic lupus erythematosus
  Temporal arteritis
Metabolic
  Acidosis
  Acute intermittent porphyria
  Electrolyte abnormalities
  Hyperthermia
  Pernicious anemia
  Wilson's disease
Neurologic
  Brain tumors (especially third ventricle)
  Cerebral syphilis
  Cerebral vascular disorders
  Combined systemic disease
  Encephalopathies (toxic, metabolic, infectious)
  Epilepsy (especially temporal lobe epilepsy)
  Essential tremor
  Huntington's disease
  Intracranial mass lesion
  Migraine headaches
  Multiple sclerosis
  Myasthenia gravis
  Organic brain syndrome
  Pain
  Polyneuritis
  Postconcussive syndrome
  Postencephalitic disorders
  Posterolateral sclerosis
  Vertigo (including Meniere's disease, and other vestibular dysfunction)
Gastrointestinal
  Colitis
  Esophageal dysmotility
  Peptic ulcer
Infectious disease
  Atypical viral pneumonia
  Brucellosis
  Malaria
  Mononucleosis
  Tuberculosis
  Viral hepatitis
Miscellaneous
  Nephritis
  Nutritional disorders
  Other malignancies (eg, oat-cell carcinoma)

evaluation of the differential diagnostic possibilities, however, includes the following considerations.[25,30] (1) In a patient with a known medical illness, the condition and its associated complications and treatment should be suspected. For example, in the asthmatic patient, hypoxia, respiratory distress, and sympathomimetic bronchodilators may all contribute to the experience of anxiety. In some patients, risk factors or predisposition, as with family history of medical illness capable of causing anxiety-like symptoms (eg, thyroid disease), may be clues to diagnosis. (2) In medical illnesses considered as mimics of anxiety, the quality of anxiety symptoms when closely examined may be different from those of primary anxiety disorders. For example, Starkman et al[31] studied 17 patients with pheochromocytoma, comparing their anxiety symptoms to those of a group of 52 patients with anxiety disorders. Most patients with pheochromocytoma did not meet criteria for panic disorder or generalized anxiety disorder; none developed agoraphobic symptoms, and their overall severity of symptoms was lower. There was a significant lack of "psychological" as opposed to physical symptoms of anxiety in most of these patients.

Harper and Roth [32] noted that patients with primary anxiety disorders were more likely to have had emotional trauma related to the onset of anxiety, daily symptoms, neurotic features, and gradual resolution of symptoms after an attack, and less likely to have loss of speech or consciousness during an episode of anxiety, than patients with anxiety associated with temporal lobe epilepsy. Thus the lack of a significant emotional experience of anxiety or the occurrence of anxiety only coincidental with particular physical events (eg, a run of ventricular tachycardia on a cardiac monitor, or spike activity on an EEG) may suggest the presence of an organic anxiety syndrome.

Evaluation directed toward the somatic system (eg, GI or cardiac) most prominently affected by anxiety symptoms may provide the greatest yield from further diagnostic investigations. (3) Characteristic features of anxiety disorders should be systematically considered: onset of anxiety symptoms after age 35, lack of personal or family history of anxiety disorders, negative childhood history, absence of significant life events heralding or exacerbating anxiety symptoms, lack of avoidance behavior, and a poor response to standard antianxiety agents all suggest the presence of an organically based anxiety syndrome.[25] (4) Even for the apparently healthy patient, particular scrutiny should be directed at more common conditions associated with anxiety: arrhythmias, thyroid abnormalities, excessive caffeine intake, and other drug use. Anxiety-like symptoms may be the first clue to a withdrawal syndrome in a patient with unreported regular sedative-hypnotic (eg, ethchlorvynol, glutethimide) or alcohol use prior to admission to the hospital. Intoxication or withdrawal from prescription or over-the-counter medication, or substances of abuse should also be suspected. Up to 2% to 3% of individuals have been reported to develop psychiatric symptoms after using prescribed or over-the-counter medication.[33]

> *Case:* A psychiatric consultation was requested from the medical service for a 31-year-old female clerk who developed "anxiety attacks" shortly after learning that she had contracted syphilis from her boy friend. She had previously experienced spontaneous "anxiety attacks" in her mid-twenties which had remitted early in a 6-month course of imipramine hydrochloride, and she had been symptom-free since. During the interview with the psychiatrist, she manifested anger and sadness about her boy friend's infidelity and her own victimization, as well as anxiety about the future of their relationship. Her "anxiety attacks," however, were different than those she had previously experienced, consisting of blurred vision; dull biparietal headaches, primarily left-sided; numbness of her extremities; and feelings of dizziness. She reported feeling anxious after the onset of these symptoms. On further questioning, the patient described a history of menstrual irregularities over the last 2 to 3 years and galactorrhea. Her prolactin level was found to be elevated, and a computed tomography (CT) scan revealed a pituitary adenoma. Surgical resection of the adenoma resulted in resolution of her anxiety attacks, although she elected to pursue psychotherapy to consider issues raised by the difficulties in her relationship.

This case serves to illustrate the following points. The presence of a prior history of an anxiety disorder, or a recent stressor, does not eliminate the need to consider medical illness in the differential diagnosis of a new or different presentation of anxiety. The patient's experience of anxiety attacks was primarily somatic, and it was fortuitous that she had a prior history of more "typical" anxiety attacks for comparison; the nature of her symptoms led to a careful exploration for neurologic disease and allowed an appropriate and timely intervention.

ANXIETY MIMICKING MEDICAL ILLNESS

The autonomic arousal associated with anxiety states allows anxiety to present as a "great imitator" of medical illness. Patients with anxiety disorders repeatedly visit their primary care doctors or "make the rounds" of a variety of medical practitioners seeking a medical diagnosis to explain their symptoms. Along the way, they may be considered "hypochondriacs," "crocks," or "just nervous" and possibly receive benzodiazepines or reassurance, but fail to be offered adequate or definitive treatment. Patients with untreated panic disorder, for example, have increased rates of alcoholism and of sedative hypnotic abuse, presumably in an attempt to self-medicate.[15,34] Sheehan et al[35] noted that 70% of patients with panic disorder in their series had been to at least ten medical practitioners without receiving diagnosis or adequate treatment: they had high somatization scores on the Symptom Checklist-90 (SCL-90) that decreased with the treatment of the panic disorder. The majority of these patients met criteria for somatization disorder, and tended to focus on the somatic symptoms of the untreated panic disorder.

Individuals with somatization disorder are nearly 100 times more likely than the general population to suffer comorbid panic disorder.[36] Of 55 patients with panic disorder referred by primary care physicians in one study, 49 (89%) initially presented with one or two somatic complaints and were misdiagnosed for months to years.[15] The three most common somatic loci of symptoms were cardiac, GI, and neurologic, with 45 (81%) of the 55 patients having a presenting pain complaint. These patients may focus on specific physical symptoms such as chest pain or diarrhea, thereby obscuring other anxiety symptoms, or may deny affective or cognitive responses to avoid the stigmatization of psychiatric illness. As noted, anxiety may also exacerbate pre-existing physical conditions such as asthma, which then become the focus of attention of both patient and physician.

The cost of unrecognized and untreated anxiety disorders in patients is high in terms of continued suffering, inefficient use of medical personnel, and costly repetitive diagnostic procedures. Clancy and Noyes[37] have documented the high rate of medical specialty consultations and procedures (most commonly cardiologic, neurologic, and GI) requested by patients with panic disorder. In one series of patients with chest pain undergoing coronary arteriography, Bass et al[38] noted that 61% of the patients with insignificant coronary disease had psychiatric morbidity on standardized interview as opposed to only 23% of those with significant coronary disease. In those with normal coronary arteries, the most common psychiatric diagnosis was anxiety neurosis. Recognition and treatment of the anxiety disorder, in some cases, may have eliminated the necessity for arteriograms. In one series,[15] panic disorder exacerbated the symptoms of patients with pre-existing medical disease and led to multiple hospitalizations—a trend that was reversed with treatment of the panic disorder. Dirks et al[39] reported that patients with chronic asthma and high levels of anxiety had more hospitalizations than asthmatic patients with physiologic illness of comparable severity but normal degrees of anxiety.

While consideration of the medical differential for anxiety is crucial, recognition and treatment of anxiety disorders is essential in preventing inefficient use of medical resources and patient exposure to costly and occasionally dangerous diagnostic and therapeutic procedures. Failure to make the pertinent psychiatric diagnosis may result in a patient continuing to "doctor shop," in the search to discover "what's really wrong with me," with repeated diagnostic procedures resonating with the patient's hypochondriacal concerns. Untreated anxiety can exacerbate symptoms of existing medical pathology and drive a cycle of escalating help-seeking behavior and hospitalization.

> *Case:* An emergency room psychiatric consultation was requested for a 35-year-old man seen acutely by cardiology six times in the past month for chest pain and tachycardia. He had been admitted to the cardiac care unit twice, where myocardial infarctions were ruled out. An extensive negative workup at another hospital had included a cardiac angiogram. After being told "there's nothing wrong with your heart, you're just nervous" and being given a prescription for diazepam, he sought emergency treatment at our institution in the hope that "they'll find out what's wrong." He had refused previous consultations with psychiatry fearing he would be dismissed as "a head case," but finally agreed to evaluation at the insistence of the medical team.
>
> He was an athletic-looking salesman in his thirties, a self-described "take charge kind of guy" without any previous psychiatric or medical history. He had a family history of hypertension and was concerned about potential "inherited heart problems." His ECG recorded a sinus tachycardia of 120 beats per minute and ST-T wave changes deemed secondary to the elevated rate. The episodic periods of anxiety, chest pain, tachycardia, diaphoresis, and hyperventilation began approximately a year earlier without clear precipitants during highway driving and had caused him to pull off the road and seek emergency medical treatment. He reported anticipating long trips with trepidation lest the episodes of chest pain be repeated.
>
> His diagnosis was panic disorder with mild agoraphobia, and treatment was initiated with alprazolam. He felt reassured that he was not "crazy," and had a definable condition for which treatment was available. The panic attacks remitted shortly thereafter, as did the patient's use of emergency medical services.

Treatment with a number of agents can dramatically relieve the spells and secondary complications of panic disorder, underscoring the importance of early diagnosis. Further, due to the physical nature of the symptoms, general medical and emergency room evaluators need to be alert to the clinical phenomena of a panic attack. Patients who describe their symptoms as "anxiety" or who evolve a major depression may be more likely to be identified as having a psychiatric disorder. Given the dramatic physical complaints in a variety of bodily systems, however, as with depression where somatic symptoms may dominate the presentation and "mask" diagnosis, an analogy may be made with missed or "masked" panic disorder.

The absent report of the affective, cognitive, or behavioral components of a panic attack can obscure the diagnosis in the face of paroxysmal physical symptoms. One case report[40] describes a patient with a symptom picture suggesting panic attack but who failed to describe the emotional experience of anxiety or panic; alexithymia, or the inability to read one's emotions, was offered as a possible mechanism for the clinical picture. The predominance of physical symptoms, or the absence of cognitive or behavioral responses, however, may not reflect "alexithymia" or a cognitive impairment, but, rather, variability in symptom expression. Some patients suffer panic attacks without experiencing a need to flee; others experience panic attacks without a sense of terror or dread, but do not necessarily lack the ability to "read" their own emotions.

Most patients with clinically significant panic attacks also suffer *limited symptom attacks* which feature only one or two physical symptoms. These may occur interspersed with major attacks and be either situational or unexpected, consisting for example, of runs of tachycardia or bouts of flushing, hyperventilation, or dizziness. Panic disorder, in its early stages, may be manifest exclusively in such minor attacks. Similarly, as antipanic therapy is effective, both unexpected and situational limited symptom attacks may be the last vestige of the disorder or continue to represent residual disorder.

For example, of the first 35 subjects randomized into a clinical trial of clonazepam versus alprazolam in the treatment of panic disorder, 33 (94%) reported having some attacks consisting of only one or two symptoms at baseline, and 50% of all attacks were limited symptom attacks. Of those subjects responding to treatment, 19% had only limited symptom attacks by study end. Inclusion in this protocol required a minimum of three major attacks in the 3 weeks prior to the study. Thus panic disorder may be evident in limited symptom attacks as a residual phenomenon, and, similarly, may manifest in this fashion as a prodrome or "mild" disorder.

As stated, patients vary in the primary "somatic locus" of anxiety distress.[30] For example, predominant panic attack symptoms may appear as cardiovascular symptoms (tachycardia, palpitations), neurologic symptoms (dizziness, paresthesias), respiratory symptoms (dyspnea), GI symptoms (diarrhea), and so forth. Recurrent limited symptom attacks may therefore be initially indistinguishable from symptoms of a number of disorders in these systems (see Table 9-3).

As noted, limited symptom attacks may be a harbinger of progression to the full syndrome, but in some cases they may also be disabling themselves and progress to such panic disorder complications as persistent anxiety, phobic avoidance, and depression.

> *Case:* A 32-year-old married factory supervisor had been out of work for 1 1/2 years due to stomach pain, nausea, and vomiting. He described his discomfort as "gnawing pains" that would occur paroxysmally followed by vomiting with little warning. In the previous 5 years he had extensive GI workups and medical management, vagotomy and pyloroplasty, and ultimately hemigastrectomy without relief of symptoms. He was totally disabled and was referred for psychiatric evaluation. The following features were noted: (1) His severe pain was paroxysmal with lower-grade persistent symptoms; (2) diazepam helped diminish but not eradicate his symptoms: (3) he was homebound and described attacks of stomach pain and vomiting only when he left his apartment as, for example, if he were to go shopping; (4) onset had followed the breakup of a relationship; (5) a major depression had evolved.
>
> On treatment with desipramine hydrochloride (coadministered with diazepam) he experienced complete symptomatic relief in 6 weeks and with maintenance treatment remained symptom-free for 5 years. He sought and found a new job following treatment and has been continuously employed for the past 5 years. As a child he recalls frequently needing to leave school because of a "nervous stomach."

This case reflects missed or masked diagnosis of panic disorder due to predominance of a limited symptom attack resembling a GI syndrome. Clues to diagnosis of panic disorder were evident, and appropriate treatment led to dramatic improvement in this disabled patient. Features reminiscent of more typical panic disorder patients were identified prior to definitive treatment including severe paroxysmal and lower-grade persistent symptoms, onset with a major life event, agoraphobic features, childhood history suggesting separation anxiety, partial relief with benzodiazepines, and secondary depression. No family history of panic attacks or agoraphobia was reported in this case.

PANIC DISORDER ASSOCIATED WITH MEDICAL ILLNESS

An association between panic disorder and other medical illnesses has been described. Katon[15] and Noyes et al[41] report an increased incidence of peptic ulcer and hypertension in patients with panic disorder. Retrospective studies by Coryell et al[42] suggest an increased risk of premature mortality from cardiac disease in men with panic disorder.

A relationship also exists between mitral valve prolapse and panic disorder. Mitral valve prolapse (MVP), usually asymptomatic, may predispose to arrhythmias, and occurs in roughly 5% to 10% of the population. Although diagnosed much more frequently in patients with panic disorder (30% – 50%) than normals or those with generalized anxiety,[43,44] the nature of the association between the disorders remains unclear. A proposed genetic linkage remains controversial.[45] Patients with panic attacks and MVP do not differ from those with panic alone in their family history of panic disorder or their response to treatment.[46]

PSYCHIATRIC ILLNESS CAUSING ANXIETY

In addition to primary anxiety disorders, anxiety symptoms may be associated with a number of other psychiatric disorders such as schizophrenia and depression.

Vague uneasiness extending to severe anxiety may either precede or accompany the symptoms of *schizophrenia*. Patients with significant degrees of anxiety may have a reduced level of functioning and manifest withdrawal superficially resembling schizophrenia. The presence of hallucinations, delusions, bizarre and disordered thinking, marked degree of social withdrawal, and characteristic premorbid personal and family history usually allows an uncomplicated differentiation of schizophrenia from anxiety disorders.

The relationship between anxiety and *depression* is complex. Weissman et al[47] report an increased prevalence of both panic disorder and depression in the families of probands with both disorders. One estimate holds that one third of patients with panic disorder, with or without agoraphobia, develop a secondary major depression and 22% have had a major depressive disorder prior to developing panic disorder[48]; the incidence of a major depressive episode in patients with panic disorder has been reported as ranging between 28% and 90% depending on the diagnostic criteria used.[49] Leckman et al[50] found 58% of a group of depressed patients had anxiety symptoms meeting DSM-III criteria for agoraphobia, panic disorder, or generalized anxiety disorder.

Although this overlap between syndromes can make the distinction between anxiety and depression difficult, a number of clinical considerations may be useful. Psychomotor retardation, persistent dysphoria, early morning awakening, diurnal variation, sense of hopelessness, and suicidal thoughts are more indicative of depression. Patients with an anxiety disorder have often not lost interest in their usual activities, but rather have lost the ability to comfortably negotiate them. They are more likely to report autonomic hyperactivity, derealization, perceptual distortions, and anxious impatience than hopelessness.[28] Advances in neurobiology at this time offer few diagnostic markers for differentiating anxiety and depressive disorders. Patients with panic disorder are less likely to nonsuppress during the dexamethasone suppression test (DST) than those patients with endogenous depression.[51] The sleep of patients with panic disorders differs from those of depressives during all-night polysomnograms.[52] There are also differences in physiologic parameters and platelet receptor binding patterns between anxious and depressed patients.[53,54]

The principle concern in differentiating depression from anxiety is not to overlook treatment with an antidepressant and, in particular, to avoid the common scenario of only prescribing a benzodiazepine for the anxiety component of a depression, leaving the depression untreated. Otherwise the frequent overlap in clinical presentation between primary depressive and primary anxiety disorders is fortunately mirrored by an overlap in therapeutic considerations.

Both disorders often have antecedents in major life events including losses, threats of loss, or interpersonal changes and upheavals, as well as major physiologic perturbations. Psychodynamic issues and psychosocial stressors may be similar.

Cognitive and behavioral strategies, on the other hand, differ if the primary problems are viewed as anxiety as opposed to depression, but antidepressant pharmacotherapy will frequently alleviate both anxious and depressive symptoms, with capability of ameliorating depression as well as comorbid panic attacks and/or generalized anxiety.

TREATMENT

The nature of the medical setting favors expedient interventions, such as drug treatment, to ease acute distress and because of the time-limited nature of medical and surgical stays. Nonetheless, as illustrated by case examples, comprehensive assessments including systematic scrutiny of psychodynamic and psychosocial factors may lead to practical interventions short of formal psychotherapy. Real and symbolic physical threats in addition to separation and loss will be the usual themes to explore in an initial interview. Disrupted relations with family members may be provocative and family interventions may prove therapeutically expedient.

For patients with persisting anxiety symptoms, behavioral and cognitive strategies, similar to those used for ambulatory patients with anxiety disorders, may be adapted to the hospitalized medical patient. With a cognitive approach, the patient with severe anxiety or panic attacks can be helped to systematically assess the reality of his worries and to view panic as catastrophic misinterpretation of otherwise benign bodily sensations.

Behavioral interventions will usually be limited to relaxation training for the generally anxious, but treatment for a phobic patient can be initiated in hospital with desensitization and, depending on the phobic stimulus, exposure techniques.

The drug treatment of anxiety essentially involves selecting agents for panic, generalized anxiety or both. As with recognizing the primacy of depression in some "anxious" patients, if the presence of panic attacks is overlooked, treatment for generalized anxiety only is likely to be inadequate and patient suffering will continue. Familiarity with panic disorder, its complications, and treatments is a necessary resource in evaluating and caring for anxious patients.

Panic Attacks

A panic attack usually lasts minutes with fairly stereotyped physical, cognitive, and behavioral components. Patients with panic disorder may experience these attacks intermittently over time or in clusters, and as stated may develop a number of complications including persistent anxiousness, phobic avoidance, depression, alcoholism, or other drug overuse.

Physical symptoms are experienced as if there is a sudden surge of autonomic, primarily sympathetic, arousal which may include cardiac, respiratory, neurologic, and GI symptoms. Cognitively, the patient feels a sense of terror, or fear of losing control, of dying, or of going crazy, and behaviorally often feels driven to flee from the setting in which the attack is experienced to a safe, secure, or familiar place or person.

The initial attack that appears to "turn on" the disorder, the "herald attack," is particularly well remembered by the patient. Subsequent attacks may be a mixture of spontaneous, unexpected attacks and those preceded by a build-up of anticipatory anxiety; the latter, called situational attacks, occur in settings where the patient might sense being at risk for panic, such as crowded places. Attacks may be "major" with four or more symptoms, or "limited symptom" attacks with fewer symptoms.

Panic disorder has its typical onset in early adult life and afflicts women three times as commonly as men. Adults with panic disorder and agoraphobia frequently have a childhood history of separation anxiety symptoms, particularly "school phobia."[55] The disorder is clearly familial and probably has a genetic basis, given a higher concordance in monozygotic compared to dizygotic twins.[56]

The onset of the disorder in a clinical population typically follows either a major life event such as a loss, threat of loss, other upheavals in work or home situations, or some physiologic event such as medical illness (eg, hyperthyroidism, vertigo), or drug use (marijuana, cocaine). For example, some patients whose first or herald attack appears triggered by a physiologic perturbation such as follows marijuana use may continue thereafter with persistent or recurrent symptoms without further drug use.

A panic attack, like an endogenous "false alarm," appears to turn on a state of vigilance or "post-panic" anxiety which resembles generalized anxiety disorder. Between attacks patients may remain symptomatic with a lower-level constant anxiousness and "anticipatory anxiety" which may crescendo into panic in certain situations or be punctuated by panic unexpectedly.

In this state of vigilance, phobic avoidance may occur as a complication. The patient may develop mild or extensive phobic avoidance, usually of travel or places of restricted escape, immediately following the onset of attacks, after a number of attacks, or never at all. In some cases the phobic avoidance evolves as a progressive constriction with the cumulative avoidance of settings where attacks have occurred.

Major depressive episodes may also complicate the course of the patient with panic disorder. The demoralization attending the sustained distress and progressive disability of panic disorder, for some, extends to a typical depression with characteristic signs and symptoms. As noted, the relationship between panic and depression is a complicated one, however. Some patients manifest no depressive symptoms; for others, it is unclear which disorder is primary as symptoms arise concurrently.

Unfortunately, alcohol use can temporarily tame the distress of panic disorder but soon yields to rebound symptoms, setting the stage for alcohol overuse.

Treatment of Panic Disorder

While early intervention offers the likelihood of preventing complications, many patients present to treatment after years of symptoms and disability. Even in the face of chronicity, however, most patients achieve substantial if not dramatic benefit with available treatments, which include antipanic pharmacotherapy and behavioral and cognitive therapies. Given the apparent primacy of the panic attack in the distress and evolution of complications of the disorder, our usual approach is to initiate antipanic medications for patients continuing to experience panic attacks, with the expectation of regression and remission of complications once the attacks have ceased. For patients with residual phobic avoidance despite prevention of panic attacks, behavioral and cognitive strategies are employed. (For some patients, behavioral and cognitive strategies are employed initially, especially where the frequency and intensity of unexpected panic are minimal, with pharmacotherapy subsequently applied if emergence or exacerbation of panic attends the behavioral program.)

Imipramine hydrochloride has well-established efficacy in panic disorder,[57] usually in the same dosage range as for treatment of depression (150–300 mg/d), but some patients may do well at lower doses. While other tricyclic antidepressants (TCAs) are probably also effective (eg, desipramine is frequently employed to decrease the anticholinergic burden), this class of agents has several drawbacks including delayed onset of benefit and treatment-emergent adverse effects. In addition to such usual TCA side effects as dry mouth, constipation, and orthostatic hypotension, panic patients are particularly prone to a sudden worsening of their disorder with the first doses. To minimize the impact of this adverse response, treatment can be initiated with very small "test" doses (eg, 10 mg of imipramine hydrochloride). If this is well tolerated, standard antidepressant dosing can be pursued; for others the adverse response typically fades over a few days allowing an upward titration of dose. For a small percentage of patients, this apparent worsening of the disorder does not subside.

The monoamine oxidase inhibitor (MAOI) phenelzine has stood up well in clinical use and controlled trials[57] and many clinicians feel MAOIs are potentially the most comprehensively effective agents for panic disorder, blocking panic attacks, relieving depression, and offering a "confidence enhancing" effect of considerable value to the patient needing to recover from vigilance and phobic avoidance. Except for postural hypotension, MAOIs are free of most of the early TCA side effects including the anxiogenic response. Unfortunately, as treatment proceeds, a variety of challenging problems emerge including insomnia, weight gain, edema, sexual dysfunction, nocturnal myoclonus, and other unusual symptoms. Further, many anxious patients are most circumspect about the dietary precautions and instructions about hypertensive crises. When treatment refusal, treatment discomfort from side effects, and treatment failure are considered, the need for a better tolerated and effective antipanic treatment is apparent. In some respects alprazolam fits this need. It has antipanic efficacy, patient acceptability, and a reasonable record of safety. In addition, it provides the speed of action which is desirable in a medical setting.

The usual dose range for most panic disorder patients on alprazolam is 2 to 8 mg/d with most achieving benefit around 4 to 6 mg. Clinical response is evident early, but lower doses are necessary to initiate treatment so that the patient can accommodate to sedation. Most patients adapt within a few days to sedating effects allowing stepwise increase to panic-blocking doses. Adaptation to sedation usually occurs without loss of therapeutic benefit, but some upward adjustment may be required after the first 2 weeks. A small percentage of patients appear particularly sensitive to the drug and experience persisting sedation despite time and careful titration. Alprazolam must be given in divided doses, usually three times a day and at bedtime, due to its relatively short duration of action.

Despite the ease of administration of alprazolam and frequently dramatic results even in the first days of treatment, clinical drawbacks include concerns about abuse and dependency, rebound symptoms between doses, withdrawal, and early relapse. The abuse potential of alprazolam is apparently similar to other benzodiazepines and varies widely among clinical populations. Most well-informed panic and phobic patients who have endured severe distress over time treat their medication with respect and understand the wisdom in maintaining the lowest effective dose; thus, unless there is evidence that a particular patient is at risk, the use of this agent appears generally safe for the disorder under consideration. As with any benzodiazepine, without controlled prescribing for targeted symptoms, inappropriate use may occur.

As a relatively short half-life benzodiazepine, the discontinuation of alprazolam, especially after long-term treatment, without a very gradual taper tailored to the individual patient's sensitivity to decreasing doses, may be followed by rebound symptoms (worsened anxiety) or a withdrawal syndrome.

With these drawbacks in mind, some clinicians initiate treatment with alprazolam and secondarily add a TCA with the goal of early taper of alprazolam and continuation treatment with imipramine, for example. For those patients who require a high-potency benzodiazepine but suffer rebound symptoms, the longer-acting high-potency benzodiazepine, clonazepam, has been effective.

With a milligram-for-milligram potency about twice that of alprazolam, clonazepam's effective dose range for panic patients will be between 1 and 5 mg/d given in morning and bedtime doses. Sedation will be the limiting factor in dose titration and is managed by initiating treatment with a low bedtime dose and titrating upward if symptoms persist and sedation resolves. Initial dose as low as 0.25 mg may be used in drug-naive patients or those particularly sensitive to benzodiazepines. Greater doses may be given at bedtime than morning if the patient is not readily accommodating to sedation, but many patients function without sedation on equal morning and bedtime doses, as with alprazolam.

The effect of a given daily dose on panic attacks and generalized anxiety will be apparent within a few days. Some patients, for unclear reasons, develop depressive symptoms on clonazepam as a treatment-emergent adverse effect. Resolution of depressive symptoms typically occurs with the introduction of a TCA; as with alprazolam, clonazepam can then be withdrawn with the expectation of a comprehensive response to the TCA. Combined treatment can again be used if anxiety symptoms break through the antidepressant treatment.

Drug Treatment of Generalized Anxiety

Benzodiazepines have been the mainstay of anxiolytic pharmacotherapy, although the clinical decision to prescribe these agents for symptom relief is a difficult one. The attitudes of individual physicians toward prescribing may be characterized as falling along a spectrum between "pharmacologic Calvinism" and "psychotropic hedonism," reflecting a personal moral stance toward prescribing medication for the relief of psychic distress. The abundant literature on antianxiety agents falls short of providing reliable measures for diagnosis and prescribing. Given the ubiquitousness of anxiety in hospital settings, the physician must frequently confront the question of whether to prescribe. The use of a benzodiazepine for the distressed, anxious patient is often a therapeutic act analogous to pain relief.

As compared with barbiturates and nonbarbiturate sedative and hypnotic agents (meprobamate, ethchlorvynol, glutethimide, methaqualone, and others), the benzodiazepines are more selectively anxiolytic, with less sedation and less morbidity and mortality in overdose and acute withdrawal. Since using a benzodiazepine represents a clinical decision to offer symptomatic relief, the critical clinical assessment is to evaluate the patient's response. The patient's coping should be enhanced in addition to and as a consequence of relief from suffering.

Choice of benzodiazepine. All available benzodiazepines are effective in treating generalized anxiety. Drug selection is based on pharmacokinetic properties which determine rapidity of onset of effect, degree of accumulation with multidosing, rapidity of offset of clinical effect, and risk of drug discontinuation syndrome.

For single or acute dosing, onset of effect is determined by the rate of absorption from the stomach and offset by distribution from plasma into lipid stores. Long half-life of any drug predicts the amount of accumulation of drug in plasma with multidosing and speed of washout upon drug discontinuation (and thus the quickness of return of symptoms or risk of rebound and withdrawal). For example, a rapidly absorbed, lipophilic agent like diazepam given acutely will have a rapid but relatively short-lived effect; with repeated dosing, however, plasma levels will be higher than a short half-life drug at steady state. The long half-life offers some tapering effect to help protect against rebound or withdrawal on discontinuation.

The clinician can choose a drug to have fast onset for greater clinical impact, slow onset to minimize sedation or spaciness, short action to allow rapid clearing, or long action to minimize interdose or posttreatment rebound symptoms (Table 9-4).

Treatment begins with low doses and upward titration. Doses vary but for usual situational anxiety should rarely exceed 30 mg of diazepam a day, or its equivalent.

Patients should expect that treatment will be of limited duration and will diminish but not eradicate the disorder. For simple phobic anxiety, occasional use is indicated. For persistent symptoms, using anxiolytics for periods of exacerbation may be effective, although patients often report sustained improvement with maintenance treatment.

Precautions in prescribing. A withdrawal syndrome, usually mild but potentially severe, depending on the dose and the duration of treatment, may follow abrupt cessation of therapy. For patients receiving usual doses for less than 4 months, during hospitalization, for example, without prior use of sedatives, the risk of an abstinence syndrome is less. In general, however, treatment is discontinued by tapering doses, gradually adjusting decrements according to patient response.

Overuse of medication and drug-seeking from multiple sources is a concern for outpatient prescribing, but with the controlled use of drugs

Table 9-4. Commonly Used Benzodiazepines in the United States

Drug	Approximate Dose Equivalence	Relative Rapidity of Onset	Relative Length of Half-Life
Alprazolam (Xanax)	1	Fast-Interim	Short-Interim
Chlordiazepoxide (Librium)	25	Intermediate	Intermediate
Clorazepate dipotassium (Tranxene)	15	Fast	Long
Diazepam (Valium)	10	Fastest	Long
Lorazepam (Ativan)	2	Intermediate	Short
Oxazepam (Serax)	30	Slower	Short
Prazepam (Centrax)	20	Slowest	Long

in hospital, particular vigilance is appropriate primarily for the patient with history of drug or alcohol abuse.

The sedative effects of benzodiazepines will be additive with other CNS depressants and plasma levels will be higher with use of certain drugs such as cimetidine. Benzodiazepines are best avoided, if possible, during pregnancy. A few patients, particularly with higher-potency benzodiazepines, are prone to increased hostility, aggressivity, and rage eruptions.

Alternatives to benzodiazepines.   Some clinicians will use low doses of neuroleptics for anxiety, without associated psychosis or delirium. This ataractic effect may yield benefit, but the clinical response may be obscured by akathisia or other neuroleptic side effects. With these drugs the duration of treatment must be restricted to days or weeks at most since availability of other effective treatments does not justify exposing the patient to risk of tardive dyskinesia.

β-Blocking drugs such as propranolol hydrochloride have proved useful in alleviating some of the peripheral autonomic symptoms of anxiety such as tremor and tachycardia. While of second- or third-line importance in treating panic attacks or more cognitively experienced symptoms (eg, worry), β-blockers are often impressively useful in social phobic syndromes and where persistent peripheral symptoms ("somatic anxiety") predominate. Agents such as atenolol which are less able to cross the blood-brain barrier, compared to propranolol, may have advantages for patients who experience fatigue or dysphoria on propranolol. Effective doses vary and treatment requires upward titration from low initial doses.

The introduction of buspirone hydrochloride appears to offer an anxiolytic or "anxioselective" agent that will allow calming without sedation or additive CNS depressant effects with other drugs. Whether buspirone will serve to treat panic attacks or severe acute anxiety will require further study, but it appears adequate for mild situational distress. With dosing roughly equivalent to usual diazepam prescribing, buspirone has not been associated with drug discontinuation syndromes. On the other hand, some patients who have prior exposure to benzodiazepines have not experienced improvement on buspirone.

There is considerable interest in the question of the efficacy of antidepressants for generalized anxiety, unassociated with panic or depression. Some reports indicate a role for TCAs,[58] for example, in diminishing persistent anxiousness. As a TCA disadvantage, the call to intervene with medication for the anxious patient in hospital typically requires a response with a more immediate-acting agent.

REFERENCES

1. Robins LN, Helger JE, Weissman MM, et al: Lifetime prevalence of specific psychiatric disorders in three sites. *Arch Gen Psychiatry* 1984; 140:949–958.
2. MacKenzie TB, Popkin MK: Organic anxiety syndrome. *Am J Psychiatry* 1983; 140:342–344.
3. Charney DS, Redmond DE Jr: Neurobiological mechanisms in human anxiety: Evidence supporting noradrenergic hyperactivity. *Neuropharmacology* 1983; 22:1531–1536.
4. Insel TR, Ninan PT, Aloi J, et al: A benzodiazepine receptor mediated model of anxiety: Studies in non-human primates and clinical implications. *Arch Gen Psychiatry* 1984; 41:741–750.
5. Huang YH, Redmond DE Jr, Snyder DR, et al: Loss of fear following bilateral lesions of the locus coeruleus in the monkey. *Neurosci Abst* 1976; 2:573.
6. Charney DS, Heninger GR: Noradrenergic function and the mechanism of action of antianxiety treatment. *Arch Gen Psychiatry* 1985; 42: 458–481.
7. Gray JA: Issues in the neuropsychology of anxiety, in Tuma AH, Maser JD (eds): *Anxiety and the Anxiety Disorders.* Hillsdale, NJ, L Erlbaum, 1985, pp 5–26.
8. Tallman JF, Gallager DW: The GABA-ergic system: A locus of benzodiazepine action. *Annu Rev Neurosci* 1985; 8:21–44.
9. Seligman MEP: Phobias and preparedness. *Behav Ther* 1971; 2:307–320.
10. Akiskal MS, McKinney WT: Overview of recent research in depression. *Arch Gen Psychiatry* 1975; 32:285–305.
11. Rodin G, Voshart K: Depression in the medically ill: An overview. *Am J Psychiatry* 1986; 143:696–705.
12. Regier D, Goldberg ID, Taube CM: The de Facto US mental health service system. *Arch Gen Psychiatry* 1978; 35:685–693.
13. Goldberg D: Detection and assessment of emotional disorders in a primary-care setting. *Int J Mental Health* 1979; 8:30–48.
14. Marsland DW, Wood M, Mayo F: Content of family practice: A data bank for patient care curriculum and research in family practice. 526, 196 patient problems. *J Fam Pract* 1976; 3:25–68.
15. Katon W: Panic disorder and somatization: Review of 55 cases. *Am J Med* 1984; 77:101–106.
16. Hollister LE: A look at the issues: Use of minor tranquilizers. *Psychosomatics* 1980; 21(suppl):4–6.
17. Weissman MM, Merikangas KR: The epidemiology of anxiety and panic disorders: An update. *J Clin Psychiatry* 1986; 47(suppl):11–17.
18. Rice RL: Symptom patterns of the hyperventilation syndrome. *Am J Med Sci* 1951; 8:691–696.
19. Wood P: DaCosta's syndrome (or effort syndrome). *Br Med J* 1941; 1:767–773.
20. Wishnie MA, Hackett TP, Cassem NH: Psychological hazards of convalescence following myocardial infarction. *JAMA* 1971; 215:1292–1296.
21. Shuckit MA: Anxiety related to medical disease. *J Clin Psychol* 1983; 44:11(section 2), 31–36.
22. Wolf S, Alma TB, Bacharach W, et al: The role of stress in peptic ulcer disease. *J Human Stress* 1979; 1:27–37.
23. Fauman MA: The central nervous system and the immune system. *Biol*

Psychiatry 1982; 17:1459–1482.

24. Greer S, Morris T, Pettingale KW: Psychological response to breast cancer: Effect on outcome. *Lancet* 1979; 2:785–787.

25. Hall RCW (ed): *Psychiatric Presentations of Medical Illness. Somatopsychic Disorders.* New York, SP Medical and Scientific Books, 1980.

26. Hall RCW, Gardner ER, Popkin MK, et al: Unrecognized physical illness prompting psychiatric admission: A prospective study. *Am J Psychiatry* 1981; 138:629–635.

27. Cavanaugh S, Wettstein RM: Prevalence of psychiatric morbidity in medical populations, in Grinspoon L (ed): *Psychiatric Update*, Washington, American Psychiatric Press, Inc., 1984, vol 3, pp 187–215.

28. Cameron OG: The differential diagnosis of anxiety: Psychiatric and medical disorders. *Psychiatr Clin North Am* 1981; 8:3–24.

29. MacKenzie TB, Popkin MK: Organic anxiety syndrome. *Am J Psychiatry* 1983; 140:342–344.

30. Rosenbaum, JF: The drug treatment of anxiety. *N Engl J Med* 1982; 306:401–404.

31. Starkman MN, Zelnick TC, Nesse RM, et al: A study of anxiety in patients with pheochromocytoma. *Arch Intern Med* 1985; 145:248–252.

32. Harper M, Roth M: Temporal lobe epilepsy and the phobic-anxiety depersonalization syndrome. *Compr Psychiatry* 1962; 3:129–151.

33. Avant RF: Diagnosis and management of depression in the office setting. *Fam Pract Recert* 1983; 5(suppl 1):41.

34. Quitkin F, Rifkin A, Kaplan T, et al: Phobic anxiety syndrome complicated by drug dependency and addiction. *Arch Gen Psychiatry* 1972; 27:159–162.

35. Sheehan DV, Ballenger J, Jacobsen E: Treatment of endogenous anxiety with phobic, hysterical and hypochondriacal symptoms. *Arch Gen Psychiatry* 1980; 37:51–59.

36. Boyd JH, Burke JD, Greenberg E, et al: Exclusion criteria of DSM III: A study of co-occurrence of hierarchy-free syndromes. *Arch Gen Psychiatry* 1984; 41:983–987.

37. Clancy J, Noyes R: Anxiety neurosis: A disease for the medical model. *Psychosomatics* 1976; 17:90–93.

38. Bass C, Wade C, Gardner WN, et al: Unexplained breathlessness and psychiatric morbidity in patients with normal and abnormal coronary arteries. *Lancet* 1983; 1:605–609.

39. Dirks JF, Schraa JC, Brown E, et al: Psycho-maintenance in asthma: Hospitalization rates and financial impact. *Br J Med Psychol* 1980; 53:349–354.

40. Jones BA: Panic attacks with panic masked by alexithymia. *Psychosomatics* 1984; 25:858–859.

41. Noyes R, Clancy J, Moenk PR, et al: Anxiety neurosis and physical illness. *Compr Psychiatry* 1978; 19:407–413.

42. Coryell W, Noyes R Jr, Howe JD: Mortality among outpatients with anxiety disorders. *Am J Psychiatry* 1986; 143:508–510.

43. Liberthson R, Sheehan DV, King ME, et al: The prevalence of mitral valve prolapse in patients with panic disorder. *Am J Psychiatry* 1986; 143:511–515.

44. Dager SR, Comess KA, Dunner DL: Differentiation of anxious patients by two dimensional echocardiographic evaluation of the mitral valve. *Am J Psy-*

chiatry 1986; 143:533–536.

45. Hickey AJ, Andrew G, Wilcken DEL: Independence of mitral valve prolapse and neurosis. *Br Heart J* 1983; 50:333–336.

46. Gorman JM, Fyer AJ, King D, et al: Mitral valve prolapse and panic disorders: Effect of imipramine, in Klein DJ, Rabkin JG (eds): *Anxiety—New Research and Changing Concepts.* New York, Raven Press, 1981, pp 317–326.

47. Weissman MM, Lechman JF, Merikangas Jr, et al: Depression and anxiety disorders in parents and children. *Arch Gen Psychiatry* 1984; 41:845–852.

48. Breier A, Charney DS, Heninger GR: Major depression in patients with agoraphobia and panic disorder. *Arch Gen Psychiatry* 1984; 41:1129–1135.

49. Lesser IM, Rubin RT: Diagnostic considerations in panic disorders. *J Clin Psychol* 1986; 47(suppl 4–10):6.

50. Leckman JF, Weissman MM, Merikangas KR, et al: Panic disorder in major depression. *Arch Gen Psychiatry* 1983; 40:1055–1060.

51. Sheehan DV, Claycomb JB, Surman OS, et al: Panic attacks and the dexamethasone suppression test. *Am J Psychiatry* 1983; 140:1063–1064.

52. Uhde TW, Roy-Byrne P, Gillin JC, et al: The sleep of patients with panic disorder. A preliminary report. *Psychiatry Res* 1984; 12:251–259.

53. Kelly D, Walter CJS: A clinical and physiological relationship between anxiety and depression. *Br J Psychiatry* 115:401–406.

54. Cameron OG, Smith CR, Hollingsworth PJ, et al: Platelet X-2 adrenergic receptor binding and plasma catecholamines in panic anxiety patients. *Arch Gen Psychiatry* 1984; 41:1144–1188.

55. Gittelman R, Klein DF: The relationship between separation anxiety and panic and agoraphobic disorders. *Psychopathology* 1984; 17(suppl 1):56–65.

56. Crowe RR: The genetics of panic disorder and agoraphobics. *Psychiatr Dev* 1985; 2:171–186.

57. Pohl R, Berchou R, Rainey JM Jr: Tricyclic antidepressants and monoamine oxidase inhibitors in treatment of agoraphobia. *J Clin Psychopharmacol* 1982; 2:399–407.

58. Kahn RJ, McNair DM, Lipman RS, et al: Imipramine and chlordiazepoxide in depressive and anxiety disorders. II. Efficacy in anxious outpatients. *Arch Gen Psychiatry* 1986; 43:79–85.

10

Borderline Patients

JAMES E. GROVES

It is not the psychodynamics of the borderline patient that troubles the staff of a general hospital; it is the behavior. Such patients wreak havoc by acting violently, polarizing the staff, refusing treatment, threatening suicide, and trying to leave the hospital against medical advice. When patients with personality or impulse disorders suffer medical illness or require surgery, the consultee does not summon the psychiatrist to provide insight into intrapsychic processes of the patient or group dynamics of the staff but to change those behaviors of the patient which interfere with the day-to-day functioning of the staff.[1] Difficulty in managing disruptive behaviors in the medical or surgical setting stems from staff-patient dissonance in three interpersonal dimensions: (1) perception of reality, (2) control of aggression, and (3) maintenance of appropriate social distance.[2]

The psychiatric consultant's role in reduction of dissonance should be direct and active, with emphasis on supporting a staff overburdened by the feelings of guilt, fear, depression, and rage,[3-7] which such patients stir up in caregivers. In the medical setting, psychoanalytic interpretations of the unconscious are destined to fail; noninterpretive behavioral approaches are the ones that work.

BORDERLINE PERSONALITY

Borderline personality is a severe, stable disorder of character "lying between" the psychoses and the neuroses in severity.[8,9] Borderline patients are characterized by impulsivity, swings from love to hate, and maddening irrationality.[10-13] They split the world into exaggerated dichotomies of good and evil. They cannot tolerate ambiguity. A middle ground does not exist. These are the patients who—by biologic flaw (intolerance to anxiety and massive oral rage) or by developmental bad luck—have never reconciled the positive and negative extremes of mental life.

Borderline patients present a symptom picture of instability in several areas: interpersonal relations, mood, and self-image.[14] They have a character disorder "without a particular behavioral specialty."[15] Table 10–1 shows the current official diagnostic criteria, but many psychiatrists have seen borderline personality as actually a subset of biologic depressive illness.[16,17] Others have seen it as a variant of better characterized traditional diagnoses, such as hysteria, sociopathy, or alcoholism.[18,19] This is not surprising, since perhaps 13% of alcoholics have borderline personality,[20] and occasionally, patients who appear to be borderline with alcoholism can become quite normal with sustained sobriety;[21] similarly, the occasional patient with major affective disorder and borderline personality will have remission of borderline characteristics when the affective disorder is treated.[22] In this same vein, sociopaths in closed social systems come to resemble borderline personalities,[23] and some borderline patients are notorious for their selfishness and disregard for the rights of others.[8,24]

Subtypes of borderline personality range from the "border with the psychoses," in which the patient is chaotic, explosive, or irrational, to the "border with the neuroses," in which the patient is a depressed,

Table 10-1. Diagnostic Criteria for Borderline Personality Disorder*

---

1. *Impulsivity or unpredictability* in at least two areas that are self-destructive, such as money, sex, gambling, drugs, shoplifting, overeating, or physical self-damage
2. A pattern of *unstable and intense interpersonal relations*, fraught with rapid shifts in attitude, idealization, devaluation, or manipulative exploitation of others
3. Inappropriate, frequently uncontrolled, or extremely *intense anger*
4. *Disturbed identity*, manifested by uncertainty about personal image, gender identity, goals, values, or loyalties, or even by transient confusion in the fundamental sense of the self
5. *Unstable mood*, with marked shifts from a normal to a depressed, anxious, or irritable mood, usually lasting for a few hours and only rarely for more than a few days
6. *Intolerance to being alone*, with frantic efforts to avoid being alone or severe depression and emptiness when alone
7. *Physical self-damage*, such as suicidal gestures, self-mutilation, recurrent accidents, or fighting
8. Chronic feelings of *emptiness or boredom*

---

* These characteristics refer to the patient's usual functioning; they are not limited to episodes of illness. They cause substantial impairment in daily living or severe emotional pain. At least five are required for the diagnosis.

Reproduced with permission from Groves JE: Borderline personality disorder. *N Engl J Med* 1981; 305:259–62. Based on *American Psychiatric Association, Diagnostic and Statistical Manual of Mental Disorders*, ed 3, Washington, DC, American Psychiatric Association, 1980.

empty clinger with a desperate need for companionship even to feel real.[25] Some patients lack a sense of their own realness and adapt like chameleons to the environment of the moment ("as-if personality").[26] But the "core borderline" is the superficially neurotic-looking person with relationships that are intense, unstable, and fleeting.[9,25,27]

Regardless of subtype, borderline patients can undergo a malignant regression and flee treatment or undergo "psychotic transference" and delusions about their caregivers.[27-29] Short episodes of delusional thinking in unstructured situations and under stress are almost pathognomonic,[8,10-13,21,25,27-29] and distinguish borderline personality from neurosis and most other personality disorders. Transient psychotic experiences are probably so characteristic of borderline personalities that some think the omission of these brief psychotic episodes from the official diagnostic criteria[14] is a mistake.[30] This similarity to schizophrenia has long bedeviled nosology,[8,26,30-32] but it has become increasingly clear that the borderline cohort representing the "border" with schizophrenia is small[22]—the "schizotypal borderline"[17,33]—and if there is a border with a biological illness, it is closer to the affective illnesses.[33-36]

Borderline personality is relatively rare, comprising possibly 1% to 5% of the psychiatric population.[21] Despite its small size, the borderline cohort stands out in the general hospital because of floridity of presentation, chronicity and severity of symptoms, and feelings of anger and helplessness stirred up in the caregivers. These patients make themselves medical and psychiatric outcasts because they ruthlessly destroy the very care they crave. They cannot tolerate paradox. Yet they keep themselves both too close and too distant from other human beings.

The psychoanalytic view of the pathogenesis of this disorder sees borderline personality as arising from failure by the individual's mother to engender coherent self-object differentiation in the first 18 months of life.[37-39] Whereas in normal development the child learns to separate from important people with sadness and with anger rather than with despair and rage, the borderline patient does not learn to tolerate the strong negative affects associated with separation[40,41] and continues into adulthood the preoedipal child's clinging, as if others were desperately needed parts of the self rather than separate persons.[24,28,32,42,43] The boundaries between the self and others are so blurred that closeness seems to threaten fusion, and separation bodes emotional starvation. The patient's relation to others is both too close and too distant. Sexuality and dependence are confused with aggression. Needs are experienced as rage. Psychoanalysts hypothesize that long-term relationships of borderline patients disintegrate because of their inability to find the optimal interpersonal distance from others. Ruthlessly dependent, they fear the very closeness they seek. They drive people away with their anger and need. There is little ability to master painful feelings or to channel needs or aggression into creative achievement. Ambivalence is not well tolerated and impulse control is poor. The borderline patient has a fragmented mental representation of the self as all bad and simultaneously as all potent; the self-view is a chaotic, crippled mixture of frightened, shameful, and grandiose images.[1]

Theories of the environmental component of borderline personality focus on neglect or exclusion of the child in the family of origin.[44,45] Psychoanalysts see as central some failure by the patient's mother (probably a borderline personality herself[46]) to catalyze the development of a coherent, stable sense of self in the infant between 6 and 24 months of age.[37-39] In normal development the 1- to 2-year old learns to separate from others with sadness rather than a paranoid tantrum; the borderline personality cannot tolerate the anxiety of separation and carries into adulthood the toddler's angry clinging. The borderline's adult relationships are called "transitional" after the "transitional object"—the beloved, soothing teddy bear or blanket that the toddler uses to remember the mother, to tolerate separations, and to bridge transitions.[47] (Interestingly, there is evidence that adults with other personality disorders for some reason did not adopt transitional objects in infancy,[48] whereas borderline personalities did. But the latter maintain rigid and maladaptive transitional relatedness into adulthood.[49]) The theory holds that the mother especially fails the child during a critical learning stage in the second year of development,[24,37-39] a time when the child learns to evoke soothing memories of the mother.[50-52] The normal child is both glad of reunion and angry at the mother for the separation just ended. The ordinary devoted mother empathizes with the child, deals with the anger equably, does not retaliate, and is in turn forgiven.[47,50] Over many such separations and reunions the child acquires an enduring sense of the lovability of the self and of the abiding patience and goodness of others, and a stable internal image of the mother. It seems, however, that the borderline patient's mother, because of her own poorly developed sense of self, does not allow the infant to get close enough; she unconsciously fears fusion with (and destruction of or by) the child. Yet she cannot let the child separate because of her own fears of being alone; on rapprochement she tends to punish and reject the child for deserting her. Apparently she converts the child into her own transitional object. Used as the imaginary playmate of the mother, the child never grows into an emotionally separate human being.[28]

Be all this as it may, all the causes of borderline personality still remain unknown. But environment and heredity both appear to have a role.[28] Innate intolerance to anxiety and some constitutional tendency toward extremes of rage are accepted even by psychoanalytic theories of borderline personality.[42] Borderline personality closely resembles aspects of traits long thought to run in families,[53-62] and the preponderance of evidence suggests that borderline personalities cluster in families with affective disorders—as many as 38% of borderline patients have first-degree relatives with some affective disorder.[63] Even if, as seems unlikely, borderline personality does not share a constitutional predisposition with affective disorder, there remains the likelihood of an inherited connection with other personality disorders,[64,65] such as narcissistic, antisocial, or passive-aggressive disorders. Two other conditions, episodic dyscontrol syndrome,[66-70] and attention deficit disorder,[71-79] have a familial predisposition and behavioral similarity to borderline personality, and there appears to be a subset of borderlines with this type of organic diathesis.[80,81]

Important for consultation-liaison management are the "primitive ego mechanisms of defense"[1,2,24,42,82-85] of the borderline patient (Table 10-2). These maladaptive cognitive operations may be all too visible during inpatient work with the borderline patient, especially splitting and projective identification. Such patients try to manage their extreme anxiety with these two primitive psychological defense mechanisms that ultimately do more harm than good.

Splitting[24] is by definition a rigid separation of positive and negative thoughts or feelings. Normal persons are ambivalent and can experience two contradictory feeling states at one time; the borderline personality characteristically shifts back and forth, entirely unaware of one feeling state while in another. Sometimes one state is rigidly held while its opposite is projected into the environment. The cause of splitting is unknown; it is said to protect the patient from the anxiety of reconciling contradictory extremes, but at the expense of the already unstable personality. In social systems[86-90] borderlines can split the staff into warring "good" and "bad" factions that unwittingly act out the patient's internal world. Projective identification[82-85] is said to consist of taking an unwanted aspect of the self, such as cruelty or envy, and ascribing it to (projecting it into) another. The patient then unconsciously pressures that person to own the projected attribute. Unaware that a self-fulfilling prophecy is being set up, the recipient complies with the projection and acts it out. These two mechanisms often complement each other, with projective identification being used to "confirm" one side of a one-sided, split view of the world.

Table 10-2. Manifestations of Primitive Defenses in Hospitalized
Borderline Patients

1. *Splitting* refers to a process of keeping apart perceptions and feelings of
   opposite quality. Staff members are divided into "all good" and "all bad" ones,
   as if the patient cannot tolerate the anxiety-producing, ambivalent notion that
   caregivers have human limits and "good" and "bad" qualities at the same time.
2. *Primitive idealization* is the tendency to see some staff as totally "good" in
   order to protect the patient from "bad" staff and painful experiences.
3. *Projective identification* is a tendency to see some staff members as "bad" as
   the patient feels. This gets translated into behavior based on the following kind
   of "logic;" "I'm bad and you take care of me. That means you're as rotten as
   I am or otherwise you wouldn't bother with me."
4. *Primitive denial* is an alternating expungement from consciousness of first one
   and then another perception of opposite quality or a wish so powerful that it
   obliterates crucial aspects of reality contradicting it. For instance, fear may
   cause the patient to deny a serious illness and flee the hospital where it might
   be treated.
5. *Omnipotence and devaluation* represent a shift between the need to establish
   a relationship with a magically powerful staff and a conviction of omnipotence
   in the self which makes all others impotent in comparison. The omnipotent
   caregivers are supposed to deliver the borderline patient from all pain. When
   this does not happen, the staff is seen as impotent and hateful.

Adapted with permission from Groves JE.[1]

While the long-term psychotherapy of the borderline patient may
involve therapeutic undoing of these defenses,[24,91] it is dangerous for a
consultant to confront such defenses willy-nilly in such a brief
encounter as a hospitalization for physical illness. It is crucial, however,
to be aware of their presence. For example, awareness of borderline
splitting will prepare the consultant to deal with the division of the
house staff into "good ones" and "bad ones." Recognition of the patient's
primitive idealization of a doctor may help the consultant prepare for the
furious devaluing which is to follow.

THE GENERAL HOSPITAL SETTING

The medical or surgical ward is a somewhat rigid social system with
its own history, boundaries, hierarchy, customs, and taboos. The introduction of a disturbing patient into this semiclosed system sometimes
places such stress on the system as to cause malfunctions in caregiving
or outright extrusion of the patient from the ward, a situation which
active psychiatric-consultation can prevent.[92-94] Psychotic and disruptive patients are exquisitely vulnerable to caregivers' ordinary imperfec-
tions in communication and consistency, and they are often remarkably

attuned to their caregivers' normal negative feelings—such as anxiety, shame, anger, and depression. Such patients are especially vulnerable to feelings of rejection.[95] After diagnosis and treatment of the patient, the consultant's first priority should be to gauge the amount of distress the staff is under. A psychologically naive house staff may regress to a helpless, frightened, or vengeful position in response to the patient's ingratitude, intractability, impulsivity, manipulativeness, dependency, entitlement, and rage.

Regression in the medical or surgical house staff may emerge as anger and disagreement among staff; it may take the form of inappropriate confrontation or rejection of the patient; or it may manifest itself as a deterioration in the patient's behavior. Regression on a ward seems to occur when there exists a large disparity between what is expected and what is found. Troublesome dissonance of this sort between patient and staff may generally occur in any or all of the following three dimensions[2]: (1) perception of reality, (2) values governing control and aggression, and (3) rules about interpersonal closeness.

The earliest and often best clue to the nature of the dissonance lies in the consultation request[96] (Table 10-3). Its wording, tone, covert and overt messages, its intensity, its timing, and the route over which it travels to reach the consultant all often reflect the dissonance between patient and staff expectations. Consultation is sought when the patient is out of touch with the staff's perception of reality. Such dissonance may range from mild, when the patient is from a different class or culture, to severe, when the patient is psychotic. When the patient is docile, the request is matter-of-fact; when the patient manifests grotesquely sexual or aggressive behavior, the consultant will receive a shrill call for help.

Consultation is sought when the patient's aggression violates staff expectations. The staff expects to be in control of the patient, who is expected to be grateful, obedient, and nondestructive. Dissonance in this dimension may range from mild, when the patient sulks, to severe, when the patient is violent or self-destructive. The tone of such a consultation request ranges from irritation to outright fear, depending on the kind of aggression the patient displays. Consultation is sought when the patient's need for closeness is different from what the staff deems appropriate. The staff expects the patient to be involved with the caregivers but to keep a certain distance. When the patient asks for repeated reassurance or when the patient makes inexhaustible or contradictory demands, a depressed, guilty request often ensues. Arrogant, peremptory consultation requests often herald a hostile-dependent-

Table 10-3. Management of the Disturbing Patient in the Medical or Surgical Setting

Type of Dissonance	Typical Consultation Request	Patient's Behaviors	Consultant's Work with the Patient	Consultant's Work with the Staff
Perception of reality	Nonspecific or confusing request for help; puzzled tone to request	Inappropriate to the realities of the illness or the milieu	Differential diagnosis of any cognitive disorder; neuroleptics and clarifying reality with the patient	Explanation of the patient's reality to the staff; modelling of "reality testing" for the staff
Control of aggression	To control or remove the patient; fearful or angry tone to the request	Menacing, self-destructive, or suicidal	Evaluation of potential danger to patient and others; search for source of the patient's panic	Recommendation of social, chemical, or physical restraint as necessary for safety of the patient
Maintenance of social distance	To take over the care of the patient; depressed or guilty tone to request	1. Dependent	1. Clarifies that some but not all of patient's needs can be realistically met	1. Gives the staff permission to say *no* to patient's most unrealistic or excessive demands
		2. Rejecting	2. Allows the patient some distance and repeatedly appeals to patient's "entitlement" and autonomous, reasonable side for cooperation	2. Diminishes staff's guilt and depression by stating the realistic impossibility of entirely satisfying the patient
		3. Manipulative (dependent *and* rejecting)	3. Sets firm, noninterpretive, nonsadistic limits on manipulation; makes an unsentimental appeal to patient's self-interest; bargains with patient	3. Serves as a forum and buffer for staff hatred toward the patient; articulates their hateful feelings *but behaves* nonsadistically

manipulative patient; depressed, tired requests may fortell an empty, clinging patient.

The primitive defenses of the patient with borderline personality can stimulate staff disagreement (Table 10-2). In order to cope with deep feelings of self-loathing, he or she may see the staff as loathsome—otherwise why would they take care of him (projective identification)? Or he or she may see staff as magically all good, to keep all the badness in the world away (primitive idealization). In order to make sense of a world in which people are both good and bad, such a patient may choose some people on the staff to be "all good" and some as "all bad" (splitting). This "explains" for the patient "why" he feels the way he does; he is caught between good and bad forces *outside* him. When the patient views the staff through his defense of splitting, he may eventually get them to behave as if it were so. The patient will tell an "all good" staff member what terrible things an "all bad" staff member has done or said or thought, and then swear the "good" one to secrecy. As less and less communication takes place and as the patient gets worse and escalates demands, the "good" staff and "bad" staff begin to disagree about the care of the patient, since the borderline may be "good" with "good" staff, and conversely. The remedy for this first depends on re-establishing open staff communication, even if it is hostile, to enable staff to get a well-rounded view of the patient. Firm, nonpunitive limit setting[86,88] (Table 10-4) is crucial for inpatient treatment of the borderline patient, because the patient has to learn that he or she cannot destroy the caregiving system or be destroyed by it, no matter how much he or she may wish this or fear it. It is a natural human instinct to confront such patients angrily, but staff should exercise precautions during in-milieu confrontations.

Avoiding confrontation of narcissistic entitlement is as important as it is difficult.[97] Borderline patients exude an offensive sense of deservedness which is always tempting for an overworked staff to confront

Table 10-4. Guidelines for In-Milieu Management of Patients with Borderline Personality

1. Acknowledge the real stresses in the patient's situation.
2. Avoid breaking down needed defenses.
3. Avoid overstimulation of the patient's wish for closeness.
4. Avoid overstimulation of the patient's rage.
5. Avoid confrontation of narcissistic entitlement.

Adapted with permission from Adler and Buie.[97]

angrily and suddenly. The point is, often the borderline patient has only this sense of entitlement to keep personality together during the multiple stresses of hospitalization. Entitlement is what hope and faith are to some normal persons. Preserving it requires a deliberate effort by an unsplit staff.

Setting limits, avoidance of confrontation, and averting overstimulation of desire for closeness and of rage are difficult to arrange on the fast-paced medical or surgical ward. Prevention of staff splitting is especially difficult because of the dense hierarchical structure. If the patient chooses the nurses to be "all bad" and the doctors to be "all good," the nurses may displace anger to the doctors but be unable to express it because of role-induced sanctions, and the doctors may see the nurses as merely incompetent—and unable to comprehend their plans, ideas, and feelings about the borderline patient. Such situations are fertile ground for the splitting patient and require concerted effort toward open communication within staff.

In general, the earlier in the borderline patient's hospitalization the consultant is called, the more overt is the reason for the consultation and the more effective the intervention; late in the hospitalization, however, the consultant may be urgently called in to see the patient for vague reasons and arrive to find the medical or surgical ward in a shambles, the patient in restraints, and the staff in bitter conflict. Usually nobody is either willing or able to say what has been going on. The patient and staff are seeking relief, not insight.

The patient has a disorganizing effect on the staff, who may regress in response to the patient's dependency, entitlement, and rage. The consultant's role in the management of such a patient should consist of a specialized type of consultee-oriented approach in which countertransference hatred and fear, typically generated in the staff by the borderline patient, are drawn away from the patient and strategically metabolized within the staff-consultant relationship. The consultant should actively promote a behavioral management practicum,[1] placed in the medical chart for reference and as a symbol of the psychiatrist's helping presence. It discusses: (a) clear communication with the patient and among staff, (b) understanding the patient's need for constant personnel, (c) dealing with the patient's entitlement without confronting needed defenses, and (d) setting firm limits on the patient's dependency, manipulativeness, rage, and self-destructive behaviors. The consultant should work to counteract feelings of helplessness in the staff, to neutralize punitive superego in the staff, and to diminish fearfulness toward the patient.

Generally, the consultant's approach should first lead directly to the consultee. The request should be elicited in person or at least on the phone because the medical record does not reveal all problems in the management of the disruptive patient. Then, the consultant should go to the head nurse to get a history of the patient's response to ward routine. Next, the consultant should read the chart and compare medication and management orders with records of medication actually administered to the patient, including medication given as occasion rises (prn). The consultant will have generated some hypotheses about the consultation and is now ready to test them in the examination of the patient. As the consultant proceeds through these steps an orderly plan emerges (Table 10-5).

Generally, the most helpful approach is the consultee-oriented model of mental health consultation[98] which involves thinking of the patient and staff as a single entity and dealing as much as possible with the strong, healthy part. The entity consists of two parts. One part, the borderline patient, has problems with object relations, pathologic behaviors exacerbated under stress, and several self-defeating and infuriating defenses, especially splitting. To prevent being split, the consultant should try to deal mainly with the healthy part, the staff. Since the staff is often closely linked in an unwilling, hateful, and guilty alliance with the patient, and its collective self-esteem is already damaged by encounters with the patient, the consultant should not damage it further by interpreting the staff's pathology.

The attempt to ally with staff rather than the patient is destined to encounter several resistances at the outset. First, the patient will be eager to engage the consultant in order to find out whether he or she is "all good" or "all bad." Second, the staff, needing the patient as a

---

Table 10-5. Order of Priorities in Consultations on Disturbing Patients

1. Physical or social restraints in emergencies—whenever the patient appears about to lose control of violent or self-destructive impulses.
2. Differential diagnosis of the disturbing patient.
3. Identification of staff-patient dissonance.
4. Treatment recommendations—psychologic and pharmacologic, short- and long-term—taking into account the ongoing medical-surgical regimen. Such recommendations should tactfully address staff-patient dissonance as well as the patient's condition.
5. Education of the consultee and staff to reduce dissonance and to lend a conceptual framework for dealing with future patients.
6. Follow-up and disposition planning adequate for the medical and psychiatric needs of the patient.

scapegoat for its sense of failure, wants the consultant to take over the care of the patient completely. Third, neither the staff nor the patient has the energy to understand what is going on; they are in pain and want relief now, preferably by removal of the patient from the ward. The consultant's job is similar in many ways to the treatment of the borderline patient in individual psychotherapy and similar to inpatient psychiatric management; what is different is that the psychiatrist is mainly working with the staff.

The alliance with the staff depends to a large extent upon previous experience with the consultant, staff's view of psychiatry, how long it takes the consultant to answer the consultation request, and how much sense the advice makes. The consultant's alliance with the borderline patient is dramatically less important in terms of outcome than the alliance with the staff. Ideally, the patient should be seen only briefly if there are enough data from corollary sources to make the diagnosis. The patient can be told that the consultant will work mainly with staff and will be seen infrequently. Aside from a brief history of the immediate stress and precipitant for the consultation request, no alliance with the patient should be sought.

Visiting the patient should be reserved for the specific purpose of the consultant's alliance with the staff. He or she goes to see the patient only (1) when a magical gesture of "taking over" is needed to comfort a desperate staff, (2) when staff members feel the consultant does not know how much they are suffering, and (3) when the staff needs a specific model or example for carrying out the consultant's recommendations, for example, limit setting.

The consultation note by its tone, specific helpful information, and description of the patient in a way the staff can immediately recognize will remain in a medical record day and night as a tangible symbol of the consultant's helping presence. It should outline the request, history, mental status at the hour of the examination, the past psychiatric history, and behavior on the ward. It should be explicit about medications, suicide, and the potential for violence. It should include specific, concrete management recommendations. For example, one might conclude a consultation note in the following fashion for a borderline patient who has been spitting in her hyperalimentation line:[1]

> *Impression:* Ms B is thought to have a chronic, severe character disorder sometimes called "borderline personality," meaning that she lies somewhere between neurosis and psychosis diagnostically and has only marginal social adjustment.
> *Recommendations:* (1) Continue haloperidol 2–10 mg orally bid prn. (2)

Have brief, *daily* staff conferences to compare notes and reach a consensus about her surgical treatment plan. (3) Try to have the same staff members work with Ms B each day; bear in mind that she tends to panic at each change of shift. (4) Set firm limits on her multiple and contradictory demands. She is quick to rage when her demands are not met and may threaten suicide. *Do not imply that Ms B does not deserve the things she demands*, but rather say over and over again that you understand what she is asking but because you feel she *deserves* the best possible care, you are going to continue to follow the course dictated by your experience and judgment. If she continues spitting in her hyperalimentation line, assure her that physical restraint will ensue. (These limits do not mean that she should not be allowed to complain but you need not tolerate more than twice as much as you would from the average patient.) (5) Carry out suicide precautions; search her luggage.

The consultant has addressed dissonance arising from the patient's version of reality, her tendency to act out, and her demandingness, neediness, and rage. The consultant has given a mandate for open communication and daily staff conferences to prevent staff splitting. Constant personnel and supportive environment are recommended. Firm limits, without challenging the patient's sense of entitlement, are set forth explicitly. The task now becomes that of seeing that recommendations are effected. There is nothing more frustrating than to labor to devise a treatment plan and then find that it is not carried out. When this happens, the consultant will find that the source of resistance is unresolved staff-patient dissonance. The consultant can ensure that recommendations are effected by systematically analyzing and reducing dissonances that baffle staff effectiveness.

Notice that nowhere in the above discussion is the inferred unconscious motivation of the patient or of the staff brought to the attention of either. This is what is meant by "noninterpretive" intervention. Psychoanalytic interpretations foster a temporary regression and have no place in the consultation with the disruptive medical/surgical patient.[1,99] Instead of interpretation, the consultant should analyze and reduce dissonance by speaking of its behavioral roots and consequences and resisting the temptation to illuminate interesting unconscious processes and conflicts.

In terms of specific recommendations, medication can be helpful. There is a growing psychopharmacologic literature on borderline patients.[100-104] (Table 10-6). Some suggest that tricyclic antidepressants may be of value in patients who resemble neurotic depressives, phobic-anxious patients, and withdrawn, obsessional patients if they appear to

Table 10-6. Pharmacologic Management of the Borderline Patient

Minor tranquilizers are acceptable antianxiety agents. They are, in fact, so acceptable that many borderline patients become dependent on them, especially on diazepam.

Antipsychotic agents are quite useful during transient psychotic episodes and, in low doses, in some chaos-ridden patients. Long-term treatment with these agents is usually unacceptable to the patient because they produce "mental numbness," and to the physician because of the risk of tardive dyskinesia.

Lithium carbonate has often been reported useful in borderline patients who have a prominent mood-cycling component to their symptom picture, and in some violence-prone patients in whom rage may represent a form of manic behavior. Lithium is toxic and risky in suicidal patients.

Tricyclic antidepressants may benefit some borderline patients—not necessarily those most depressed or having vegetative symptoms of depression. These agents help with anxiety and insomnia. There is no particular pattern of symptoms that predicts a favorable response. Tricyclic antidepressants may be contraindicated in the violent patients discussed above, because manic or violent episodes may be provoked. These drugs are toxic in overdosage.

Monoamine oxidase inhibitor antidepressants are currently fashionable for a trial in "atypical" depressions and especially in borderline patients with hypersensitivity to rejection and an avoidant, phobic component to their presentation. Despite the intimidating dietary restrictions required with these drugs, they may be uniquely useful in borderlines (and others) with phobias. Suicide is easily effected with these drugs.

Reproduced with permission from Groves JE: Borderline personality disorder. *N. Engl J Med* 1981; 305:259–262.

have a phasic mood disorder. At the other end of the spectrum are the chaotic, inappropriate, negative, and hostile patients and the extremely labile patients. For such patients, antipsychotic medication may be valuable.[102] Some suggest lithium carbonate also is of value in dampening mood swings in such patients or suggest monoamine oxidase inhibitors may be useful for those who resemble "hysteroid dysphoric" patients.[104] The psychopharmacologic management of the borderline patient is a source of controversy. Opinions abound but controlled studies do not exist.

On a medical or surgical ward nonpsychotic disruptive patients are usually given sedative-hypnotics. If such a regimen is not effective it tends to tantalize and anger the patient and staff. The upshot of such a trial may be a patient who is more out of control on medication than off or a patient who is moving toward habituating doses of sedative-hypnotics. If the patient does not respond well to hypnotics or if reality-testing or impulse control are marginal, an antipsychotic agent in adequate dosages should be begun without delay.

Dissonance arising when the patient is out of touch with the staff's reality is reduced when the consultant explains the nature of the dissonance to the staff and when the staff tests reality for the patient: The term "reality testing" is much bandied about but staff may nonetheless try to humor the patient owing to a fear that to challenge paranoid thinking or delusional notions will make the patient worse. The consultant may need to model reality testing for the staff.[2]

PATIENT I don't trust you.
CONSULTANT Why should you—you've never seen me before. I'm Dr Smith. Dr Jones asked me to help you with your anxiety.
PATIENT Dr Jones hates me.
CONSULTANT Dr Jones is irritated with your pulling out your intervenous tubing, but he isn't going to harm you.
PATIENT You're like all of them—want to kill a guy.
CONSULTANT You're wrong about that. We want to help you get over this infection.
PATIENT Bullshit!
CONSULTANT No bullshit.

Dissonance arising when the patient has different values governing control and aggression is typically reduced when the consultant defines the range of appropriate responses to patient anger, from supporting the sulking patient or giving in to a mildly overcontrolling patient, to absolute limits on a violent patient. The staff fear overreacting and the consultant reduces their anxiety by outlining the management of varying degrees of aggression. Control of violent and aggressive behavior is an issue in treating only a small minority of patients in the general hospital. Disruptions are mostly born of self-protective or fearful impulses in the confused or delirious patient. Rarely, however, will a patient become dangerous. And in these rare instances, the most common warning is fear; someone becomes scared of the patient. Staff almost never fear delirious behavior, controllable anger, or senile pique but they do tend to become edgy, then wary, and then frightened of violence. This intuition in the caregivers is often all the warning the consultant gets before an explosion. Ominous signs in the patient are (1) rapidly increasing demandingness, (2) more frequent and intense anger, especially with abusive language, (3) mounting agitation and paranoia, and (4) an implacable, irrestible crescendo of menace. _Before_ any decision about physical restraint of the potentially violent patient is made, hospital security guards should be _standing by_ on the ward. This is a _first_ step in the decision-making process. Security can always be dismissed with thanks after standing by, but to delay summoning help until _after_ such a decision risks panicking the paranoid or borderline patient, who may have an uncanny ability to sense an impending confrontation.

Dissonance arising when the patient's need for closeness seems inappropriate to the staff is often effectively reduced when the consultant gives the staff permission to say no to a patient who demands too much. Giving is a familiar role for caregivers but they may feel guilty when they cannot satisfy all the patient's needs. Much of this type of dissonance arises when the staff feels trapped between a sense of obligation to give and an angry desire to withhold.

Pathologic dependency presents in one of its extremes as *manipulativeness*—an intense, convert, contradictory, self-defeating attempt to get needs met.[1,3] It is the behavioral manifestation of a need by the patient to get close to but at the same time to maintain safe distance from sources of emotional support. (Occasional patients feel so empty that, paradoxically, to get needs met threatens them with engulfment; they are so famished that closeness may actually make them feel merged with someone else and therefore not really alive.) Such patients seem to have a deathly fear of that which they most crave. In limit-setting confrontations with manipulative, entitled patients the consultant may have to model the firmness, repetition, and appeal to the patient's sense of entitlement (rather than an assault on it) for the caregiving staff:

CONSULTANT . . . Now what is this about your not taking the antibiotics that Dr Black has prescribed?

PATIENT I am not gonna talk especially with *that* one here. Listen, I don't like her face and you can't force me, force this crap down my throat!

CONSULTANT Well, you don't have to like this lady here, and there's no particular reason why you should have to like *me* either, but there are several very good reasons why you should take your antibiotics that Dr Black has prescribed for you.

PATIENT Yeah, well, I'm not going to take that damn stuff. Get me a lawyer! I know my rights!

CONSULTANT You have every right to the very best medical care we can give you. Why is it that you feel so strongly against the antibiotics that Dr Black has prescribed for you?

PATIENT It's no good and, besides, Dr. Green said I oughtn't ever take antibiotics.

CONSULTANT Dr. Green said you should *never* take antibiotics? *Really?*

PATIENT He said they'd kill me.

CONSULTANT Really? How come?

PATIENT [*Shouts*] Are you saying that Dr. Green is a liar?

[*Here the consultant realizes that he is overstimulating the rage of the patient and allowing himself to be split against Dr Green. He*

> *decides to lead back to an appeal to the patient's sense of entitlement.*]
>
> CONSULTANT Dr. Green...was he your doctor from before?
>
> PATIENT Best damn doctor I ever had and one million times better than the rest of you put together!
>
> CONSULTANT Sounds like you like him a lot. He saw you through that other time you were in hospital?
>
> PATIENT Yes.
>
> CONSULTANT And at that time you didn't need antibiotics.
>
> PATIENT Listen, goddammit, I am not going to take that crap!
>
> CONSULTANT Well, the reason I ask is that you now have a fever from this infection and we on the staff feel that you deserve to have it treated in the best way possible.
>
> PATIENT Dr Black, what does she know?
>
> CONSULTANT Well, we *all* feel—
>
> PATIENT I am not...look, Dr Green said that I shouldn't take antibiotics.
>
> CONSULTANT —that you deserve the best possible treatment of this infection. I'm sure that if Dr Green were here now he would *want* you to have the very best possible treatment of this infection, that he would agree that you deserve—
>
> PATIENT Well get him here. Get him on the phone.
>
> CONSULTANT —would agree that you deserve—
>
> PATIENT Well, call him up. Get him on the phone.
>
> CONSULTANT I can't. [*Pauses.*] Don't you think that if Dr Green knew you were suffering from an infection that he would want you to have antibiotics, that he would want you to get the very best treatment, which you deserve.
>
> PATIENT No.
>
> CONSULTANT You don't feel you deserve the best possible care of this infection?
>
> PATIENT Get her out of here! I don't like her face.
>
> CONSULTANT We're going to leave you now for a little while and I hope that you'll think it over and allow yourself to have the kind of good medical care you're entitled to.

The consultant has to keep uppermost in mind the appeal to the entitlement and not get drawn into logical or illogical arguments. Moreover, it is important to avoid interpreting the resistance to cooperation as a fear of dependency needs, a tactic which would at best leave the patient somewhat bewildered. Repetition is crucial. Encounters to engage compliance often have to be repeated two or three times at ten-minute intervals before the patient agrees, for instance, to take medication.

Dependent, manipulative patients stir up sadism in the caregivers which inhibits the setting of firm, effective limits. The staff on a medical or surgical ward routinely and effectively help most patients establish better contact with reality, aid them in finding appropriate interpersonal distance, and suffer with and support them when they are angry and sad. What is it about the disturbing patient which so compromises these intuitive functions in the staff?

Regression in the staff under the pressures of the borderline patient's character pathology is probably at least partly due to the subtlety of the patient's distortions of reality and the grossness of the patient's dependency and rage. The caregiver's ideal[5] is "to know all, to love all, to heal all" and especially alien to the caregiver is to harbor malice and aversion—hatred—toward sick people. But the borderline patient can generate a lively sense of sadism because unceasing demands make us feel guilty and worthless and unremitting anger makes us feel frightened and hurt. It is probably the *additional* heavy burden of having to deny or disown from the self such unwanted, hateful, and sadistic feelings that most compromises the staff's effective functioning. The consultant's best strategy, then, is to create a noninterpretive relationship with the staff in which such negative feelings can be acknowledged and dealt with.

The consultant does this by supporting the staff's collective self-esteem by reinforcing strengths rather than pointing out weaknesses, by teaching, by lending a conceptual framework to mitigate anxiety, by modelling interactions that encourage identification with an effective clinician, and—most of all—by matter-of-factly stating that such patients stir up hatred even in the best of caregivers.

> CONSULTANT Now let me see if I understand...you don't feel you're getting anywhere with her because—because why?
>
> STAFF A Well, it's just that—oh heck—all the things we've just talked about. She's bitchy, she's a liar. She's manipulative. She doesn't listen. She tells lies about us.
>
> CONSULTANT And the team meetings?
>
> STAFF A Well, they've helped a certain extent—at least we're not at each other's throats. At least we can compare notes and sort out the lies... but we—or at least *I* can't get anywhere.
>
> CONSULTANT Even though the meetings have helped and her behavior has settled down, you don't *feel* like you're getting anywhere.
>
> STAFF A I can't do it—I mean, can't get her to do what's best for her, can't get her to listen to me—I mean, it's not like I'm wanting to punish her, not like I *want* her to suffer with the dressing changes and so on—but like she won't mind me and acts like I'm *trying* to hurt her——
>
> STAFF B She's just the same with me! I mean, like you go near her and she yells the roof down. I can't stand it any more. I just don't go near her any more because I don't like being accused of deliberately hurting her.

CONSULTANT So everybody feels the same way—she won't listen, she lies, and she makes us feel like we're deliberately hurting her. [*Pause.*] Sounds like she needs a *spanking*. . . .
[*Pause, then A and B laugh explosively.*]
STAFF A I'm glad *you* said that, not me!
STAFF B I've thought that myself!
CONSULTANT Well, we've all thought it. She makes me mad as hell. You folks work your guts out but she makes you feel like you're sadists or something. She's the kind of patient who makes us *wish* something bad would happen to her—or makes us stay away from her, as you have. [*Nods to B.*]
STAFF A You know, if she didn't make me so mad at her, I think I wouldn't mind so much that she doesn't listen or tells lies.
CONSULTANT Exactly! She makes us mad and stirs up rejecting feelings —feelings of hate that are perfectly normal in dealing with this type of patient—and as a consequence, we feel guilty, feel like we are bad somehow for having these normal feelings of anger.
STAFF B But what do we do to get rid of the angry feelings?
CONSULTANT I'm not sure we *can* "get rid" of the hate she causes us to feel—all we can do is not let it interfere with our job with her—you know, she's pulling what I like to call the "skunk maneuver." [*A and B laugh.*] You know what I mean: her behavior makes us so mad that she "stinks" us away—I try *not* to deny the bad smell but, even knowing that I'm very angry, keep on trying to do my job, keep on setting firm, consistent limits.

Whenever the staff brings even a hint of negative reference to the patient, the consultant can recognize it by saying something like, "Yeah, these patients *are* manipulative and irritating as hell!" Or, "Everybody dislikes dealing with this kind of patient—I know *I* do." This personalization, juxtaposed with the consultant's own *nonsadistic behavior toward the patient*, legitimizes hostility toward the patient but shares it among the staff rather than inflicting it upon the patient.

Termination of the hospitalization of the pathologically dependent patient is fraught with hazard. The patient may not only intensify disruptive behavior to prolong the hospital stay but—simultaneously—try to leave prematurely. The borderline patient may secretly infect dressings or intravenous lines with saliva or feces and develop a fever while threatening to leave the hospital against advice. Or the patient may increase suicidal gestures, such as wrist-slashing,[105] in order to manipulate the staff. Firm limits on sabotage and elopement should be discussed with the staff. Around termination, they should be more observant of the patient and more visible and firm. A specific discharge date should be set and firmly adhered to[105] despite the predictable worsening in the patient's psychological status.

After the patient has left, it is good for the consultant to return to the ward once more to review the treatment of the patient and to share some of the consultant's own feelings.[1] In this way, the consultant not only "terminates" with the staff but prepares the way for future work with the next borderline patient who comes to the ward.

REFERENCES

1. Groves JE: Management of the borderline patient on a medical or surgical ward: the psychiatric consultant's role. *Int J Psychiatry Med* 1975; 6:337–348.
2. Groves JE: Psychotic and borderline patients, in Hackett TP, Cassem NH (eds): *The MGH Handbook of General Hospital Psychiatry*, ed 1. St Louis, CV Mosby Co, 1978, pp 174–208.
3. Groves JE: Taking care of the hateful patient. *N Engl J Med* 1978; 298:883–887.
4. Stoudemire A, Thompson TL II: The borderline personality in the medical setting. *Ann Intern Med* 1982; 96:76–79.
5. Maltsberger JT, Buie DH: Countertransference hate in the treatment of suicidal patients. *Arch Gen Psychiatry* 1974; 30:625–633.
6. Adler G: Valuing and devaluing in the psychotherapeutic process. *Arch Gen Psychiatry* 1970; 22:454–461.
7. Adler G: Helplessness in the helpers. *Br J Med Psychol* 1972; 45:315–326.
8. Knight RP: Borderline states. *Bull Menninger Clin* 1953; 17:1–12.
9. Grinker RR: Neurosis, psychosis, and the borderline states, in Freedman AM, Kaplan HI, Sadock BJ (eds): *Comprehensive Textbook of Psychiatry*, ed 2. Baltimore, Williams & Wilkins Co, 1975, pp. 845–850.
10. Sheehy M, Goldsmith L, Charles E: A comparative study of borderline patients in a psychiatric outpatient clinic. *Am J Psychiatry* 1980; 137: 1374–1379.
11. Perry JC, Klerman GL: Clinical features of the borderline personality disorder. *Am J Psychiatry* 1980; 137:165–173.
12. Perry JC, Klerman GL: The borderline patient: a comparative analysis of four sets of diagnostic criteria. *Arch Gen Psychiatry* 1978; 35:141–150.
13. Gunderson JG, Kolb JE: Discriminating features of borderline patients. *Am J Psychiatry* 1978; 35:792–796.
14. American Psychiatric Association: *Diagnostic and Statistical Manual of Mental Disorders*, ed 3. Washington, DC American Psychiatric Association, 1980.
15. Mack JE: Afterword, in Mack JE (ed): *Borderline States in Psychiatry*. New York, Grune & Stratton, Inc, 1975, pp 135–138.
16. Klein DF: Psychopharmacology and the borderline patient, in Mack JE (ed): *Borderline States in Psychiatry*. New York, Grune & Stratton Inc, 1975, pp 75–91.
17. Stone MH: *The Borderline Syndrome: Constitution, Personality, and Adaptation*, New York, McGraw-Hill Book Co, 1980.
18. Guze SB: Differential diagnosis of the borderline personality syndrome, in Mack JE (ed): *Borderline States in Psychiatry*. New York, Grune & Stratton,

Inc, 1975, pp 69–74.

19. Welner A, Liss JL, Robins E: Personality disorder. II. Follow-up. *Br J Psychiatry* 1974; 124:359–366.

20. Nace EP, Saxon JJ, Shore N: A comparison of borderline and nonborderline alcoholic patients. *Arch Gen Psychiatry* 1983; 40:54–56.

21. Vaillant GE, Perry JC: Personality disorders, in Kaplan HI, Freedman AM, Sadock BJ (eds): *Comprehensive Textbook of Psychiatry*, ed. 3. Baltimore, Williams & Wilkins Co, 1980, pp 1562–1590.

22. Pope HG, et al: The validity of DSM-III borderline personality disorder. *Arch Gen Psychiatry* 1983; 40:23–30.

23. Vaillant GE: Sociopathy as a human process. *Arch Gen Psychiatry* 1975; 32:178–183.

24. Kernberg O: *Borderline Conditions and Pathological Narcissism.* New York, Jason Aronson, Inc, 1975.

25. Grinker RR, Werble B, Drye R: *The Borderline Syndrome: a Behavioral Study of Ego-Functions.* New York, Basic Books, Inc, 1968.

26. Deutsch H: Some forms of emotional disturbance and their relationship to schizophrenia. *Psychoanal Q* 1942; 11:301–321.

27. Gunderson JG, Singer MT: Defining borderline patients: an overview. *Am J Psychiatry* 1975; 132:1–10.

28. Groves JE: Current concepts in psychiatry: borderline personality disorder. *N Engl J Med* 1981; 305:259–262.

29. Kolb JE, Gunderson JG: Diagnosing borderline patients with a semi-structured interview. *Arch Gen Psychiatry* 1980; 37:37–41.

30. Gunderson JG: The relatedness of borderline and schizophrenic disorders. *Schizophr Bull* 1979; 5:17–22.

31. Gunderson JG, Carpenter WT, Strauss JS: Borderline and schizophrenic patients: a comparative study. *Am J Psychiatry* 1975; 132:1257–1264.

32. Modell A: Primitive object relationships and the predisposition to schizophrenia. *Int J Psychoanal* 1963; 44:282–292.

33. McGlashan TH: The borderline syndrome, is it a variant of schizophrenia or affective disorder? *Arch Gen Psychiatry* 1983; 40:1319–1323.

34. Stone MH: Borderline syndromes: a consideration of subtypes and an overview, directions for research. *Psychiatr Clin North Am* 1981; 4:3–24.

35. Akiskal HS: Subaffective disorders: dysthymic, cyclothymic, and bipolar II disorders in the "borderline" realm. *Psychiatr Clin North Am* 1981; 4:25–60.

36. Carroll BJ, et al: Neuroendocrine evaluation of depression in borderline patients. *Psychiatr Clin North Am* 1981; 4:89–100.

37. Mahler MS: *On Human Symbiosis and the Vicissitudes of Individuation.* New York, International Universities Press, 1968.

38. Kernberg OF: Early ego integration and object relations. *Ann NY Acad Sci* 1972; 193:233–247.

39. Shapiro ER: The psychodynamics and developmental psychology of the borderline patient: a review of the literature. *Am J Psychiatry* 1978; 135:1305–1315.

40. Zetzel (Rosenberg) E: Anxiety and the capacity to bear it. *Int J Psychoanal* 1949; 30:1–12.

41. Winnicott DW: The capacity to be alone. *Int J Psychoanal* 1958; 39:

416–420.

42. Kernberg O: Structural derivatives of object relationships. *Int J Psychoanal* 1966; 47:236–253.

43. Kernberg O: The treatment of patients with borderline personality organization. *Int J Psychoanal* 1968; 49:600–619.

44. Walsh F: Family Study 1976: 14 new borderline cases, in Grinker RR, Werble B (eds): *The Borderline Patient.* New York, Jason Aronson, Inc, 1977, 157–177.

45. Gunderson JG, Kerr J, Englund DW: The families of borderlines: a comparative study. *Arch Gen Psychiatry* 1980; 37:27–33.

46. Masterson JF: The borderline adult: therapeutic alliance and transference. *Am J Psychiatry* 1978; 135:437–441.

47. Winnicott DW: *Playing and Reality.* New York, Basic Books, Inc, 1971.

48. Horton PC, Louy JW, Coppolillo HP: Personality disorder and transitional relatedness. *Arch Gen Psychiatry* 1974; 30:618–622.

49. Arkema PH: The borderline personality and transitional relatedness. *Am J Psychiatry* 1981; 138: 172–177.

50. Adler G, Buie DH: Aloneness and borderline psychopathology: the possible relevance of child developmental issues. *Int J Psychoanal* 1979; 60:83–96.

51. Robertson J, Robertson J: Young children in brief separation: a fresh look. *Psychoanal Study Child* 26:264–315, 1971.

52. Fraiberg S: Libidinal object constancy and mental representation. *Psychoanal Study Child* 1969; 24:9–47.

53. Hutchings B, Mednick SA: Registered criminality in the adoptive and biological parents of registered male adoptees, in Fieve RR, Brill H, Rosenthal D (eds): *Genetic Research in Psychiatry,* New York, International Universities Press, 1974, pp 105–24.

54. Bohman M: Some genetic aspects of alcoholism and criminality. *Arch Gen Psychiatry* 1978, 35:269–276.

55. Cadoret RJ, Cain CA, Grove WM: Development of alcoholism in adoptees raised apart from alcoholic biologic relatives. *Arch Gen Psychiatry* 1980; 37:561–563.

56. Frances RJ, Timm S, Bucky S: Studies of familial and nonfamilial alcoholism. I. Demographic studies. *Arch Gen Psychiatry* 1980; 37: 564–566.

57. Stone MH: The borderline syndrome: evolution of the term, genetic aspects, and prognosis. *Am J Psychother* 1977; 31:345–365.

58. Siever LJ, Gunderson JG: Genetic determinants of borderline conditions. *Schizophr Bull* 1979; 5:59–86.

59. Miner GD: The evidence for genetic components in the neuroses. *Arch Gen Psychiatry* 1973; 29:111–118.

60. Crowe RR: An adoption study of antisocial personality. *Arch Gen Psychiatry* 1974; 31:785–791.

61. Goodwin DW, et al: Drinking problems in adopted and non-adopted sons of alcoholics. *Arch Gen Psychiatry* 1974; 31:164–169.

62. Winokur G, Crowe RR: Personality disorders, in Freedman AM, Kaplan HI, Sadock BJ (eds): *Comprehensive Textbook of Psychiatry,* ed 2. Baltimore, Williams & Wilkins Co, 1975, pp 1279–1297.

63. Soloff PH, Millward JW: Psychiatric disorders in the families of borderline

patients. *Arch Gen Psychiatry* 1983; 40:37–44.

64. Rinsley DB: Dynamic and developmental issues in borderline and related "spectrum" disorders. *Psychiatr Clin North Am* 1981; 4:117–132.

65. Torgersen S: Genetic and nosological aspects of schizotypal and borderline personality disorders. *Arch Gen Psychiatry* 1984; 41:546–554.

66. Monroe RR: *Episodic Behavioral Disorders, a Psychodynamic and Neurophysiologic Analysis.* Cambridge, Harvard University Press, 1970.

67. Robins LN: *Deviant Children Grown Up: Sociologic and Psychiatric Study of Sociopathic Personality.* Baltimore, Williams & Wilkins Co, 1966.

68. Mark VH, Ervin FR: *Violence and the Brain.* New York, Harper & Row Publishers, Inc, 1970.

69. Detre TP, Jarecki HG: *Modern Psychiatric Treatment.* Philadelphia, JB Lippincott Co, 1971.

70. Bach-y-Rita G, et al: Episodic dyscontrol: a study of 130 violent patients. *Am J Psychiatry* 1971; 127:1473–1478.

71. Cantwell DP: Psychiatric illness in families of hyperactive children. *Arch Gen Psychiatry* 1972; 27:414–417.

72. Morrison JR, Stewart MA: A family study of the hyperactive child syndrome. *Biol Psychiatry* 1971; 3:189–195.

73. Morrison JR, Stewart MA: The psychiatric status of the legal families of adopted hyperactive children. *Arch Gen Psychiatry* 1973; 28:888–891.

74. Mann HB, Greenspan SI: The identification and treatment of adult brain dysfunction. *Am J Psychiatry* 1976; 133:1013–1017.

75. Quitkin FM, Klein DF: Two behavioral syndromes in young adults related to possible minimal brain dysfunction. *J Psychiatr Res* 1969; 7:131–142.

76. Mendelson W, Johnson N, Stewart MA: Hyperactive children as teenagers: a follow-up study. *J Nerv Ment Dis* 1971; 153:273–279.

77. Richmond JS, Young JR, Groves JE: Violent dyscontrol responsive to *d*-amphetamine. *Am J Psychiatry* 1978; 135:365–366.

78. Wood DR, et al: Minimal brain dysfunction in adults. *Arch Gen Psychiatry* 1976; 33:1453–1460.

79. Morrison JR, Minkhoft K: Explosive personality as a sequel to the hyperactive-child syndrome. *Compr Psychiatry* 1975; 16:343–348.

80. Andrulonis PA, et al: Organic brain dysfunction and the borderline syndrome. *Psychiatr Clin North Am* 1981; 4:47–66.

81. Andrulonis PA, et al: Borderline personality subcategories. *J Nerv Ment Dis* 1982; 170:670–679.

82. Kernberg O: Borderline personality organization. *J Am Psychoanal Assoc* 1967; 15:641–685.

83. Ogden TH: On projective identification. *Int J Psychoanal* 1979; 60:357–373.

84. Kernberg O: Neurosis, psychosis and the borderline states, in Kaplan HI, Freedman AM, Sadock BJ (eds): *Comprehensive Textbook of Psychiatry,* ed. 3. Baltimore, Williams and Wilkins Co, 1980, pp 1079–1092.

85. Nadelson T: Borderline rage and the therapist's response. *Am J Psychiatry* 1977; 134:748–751.

86. MacVicar K: Splitting and identification with the aggressor in assaultive borderline patients. *Am J Psychiatry* 1978; 135:229–231.

87. Main TF: The ailment. *Br J Med Psychol* 1957; 30:129–145.

88. Adler G: Hospital treatment of borderline patients. *Am J Psychiatry* 1973;

130:32–35.
89. Burnham DL: The special-problem patient: victim or agent of splitting? *Psychiatry* 1966; 29:105–122.
90. Stanton AH, Schwartz MS: *The Mental Hospital*. New York, Basic Books, Inc, 1954.
91. Kernberg O: Structural interviewing. *Psychiatr Clin North Am* 1981; 4:169–195.
92. Reding GR, Maguire B: Nonsegregated acute psychiatric admissions to general hospitals—continuity of care within the community hospital. *N Engl J Med* 1973; 289:185–189.
93. Meyer E, Mendelson M: Psychiatric consultation with patients on medical and surgical wards: patterns and processes. *Psychiatry* 1961; 24:197–220.
94. Lipowski ZJ: Consultation-liaison psychiatry: an overview. *Am J Psychiatry* 1974; 131:623–630.
95. Reich P, Kelly MJ: Suicide attempts by hospitalized medical and surgical patients. *N Engl J Med* 1976; 294:298–301.
96. Kucharski A, Groves JE: The so-called "inappropriate" consultation request on a medical or surgical ward. *Int J Psychiatry Med* 1976–1977; 7:209–220.
97. Adler G, Buie DH: The misuses of confrontation with borderline patients. *Int J Psychoanal Psychother* 1972; 1:109–120.
98. Caplan G: *The Theory and Practice of Mental Health Consultation*. New York, Basic Books, Inc, 1970.
99. Gordon C, Beresin E: Conflicting models for the inpatient management of borderline patients. *Am J Psychiatry* 1983; 140:979–983.
100. Klerman GL: Atypical affective disorders, in Kaplan HI, Freedman AM, Sadock BJ (eds): *Comprehensive Textbook of Psychiatry*, ed 3. Baltimore, Williams & Wilkins Co, 1980, pp 1339–1342.
101. Cole JO: Drug therapy of borderline patients. *McLean Hosp J* 1980; 5:110–125.
102. Brinkley JR, Beitman BD, Friedel RO: Low-dose neuroleptic regimens in the treatment of borderline patients. *Arch Gen Psychiatry* 1979; 36:319–326.
103. Klein DF: Psychopharmacological treatment and delineation of borderline disorders, in Hartocollis P (ed): *Borderline Personality Disorders: The Concept, the Syndrome, the Patient*. New York, International Universities Press, 1977, pp 365–383.
104. Liebowitz MR, Klein DF: Interrelationship of hysteroid dysphoria and borderline personality disorder. *Psychiatr Clin North Am* 1981; 4:67–88.
105. Grunebaum HU, Klerman GL: Wrist slashing. *Am J Psychiatry* 1967; 124:527–534.

11

Psychotic Patients

JAMES E. GROVES and THEO C. MANSCHRECK

"He can't stay here—he's crazy!"
— *House officer to consultant.*

The psychotic patient with a serious physical illness can become a hospital orphan. In practice, patients with a combination of serious psychiatric and somatic illnesses tend to remain on general hospital wards because life-threatening medical or surgical conditions overrule other considerations. Often the psychiatric consultant must coordinate the treatment and effect the behavioral management of the psychotic patient. This chapter is a practicum for the consultant who becomes responsible for such situations. The two general areas of the consultant's work are (1) the patient and (2) the consultee and house staff. Neglect of either area rapidly undermines the other.

THE PATIENT

Work with the patient begins with differential diagnosis; intelligent differential diagnosis begins with an awareness of the multiple manifestations and many causes of disorders of behavior and thinking. Initial discriminations are made among conditions that fall into the following categories:

1. A formal or content disorder of thinking as shown on mental status examination
2. Acute onset, rapid deterioration, and sudden personality change without history of similar episodes
3. Impairment of consciousness, orientation, memory, perception, or intellectual function (eg, verbal, spatial, or arithmetical abilities)
4. Physical, neurologic, or laboratory abnormalities

Illnesses that present symptoms in the first and second categories, but not in the third and fourth, tend to have nonorganic diagnoses, eg, schizophrenia. It is important to be aware, however, that a catastrophic deterioration of personality in persons previously functioning at a high level (category 2) often signifies an organic illness such as encephalitis. When abnormalities in intellect (category 3) are found, especially when there are also physical, neurologic, or laboratory abnormalities, the clinician's suspicion of organic causes of psychosis should be increased. "Psychosis" is used here in its broadest sense as any state in which the patient is out of touch with reality. In Table 11-1 is a list of conditions in which the patient may appear psychotic.

Table 11-1. Diagnostic Possibilities When the Patient Appears out of Touch with Reality

Psychiatric
Schizophrenia, acute or chronic
Manic-depressive illness, manic or
  depressed
Personality disorders (eg, borderline)
Stress (reactive) disorders
  (eg, traumatic war neurosis)
Episodic dyscontrol
Ganser's syndrome

Neurologic
Head trauma
Space-occupying lesions (eg, tumors,
  hydrocephalus)
Vascular lesions (eg, infarcts,
  hemorrhages)
Seizure disorders, especially
  psychomotor seizures
Degenerative diseases (eg,
  Alzheimer's, Pick's, and
  Huntington's diseases)
Infections of the CNS

Endocrine
Thyroid disorders
Parathyroid disorders
Adrenal dysfunction
Pituitary dysfunction
Diabetes mellitus

Metabolic
Fluid and electrolyte imbalance
Respiratory failure
Cardiac failure
Hepatic failure
Renal failure

Hypoglycemia, hyperglycemia,
  ketoacidosis
Porphyria
Wilson's disease
Folate-responsive homocystinuria
Adult phenylketonuria
Periodic catatonia

Deficiency states
Pernicious anemia
Beriberi, Wernicke-Korsakoff
  syndrome
Pellagra
Pyridoxine deficiency

Postoperative states
Postoperative delirium
Postoperative psychosis
Postoperative depression

Systemic illnesses
Carcinomatosis
Infections (bacterial, fungal,
  parasitic)
Viral syndromes, hepatitis,
  mononucleosis
Starvation, dehydration, exposure,
  heatstroke
Collagen and autoimmune diseases

Abstinence phenomena
Alcohol withdrawal, delirium
  tremens
Barbiturate withdrawal
Narcotic withdrawal

Intoxications
  Alcohol (eg, hallucinosis, pathologic
    intoxication)
  Barbiturates
  Hallucinogens (eg, amphetamines,
    LSD, mescaline, THC, and
    phencyclidine hydrochloride)
  Opiates, especially cocaine
  Heavy metals
  Bromide
  Organic phosphates (insecticides)
  Anticholinergic compounds
  Carbon monoxide
  Carbon disulfide, other industrial
    agents

Unwanted effects of medication
  Antipsychotics ("psychotoxic" or
    "paradoxical" reactions and/or
    akathisia)

Sedative-hypnotics
Antidepressants
Lithium carbonate
Disulfiram
Levodopa
Analgesics (narcotics, pentazocine)
Anticonvulsants
Antituberculous drugs (isoniazid,
  cycloserine)
Antiinflammatory agents
  (indomethacin, phenylbutazone)
Antihypertensive agents (especially
  those containing reserpine and
  methyldopa)
Cardiac drugs (digitalis,
  procainamide hydrochloride,
  propranolol hydrochloride)
Idiosyncratic reactions to almost any
  medication

Differential Diagnosis of Psychotic Conditions

Schizophrenia. The third edition of the *Diagnostic and Statistical Manual of Mental Disorders* of the American Psychiatric Association (DSM-III[1]) provides the following definition of schizophrenia:

> The essential features of this group of disorders are: the presence of certain psychotic features during the active phase of the illness, characteristic symptoms involving multiple psychological processes, deterioration from a previous level of functioning, onset before age 45, and a duration of at least six months. The disturbance is not due to an Affective Disorder or Organic Mental Disorder. At some phase of the illness Schizophrenia always involves delusions, hallucinations, or certain disturbances in the form of thought.

The new definition (Table 11-2) contains several aspects.[2] First of all, there is an explicit view that schizophrenia is an idiopathic syndrome with heterogeneous causes. Second, there is a more balanced emphasis on symptoms and course factors because neither alone sufficiently distinguishes the schizophrenic group.[3,4] Third, the criteria narrow the boundaries of schizophrenia as defined by Bleuler in 1911[5] and the DSM-II in 1968.[6] Fourth, the requirement that affective and organic mental disorders be ruled out makes schizophrenic disorder a diagnosis of exclusion. And finally, the traditional phenomenologic subtypes (eg, paranoid, catatonic, and hebephrenic) have been de-emphasized, owing largely to lack of validation.[7] There is no diagnostic laboratory test for

Table 11-2. Diagnostic Criteria for Schizophrenic Disorders

I. At least one of the following during a phase of the illness:
  A. Bizarre delusions (content is patently absurd and has no possible basis in fact), such as delusions of being controlled, thought broadcasting, thought insertion, or thought withdrawal.
  B. Somatic, grandiose, religious, nihilistic, or other delusions without persecutory or jealous content.
  C. Delusions with persecutory or jealous content if accompanied by hallucinations of any type.
  D. Auditory hallucinations in which either a voice keeps up a running commentary on the individual's behavior or thoughts or two or more voices converse with each other.
  E. Auditory hallucinations on several occasions with content of more than one or two words, having no apparent relation to depression or elation.
  F. Incoherence, marked loosening of associations, markedly illogical thinking, or marked poverty of content of speech if associated with at least one of the following:
    1. Blunted, flat, or inappropriate affect.
    2. Delusions or hallucinations.
    3. Catatonic or other grossly disorganized behavior.
II. Deterioration from a previous level of functioning in such areas as work, social relations, and self-care.
III. Duration: continuous signs of the illness for at least 6 months at some time during the person's life, with some signs of the illness at present. The 6-month period must include an active phase during which there are symptoms from I, with or without a prodromal or residual phase.
IV. The full depressive or manic syndrome, if present, developed after any psychotic symptoms, or was brief in duration relative to the duration of the psychotic symptoms in I.
V. Onset of prodromal or active phase of the illness before age 45.
VI. Not due to any organic mental disorder or mental retardation.

Reprinted from the American Psychiatric Association's *Diagnostic and Statistical Manual of Mental Disorders*, ed 3.

schizophrenic disorder; for the diagnosis to be made, the patient's condition must fulfill the DSM-III criteria. A period of at least 6 months of continuous signs of the illness is essential for diagnosis, and the illness must include an active phase with prominent psychotic symptoms and may or may not include a prodromal or residual phase (Table 11-3).

A residual phase usually follows the active phase. Its clinical picture may be similar to that of the prodromal phase, with the possible addition of lingering delusions and hallucinations or more pronounced difficulties in role functioning, affect, and volition.

Careful differential diagnosis is essential; it is well known that many diseases mimic features of schizophrenia.[8] Moreover, no single feature of

Table 11-3. Prodromal or Residual Symptoms of Schizophrenia

1. Social isolation or withdrawal
2. Marked impairment in role functioning as wage-earner, student, or homemaker
3. Markedly peculiar behavior (eg, collecting garbage, talking to oneself in public, or hoarding food)
4. Marked impairment in personal hygiene and grooming
5. Blunted, flat, or inappropriate affect
6. Digressive, vague, overelaborate, circumstantial, or metaphorical speech
7. Odd or bizarre ideation, or magical thinking (eg, superstitiousness, clairvoyance, telepathy, "sixth sense," "others can feel my feelings," overvalued ideas, ideas of reference)
8. Unusual perceptual experiences (eg, recurrent illusions, sensing the presence of a force or person not actually present)

the illness is unique to it.[9-11] Unfortunately, many physicians ignore these facts and tend to diagnose any flagrant psychosis as "acute schizophrenia." On the other hand, certain symptoms appear to be highly discriminating, particularly thought insertion, broadcasting, withdrawal, delusions of control, and certain types of auditory hallucinations.[12,13]

Organic mental disorders often present with features that suggest a schizophrenic disorder. For example, phencyclidine hydrochloride or amphetamine intoxication may induce a similar clinical condition (organic delusional syndrome). The presence of disorientation; memory impairment; visual and other types of hallucinations in the absence of auditory hallucinations; abrupt changes in mental state, mood, or personality; and failure to respond to treatment should spur the search for known organic causes.

Other psychiatric disorders must also be excluded, especially manic and psychotic depressive disorders; paranoid disorders in which prominent hallucinations, incoherence, or bizarre delusions are generally absent; and schizophreniform disorders, which by definition have a duration of less than 6 months, and in which prognosis is generally more favorable. Mental retardation, certain personality disorders, and factitious conditions must also be considered.

The course of schizophrenic disorders varies greatly, but recurrent episodes of active psychosis and persistent impairment are common.[11] Impairments fall into two main groups which often overlap, have varying degrees of severity, and may fluctuate widely. One group consists of symptoms associated with active psychosis, including the disabling effects of incoherence and unpredictable associations in speech, chronic delusions, and hallucinations. The other and most characteristic group consists of apathy, lack of ambition, slowed, impoverished thought, underactivity, and withdrawal. Although both groups are disabling, the second group, not surprisingly, is associated with poor social performance.[13]

Prognosis has improved somewhat, largely as a result of the benefits of antipsychotic medication in alleviating and preventing episodes of active psychosis.[14] Full recovery is uncommon and usually occurs within the first 2 years; after 5 years of illness, few patients recover.

The cause of schizophrenic disorders remains obscure. Nevertheless, evidence from clinical, genetic, epidemiologic, and biochemical investigations is consistent with the concept that schizophrenia is a disease. Numerous diseases mimic schizophrenia, including the psychoses associated with brain disease, especially temporal-lobe epilepsy,[15] intoxication disorders (eg, with amphetamine and phencyclidine),[16,17] and metabolic illness (eg, porphyria).[8] Reports of electrodermal dysfunction, changes in EEG-evoked response,[18] differences in cerebral blood flow activity,[19] neurologic soft signs,[20] motor abnormalities,[21] disturbances in smooth-pursuit eye tracking[22] and optokinetic nystagmus,[23] and radiographic evidence of anatomical abnormalities[24] (especially ventricular enlargement), and sensory and cognitive deficits[25,26] have strengthened the view that schizophrenic disorder is a disease.

Consistent with that concept is the observation that whereas the lifetime risk of schizophrenic disorder in the general population is about 1%, genetic studies indicate that the risk increases with the degree of biologic relatedness to an affected family member.[27,28] The mode of transmission is unclear. Monogenic (autosomal dominance with reduced penetrance) and polygenic theories appear to be partly supported by available evidence. Yet, large numbers of schizophrenic patients have no identifiable family members with the disorder. Studies of social class have demonstrated a disproportionate rate of schizophrenia in lower-class families, and the increase cannot be explained solely in terms of a downward social drift among schizophrenics.[14] The study of family relationships has also been voluminous,[14] but although it appears that families of schizophrenics have a wide range of deviancies, the direction of causal influence is unclear. Some studies suggest that parental difficulties may be the result of living with disturbed children, in contrast to the more popular view that parents' problems promote maladjustment in their offspring.[29]

The study of biochemical aspects of schizophrenia has been influenced by new advances in neurosciences and by increased attempts to relate clinical to neurobiologic features. The hypothesis that certain central dopaminergic systems may be overactive in schizophrenia remains the main beacon for current investigations.[30] The consistent antidopamine effects of available antipsychotic drugs (phenothiazines, butyrophenones, thioxanthenes, dibenzoxazepines, and dihydroindolones) and the psychotic effects of dopamine-stimulating drugs such as amphetamine have supported this view. Antipsychotic drugs are thought to work on the basis of dopamine-receptor antagonism, particularly in the mesolimbic dopamine system.[31]

The connection between dopamine and the clinical phenomena of schizophrenia is not clear. The fact that antipsychotic drugs are useful in the treatment of affective, drug-induced, and organic psychoses suggests that dopamine disturbances are not unique to schizophrenia. Certainly the "positive" symptoms of active schizophrenia (delusions, hallucinations, and certain aspects of disturbed thinking) are responsive to these agents. Yet, interestingly, the "negative" symptoms (flat affect, loss of drive, and impoverished thought) are probably little affected by drugs; because of their association with intellectual changes and increased ventricular size, these symptoms may represent a subtype of schizophrenic disorder.

Antipsychotic medications are particularly successful in improving symptoms associated with the active phase, including hallucinations, verbal incomprehensibility, delusions, agitation, perplexity, insomnia, and anxiety. Patients receiving maintenance antipsychotic medication relapse less often than those treated with placebo. Moreover, the prophylactic value of antipsychotic drugs may be enhanced with counseling and rehabilitative interventions.[32]

Yet, the limitations of antipsychotic drugs are becoming increasingly apparent.[33] For example, many patients recover from the acute phase of illness but do not satisfactorily readjust to the demands of their previous routine. Residual symptoms, subtle deficiencies in cognitive and motor performance, and affective response may simply be refractory to these agents. The reasons that many patients (up to 30% or more) do *not* relapse while taking a placebo also remain unclear.[33] Limitations on the use of antipsychotic medications are their multiple and frequent side effects, notably extrapyramidal disturbances and tardive dyskinesia. The latter remains only partially understood and is difficult to treat.

To offer traditional psychotherapy as the only treatment for schizophrenic disorder is generally regarded as inadequate and negligent. Psychoanalysis and other insight-oriented psychotherapies have little demonstrated value in this illness.[14] On the other hand, the doctor-patient relationship is as critical to successful treatment as it is anywhere in medicine. Its aims are monitoring the course of illness, encouraging social relations, developing interests, maintaining employment, and helping the patient and family to understand the illness.

Schizophrenic patients generally receive less than optimal medical care, partly because of reluctance to use services, inability to express specific complaints clearly, and the physician's tendency to attribute vague somatic complaints to the psychopathology. These problems are vital: schizophrenic patients on the average are more likely to die at an early age and may be more likely to die of the complications of routine medical illness.[34]

Affective disorders. Disorders of mood are discussed more fully elsewhere. For differential diagnosis of the psychotic conditions, suffice it to say that manic-depressive illness presenting with either depression or mania may resemble schizophrenia. Dysphoric mood, vegetative signs and symptoms of depression—such as weight loss, early morning awakening, loss of libido, and diurnal mood variation—along with guilt, rumination, agitation, or psychomotor retardation, all strongly indicate a diagnosis of affective illness. Sometimes paranoid thinking is associated with depressive illness and there may be hallucinations and delusions; usually, however, there is a tinge of guilt or self-reproach with these. The patient will be convinced of wrongdoing, bodily damage, or a terminal condition, such as cancer. In manic psychosis, there is usually paranoia and almost always elation or irritation. The affect is labile and sometimes inappropriate. Speech displays flight of ideas—rapid jumping from topic to topic so that connections are usually apparent and sometimes related to external stimuli, unlike loose associations, in which connections are illogical or bizarre. The manic patient is frequently amusing, charming, or touching, and does not seem as alien to the examiner as the schizophrenic patient.

Borderline personality. This disorder is discussed more fully in chapter 10. A psychotic episode is not uncommonly seen in borderline personality disorder, but it is usually of short duration. In the differential diagnosis of borderline personality and psychosis, several other diagnostic entities deserve consideration. Posttraumatic stress disorder, or traumatic war neurosis,[35-37] may present similar symptoms, but it occurs in combat veterans and, in its classical presentation, the patient's prewar adjustment is said to have been good. In contrast, the borderline patient's history of maladjustment goes back to childhood or early adolescence. The episodic dyscontrol syndrome, which is usually synonymous with "explosive personality," is also similar to borderline personality.[38-43] Such individuals, usually male, come to attention because of gross outbursts of rage and verbal or physical abusiveness.

These outbursts are sudden, intense, and in response to various gradations of provocation ranging from minimal to massive. Between episodes, the individual may exhibit some social maladjustment but sometimes exhibits quite ordinary behavior or is even deeply repentant at these losses of control. Clearly, dyscontrol is multietiological. When large cohorts of nonpsychotic violent patients are studied,[44] a small percentage is found to have temporal lobe epilepsy, a larger percentage has "seizure-like" episodes, and a larger percentage has pathologic intoxications with alcohol.[43] About half of these patients, however, have no such obvious explanation and fall into a mixed group which may contain persons with psychosis or seizures or persons with borderline or antisocial personality. Monroe's schema[40] for classifying episodic behavioral disorders has great appeal because such conditions are arranged along a continuum ranging from disorganized, amorphous, uncoordinated attacks on the nearest object at hand (ictal), through conditions in which there is a period of increasing tension and internal struggle preceding the explosive attack, after which an enormous sense of relief supervenes (impulse dyscontrol), to conditions in which there is unconscious conflict and considerable neutralization of the aggressive act by ego defense mechanisms (acting out). Depending on where along the continuum the dyscontrolled acts fall, Monroe recommends pharmacologic treatment with anticonvulsants, benzodiazepines, or a combination of the two.[40]

There is a body of evidence that implicates hereditary factors and organic brain disorders in the etiology of impulsive and dyscontrolled behavior. For instance, adoption studies suggest that a criminal biological father's offspring who are reared by a noncriminal adoptive father are more likely to become criminal than those of a noncriminal biological father whose offspring are reared by a criminal adoptive father.[45,46] Persons with antisocial behavior have a high prevalence of abnormal EEG findings and of "soft neurological signs" similar to those accompanying "minimal brain damage."[42] Finally, there is evidence suggesting that attention deficit disorder ("hyperkinetic syndrome") in childhood, which is often part of the family history,[47,49] may go on to be associated with delinquency and episodic dyscontrol in adulthood.[50-52] Moreover, amphetamines or tricyclic antidepressants not only benefit hyperactive children, but may also ameliorate impulsive and dyscontrolled behavior in adults.[53-55]

Psychopharmacologic Management

Although psychopharmacology is discussed in more detail in chapters 26 and 27, a few basic points are worth attention here:

1. The consultant should be knowledgeable about one or two drugs from each class—the sedative hypnotics, the antipsychotics, the antidepressants, lithium, and the antiparkinsonian drugs—rather than lightly conversant with myriad drugs.
2. Pharmacologic control, if indicated, of disruptive behavior is crucial for the safety of the patient, of fellow patients, and of the staff. Undermedication—especially with inadequate supervision of the patient—is typically far more hazardous than the commonly feared "overdosing" of a patient.
3. Drug interactions are to be avoided whenever possible. A risk for psychotic patients on pressors is "epinephrine reversal" and hypotension with phenothiazines. Another, for patients taking antihypertensive medication, is hypotension or hypertension with antidepressants.
4. Route of administration deserves attention: benzodiazepines are absorbed much better orally than intramuscularly (IM), unlike most other psychoactive drugs.
5. Illness-drug interactions require forethought. Antidepressants are particularly taxing to the cardiovascular system and often require so long for effect that electroconvulsive therapy (ECT) should be considered as a safer alternative for consenting severely depressed individuals (and even some with other psychotic illnesses), provided the patient is free of CNS pathology. The serum half-life of tranquilizers is prolonged in patients with liver disease. Especially troublesome are the benzodiazepines because they are often given routinely and signs of overdose may not become apparent until several days after the first administration.
6. Careful attention to the dose of antipsychotic medications is necessary because clinical response (and probably serum levels[56]) vary widely from patient to patient and from dose to dose.
7. Whenever a psychotic illness is thought to be caused by a neurologic, toxic, metabolic, or endocrine condition, treatment of the underlying condition should—if at all possible—be carried out without resort to psychopharmacologic controls in order not to confuse the clinical picture.

THE CONSULTEE AND HOUSE STAFF

The 4-year experience of Reding and Maguire[57] in managing acute psychiatric admissions to a general hospital in which psychiatric patients were not segregated from medical and surgical patients demonstrates the utter necessity for the intensive collaboration of the psychiatric consultant and the attending physician and nursing staff. The consultant in their hospital was not only readily available to the consultee but also gave particular attention to the nursing staff's education in the psychological management of the patient and to apprehensions regarding the potentially disruptive patient. The study reported on 344 admissions for acute psychiatric disorders spanning more than 4000 patient-in-hospital days; 40% of these patients were acutely schizophrenic or paranoid and 25% were psychotically depressed or suicidal. During this time not one homicidal or suicidal attempt was made and only seven patients had to be transferred to a psychiatric hospital.

The 7-year experience of Reich and Kelly[58] showed that suicide attempts on medical and surgical wards correlated not so much with depression in serious medical illness such as cancer, but rather with anger over loss of social supports in patients with personality disorders and psychosis. Of 17 suicide attempts, 15 occurred in a clinical setting in which the patient's experience was of being abandoned—during failing treatment, imminent discharge, dispute with the staff, or staff holiday.

The consultant can conceptualize the psychiatric consultation in several different ways. Meyer and Mendelson[59] see consultations as issuing from a feeling of uncertainty in the consultee, coupled with a sense of responsibility. If a patient throws a drinking glass while experiencing delirium tremens, the consultee has the sense of responsibility but not the uncertainty; the patient is exhibiting common behavior for a common condition. Identical behavior by a patient who has an undiagnosed illness is much more likely to precipitate a high anxiety request for consultation. Caplan[60] sees as determinants for consultation requests in community health centers feelings in the consultee of "(a) lack of knowledge, (b) lack of skill, (c) lack of self-confidence, or (d) lack of professional objectivity." Something about the patient's illness or behavior causes the consultee to feel inadequate to the situation. Lipowski[61] finds that psychiatric consultation requests occur (1) when no convincing organic cause can be found for somatic complaints, (2) when there is a change in the patient's habitual behavior, (3) when the patient has a recognizable psychiatric illness for which the consultee seeks management recommendations, and (4) when the patient displays deviant illness behavior, such as self-destructive noncompliance with medical advice, excessive dependence, gross denial of illness, a given-up attitude, factitial illness, or suicidal threats or attempts.

Bibring[62] has noted that when problems occur between physicians and patients it is not so much that physicians may not understand the patients but that the physicians may not understand their own reactions to the patients. Bibring and Kahana[63,64] discuss several personality types and the typical reactions of each to the stress of illness: the dependent patient asks for unlimited attention; the overorderly patient is obsessed about details; the overanxious, overinvolved patient is intense and dramatic; the long-suffering, martyrlike patient rejects comforting; guarded and aggrieved, overindependent, and aloof, fearful patients appear quarrelsome, hostile, or disdainful. For Bibring and Kahana, the work of the consultant is to recognize the wishes and fears that underlie such behaviors and to advise the staff about coping with them.[63,64]

These several conceptual schemata treat the physician-patient-staff relationship as a system into which the psychiatrist is summoned for information or expertise. They acknowledge that the consultant's best work with the patient may be in vain without equally careful work with the staff. They imply the presence of dysfunction in consultee and staff that sunders them from customary effective functioning when the patient's behavior becomes a source of staff distress. The approach to consultation described in this chapter is based on the examination of behavior rather than personality because it is not the personality of the patient that is bothersome to the staff. It is the behavior.

The psychotic patient puts the staff off; schizophrenic patients, for example, are often strange, sometimes violent, and always frightened, and their odd behaviors and eery thinking alienate caregivers. One of the first steps in the management of such a patient in the medical or surgical context is for the consultant to demonstrate control over the patient's psychiatric symptoms by means of medication and social structuring. Seeing the consultant do this gives staff a feeling of control. In the following discussion, schizophrenia will serve as an example for the management of psychotic patients.

Because psychotic disorders represent a group of illnesses with varied presentations, consultation for the hospitalized patient calls for diagnostic review followed by both medical and psychological strategies. The consultant should determine and document the accuracy of the diagnosis, the phase of the illness, and the current level of psychopathology (Table 11-4). Discussion with the physician who follows the patient outside the hospital usually answers most questions and provides a highly efficient method of anticipating management issues in the care of the patient. These data constitute the basis for further evaluation and intervention.

Two common conditions, schizophrenia in remission and acute

Table 11-4. The Consultant's Role During Phases of Schizophrenic
Disorders

Active Phase
   Characterized by psychotic symptoms: delusions, hallucinations, derailment,
   incoherence, poverty of content of speech, markedly illogical thinking, grossly
   disorganized or catatonic behavior. Specific symptoms are noted in Table 11-2.
   Consultant problem: early diagnosis; prompt, effective medical intervention;
   staff education.

Prodromal Phase
   Characterized by clear deterioration in previous level of functioning; a phase of
   variable length and occasionally vague beginnings. This and the residual phase
   may or may not occur as part of schizophrenic disorders. Symptoms are listed in
   Table 11-3.
   Consultant problem: recognition of impending disorder, thorough evaluation
   and careful follow-up with staff.

Residual Phase
   Characterized by same features as prodromal phase, but occurs after an active
   phase of the illness. Disturbed thinking and impaired role functioning are more
   common. Occasional psychotic symptoms but without strong affective
   accompaniment are present.
   Consultant problem: watchful maintenance of remission; staff support.

---

psychosis, usually require advising staff on pharmacologic approaches.
Patients in remission from schizophrenic psychosis usually are on
maintenance medication and require continuation of drug treatment;
they need a careful review of the medication history, response to
treatment, side effects, compliance, and routes of administration.
Admission to hospital and the stresses of medical and surgical illness can
cause heightened arousal and early signs of relapse into psychosis, such
as poor sleep, anxiety, irritability, gloomy mood, and withdrawn behavior. These patients may need increased doses of maintenance medications to prevent decompensation into active psychosis.

It is important to be aware of the patient's history of handling
stressful situations. Some may have resorted to suicidal behavior or to
the use of alcohol and drugs. Awareness of these potential reactions may
permit their early recognition. The occurrence of acute active psychosis
or the worsening of mild residual psychotic symptoms may bring the
patient to the attention of the consultant. In active psychosis the need to
initiate treatment rapidly may be paramount not only for the patient but
for staff and other patients as well. Such patients can be difficult for staff
to manage because of their gross confusion, intrusive and loud behavior,

lack of judgment, and profound apprehension. Indicated here are antipsychotic medications, the most acceptable and conservative form of treatment; but if it is unclear whether psychosis is due to schizophrenic disorder or to an affective illness, it may be useful to try sedating medications, such as benzodiazepines, to determine whether anxiety and behavioral lability are the main features of the illness and also to allow time for further diagnostic evaluation. Another approach is to use the short acting antipsychotic droperidol, which has been successfully employed in anesthesia and is now recognized as a safe approach to early diagnostic management of the psychotic patient. Others have employed intravenous (IV) haloperidol with some success in the rapid alleviation of active psychosis in medically hospitalized psychotic patients.

Pharmacologic interventions are critical, but it is also essential that the consultant help staff master psychological management principles as well. In general, the goal of psychological and drug treatment is to avoid psychosis or to minimize it. A related goal is to effect optimal medical care efficiently. Indeed most schizophrenic patients do well in medical and surgical settings. However, there are certain principles which remain fundamental for successful hospitalization. First and foremost is the importance of the doctor-patient relationship. Because schizophrenic patients are often frightened or act in peculiar ways and can alienate staff and other patients with their eccentricity and irritability, there is a need for a conscious effort at an appropriate doctor-patient relationship: *The staff should show a caring attitude but not smother the patient with good will.* Appropriate distance is easier for the patient to deal with and does not add to the stress of hospitalization. This relationship, though limited in time and depth, is still necessary for the hospitalization to work, and for the doctor to elicit essential cooperation and compliance from the patient. The patient's attitude is influenced by the schizophrenic illness and also by previous experiences with physicians and other health care professionals.

Communication with the patient is as critical as it is anywhere in the rest of medicine, and the consultant provides a model for the staff in this. In the hospital, inadequate communication with the schizophrenic patient can lead to more serious consequences than with other patients because of the marked distortion and difficulty with compliance that result. *The staff should be helped to provide simple, repetitive, and direct statements, frank and free of jargon.* The staff and treating physician should not try to humor the patient but rather should make sure that the patient understands fully what is being said. The best and most effective way to do so is to keep matters simple and check for understanding, if necessary repeatedly.

Another issue in the psychological treatment of psychotic inpatients is the management of their suffering. Schizophrenic patients, for instance, often react to sources of difficulty not by complaining but through increased agitation, worry, insomnia, and the like. If the doctor is not used to eliciting new complaints or checking for old ones, the patient may not communicate them.

Especially is it important for the consultant to show the consultee how to monitor side effects of medication. The antipsychotic medications produce multiple side effects as do the antiparkinsonian agents with which they are often prescribed. Anticholinergic side effects may have several consequences and are associated with both types of medications. For patients at bed rest, constipation may develop. Occasionally, dry mouth, blurred vision, and urinary retention lead to problems. It is, of course, critical to anticipate the multiple motor side effects of anti-psychotic drugs. There are four to consider, any one of which can be distrubing and stressful. Extrapyramidal side effects include drug-induced parkinsonism, akathisia, and acute dystonias. Each tends to occur early in treatment, that is, generally within the first days up to 6 weeks, but they may occur later in the course of treatment as well. These side effects sometimes respond to the reduction of antipsychotic medication or the administration of anticholinergic drugs, although akathisia is often difficult to conquer. Tardive dyskinesia usually occurs late in antipsychotic treatment and often appears when it is discontinued. It is a difficult disorder to treat and should probably be evaluated by the psychiatric consultant.

Another area of suffering is sleep disturbance. Sleep difficulties may be a sign of impending psychosis or unbearable anxiety which may lead to psychosis. The consultant needs to determine whether sleep medication is appropriate or whether the patient's medications need to be altered. Another concern is pain. Many schizophrenic patients have altered experiences of pain and in some cases appear to adapt well to pain that other patients might find intolerable. Nevertheless, the key is to be certain the patient is comfortable. Yet another area of concern is the nutrition of the patient. If the schizophrenic patient is not eating, an important consideration is whether the patient is experiencing un-detected psychosis; specifically, the complaint may have nothing to do with appetite but rather a concern that the food is being poisoned.

Extended convalescence presents issues similar to those of acute care. Patients who stay in the hospital for prolonged periods will have more difficult adjustments to make and will need to be thoughtfully appraised with respect to their capacity to adapt. All side effects and related issues throughout rehabilitation will require periodic review.

Of crucial importance in the psychological treatment of schizophrenic inpatients is the patient's relationship with the staff. The most important techniques are to implement sound medical intervention with the patient, a good doctor-patient relationship, and clear and simple communication and communication channels. It is a fact that stimulation—whether noise, crowding, or sudden changes in the social structure—has enormous impact on the psychotic patient. The reduction of unnecessary stimulation can be addressed by close consultation between consultant and staff. The consultant may pay particular attention to those factors which tend to increase the risk for active psychosis, even among the most stable patients. These include social isolation, based on patient or staff withdrawal; lack of adequate communication about the medical condition and guidance as to its treatment; interference with sleep; and interruption of daily routine. Naturally, some discomfort, stress, and stimulation cannot be avoided in hospital.

The consultant also should anticipate the needs of the staff in order to short circuit common problems that lead to hazardous consequences. Careful, practical discussion with staff about these management problems, direct, thorough responses to their questions and apprehensions, and clear guidelines about what to expect, when to expect it, and how to get help cement the consultant's alliance with staff. Concrete suggestions and specific guidance cut through the staff's uncertainty and reinforce their skills in caring for the psychotic patient.

REFERENCES

1. American Psychiatric Association: *Diagnostic and Statistical Manual of Mental Disorders*, ed 3. Washington, DC, American Psychiatric Association, 1980.
2. Manschreck TC: Schizophrenic disorders. *N Engl J Med* 1981; 305:1628–1632.
3. Pope HG Jr, Lipinski JF Jr: Diagnosis in schizophrenia and manic-depressive illness: a reassessment of the specificity of "schizophrenic" symptoms in the light of current research. *Arch Gen Psychiatry* 1978; 35:811–828.
4. World Health Organization: *Report of the International Pilot Study of Schizophrenia*. Geneva, World Health Organization, 1973.
5. Bleuler E: *Dementia Praecox or the Group of Schizophrenias*. Zinkin J (trans). New York, International Universities Press, 1950.
6. American Psychiatric Association: *Diagnostic and Statistical Manual of Mental Disorders*, ed 2. Washington, DC, American Psychiatric Association, 1968.
7. Carpenter WT Jr, Bartko JJ, Carpenter CL, et al: Another view of schizophrenia subtypes: a report from the international pilot study of schizophrenia. *Arch Gen Psychiatry* 1976; 33:508–516.
8. Reid AA: Schizophrenia—disease or syndrome? *Arch Gen Psychiatry* 1973;

28:863–869.

9. Gelenberg AJ: The catatonic syndrome. Lancet 1976; 1:1339–1341.
10. Manschreck TC, Petri M: The paranoid syndrome. Lancet 1978; 2:251–253.
11. Hamilton M (ed): Fish's Schizophrenia, ed 2. Bristol, England, John Wright, 1976.
12. Scharfetter C, Moerbt H, Wing JK: Diagnosis of functional psychoses: comparison of clinical and computerized classifications. Arch Psychiatr Nervenkr 1976; 222:61–67.
13. Wing JK: Reasoning about Madness. New York, Oxford University Press, 1978.
14. Neale JM, Oltmanns TF: Schizophrenia. New York, John Wiley & Sons, Inc, 1980.
15. Davison K, Bagley CR: Schizophrenia-like psychoses associated with organic disorders of the central nervous system: a review of the literature, in Herrington RN (ed): Current Problems in Neuropsychiatry. Ashford, England, Headley Press, 1969, pp 113–184.
16. Ellinwood EH Jr: Amphetamine psychosis. I. Description of the individuals and process. J Nerv Ment Dis 1967; 144:273–283.
17. Allen RM, Young SJ: Phencyclidine-induced psychosis. Am J Psychiatry 1978; 135:1081–1084.
18. Spohn HE, Patterson T: Recent studies of psychophysiology in schizophrenia. Schizophr Bull 1979; 5:581–611.
19. Ingvar DH, Franzén G: Distribution of cerebral activity in chronic schizophrenia. Lancet 1974; 2:1484–1486.
20. Tucker GJ, Campion EW, Silberfarb PM: Sensorimotor functions and cognitive disturbance in psychiatric patients. Am J Psychiatry 1975; 132: 17–21.
21. Manschreck TC, Maher BA, Rucklos ME, et al: Disturbed voluntary motor activity in schizophrenia. Psychol Med 1982; 73–84.
22. Holzman PS, Levy DL: Smooth pursuit eye movements and functional psychoses: a review. Schizophr Bull 1977; 3:15–27.
23. Latham C, Holzman PS, Manschreck TC: Optokinetic nystagmus and pursuit eye movements in schizophrenia. Arch Gen Psychiatry 1981; 38:997–1003.
24. Weinberger DR, Torrey EF, Neophytides AN, et al: Lateral cerebral ventricular enlargement in chronic schizophrenia. Arch Gen Psychiatry 1979; 36:735–739.
25. Siegel C, Waldo M, Mizner LE, et al: Deficits in sensory gating in schizophrenic patients and their relatives. Arch Gen Psychiatry 1984; 41:607–612.
26. Braff DL, Saccuzzo DP: The time course of information-processing deficits in schizophrenia. Am J Psychiatry 1985; 142:170–174.
27. Tsuang MT, Vandermey R: Genes and the Mind: Inheritance of Mental Illness. New York, Oxford University Press, 1980.
28. Kety SS, Rosenthal D, Wender PH, et al: Mental illness in the biological and adoptive families of adopted individuals who have become schizophrenic: a preliminary report based on psychiatric interviews, in Fieve RR, Rosenthal D, Brill H (eds): Genetic Research in Psychiatry. Baltimore, Johns Hopkins Press, 1975, pp 147–165.
29. Hirsch SR, Leff JP: Abnormalities in Parents of Schizophrenics. London,

Oxford University Press, 1975.
30. Bowers MB Jr: Biochemical processes in schizophrenia: an update. *Schizophr Bull* 1980; 6:393–403.
31. Snyder SH: Dopamine receptors, neuroleptics, and schizophrenia. *Am J Psychiatry* 1981; 138:460–464.
32. Hogarty GE: Aftercare treatment of schizophrenia: current status and future direction, in van Praag HM (ed): *Management of Schizophrenia: Biological and Sociological Aspects.* Assen, The Netherlands, Van Gorcum, 1979, pp 19–36.
33. Vaughn CE, Leff JP: The influence of family and social factors on the course of psychiatric illness: a comparison of schizophrenic and depressed neurotic patients. *Br J Psychiatry* 1976; 129:125–137.
34. Tsuang MT, Woolson RF, Fleming JA: Premature deaths in schizophrenia and affective disorders: an analysis of survival curves and variables affecting the shortened survival. *Arch Gen Psychiatry* 1980; 37:979–983.
35. Van Putten T, Emory WH: Traumatic neuroses in Vietnam returnees—a forgotten diagnosis? *Arch Gen Psychiatry* 1973; 29:695–698.
36. Haley SA: When the patient reports atrocities. *Arch Gen Psychiatry* 1974; 30:191–196.
37. Fox RP: Narcissistic rage and the problem of combat aggression. *Arch Gen Psychiatry* 1974; 31:807–811.
38. Pincus JH, Tucker GJ: *Behavioral Neurology.* London, Oxford University Press, 1974, chapters 1–4.
39. Winokur G, Crowe RR: Personality disorders, in Freedman AM, Kaplan HI, Sadock BJ (eds): *Comprehensive Textbook of Psychiatry,* ed 2. Baltimore, Williams & Wilkins Co, 1975, pp 1279–1297.
40. Monroe RR: *Episodic Behavioral Disorders, a Psychodynamic and Neurophysiologic Analysis.* Cambridge, Harvard University Press, 1970.
41. Robins LN: *Deviant Children Grown Up: Sociologic and Psychiatric Study of Sociopathic Personality.* Baltimore, Williams & Wilkins Co, 1966.
42. Mark VH, Ervin FR: *Violence and the Brain.* New York, Harper & Row Publishers Inc, 1970.
43. Detre TP, Jarecki HG: *Modern Psychiatric Treatment.* Philadelphia, JB Lippincott Co, 1971.
44. Bach-y-Rita G, Lion JR, Climent CE, et al: Episodic dyscontrol: a study of 130 violent patients. *Am J Psychiatry* 1971; 127:1473–1478.
45. Crowe RR: An adoption study of antisocial personality. *Arch Gen Psychiatry* 1974; 31:785–791.
46. Hutchings B, Mednick SA: Registered criminality in the adoptive and biological parents of registered male adoptees, in Fieve RR, Brill H, Rosenthal D (eds): *Genetic Research in Psychiatry.* New York, New York University Press, 1974.
47. Cantwell DP: Psychiatric illness in families of hyperactive children. *Arch Gen Psychiatry* 1972; 27:414–417.
48. Morrison JR, Stewart MA: A family study of the hyperactive child syndrome. *Biol Psychiatry* 1971; 3:189–195.
49. Morrison JR, Stewart MA: The psychiatric status of the legal families of adopted hyperactive children. *Arch Gen Psychiatry* 1973; 28:888–891.
50. Mann HB, Greenspan SI: The identification and treatment of adult brain

dysfunction. *Am J Psychiatry* 1976; 133:1013–1017.

51. Quitkin FM, Klein DF: Two behavioral syndromes in young adults related to possible minimal brain dysfunction. *J Psychiatr Res* 1969; 7:131–142.

52. Mendelson W, Johnson N, Stewart MA: Hyperactive children as teenagers: a follow-up study. *J Nerv Ment Dis* 1971; 153:273–279.

53. Richmond JS, Young JR, Groves JE: Violent dyscontrol responsive to d-amphetamine. *Am J Psychiatry* 1978; 135:365–366.

54. Wood DR, Reimherr FW, Wender PH, et al: Minimal brain dysfunction in adults. *Arch Gen Psychiatry* 1976; 33:1453–1460.

55. Morrison JR, Minkhoft K: Explosive personality as a sequel to the hyperactive-child syndrome. *Compr Psychiatry* 1975; 16:343–348.

56. Rivera-Calimlim L, Nasrallah H, Strauss J, et al: Clinical response and plasma levels: effect of dose, dosage schedules, and drug interaction on plasma chlorpromazine. *Am J Psychiatry* 1976; 133:646–652.

57. Reding GR, Maguire B: Nonsegregated acute psychiatric admissions to general hospitals—continuity of care within the community hospital. *N Engl J Med* 1973; 289:185–189.

58. Reich P, Kelly MJ: Suicide attempts by hospitalized medical and surgical patients. *N Engl J Med* 1976; 294:298–301.

59. Meyer E, Mendelson M: Psychiatric consultation with patients on medical and surgical wards: patterns and processes. *Psychiatry* 1961; 24:197–220.

60. Caplan G: *The Theory and Practice of Mental Health Consultation.* New York, Basic Books, Inc, 1970.

61. Lipowski ZJ: Consultation-liaison psychiatry: an overview. *Am J Psychiatry* 1974; 131:623–630.

62. Bibring GL: Psychiatry and medical practice in a general hospital. *N Engl J Med* 1956; 254:366–372.

63. Bibring GL, Kahana RJ: *Lectures in Medical Psychology.* New York, International Universities Press, 1968.

64. Kahana RJ, Bibring GL: Personality types in medical management, in Zinberg NE (ed): *Psychiatry and Medical Practice in a General Hospital.* New York, International Universities Press, 1964.

12

Depression

NED H. CASSEM

Commonest among psychiatric disorders, depression sufficient to warrant professional care affects from 4% to 6% of the general population.[1] Although this condition ranks first among reasons for psychiatric hospitalization (23.3% of total hospitalizations), it has been estimated that 80% of all persons suffering from it are either treated by nonpsychiatric personnel or are not treated at all.[2]

Depression is often seen in general medical practice and studies estimate that from 22% to 32% of all medical inpatients show at least mild depression.[3–6] At Massachusetts General Hospital (MGH) the psychiatric consultant called to see a medical patient will make a diagnosis of major depression in about 20% of cases, making depression the commonest problem presented for diagnostic evaluation and treatment.

Failure to treat depression leaves the patient at even higher risk for further complications and death. Proceeding to cardiac surgery while in a state of major depression, for example, is known to increase the chances of a fatal outcome.[7] Even in outpatient depressed patients the risks of mortality, chiefly due to cardiovascular disease, are more than doubled.[8] There remains a clinical sense, moreover, that any seriously ill person who has neurovegetative symptoms, and who has given up and wishes he were dead, is going to do worse than if he had hope and motivation. Some investigators have been able to demonstrate that the immune defenses, specifically lymphocyte function, of patients become defective with the onset of depression.[9,10] The psychiatric consultant cannot wait for theoretical settlement of these fascinating questions. Major depression, even if the patient were healthy in every other way, is misery requiring treatment. When a person already seriously ill becomes depressed as well, failure to recognize and treat the disorder is even more unfortunate.

MAKING THE DIAGNOSIS OF DEPRESSION

Major depression almost always requires drug treatment or occasionally electroconvulsive therapy (ECT). Since this is the case, the first question becomes: What is *major* depression in the medically ill and how is it diagnosed? The American Psychiatric Association's *Diagnostic and Statistic Manual* (DSM-III)[11] criteria for major depression should be applied to the patient with medical illness in the same way as they are to a primary psychiatric patient. This immediately creates an academic difficulty, since one of the exclusion criteria in DSM-III, that the dysphoria not be due to any organic mental disorder, could be interpreted as excluding a diagnosis of major depression in any patient with a pre-existing medical illness. A stroke in the left hemisphere, for example, is commonly followed by a syndrome clinically indistinguishable from major depression. According to the earlier distinction between primary and secondary depression, such a patient could be diagnosed as having a *secondary* depression. (That is, the depressive episode occurred later in time than the stroke and is therefore called "secondary.") This distinction is not available in DSM-III. One could call it *organic affective disorder*, particularly in the case of a stroke, where a cause-effect relationship is more clear. Nevertheless, a patient does not have to meet the full criteria for major depression in order to be diagnosed as organic affective disorder (only two or more of the same eight criteria need be met instead of four or more). This dilemma is further confused when no cause-effect relationship is clear—as when a patient sustains myocardial infarction (MI) and later develops the syndrome of major depression. Our recommendation is to represent the clinical reality as accurately as possible by the diagnosis. Therefore, when the patient meets full criteria for *major depression*, this diagnosis should be given.

Diagnosis is crucial to treatment. Three critical questions face the consultant at the outset: (1) On clinical examination does the patient manifest depression? (2) If so, is it due to an organic cause that can be treated or reversed? (3) Is the depression one which will respond to drugs? A frequent question put to the consultant by fellow physicians is what depression is the kind that drugs will alleviate. The best answer is that depression which meets the criteria for major depression.

Major Depression

Depression, one of those words used by most to describe even minor and transient mood fluctuations, has the misfortune of overused words: It is seen everywhere, often thought to be normal, and therefore likely to be dismissed even when it is serious. This applies all the more to a patient with serious medical illness: The man has cancer, therefore his depression is "appropriate." "Depression" in this text is used to denote the disorder of major depression. As such it is a seriously disabling condition for the patient, capable of endangering him even to death, and never appropriate. There are many instances of minor depression, usually referred to here as "despondency," which will be discussed below.

Two assumptions are made here: (1) This depressive syndrome in medically ill patients shares the pathophysiology of (primary) major affective disorder, and (2) proper diagnosis is made by applying the same criteria. Since far less epidemiologic information is available on depression in the medically ill, the requirement that the dysphoria be present for 2 weeks should be regarded as only a rough approximation for medically ill patients. Eight symptoms are presented by DSM-III, of which at least four are required to make the diagnosis of major depressive episode.

1. Poor appetite or significant weight loss (when not dieting) or increased appetite or significant weight gain
2. Insomnia or hypersomnia
3. Psychomotor agitation or retardation
4. Loss of interest or pleasure in usual activities, or decrease in sexual drive not limited to a period when delusional or hallucinating
5. Loss of energy; fatigue
6. Feelings of worthlessness, self-reproach, or excessive or inappropriate guilt
7. Complaints or evidence of diminished ability to think or concentrate, such as slowed thinking, or indecisiveness not associated with marked loosening of associations or incoherence
8. Recurrent thoughts of death, suicidal ideation, wishes to be dead, or suicide attempt.

But if the patient has a medical illness like advanced cancer, how can one attribute anorexia or fatigue to something other than the malignant disease itself? This legitimate concern highlights the complexity of the clinical situation, although it is worth remembering that if the consultee requested psychiatric consultation, the patient's symptoms were probably judged to have been in excess of the effects of the disease process. Sometimes the consultee will put in the consultation without being confident of this but hoping that the consultant can locate some psychiatric symptomatology which can be treated, thereby relieving the patient of distress which current treatment has been unable to alter.

The first help comes from discovery of symptoms that are more clearly the result of major depression, such as the presence of self-reproach ("I feel worthless"), the wish to be dead, or psychomotor retardation (few medical illnesses of themselves produce psychomotor retardation; hypothyroidism is one of them). Insomnia or hypersomnia can also be helpful, although the patient may have so much pain, dyspnea, or frequent clinical crises that sleep is impaired by these events. Although libidinous interests may not be high in an intensive care unit (ICU) patient, some form of interest can usually be assessed—as when talk gets around to children or grandchildren, key interests, or people. Do they still find that their interest quickens or is blunted? The ability to think or concentrate, like the other symptoms, needs to be specifically asked about in every case.

A second help for diagnosis is to free the search for specific neurovegetative symptoms from the patient's own misconceptions of depression. This label is often viewed as signifying some inner loss of courage or motivation, often with the fear that the patient's physician asked for psychiatric consultation because the symptoms were thought to be "in my head" or even the result of malingering. Depression is as much a somatic as a psychic disorder. Some patients who readily recognize a feeling like sadness mistakenly assume they should automatically "know" when they are depressed. This is no more logical than the assumption that one should know, in the presence of multiple symptoms, that one has systemic lupus. (Moreover, some individuals lack awareness of even simple feelings like sadness.) The somatic manifestations of depression (insomnia, restlessness, anhedonia, etc) may even be construed as proof by patients that they have no "psychic" illness. "No, doctor, no way am I depressed; if I could just get rid of this pain everything would be fine." Persistence and aggressive questioning are required to elicit the presence or absence of the eight symptoms.

If the history establishes six of eight symptoms, the consultant may not be certain that three of them have anything to do with depression but may just as likely stem from the medical illness itself. In this case one must make a judgment whether there is anything in the treatment of the primary medical condition which can be improved. Of course, if the patient were found to be clinically hypothyroid, the treatment of choice would not be antidepressants but judicious thyroid replacement. Usually, however, everything is being done for the patient to alleviate the symptoms of the primary illness. If this appears to be the case, our recommendation is to make the diagnosis of major depression and proceed with treatment.

Further confirmation of a diagnosis of major depression can be made with relative ease and safety by giving the patient a psychostimulant. Dextroamphetamine (not the sustained release preparation) or methyl-phenidate hydrochloride can be used. The starting dose of dextroamphetamine sulfate (Dexedrine) in medically ill patients is usually 5 or 10 mg, given once in the morning before breakfast. It is given once because the half-life varies between seven and 30 hours; late administration can cause insomnia. The starting dose of methylphenidate hydrochloride for the same type of probe is also 5 to 10 mg, but it should be given at least twice a day, for example, at 8 AM and 2 PM. The half-life is short, from two to four hours, and in some cases the patient may benefit from a third dose. When there is concern that the stimulant might in some way worsen the patient's condition, for example, specifically elevate the blood pressure of the hypertensive patient (as in the depressed renal failure patient with a pressure of 230/110 mmHg despite antihypertensive medications) or the cardiac patient with arrhythmias, one can start with an initial dose of 2.5 mg of either drug and carefully check vital signs over the next four hours. When successful the test is quite dramatic: Nurses, family, and sometimes even the patient comment on how much better they feel. Failure should not be pronounced until the dose has been successively increased (eg, 5 mg the first day, 10 mg the second, and 15 mg the third day) to the point that recognizable effects are reported by the patient, such as "I feel nervous and on edge today but not better." A further discussion of psychostimulants occurs below.

At some point in the future the dexamethasone suppression test (DST) may prove useful in routine diagnosis of major depression. Any acute medical illness, even acute stress, can produce a (false-positive) failure to suppress cortisol when the DST is used. Since there is a general consensus that the DST should not be used routinely for diagnosis even in primary psychiatric patients,[12,13] its use and interpretation remain even more obscure when the patient in question has been hospitalized for a primary medical illness.

States Commonly Mislabeled "Depression"

Up to one third of patients referred for depression will, on clinical examination, have neither major nor minor depression. By far the commonest diagnosis found among these mislabeled referrals at the MGH has been an organic mental syndrome. A quietly confused patient often looks depressed. The patient with dementia or with a frontal lobe syndrome due to brain injury can lack spontaneous initiative and thus appear depressed. Only the complete physical and mental status examinations reveal the telltale abnormalities.

Although much less common, mental retardation may also be mistaken for depression, especially when failure to grasp or comply with complex instructions make no sense to those caring for the patient ("He seems not to care"). If suspected, mental retardation can be confirmed by history from family or past records and/or by formal intelligence testing.

Another unrecognized state sometimes called depression by the consultee and easier for the psychiatrist to recognize is anger. The patient's physician, realizing that the patient has been through a long and difficult illness, may perceive reduction in speech, smiling, and small talk on the patient's part as depression. The patient may thoroughly resent the illness, be irritated by therapeutic routines, and be fed up with the hospital environment, but, despite interior fuming, remain reluctant to discharge overt wrath in the direction of the physician or nurses.

Excluding Organic Causes of Depression

When clinical findings confirm that the patient's symptoms are fully consistent with major depression, the consultant is still responsible for the differential diagnosis of this syndrome. Could the same constellation of symptoms be due to medical illness or its treatment? The psychiatrist functions here as the last court of appeal. Should the patient's symptoms be due to an as yet undiagnosed illness, the last physician with the chance of detecting it is the consultant. Differential diagnosis in this situation is qualitatively the same as that described for excluding the organic causes of delirium (see chapter 6). With depression, while the same process should be completed, certain conditions more commonly produce depressive syndromes and are worthy of comment.

A check on the medications which the patient is currently receiving will generally tell the consultant whether or not the patient is receiving something which might cause a change in mood. Ordinarily one would like to establish that a relationship between the onset of depressive symptoms and either the start of or a change in the medication occurred. If such a connection can be established, the simplest course would be to stop the agent and monitor the patient for improvement. When the patient requires continued treatment, as for hypertension, the presumed offending agent can be changed—with the hope that the change to another antihypertensive will be followed by resolution of depressive symptoms. When this fails or when clinical judgment warrants no change in medication, it may be necessary to start an antidepressant along with the antihypertensive (see chapter 27) drug. Table 12-1 presents drugs more commonly associated with the production of a depressive syndrome.

Abnormal laboratory values should never be missed and may provide the clues to an undiagnosed abnormality responsible for the depressive

Table 12-1.

Antihypertensives	Cimetidine
Reserpine	Barbiturates
Methyldopa	Benzodiazepines
Thiazides	β-blockers, esp. propranolol
Spironolactone	hydrochloride
Clonidine hydrochloride	Metoclopramide hydrochloride
Oral contraceptives	Cocaine
Steroids and ACTH	Amphetamine

symptoms. Laboratory values necessary for the routine differential diagnosis in psychiatric consultation are given in chapter 6. A work-up is not complete if the evaluation of thyroid and parathyroid function is not included.

Many medical illnesses have been associated with depressive symptoms. The list is extensive and for all practical purposes can be included with the list of medical illnesses which can cause delirium (see chapter 6). For more than 50 years[14] carcinoma of the pancreas has been noted to show frequent association with psychiatric symptoms, especially depression, which in some cases seems to be the first manifestation of the disease. Using a group of gastric cancer patients as control, Holland et al[15] in a prospective study demonstrated that pancreatic cancer patients reported significantly more psychiatric disturbance, depression included, than did gastric cancer patients. The DSM-III criteria were not used. Whether the increase in psychiatric symptoms is due to the grim prognosis of pancreatic cancer (though depression has often been demonstrated before the patient or physician knew the diagnosis) or to a humoral process initiated by the malignancy is unclear. Pomara and Gershon[16] reported a case of treatment-resistant, DST-positive depression in which the patient was eventually diagnosed to have pancreatic carcinoma. After excision the response to antidepressants was improved and the DST normalized. Although the ability of pancreatic cancer to induce major depression still awaits scientific confirmation, the clinical lore justifies its inclusion in the differential diagnosis for organic causes of psychiatric symptoms. Patients with hereditary pancreatitis, inherited by autosomal dominance, are predisposed to develop cancer of the pancreas, so that for them gastrointestinal (GI) symptomatology is an essential subject of inquiry.

Most other illnesses included in the differential diagnosis seem capable of causing either depressive or delirious symptoms. For this reason the differential list to be considered for any medical illness producing psychiatric symptoms must be comprehensive. We see no advantage in limiting the list or changing it to match each psychiatric disorder. However, quite pertinent to the consultant is a brief discussion of those conditions more frequently associated with symptoms of major depression—symptoms often so severe that antidepressant therapy is an essential contribution to restoring the patient's sense of well being.

Stroke. Direct injury to the brain can produce regular changes of affect which progress to a full syndrome of major depression. One model for this is the cerebrovascular accident (CVA), now shown by Robinson et al,[17] and others to be often followed by major depression. According to these studies, when the stroke is unilateral, major depression will occur in about 60% of patients with a left hemisphere lesion and in about 15% of patients with a right hemisphere lesion. The depression will appear within the acute period in about two thirds of patients destined to suffer it, with the remainder developing it by the sixth month. If left untreated, this severe depression will last at least 8 to 9 months. Moreover, the severity of the depression is directly related to the distance of the injury from the frontal pole (correlation for left frontal pole = $-.92$, for right = $.76$), that is, the closer the insult to the left frontal pole, the more depressed the patient will be. This is not a function of aphasia, which can exist without depression, just as depression can be found in the absence of aphasia. The authors also found that the relationship between severity and location remained strong when intellectual and physical impairment, quality of social supports, and age were taken into account. Further work by the same group established the same relationship between location of injury and severity of depression in patients with traumatic brain injury other than stroke, patients with bilateral brain injury, and even in left-handed patients with similar lesions.

Right hemisphere lesions deserve special diagnostic attention. As noted above, the closer the lesion is to the occipital pole, the more likely the patient is to be depressed. But when the lesion was in the right anterior location, the mood disorder tended to be an apathetic, indifferent state associated with "inappropriate cheerfulness." The patient, however, seldom *looks* cheerful, and may have complaints of loss of interest or even worrying. This disorder was found in six of 20 patients with single right hemisphere strokes (and in none of 28 patients with single left hemisphere lesions).

Prosody is also at risk in right hemisphere injury. Ross and Rush[18] focused clinical attention on the presentation of *aprosodia* (lack of "prosody" or inflection, rhythm, and intensity of expression) when the right hemisphere is damaged. Such a patient could appear quite depressed and be so labeled by staff and family, but simply lack the neuronal capacity to express and/or recognize emotion. These authors compared aprosodias to the aphasias that occur when corresponding sites in the left hemisphere are damaged. If one stations oneself out of the patient's view, selects a neutral sentence (eg, "The book is red"), asks the patient to identify the mood as mad, sad, frightened, or elated, and then declaims the sentence with the emotion to be tested, one should be able to identify those patients with a receptive aprosodia. Next the patient is presented with facial portrayals of the same emotions and asked to identify them (thereby separating visual from auditory clues). The patient can be then asked to portray facial or vocal expressions for the same emotions in order to test for the presence of an expressive aprosodia. There is no reason why a stroke patient cannot suffer from both aprosodia and depression, but separate diagnostic criteria and clinical examinations exist to recognize each one.

Because stroke is among the most disabling of injuries, the danger of labeling major depression associated with it as "appropriate" is extremely high, since, when it is so labeled, one can almost assume that treatment of the depression with antidepressants will not occur.

When depressed stroke patients are treated with appropriate drugs, they respond well. In a randomized, double-blind study of depressed stroke patients Lipsey et al[19] demonstrated a significant response to therapeutic plasma levels of nortriptyline hydrochloride after 6 weeks of treatment. Without treatment the depression is quite likely not to remit for 9 months.

The subcortical dementias. Parkinson's disease and Huntington's disease commonly include major depression within their symptomatology. The latter may present with a major depression prior to the onset of either chorea or dementia.[20] Diagnosis is made clinically, as described above. Some reports note that as depression is treated in the patient with Parkinson's disease, the parkinsonian symptoms will also improve, and may do so before the depressive symptoms subside. This is especially striking in case reports in which ECT was used,[21,22] although the same improvement has been reported after tricyclic antidepressants. Treatment of major depression in either disease may increase the comfort of the patient and is always worth a try. Huntington's patients may be sensitive to the anticholinergic side effects of tricyclics (though not invariably) so that the less anticholinergic drugs should be tried first.

Another subcortical dementia worth noting is Binswanger's encephalopathy, a state of white matter demyelination presumably based on arteriosclerosis, presenting with an abulic withdrawn state and a paucity of focal neurologic findings. Whenever affective symptoms are discovered on clinical examination a trial of antidepressant medication may produce striking relief for the patient. This supposedly rare condition is no exception.[23]

The encephalopathy caused by the HTLV-III virus, particularly in its earlier manifestations, produces a syndrome which verges on and often becomes major affective disorder. Depression can exist, as can mania or hypomania, in more advanced stages of the infection or with some of the opportunistic infections suffered by patients with AIDS-related complex (ARC) or acquired immunodeficiency syndrome (AIDS). The subtle impairment of concentration and attention is often the first sign noticed by the sufferer of the illness, but these symptoms will be followed by mild memory impairment, lethargy, loss of libido, and social withdrawal. Marked psychomotor retardation may be present.[24-28] At least in the earlier stages and often in the more advanced instances of infection, whether with the HTLV-III virus itself or with one of the opportunistic infections of the CNS, a dramatic response can occur to antidepressive treatment. Our current recommendation is to start with dextroamphetamine sulfate, 5 to 10 mg once in the morning, as described below. Table 12-2 presents the CNS complications of AIDS.

CHOICE OF APPROPRIATE ANTIDEPRESSANT TREATMENT

In chapters 26 and 27 the properties, side effects, dosages, and drug interactions of antidepressant medications are discussed in detail. These principles hold for the specific setting of consultation as they do when used in the treatment of primary depression. Although there has been concern that medically ill, depressed patients will not respond well to antidepressants,[29] our experience is encouraging. Whenever major depression is diagnosed, the effort to alleviate the clinical symptoms almost always includes somatic treatments. The consultant who understands the interactions of the antidepressants with illness and other drugs is best prepared to prescribe these agents effectively.[30]

Electroconvulsive therapy (ECT) remains the single most effective somatic treatment of depression. Recent nationwide review has only sustained its merit. Indications for its use are discussed in chapter 13.

Prescribing Antidepressants for the Medically Ill

Since the cardiac patient generates the most concern in the use of antidepressant drugs, a specific approach to prescribing safely for this patient is emphasized here. Ever since sudden death in cardiac patients was first associated with amitriptyline hydrochloride,[31,32] physicians

Table 12-2. CNS Complications of Acquired Immunodeficiency
Syndrome

Infectious complications
  Viral
    Cytomegalovirus
    Herpes simplex I and II
    Herpes zoster
    Papovavirus (progressive multifocal leukoencephalopathy)
    HTLV-III dementia
  Bacterial
    Mycobacterium avium intracellulare
    M tuberculosis hominis
    Nocardia
    Listeria monocytogenes
  Fungal
    Candida
    Cryptococcus neoformans
    Histoplasma capsulatum
    Coccidioides immitis
    Aspergillus
    Blastomyces dermatitidis
  Protozoa
    Toxoplasma gondii
Noninfectious complications
  Neoplasms
    Primary CNS lymphoma
    Kaposi's sarcoma
    Metastatic lymphoma
  Vascular
    Marantic endocarditis
    Cerebral hemorrhage
Peripheral neuropathy
Retinopathy

Adapted with permission from Harris et al.[28]

have tended to fear the use of tricyclics when cardiac disease is present. Fowler and et al[33] emphasized that life-threatening arrhythmias can occur even in patients free of cardiac disease. What guidelines, then, can one use in order to prescribe these agents safely for depressed patients with medical illness?

Depression itself is a life-threatening disease and should be treated. Choice of agent often takes its clinical starting point on whether the patient is especially troubled by insomnia. The sedative potency of the available ten "cyclic" antidepressants can generally be predicted by their antihistaminic property, specifically their in vitro affinity for the histamine$_1$ receptor. Table 12-3 gives these values.[34,35]

The antihistaminic property of these drugs gives a reasonably good estimate of their sedative properties. Trazodone, shown in Table 12-3 to have very low affinity for the H$_1$ receptor, is actually rather sedating in clinical use. This same property can also be used to predict how much weight gain may be associated with the antidepressant. Those troubled by obesity may be at additional risk if treated with those agents higher on the list. Alprazolam, a triazolobenzodiazepine reported to have antidepressant as well as antianxiety effects, is relatively sedating, though it is not a potent antihistamine in its own right. Even though the manufacturer does not include depression among indications for alprazolam use, and even though clinicians voice doubts about its efficacy, double blind, placebo controlled studies continue to support its antidepressant effectiveness.[36] The MAOIs generally have low sedative potency, although phenelzine sulfate can produce patient complaints of drowsiness.

All antidepressants in the cyclic and MAOI categories usually correct the insomnia of depression, a therapeutic effect not thought to be related

Table 12-3. Sedative and Antihistaminic Properties of Antidepressant Drugs

Agent	H$_1$ Receptor Affinity	Sedative Potency
Doxepin	3100*	High
Amitriptyline	770	High
Imipramine	10	Moderate
Trimipramine	1000	High
Protriptyline	2.9	Low
Nortriptyline	14	Moderate
Desipramine	0.4	Low
Amoxapine	15	Moderate
Maprotiline	100	High
Trazodone	1.4	High
Monoamine Oxidase Inhibitors (MAOIs)		Low
Alprazolam		High
Antihistaminic reference		None
Diphenhydramine hydrochloride	4	

*Units are affinities expressed as $10^{-7} \times 1/K_B$, where K_B = equilibrium dissociation constant in molarity.

to their effects on brain histamine. Therefore this discussion highlights a sedative effect of the drugs which occurs in addition to and independent of these agents' ability to correct the specific sleep disturbances of major depression (eg, to lengthen rapid eye movement [REM] latency).

Occasionally the consultant may come upon a patient in whom antihistamines have been tried and failed to achieve therapeutic effect, such as in the treatment of an allergic rash or the itching associated with uremia. Since doxepin hydrochloride is the most potent antihistamine in clinical medicine, a trial of even 5 mg may provide relief not available with a weaker antihistamine.

Threatening the successful use of antidepressants is the occurrence of unwanted side effects. In general these side effects can be summarized as belonging to three groups: (1) orthostatic hypotension, (2) anticholinergic side effects, and (3) cardiac conduction effects. Once these three side effects are understood for each of the antidepressants, safe clinical prescription of the drugs is far more likely.

Orthostatic hypotension. It would be nice were orthostatic hypotension directly related to each drug's in vitro affinity for the α_1-noradrenergic receptor, but this is not the case. Table 12-4 presents the drugs with a clinical rating of their respective likelihoods of causing an orthostatic fall in blood pressure.

In general, among the tricyclics tertiary amines are more likely to cause an orthostatic fall in blood pressure than are secondary amines. For reasons which are not clearly understood, imipramine is the tricyclic most commonly associated with clinical mishaps, such as falling and sustaining a fracture or head injury. The orthostatic effect appears earlier than the therapeutic effect for imipramine, and will be objectively verifiable at less than half the therapeutic plasma level. Hence the drug may have to be discontinued long before a therapeutic plasma level is reached. On the other hand, once postural symptoms develop, increasing the dose of antidepressant is not likely to make the symptoms worse.

Often one can detect which patient is susceptible to this fall in blood pressure simply by testing the orthostatic fall in systolic pressure before starting the drug. The patient whose systolic pressure falls more than 15 mmHg on rising from a lying to a standing position is likely to sustain a fall about twice that after starting imipramine. Naturally, younger patients may tolerate a fall in pressure more easily than older, so an orthostatic fall in pressure may not produce symptoms or symptoms serious enough to require discontinuation of the drug. In patients who are medically ill, however, sensitivity to side effects tends to be higher. Some have noted that, even though the objective fall in standing pressure

Table 12-4. Orthostatic Potencies of Antidepressant Drugs

Agent	α_1-Receptor Affinity*	Orthostatic Potential
Doxepin	4.2[†]	Moderate
Amitriptyline	3.7	Moderate
Imipramine	1.1	High
Trimipramine	4.2	Moderate
Protriptyline	0.75	Low
Nortriptyline	1.6	Low
Desipramine	0.75	Low
Amoxapine	2.0	Low
Maprotiline	1.1	Low
Trazodone	2.8	Moderate
MAOIs		High
Alprazolam		None
Antihypertensive reference Prazosin hydrochloride	1640.0	None

* From Richelson.[34,35]
[†] See footnote to Table 12-3 for description of units.

will continue for several months, some patients with initial symptoms accommodate subjectively and no longer complain of the side effect. As can be seen from the list, choice of a secondary amine is the easiest way to avoid orthostatic hypotension.[37] There is some clinical consensus that nortriptyline is the tricyclic least likely to cause the side effect. Trazodone, one of the newer agents, will produce a hypotensive effect more often than the secondary amines; hence it has no advantage when this side effect is considered.

Monoamine oxidase inhibitors are notorious for causing orthostatic hypotension; in fact, this is the commonest troublesome side effect. Phenelzine and tranylcypromine sulfate will produce the orthostatic effect about as often as imipramine. Nor can the clinician, when prescribing an MAOI, be confident that the predrug fall in orthostatic blood pressure will successfully predict those patients especially at risk. The orthostatic effect (and therefore the postural symptoms) usually occurs only 2 to 4 weeks after the patient has been taking the MAOI.

Alprazolam has not been associated with orthostatic hypotension.

Anticholinergic effects. The anticholinergic effects of tricyclics cause many nuisances for patients. Urinary retention, constipation, dry mouth, confusional states and tachycardia are the commonest. The increase in heart rate is a sinus tachycardia resulting from the ability of the drugs to oppose vagal tone on the heart. As many as 30% of a group of normal individuals will respond with tachycardia to amitriptyline.[38] This side effect correlates nicely with the in vitro affinity of each drug for the acetylcholine muscarinic receptor, presented in Table 12-5.[39] As seen in the table, amitriptyline is the most anticholinergic of the antidepressants, with protriptyline a rather close second. These agents will regularly cause tachycardia in medically ill patients, and one should check the heart rate as the dose is increased. If significant tachycardia results, another agent may have to be used. Many hospitalized patients, particularly those with ischemic heart disease, are already being treated with β-adrenergic blockers, such as propranolol. When this is the case, the β-blocker will usually protect the patient from developing a significant tachycardia.

All the cyclic agents except trazodone are significantly anticholinergic. If one switches from, for example, imipramine to desipramine because the patient developed urinary retention, the patient is quite likely to develop retention again on desipramine. The newer agents amoxapine and maprotiline are not significantly less anticholinergic in clinical use than desipramine. Trazodone is almost devoid of activity at

Table 12-5. Anticholinergic Potencies of Antidepressant Drugs

Agent	Muscarinic Receptor Affinity	Anticholinergic Potency
Doxepin	1.3*	High
Amitriptyline	5.5	Very high
Imipramine	1.1	High
Trimipramine	1.7	High
Protriptyline	4.0	Very high
Nortriptyline	0.7	Moderate
Desipramine	0.5	Moderate
Amoxapine	0.1	Moderate
Maprotiline	0.2	Moderate
Trazodone	0.0003	Very low
MAOIs	<0.00001	None
Alprazolam		None
Anticholinergic reference Atropine	48.0	

* See footnote to Table 12-3 for description of units.

the muscarinic receptor site, and it is a worthwhile choice when another agent has caused unwanted anticholinergic side effects.

The MAOIs are without activity at the acetylcholine muscarinic receptor; hence they can also be useful alternatives when these side effects impair access of a patient to an antidepressant. Alprazolam similarly lacks significant anticholinergic activity.

Cardiac conduction effects. All tricyclics appear to prolong ventricular depolarization. This will tend to produce on the ECG a lengthening of the PR and QRS intervals, as well as the QT interval, corrected for heart rate (QT-c). When the main effect of these agents is measured by His bundle electrocardiography, it is the H-V portion of the recording that is preferentially prolonged. That is, these drugs tend to slow the electrical impulse as it passes through the specialized conduction tissue known as the His-Purkinje system. This makes them resemble in action the class IA antiarrhythmic drugs such as quinidine and procainamide hydrochloride. In practical terms, this means that the depressed cardiac patient with ventricular premature contractions, when started on an antidepressant such as imipramine, is likely to receive a reduction in the ventricular irritability.

Ordinarily, this property will not pose a problem for the cardiac patient who does not already have disease in his conduction system. The patient who already has conduction system disease, however, is the patient one needs to be most concerned about. First-degree heart block and right bundle-branch block (BBB) are the mildest forms of pathology, and ordinarily should not pose a problem for antidepressant treatment. When the patient's disease is bifascicular block, BBB with prolonged PR, alternating BBB, or second- or third-degree atrioventricular (AV) block, extreme caution is necessary in treating the depression. Cardiology consultation will almost always already be present for the patient. Electrolyte abnormalities, particularly hypokalemia or hypomagnesemia, increase the danger to these patients and require careful monitoring.

Occasionally the question will arise clinically whether one of the cyclic agents is less likely than another to cause a quinidinelike prolongation in conduction, particularly when the patient already shows some intraventricular conduction delay. There is some evidence that the hydroxy metabolites of the traditional tricyclics are more specifically related to the production of slowing in A-V conduction,[40] possibly more so in elderly patients. Some clinicians continue to feel that doxepin is less likely than, say, imipramine, to prolong cardiac conduction even though the literature reviews present reasonable evidence to refute this.[41] Early His bundle electrographic studies of patients who had taken overdoses of tricyclics indicated that those who had overdosed on doxepin did not show the same H-V prolongation in their recordings as occurred with other tricyclics. Disputes remain because no plasma levels of doxepin were reported. Our clinical bias is that doxepin has less tendency to alter cardiac conduction, but the consultant must remember that patients with pre-existing abnormalities of cardiac conduction require appropriate clinical vigilance to protect them from further aggravation of their cardiac condition. Amoxapine has likewise been touted to have fewer cardiac side effects, again based on patients who had taken overdoses. Although these patients were noted to have suffered seizures, coma, and acute renal failure, the authors thought it worth nothing that no cardiac toxicity resulted.[42,43] But atrial flutter–fibrillation has been reported in patients taking amoxapine.[44,45]

Trazodone also has been defended in a thorough review by Ayd[46] as holding promise for being less cardiotoxic than other cyclic antidepressant drugs. This is worth remembering when one meets the depressed patient with heart disease, particularly the elderly patient in whom heightened sensitivity to all side effects is a concern. However, even though trazodone is said not to prolong conduction in the His-Purkinje system, aggravation of pre-existing ventricular irritability has been reported to have been aggravated by trazodone.[47] Hence, clinical caution cannot be abandoned.

How then should the consultant approach the depressed patient with conduction disease? Depression can itself be life-threatening and more damaging to cardiac function than a drug. It must be treated. One therefore might begin with a psychostimulant. Should the patient show a positive response, the stimulant can be continued as long as it is helpful. By starting with a very low dose (2.5 mg of either dextroamphetamine or methylphenidate hydrochloride), one is reasonably assured that no toxicity will result. The fragile patient can be monitored for heart rate and blood pressure responses at hourly intervals after receiving the drug, up to four hours. If no beneficial response is noted, the next day the dose should be raised to 5 mg (our usual starting dose), then to 10, 15, and 20 mg on successive days, if necessary. One should be able to see *some* response to the stimulant, even a negative one (usually that the patient is made to feel more tense, "wired," or agitated) so that a clear response can be demonstrated. (It makes little sense to stop a stimulant trial without seeing any response unless the patient can report some subjective verification of a drug effect. Of course, an adverse elevation of heart rate or blood pressure is a reason for stopping the trial.)

When would one then add another antidepressant? The commonest clinical reason is the persistence of insomnia, which stimulants do not relieve. Next would be when the clinical plateau of the positive response to stimulants remains at an unacceptably low level (ie, the depression does not continue to clear). In this case, if the patient has cardiac conduction problems and persistent insomnia, doxepin or trazodone can be started, but with a small dose, such as 10 to 25 mg of doxepin hydrochloride or 25 to 50 mg of trazodone hydrochloride the first night. The degree of clinical vigilance must match the clinical precariousness of the patient. If he has shifting bundle-branch block and compromised ventricular function, he will require a cardiac monitor (though such a patient will probably already be monitored in this way). Discussion of the type and intensity of monitoring takes place with the consultee.

The role of the psychiatric consultant is to recommend aggressive treatment for depression, with the consultee helping to decide what means are appropriate to detect possible side effects. If the patient's conduction were so unstable that no cyclic drug was appropriate, then a MAOI would be an excellent choice, provided the patient can tolerate the orthostatic hypotension which may result. The adage "start low, go slow," which is so appropriate in the treatment of elderly patients, is also a good rule for medically unstable patients. If the depression has left the patient dangerously suicidal or catatonic, ECT is the treatment of choice. When an antidepressant can be used, monitoring must take into account both the development of a steady state (which may take around five half-lives of the drug) and the rate at which the dose is being increased. When the patient requires rapid, for example, daily dose increase, then a daily rhythm strip may be necessary, as well as another five half-lives after reaching that level thought to represent the therapeutic dose. Plasma levels are especially useful when a 3- to 4-week drug trial is judged worthwhile. Reliable levels have been established only for nortriptyline hydrochloride (50–150 ng/mL), desipramine hydrochloride ($\geq$125 ng/mL) and imipramine hydrochloride ($\geq$200 ng/mL).

Myocardial depression.   Do antidepressant drugs depress left ventricular function? The best answers to this question have been provided by Giardina et al[48] and Raskind et al.[49] Left ventricular ejection fractions were measured before and during imipramine, doxepin, and nortriptyline treatment of cardiac patients with major depression. These tricyclics showed no adverse effects on ventricular function, even in patients who demonstrated impaired ventricular function before drug treatment. Glassman et al[50] have also reported safe use of antidepressants in patients with congestive heart failure.

Psychostimulant use.   A recently published study reviews the MGH experience with the use of dextroamphetamine and methylphenidate in depressed medically ill patients.[51] The use of psychostimulants as predictors of response to antidepressant drugs is well known.[52] Their use as therapeutic agents was gradually discontinued several years ago,[53] but when patients with symptoms of major and minor depression continued to respond to stimulants, often achieving remission of their symptoms, these agents became independent antidepressants in our consultation practice. Their effects on heart rate and blood pressure have been found to be trivial, even though any patient with hypertension or unstable cardiac rhythm requires monitoring of vital signs when started on these agents. The commonest fear expressed about their use was that they would reduce appetite in patients who were already anorexic either from their illness or their depression or both. Not a single case of interference with appetite was found associated with the use of these drugs. In several instances, increased appetite was reported by the patients—another striking and important benefit associated with their use.

Finally, in those patients who suffered both depressive symptoms and either dementia or an organic brain syndrome (eg, head injury), there was a fear that use of a stimulant would result in agitation, confusion, or psychosis. In 17 patients with an associated diagnosis of dementia, only two showed a worsening of confusion, which disappeared within 24 hours of discontinuing the drug. Hence our practice is now to begin with a stimulant. If it helps (as it did to a moderate or marked degree in 48% of the patients), it will do so within a short time: about 93% of the patients who responded positively reached their maximum benefit by the second day. As long as it helps, the stimulant is maintained. Tolerance was not found in our patient sample. The same dose of stimulant was therefore maintained until the depressive symptoms had cleared or the patient was discharged. A small group of patients were discharged with instructions to continue taking the agent at home. The majority stopped the medication within 2 to 3 weeks. A few continued for 1 year or longer.

There is a strong bias against stimulants, dextroamphetamine more so than methylphenidate, because of associated street abuse. In the MGH review cited, neither tolerance nor abuse was found in the patients for whom these agents were prescribed.

How long antidepressants need to be maintained in major depression associated with medical illness is not known. Even though patients with primary affective disorder should be maintained on their antidepressant for longer than 6 months, the same requirement is not clear for major depression in the medical setting. One clinical rule of thumb, however, would be that when the syndrome of major depression appears to have been induced by direct brain injury (stroke, head trauma), the maintenance of antidepressant medication should exceed 6 months. For other patients, for example, a patient with a prolonged hospitalization after surgery who becomes depressed, stopping the antidepressant within 1 to 2 weeks after the depressive syndrome has remitted has not seemed to have been followed by relapse.

Secondary Mania

Occasionally one will be asked to see a patient with mania or hypomania of 1 (or more) week's duration, in whom no prior history of affective disorder can be obtained. Described by Krauthammer and Klerman,[54] this phenomenon results from an organic dysfunction. Table 12-6 lists the causes of secondary mania. The emergence of mania or hypomania usually signifies the presence of bipolar affective disease, but cases such as those in Table 12-6 continue to accumulate in the literature, indicating that alteration of brain states can lead to a clinical picture indistinguishable from primary mania.

Use of Lithium Carbonate in the Medically Ill

The treatment of secondary mania is the same as that for primary mania (see chapter 26). Neuroleptics and lithium carbonate are required

Table 12-6. Reported Causes of Secondary Mania

Drugs	Corticosteroids, isoniazid, procarbazine hydrochloride, LSD, sympathomimetics, levodopa, cyproheptadine hydrochloride, thyroxine, L-glutamine, tolmetin, alprazolam, metrizamide, propafenone, captopril, yohimbine, alcohol intoxication
Drug withdrawal	Clonidine hydrochloride
Metabolic	Hemodialysis, postoperative state, hyperthyroidism, vitamin B_{12} deficiency
Infection	Influenza, Q fever, post-St Louis type A encephalitis, cryptococcosis
Neoplasm	Meningiomas, gliomas, thalamic metastases
Epilepsy	Right temporal focus
Surgery	Right hemispherectomy
Cerebrovascular accident	Thalamic stroke
Other	Cerebellar atrophy

Data from Greenberg and Brown[55] and Harsch et al.[56]

in most cases. A word of caution is due when lithium is used in elderly patients or patients with cardiac disease. On the ECG of a patient taking lithium one will see T wave flattening in about 50% of cases, but this is benign and a reversible phenomenon. Lithium appears to have some inhibitory effects on impulse generation and transmission within the atrium. Hence the reports of adverse cardiac effects of lithium have been those of sinus node dysfunction and first-degree AV block.[57–59] Since the elderly seem particularly prone to these effects, caution is essentially reserved for them and for patients who have pre-existing disturbances of atrial conduction.[60]

A further caution about lithium's toxicity when combined with other agents comes from a report by Lyman et al[61] in which 100 patients with small cell bronchogenic carcinoma were randomly assigned to receive either lithium (because it had been shown to reduce the incidence of infection in a similar group of patients) or placebo. All patients received treatment which included doxorubicin and, with it, cyclophosphamide and mediastinal radiation, both of which can increase the doxorubicin-associated heart failure in patients over 70 years of age. In patients with pretreatment cardiovascular abnormalities (by history, examination, or ECG) the combination of lithium and theophylline bronchodilators was significantly associated with sudden death, which occurred in 13 patients, 11 of whom were on lithium. There was a strong interaction between lithium and bronchodilator use, such that each agent alone could not be shown to make a significant independent contribution to sudden death. Of course, small-cell bronchogenic carcinoma is rapidly lethal in itself (lack of tumor response to treatment was itself the most powerful predictor of death).

The severity of illness in such a group of patients justifies the heightened concern every clinician has when any treatment is under-taken. Ordinarily lithium's effects on the heart can be assumed to be benign, but as any serious illness becomes more complicated and treatments increase, patients are at greater risk. Nor can it be forgotten that mania, like depression, can seldom be tolerated either by the patient or by his caregivers. Whether the alternative treatments such as calcium channel blockers or adjunctive measures such as lorazepam are as useful in secondary mania as in primary mania remains to be established.

Thioridazine

A final caution about cardiovascular toxicity should include discussion of thioridazine. Notorious among neuroleptics for its potential cardiac side effects, this drug should not be used in combination with tricyclic antidepressants unless there is a very special need. It, too, possesses quinidinelike properties, has been associated with reports of sudden death which antedate similar reports with tricyclics,[62] and was more recently implicated in the causation to torsade de pointes ventricular tachycardia.[63] Thioridazine's uniquely high anticholinergic properties (roughly equivalent in vitro to desipramine) can be troublesome as well. However, this very property might make it particularly useful to treat the delirium of a patient with Parkinson's disease. As little as 5 to 10 mg can be helpful in such a patient. Again relevant is the caution to avoid hypokalemia and hypomagnesemia which pose special hazards for cardiac rhythm disturbances.

Other DSM-III Diagnoses of Depression

Organic affective syndrome.   When the etiology of depressed mood is an organic factor, such as an antihypertensive drug or a stroke, the resulting depression can be referred to as *organic affective syndrome* (293.83) if at least two of the eight criteria mentioned above are met. Our recommendation is that when four or more criteria are met, the diagnosis of major depression be used and when two or three only are reached, organic affective syndrome be the label. Treatment of organic affective syndromes is a matter of clinical judgment; whenever the clinician prefers to use antidepressant medication, the same categories of drugs mentioned with major depression are useful.

Psychological factors affecting physical condition.   Use of the diagnosis *psychological factors affecting physical condition* (316.00) occurs when a physical disorder is known to be affected by emotional states. For example, if a person were to become despondent, psoriasis or migraine might worsen. In a true sense, the course of nearly any physical condition could be judged to worsen or become prolonged because of the patient's emotional state. This diagnosis is not used when a somatoform disorder is present.

Adjustment disorder with depressed mood.   When the patient does not meet the criteria for major depression, the diagnosis of *adjustment disorder with depressed mood* (309.00) is most commonly the appropriate one. As mentioned above, the term depression is appropriately reserved for major depression. But despondency is omnipresent in the sick, so that its understanding and common-sense remedies deserve attention.

DESPONDENCY CONSEQUENT TO SERIOUS ILLNESS

Despondency in serious illness appears to be a natural response and is here regarded as the psychic damage done by the disease to the patient's self-esteem. Bibring's definition of depression is a "response to narcissistic injury."[64] The response is here called "despondency" and not depression because depression is reserved for those conditions that meet the research criteria of primary or secondary affective disorder. In any serious illness, then, the mind sustains an injury of its own, as though the illness, for example, myocardial infarction, produces an ego infarction. Even when recovery of the diseased organ is complete, recovery of self-esteem appears to take somewhat longer. In myocardial infarction patients, for example, while the myocardial scar has fully formed in 5 to 6 weeks, recovery of the sense of psychological well-being seems to require 2 to 3 months.

Management of the Acute Phase of Despondency

A mixture of dread, bitterness, and despair, despondency presents the self as broken, scarred, ruined. Work and relationships seem jeopardized. Now it seems to the patient too late to realize career or personal aspirations. Disappointment with both what has and has not been accomplished haunts the individual, who may now feel old and a failure. Concerns of this kind become conscious very early in acute illness and their expression may prompt consultation requests as early as the second or third day of hospitalization.[65]

Management of these illness-induced despondencies is divided into acute and long-term phases. In the acute phase, the patient is encouraged but never forced, to express such concerns. The extent and detail are determined by the individual's need to recount them. Many patients are upset to find such depressive concerns in consciousness and even worry that this signals a "nervous breakdown." It is therefore essential to let patients know that such concerns are the normal emotional counterpart of being sick, and that even though there will be "ups and downs" in their intensity, these concerns will probably disappear gradually as health returns. It is also helpful for the consultant to be familiar with the rehabilitation plans common to various illnesses, so that patients can also be reminded, while still in the acute phase of recovery, that plans for restoring function are being activated.

Paradoxically, many of the issues discussed in the care of the dying patient (chapter 17) are relevant here. Heavy emphasis is placed on maintaining the person's sense of self-esteem. Self-esteem often falters in seriously ill persons even though they have good recovery potential. Hence efforts to learn what the sick person is like can help the consultant alleviate the acute distress of a damaged self-image. The consultant should learn any "defining" traits, interests, and accomplishments of the patient so that the nurses and physicians can be informed of them. For example, after learning that a woman patient had been a star sprinter on the national Polish track team preparing for the 1940 Olympics, the consultant relayed this both in the consultation note and by word of mouth to her caregivers. "What's this I hear about your having been a champion sprinter?" became a common question that made her feel not only unique, but appreciated. The objective is to restore to life the real person within the patient who has serious organic injuries or impairment.

Few things are more discouraging for the patient, staff, or consultant than no noticeable sign of improvement. When there is no real progress, all the interventions discussed in chapter 17 are necessary. At other times progress is being made but so slowly that the patient cannot feel it in any tangible way. By using his ingenuity the consultant may find a way to alter this. Many of the suggestions below apply, and a knowledge of the physiology of the illness is essential. However, psychological interventions can also be helpful. For example, getting a patient with severe congestive heart failure out of bed and into a reclining chair (known for 25 years to produce even less cardiovascular strain than the supine position)[66] can provide reassurance and boost confidence. For some patients with severe ventilatory impairments and difficulty weaning from the respirator, a wall chart depicting graphically the time spent off the ventilator each day (one gold star for each five-minute period) is encouraging. Even if the patient's progress is slow, the chart documents and dramatizes each progressive step. Of course, personal investment in very ill persons may be far more therapeutic in itself than any gimmick, but such simple interventions have a way of focusing new effort and enthusiasm on each improvement.

Management of Postacute Despondencies: Planning for Discharge and After

Even when the patients are confident their illness is not fatal, they usually become concerned that it will cripple them. As noted, psychological "crippling" is a normal hazard with organic injury. Whether the patient is an employable uncomplicated myocardial infarction patient or a chronic emphysematous "panter" with carbon dioxide tension of 60 mmHg, only restoration of self-esteem can protect him from emotional incapacitation. Even when the body has no room for improvement, the mind can usually be rehabilitated.

Arrival home from the hospital often proves to be a vast disappointment. The damage due to illness has been done, acute treatment is completed, and health professionals are far away. Weak, anxious, and demoralized, the patient experiences a "homecoming depression."[67] Weakness is a universal problem for any individual whose hospitalization required extensive bed rest; in fact, it was the symptom most complained of by one group of postmyocardial infarction patients visited in their homes.[67] Invariably the individuals attribute this weakness to the damage caused by the disease (to heart, lungs, liver, etc). However, a large part of this weakness is due to muscle atrophy and the systemic effects of immobilization. Bed rest, a disease in itself, includes among its ill effects venous stasis with threat of phlebitis, embolism, orthostatic hypotension, a progressive increase in resting heart rate, loss of about 10% to 15% of muscle strength per week (due to atrophy), and reduction of about 20% to 25% in maximal oxygen uptake capacity in a 3-week period. This was dramatically illustrated by the study of Saltin et al[68] of five healthy college students who, after being tested in the laboratory, were placed on 3 weeks' bed rest. Three of the men were sedentary and two were trained athletes. As shown in Figure 12-2, after the period of bed rest, it took the three sedentary men 8, 10, and 13 days to regain their pre–bed rest maximal oxygen uptake levels, whereas it took the two athletes 28 and 43 days to reach their initial values. The better the patient's condition, the longer it takes for the recovery of strength. Entirely unaware of the physiology of muscle atrophy, patients mistakenly believe that exercise, the only treatment of atrophy, is dangerous or impossible.

Fear can be omnipresent following discharge from the hospital. Every least bodily sensation, particularly in the location of the affected organ, looms as an ominous sign of the worst—recurrence (myocardial infarction, malignancy, GI bleeding, perforation, or other), metastatic spread, (another) infection, or some new disaster that will cripple the individual even further. Most of the alarming symptoms felt in the early posthospital days are so trivial that they would never have been noticed before, but the threshold is far lower now and patients may find any unusual sensation a threat. When the alarm has passed, they may then feel foolish or even disgusted with themselves for being hypochondriacal. It helps to know in advance that such hypersensitivity to bodily sensations commonly occurs, that it is normal, and that it is time-limited. Though there are wide ranges in the time it takes for this problem to disappear, a well-adjusted patient who has an uncomplicated myocardial infarction requires from 2 to 6 months for these fears to resolve (far more time than the recovery of the myocardium). With specific measures, this time may be shortened.

Whether the person can improve a physical function like oxygen

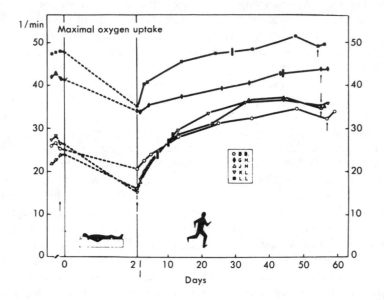

Figure 12-2. Maximal oxygen uptake in sedentary and athletic men after 3 weeks' bed rest.

consumption (eg, patients with myocardial infarction or GI bleeding) or cannot do so at all (eg, a person with chronic obstructive lung disease), the mental state is basically the same—a sense of imprisonment in a damaged body that is unable to sustain the everyday activities of a reasonable life. The illness has mentally crippled the individual. Horizons have shrunk drastically, so that the person may feel literally unable or afraid to leave the house, walk across a room, or stray far from the phone. Moreover, such people are likely to regard routine activities like walking, riding a bike, or raking leaves as too exhausting or dangerous. For some individuals, life comes to a near standstill.

The best therapy for such psychological constriction is a program that emphasizes early and progressive mobilization in the hospital and exercise after discharge. A physician might naturally be wary of prescribing this for a person with severe chronic obstructive pulmonary disease who is dyspneic while walking at an ordinary pace. However, Alpert et al [69] studied five such patients, measuring pulmonary function and performing catheterization of the right side of the heart before and after an 18-week physical training program. Even though the investigators found that cardiopulmonary functions were essentially unaltered by physical conditioning, these patients reported great improvement in subjective exercise tolerance. Objective bicycle exercise tolerance increased as much as a thousand-fold in all five persons examined. Several self-imposed restrictions (eg, never being far from an oxygen tank) were dramatically relieved. The psychiatric consultant should be aware that chronic pulmonary patients considered to have "irreversible" disease can be significantly helped by a specific rehabilitation program.[70–73]

Progress in writing exercise regimens for the recuperation period has been greatly helped by the definition and use of the metabolic equivalent (MET). One MET is defined as the energy expenditure per kilogram per minute of the average 70 kg person sitting quietly in a chair. This amounts to about 1.4 calories per minute or 3.5 to 4.0 mL of oxygen consumed per kilogram per minute. Table 12-7 lists activities for which measurements in MET have been determined.[74] For example, after recovery from uncomplicated myocardial infarction, the average middle-aged person is capable of performing at a level of 8 to 9 MET. This includes running at 5.5 mph (jogging slightly faster than 11-minute miles), cycling at 13 mph, skiing at 4 mph, noncompetitive squash, and handball, fencing, and vigorous basketball. If, however, less than ordinary activity produces symptoms, then the capacity of the post-coronary patient is nearer 4 MET. Despite obvious impairment, this level of capacity includes swimming the breast stroke at 20 yd/min, cycling at 5.5 mph, walking up a 5% incline at 3 mph, playing table tennis, golf (carrying clubs), badminton, lawn tennis doubles, and raking leaves. For the patient these are carefully computed, quantitated capacities. A list of activities quantified in MET is far more concrete and specific than statements such as, "Use your own judgment," or, "Do it in moderation." Instead, the patient can be given a list and told to select activities up to a specific level of MET. The physician who wishes to determine a tolerable level can use such devices as the step test, treadmill, and bicycle ergometer for which energy demand in MET at different levels has already been determined. Handy charts can be obtained from the American Heart Association manual.[75]

Activity levels can be gradually increased whenever appropriate. Patients should take responsibility for the extra costs that emotional involvement may require. For example, they could be told, "I now move you to a level of activity of 5 MET. You will find at this level all the

Table 12-7. Energy Expenditure per Kilogram per Minute (MET) in the Average 70 kg Individual

Activity	MET
Self-Care	
Rest, supine	1
Sitting	1
Standing, relaxed	1
Eating	1
Conversation	1
Dressing, undressing	2
Washing hands, face	2
Using bedside commode	3
Walking, 2.5 mph	3
Showering	3.5
Using bedpan	4
Walking downstairs	4.5
Walking, 3.5 mph	5.5
Propulsion, wheelchair	2
Ambulation with braces and crutches	6.5
Industrial Activities	
Watch repairing	1.5
Armature winding	2.0
Radio assembly	2.5
Sewing at machine	2.5
Bricklaying	3.5
Plastering	3.5
Tractor ploughing	3.5
Wheeling barrow, 115 lb, 2.5 mph	4.0
Horse ploughing	5.0
Carpentry	5.5
Mowing lawn by hand	6.5
Felling tree	6.5
Shoveling	7.0
Ascending stairs with 17 lb load at 27 ft/min	7.5
Planing	7.5
Tending furnace	8.5
Ascending stairs with 22 lb load at 54 ft/min	13.5
Housework Activities	
Hand sewing	1
Sweeping floor	1.5
Machine sewing	1.5
Polishing furniture	2
Peeling potatoes	2.5
Scrubbing, standing	2.5
Washing small clothes	2.5
Kneading dough	2.5

Table 12-7.—continued

Activity	MET
Scrubbing floors	3
Cleaning windows	3
Making beds	3
Ironing, standing	3.5
Mopping	3.5
Wringing by hand	3.5
Hanging wash	3.5
Beating carpets	4
Recreational Activities	
Painting, sitting	1.5
Playing piano	2
Driving car	2
Canoeing, 2.5 mph	2.5
Horseback riding, slow	2.5
Volley ball	2.5
Bowling	3.5
Cycling, 5.5 mph	3.5
Golfing	4
Swimming, 20 yd/min	4
Dancing	4.5
Gardening	4.5
Tennis	6
Trotting horse	6.5
Spading	7
Skiing	8
Squash	8.5
Cycling, 13 mph	9

Reproduced with permission from Cassem and Hackett.[74]

activities that your heart (or lungs or body) are physically capable of performing. Activities you enjoy are the best. Remember that getting emotionally upset or very competitive during activity increases the energy cost to your heart (lungs, body, etc). If you cannot do some of these things without getting all worked up, you will have to ease off; only you can judge that. But you now know that you are physically capable of performing at 5 MET." In this statement vagueness remains, but only in the area of subjective emotions. Patients not only experience their emotions physically and mentally but also should be aware of them, whereas they cannot detect changes in their left ventricular end-diastolic pressure or arterial oxygen saturation. Moreover, emotional self-control is a fair request to make of patients who, although not responsible for detecting a rising wedge pressure on the tennis court, must try to control rising killer instincts.

In any serious illness where there are likely to be so many "don't's" constricting the patient's world, an exercise regimen provides something to do that widens the space of existence. If a patient were limited by a maximum tidal volume of 13 L/min, an exercise program could not increase it, but it would help him to see that even within those limits he can increase (at least) subjective exercise tolerance, venture farther (eg, away from oxygen), and, one hopes, experience increased freedom. Some patients suffer illnesses in which reserves wax and wane (the cancer patient with remissions and exacerbations, aplastic anemia patients between transfusions). They may view life energy as a fixed quantity that is used up by activity little by little; thus they fear activity. The psychological benefits of exercise are such that activities should bring some sense of renewed vitality (improved sleep and appetite are common effects) rather than a sense of depletion or exhaustion. As hematocrit decreases (or blood urea nitrogen increases), capacity for exercise decreases. To continue exercising, such a person could set as a target a heart rate that was commonly experienced while exercising at his prescribed level of MET, or time and distance could be decreased accordingly. When his chronic congestive heart failure worsened, one man simply returned to the scene of his exercising, changed into his exercise gear, and sat talking with the regulars before returning home.

Just as getting sick is depressing, so is lack of progress in getting well. This normal despondency can further retard recovery. Self-esteem is restored by the methods described in chapter 17. Yet it is also restored by recovery of the body. The consultant who continuously studies the iatrogenic and reversible aspects of physical abnormality and the mythical obstacles to recovery can more effectively contribute to the shortening of convalescence and the rehabilitation of self-esteem.

REFERENCES

1. Myers JK, Weissman MM, Tischler GL, et al: Six-month prevalence of psychiatric disorders in three communities. *Arch Gen Psychiatry* 1984; 41:959–967.
2. Regier DA, Goldberg ID, Taube CA. The de facto U.S. Mental Health Services systems. *Arch Gen Psychiatry* 1978; 35:685.
3. Moffic HS, Paykel ES: Depression in medical in-patients. *Br J Psychiatry* 1975; 126:346.
4. Stewart JA, Drake F, Winokur G: Depression among medically ill patients. *Dis Nerv System* 1965; 26:479–485.
5. Schwab JJ, Bialow M, Brown JM, et al: Diagnosing depression in medical

inpatients. *Ann Intern Med* 1967; 67:695–707.

6. Cavanaugh SVA: Diagnosing depression in the hospitalized patient with chronic medical illness. *J Clin Psychiatry* 1984; 45:13–16.

7. Tufo HM, Ostfeld AM, Shekelle R: Central nervous system dysfunction following open-heart surgery. *JAMA* 1970; 212:1333.

8. Rabins PV, Harvis K, Koven S: High fatality rates of late-life depression associated with cardiovascular disease. *J Affective Dis* 1985; 9:165–167.

9. Schleifer SJ, Keller SE, Siris SG, et al: Depression and immunity: lymphocyte function in ambulatory depressed patients, hospitalized schizophrenic patients, and patients hospitalized for herniorrhaphy. *Arch Gen Psychiatry* 1985; 42:129–133.

10. Kronfol Z, Nasrallah HA, Chapman S, et al: Depression, cortisol metabolism and lymphocytopenia. *J Affective Dis* 1985; 9:169–173.

11. American Psychiatric Association: *Diagnostic and Statistical Manual of Mental Disorders* (3rd ed). Washington, American Psychiatric Association, 1980.

12. Hirschfield RMA, Koslow SH, Kupfer DJ: The clinical utility of the dexamethasone suppression test in psychiatry. *JAMA* 1983; 250:2172–2174.

13. Arana GW, Baldessarini RJ, Ornsteen M: Dexamethasone suppression test for diagnosis and prognosis in psychiatry. *Arch Gen Psychiatry* 1985; 42:1193–1204.

14. Yaskin JD: Nervous symptoms at earliest manifestations of carcinoma of the pancreas. *JAMA* 1923; 96:1664–1668.

15. Holland JC, Korzun AH, Tross S, et al: Comparative psychological disturbance in patients with pancreatic and gastric cancer. *Am J Psychiatry* 1986; 143:982–986.

16. Pomara N, Gershon S: Treatment-resistant depression in an elderly patient with pancreatic carcinoma: Case report. *J Clin Psychiatry* 1984; 45:439–440.

17. Robinson RG, Lipsey JR, Price TR: Diagnosis and clinical management of post-stroke depression. *Psychosomatics* 1985; 26:769–778.

18. Ross ED, Rush AJ: Diagnosis and neuroanatomical correlates of depression in brain-damaged patients. *Arch Gen Psychiatry* 1981; 38:1344–1354.

19. Lipsey JR, Robinson RG, Pearlson GD, et al: Nortriptyline treatment of post-stroke depression: A double-blind study. *Lancet* 1984; 1:297–300.

20. Folstein SE, Abbott MH, Chase GA, et al: The association of affective disorder with Huntington's disease in a case series and in families. *Psychol Med* 1983; 13:537–542.

21. Asnis G: Parkinson's disease, depression, and ECT: A review and case study. *Am J Psychiatry* 1977; 134:191–195.

22. Holcomb HH, Sternberg DE, Heninger GR: Effects of electroconvulsive therapy on mood, Parkinsonism, and tardive dyskinesia in a depressed patient: ECT and dopamine systems. *Biol Psychiatry* 1983; 18:865–873.

23. Summergrad P: Depression in Binswanger's encephalopathy responsive to tranylcypromine: Case report. *J Clin Psychiatry* 1985; 46:69–70.

24. Snider WD, Simpson DM, Nielsen S, et al: Neurological complications of acquired immune deficiency syndrome: Analysis of 50 patients. *Ann Neurol* 1983; 14:403–418.

25. Shaw GM, Harper ME, Hahn BH, et al: HTLV III infection in brains of children and adults with AIDS encephalopathy. *Science* 1985; 227:177–182.

26. Ho DD, Rota TR, Schooley RT, et al: Isolation of HTLV-III from cerebro-spinal fluid and neural tissues of patients with neurologic syndromes related to the acquired immunodeficiency syndrome. *N Engl J Med* 1985; 313: 1493–1497.

27. Holland JC, Tross S: The psychosocial and neuropsychiatric sequelae of the acquired immunodeficiency syndrome and related disorders. *Ann Intern Med* 1985; 103:760–764.

28. Harris AA, Segreti J, Levin S: Central nervous system infections in patients with the acquired immune deficiency syndrome (AIDS). *Clin Neurophar-macol* 1985; 8:201–210.

29. Popkin MK, Callies AL, Mackenzie TB: The outcome of antidepressant use in the medically ill. *Arch Gen Psychiatry* 1985; 42:1160–1163.

30. Jefferson JW: Biologic treatment of depression in cardiac patients. *Psychoso-matics* 1985; 26:31–38.

31. Coull DC, Crooks J, Dingwall-Fordyce I, et al: Amitriptyline and cardiac disease: risk of sudden death identified by monitoring system. *Lancet* 1970; 2:590–591.

32. Robinson DS, Barker E: Tricyclic antidepressant cardiotoxicity. *JAMA* 1976; 236:1089–1090.

33. Fowler NO, McCall D, Chou T, et al: Electrocardiographic changes and cardiac arrhythmias in patients receiving psychotropic drugs. *Am J Cardiol* 1976; 37:223–230.

34. Richelson E: Pharmacology of antidepressants used in the U.S. *J Clin Psychiatry* 1982; 43 (No. 11, section 2):4–11.

35. Richelson E: Are receptor studies useful for clinical practice? *J Clin Psy-chiatry* 1983; 44 (No. 9, section 2):4–9.

36. Overall JE, Biggs J, Jacobs M, et al: Comparison of alprazolam and imipramine for treatment of outpatient depression. *J Clin Psychiatry* 1987;48:15–19.

37. Glassman AH: Cardiovascular effects of tricyclic antidepressants. *Ann Rev Med* 1984; 35:503–511.

38. Jefferson JW: A review of the cardiovascular effects and toxicity of tricyclic antidepressants. *Psychosom Med* 1975; 37:160–179.

39. Cassem NH. Cardiovascular effects of antidepressants. *J Clin Psychiatry* 1982; 43 (No. 11, section 2):22–28.

40. Young RC, Alexopoulos GS, Chamoian CA, et al: Plasma 10-hydroxynor-triptyline and ECG changes in elderly depressed patients. *Am J Psychiatry* 1985; 142:866–868.

41. Luchins DJ: Review of clinical and animal studies comparing the cardio-vascular effect of doxepin and other tricyclic antidepressants. *Am J Psychiatry* 1983; 140:1006–1009.

42. Kulig K, Rumack BH, Sullivan JB Jr, et al: Amoxapine overdose: Coma and seizures without cardiotoxic effects. *JAMA* 1982; 248:1092–1094.

43. Pumariega AJ, Muller B, Rivers-Bulkeley N: Acute renal failure secondary to amoxapine overdose. *JAMA* 1982; 248:331–341.

44. Zavodnick S: Atrial flutter with amoxapine: A case report. *Am J Psychiatry* 1981; 138:1503–1505.

45. Murray GB: Atrial fibrillation/flutter associated with amoxapine: Two case reports. *J Clin Psychopharmacol* 1985; 5:124–125.

46. Ayd FJ Jr: Trazodone cardiac effects. *Int Drug Ther Newsletter* 1985;

20:29–32
47. Pohl R, Bridges M, Rainey JM Jr, et al: Effects of trazodone and despiramine on cardiac rate and rhythm in a patient with preexisting cardiovascular disease. *J Clin Psychopharmacol* 1986;6:380–381.
48. Giardina E-GV, Bigger JT Jr, Johnson LL: The effect of imipramine and nortriptyline on ventricular premature depolarizations and left ventricular function, abstract. *Circulation* 1981; 64 (suppl):IV–316.
49. Raskind M, Veith RC, Barnes R, et al: Cardiovascular and antidepressant effects of imipramine in the treatment of secondary depression in patients with ischemic heart disease. *Am J Psychiatry* 1982; 139:1114–1117.
50. Glassman AH, Johnson LL, Giardina E-GV, et al: The use of imipramine in depressed patients with congestive heart failure. *JAMA* 1983; 250:1997–2001.
51. Woods S, Tesar GE, Murray GB, et al: Psychostimulant treatment of depressive disorders secondary to medical illness. *J Clin Psychiatry* 1986; 47:12–15.
52. Van Kammen DP, Murphy DL: Prediction of imipramine antidepressant response by a one-day amphetamine trial. *Am J Psychiatry* 1978; 135:1179–1184.
53. Tesar GE. The role of stimulants in general medicine. *Drug Ther* 1982; 12:186–195.
54. Krauthammer C, Klerman GL: Secondary mania. *Arch Gen Psychiatry* 1978; 35:1333–1339.
55. Greenberg DB, Brown GL: Mania resulting from brain stem tumor. *J Nerv Ment Dis* 1985; 173:434–436.
56. Harsch HH, Miller M, Young LD: Induction of mania by L-dopa in a nonbipolar patient. *J Clin Psychopharmacol* 1985; 5:338–339.
57. Wellens H, Cats VM, Durren D: Symptomatic sinus node abnormalities following lithium carbonate therapy. *Am J Med* 1975; 59:285–287.
58. Wilson J, Kraus E, Bailas M, et al: Reversible sinus node abnormalities due to lithium carbonate therapy. *N Engl J Med* 1976; 294:1222–1224.
59. Mitchell JE, MacKenzie TB: Cardiac effects of lithium therapy in man. *J Clin Psychiatry* 1982; 43:47–51.
60. Roose SP, Bone S, Haidorfer C, et al: Lithium treatment in older patients. *Am J Psychiatry* 1979; 136:843–844.
61. Lyman GH, Williams CC, Dinwoodie WR, et al: Sudden death in cancer patients receiving lithium. *J Clin Oncol* 1984; 2:1270–1274.
62. Richardson HL, Graupner KI, Richardson ME: Intramyocardial lesions in patients dying suddenly and unexpectedly. *JAMA* 1966; 195:254–260.
63. Kemper AJ, Dunlap R, Pietro DA: Thioridazine-induced torsade de pointes. *JAMA* 1983; 249:2931–2934.
64. Bibring E: The mechanism of depression, in Greenacre P (ed): *Affective Disorders: Psychoanalytic Contributions to Their Study*. New York, International Universities Press, 1953, pp 13–48.
65. Cassem NH, Hackett TP: Psychiatric consultation in a coronary care unit. *Ann Intern Med* 1971; 75:9–14.
66. Levine SA, Lown B: "Armchair" treatment of acute coronary thrombosis. *JAMA* 1952; 148:1365.
67. Wishnie HA, Hackett TP, Cassem NH: Psychologic hazards of convalescence following myocardial infarction. *JAMA* 1971; 215:1292–1296.
68. Saltin B, Blomqvist G, Mitchell JH, et al: Response to exercise after bed rest

and after training. *Circulation* 1968; 38 (suppl 7):1–78.

69. Alpert JS, Bass H, Szucs MM, et al: Effects of physical training on hemodynamics and pulmonary function at rest and during exercise in patients with chronic obstructive pulmonary disease. *Chest* 1974; 66: 647–651.

70. Unger KM, Moser KM, Hanser P: Selection of an exercise program for patients with chronic obstructive pulmonary disease. *Heart Lung* 1980;9:68–76.

71. Pardy RL, Rivington RN, Despas PJ, et al: Inspiratory muscle training compared with physiotherapy in patients with chronic airflow limitation. *Am Rev Respir Dis* 1981;123:421–425.

72. Gift AG, Plaut SM, Jacox A: Psychologic and physiologic factors related to dyspnea in subjects with chronic obstructive pulmonary disease. *Heart Lung* 1986;15:595–602.

73. Andrews JL Jr: Pulmonary rehabiliation. *Prac Cardiol* 1986;12:127–137.

74. Cassem NH, Hackett TP: Psychological aspects of myocardial infarction. *Med Clin North Am* 1977; 61:711–721.

75. American Heart Association: Exercise testing and training of individuals with heart disease or at high risk for its development. Dallas, American Heart Association, 1975.

13

Electroconvulsive Therapy in the General Hospital

CHARLES A. WELCH

Electroconvulsive therapy (ECT) remains an indispensable treatment in the general hospital because of the large percentage of depressed patients who fail either to improve with drugs or to tolerate their side effects. There has been some improvement in drug response rates with monitoring of blood levels and newer agents, but for 15% to 20% of depressed patients, effective drug treatment is still unattainable. These patients carry a grim prognosis if they remain depressed, with a 36% mortality at 31 months,[1] and even higher mortality in the elderly. Consequently, the recent direction of ECT practice has been toward reducing side effects and improving efficacy, rather than discontinuing its use.

INDICATIONS

The symptoms which predict a good response to ECT are those of major depression: anorexia, weight loss, early morning awakening, impaired concentration, pessimistic mood, motor restlessness, speech latency, constipation, and somatic or self-deprecatory delusions.[2] The cardinal symptom is the acute loss of interest in activities which formerly gave pleasure. These are exactly the same symptoms which constitute the indication for antidepressant drugs and at the present time there is no way to predict which patients will ultimately be unresponsive to drugs. The definition of drug failure varies with the individual patient; young, healthy, nonsuicidal patients can safely receive four or more different drug regimens before moving to ECT, while older patients may be unable to tolerate more than one drug trial without serious morbidity.

Most patients receive a trial of medication first, but the following groups may receive ECT as a primary treatment.

1. Severely malnourished, dehydrated, and exhausted patients who are medically at risk should be treated without further delay.

261

2. Patients with complicating medical illnesses such as cardiac arrhythmia are usually more safely treated with ECT than with antidepressants.

3. In the delusionally depressed, tricyclics yield a response rate no better than placebo,[3] while ECT yields a response rate in the range of 90%.[4] Preliminary data indicate that a tricyclic-neuroleptic combination may also be quite effective in delusional depression,[5] but it should be reserved for younger patients because of the severity of side effects.

4. Catatonic patients whose underlying diagnosis is affective disorder are very responsive to ECT. Approximately two thirds of catatonics in the general hospital population suffer from affective disorder,[6] and prompt treatment is essential because of the severity of complications, including contractures, pneumonia, and venous emboli.

5. Patients who have been unresponsive to medication during previous episodes may be justifiably treated with ECT.

Schizophrenia often improves for several weeks following ECT, but the long-term course of the illness is not usually altered by the treatment. However, a subgroup of young psychotic patients, conforming to the "schizophreniform" profile (acute onset, family history of affective disorder, affective intactness) often show sustained improvement.[7]

Mania is also responsive to ECT,[8] but because of the effectiveness of drug therapy, ECT is rarely used. To date there have been no prospective comparisons of drugs and ECT in the treatment of mania.

CONTRAINDICATIONS

There are few absolute contraindications to ECT. Increased intracranial pressure may be exacerbated by the seizure resulting in mechanical brainstem injury. Digitalis toxicity may potentiate the vagal bradycardia following the seizure, resulting in bradycardic arrest. On the other hand, ECT has been safely given to patients with a wide variety of other medical conditions, including pregnancy, intracranial tumor or aneurysm, old cerebral infarction, carotid stenosis, seizure disorder, marginally compensated congestive heart failure, cardiac arrhythmias, hypertension, and endocrine disorders. The risk of ECT is low when properly performed, with a reported mortality of 4.5 per 100,000 treatments.[9] The last 800 patients at Massachusetts General Hospital (MGH) included over 50 patients with cardiac disease who were treated without fatalities. Other centers also report successful treatment of severely ill patients, with appropriate medical precautions.[10]

TECHNIQUE

The routine pre-ECT work-up includes a thorough medical history and physical examination, with chest films, ECG, urinalysis, complete blood count, blood sugar, BUN, and electrolytes. Additional studies are indicated for specific problems. For instance, with impaired cognition a metabolic screen, computed tomography (CT) scan, and EEG should usually be added to the above.

It is essential that the patient's medical condition be optimized prior to starting treatment. Dosage of ongoing medications such as digitalis, insulin, antihypertensives, and diuretics should be assessed. Elderly patients often arrive at the general hospital severely malnourished and dehydrated, and ECT is contraindicated until they have had four to five days of rehydration, with alimentation via feeding tube if necessary.

The main surgical recovery room has become the commonest location for administering ECT in the general hospital. In the early morning it is generally quiet but provides adequate equipment and staff for any emergency. With the acuity of medical illness now seen in most general hospitals, it is no longer advisable to perform ECT in an isolated treatment room. Anesthesia is usually methohexital sodium and succinylcholine chloride each at approximately 1 mg/kg, and is administered by an anesthesiologist, with ventilation via Ambu bag with oxygen. Moderate hyperventilation lowers the seizure threshold and reduces cognitive side effects.

Electrocardiographic monitoring is now used routinely, and is mandatory in patients with known cardiac disease. Up to 30% of patients have been reported to experience ectopy during ECT, but lasting ECG changes are rare.[11]

Blood pressure fluctuations present a more difficult problem. Occasional patients, particularly the elderly or those with pre-existing hypertension, develop marked hypertension for five to ten minutes immediately after the stimulus. If this exceeds systolic of 240 mmHg or diastolic of 120 mmHg, it should be treated with intravenous (IV) antihypertensives. Nitroglycerine, infused at 0.5 to 3.0 µg/kg/min,[12] or Nitroprusside, infused at 1–5 µg/kg/min,[13] are two effective antihypertensives. Nitroglycerine dilates both venous and arterial systems and causes less abrupt changes in blood pressure, making it appropriate for moderate hypertension. It may be used with frequent manual blood pressure monitoring. Nitroprusside acts on the arterial system but is a more potent agent, making it preferable for severe cases. Intra-arterial blood pressure monitoring is advisable when first used, but once dose requirements have been established manual measurement may be sufficient. Care must be taken not to overtreat, since the hypertensive phase is normally followed by a shift to mild hypotension 15 to 20 minutes after the seizure in most patients. In cases with pre-existing baseline hypertension, treating it adequately prior to a course of ECT usually reduces the problems encountered during the treatment. Premedication with beta blockers appears to be very effective in blunting hypertension during treatment.

A nurse should be present to monitor vital signs during the treatment and for 30 minutes thereafter. The period of highest risk is five to ten minutes after treatment, and an experienced staff person certified in cardiopulmonary resuscitation (CPR) should give undivided attention to monitoring airway, vital signs, and agitation during this period of recovery.

Unilateral nondominant electrode placement is associated with markedly less confusion and memory impairment than bilateral placement.[14] Furthermore, there is a growing body of evidence that unilateral stimulation, when performed under optimal conditions, is just as effective as bilateral for most patients.[15,16] It is important that the stimulus be above seizure threshold, that skin contact be meticulously prepared with saline or alcohol, and that there be no concurrent anticonvulsant medications such as flurazepam hydrochloride. When patients fail to respond to 12 unilateral ECTs, switching to bilateral placement is warranted, provided the diagnosis of major depressive illness remains solid.[17]

Although sine wave stimulus has been more commonly used in the past, brief pulse wave form is more efficient at inducing seizure activity, requiring less than a third as much current. There is also some reduction in posttreatment confusion and memory impairment,[18] and brief pulse is gradually becoming the standard ECT wave form in the United States. In addition to being more efficient, the newer brief pulse instruments have built-in limits to prevent excessive stimulus, offering an important advantage over older instruments.

Generalization of the seizure to the entire brain is essential for efficacy.[19] The simplest way to monitor seizure generalization is by inflating a blood pressure cuff on the arm above systolic pressure just prior to injection of the succinylcholine. The peripheral convulsion can then be observed unmodified in the hand. In unilateral ECT the cuff is placed on the arm ipsilateral to the stimulus. Some ECT instruments have a built-in single-channel EEG monitor but this is not a reliable indicator of full seizure generalization since partial seizures may also generate a classical seizure tracing.

The average number of ECTs necessary to treat major depression is consistently reported between six and 12 treatments, but occasional patients may require up to 30. The customary timing is three sessions per week with one full seizure per session. The use of more than one seizure per session (multiple monitored ECT) has no proven advantages. The most objective comparison of single and multiple ECT was performed by Fink, who concluded: "Multiple ECT carried more risks and fewer benefits than conventional ECT for our patients."[20]

ADVERSE EFFECTS

The most important side effect of ECT is anterograde memory impairment, which for the typical unilateral patient is mild and lasts for several weeks after the last treatment. Retrograde amnesia is generally limited to events immediately prior to the treatment. However, severe organic brain syndromes occasionally occur following ECT, and are usually associated with bilateral placement, high intensity stimulus, or pre-existing cognitive deficit. Although there is no clear evidence for structural damage secondary to ECT,[21] it appears that occasional patients continue to show cognitive deficits up to 6 months after treatment.[22]

MAINTENANCE MEDICATION

Following successful treatment the risk of relapse is over 50% at 12 months without maintenance medication.[23] Amitriptyline hydrochloride, imipramine hydrochloride, phenelzine sulfate, tranylcypromine sulfate, and lithium carbonate have all been shown to reduce the relapse rate to 10% to 15% at 12 months. Statistically, they appear equally effective, and the choice should be based on underlying diagnosis and prior drug response. The use of maintenance ECT (one treatment per month for the indefinite future) is widely practiced, but usually reflects failure to adequately apply appropriate drug therapy.

CONCLUSION

The use of ECT has become increasingly specific in recent years and the era of widespread abuse and overuse of the treatment is thankfully over. However, standards of practice remain unregulated, and in spite of increasing technical complexity there are still no qualifying tests for practitioners. In the coming era of prospective payment and "cost-effective" treatment, there is a danger that ECT will again be used with inadequate discretion, in the search for prompt treatment results. Nevertheless, it remains a safe and lifesaving treatment for hundreds of thousands of patients who without it would probably not recover from major depression.

REFERENCES

1. Huston PE, Locher LM: Involutional psychosis: Course when untreated and when treated with EST. *Arch Neurol Psychiatry* 1948; 59:385–394.
2. Carney MWP, Roth M, Garside RF: The diagnosis of depressive syndromes and the prediction of ECT response. *Br J Psychiatry* 1965; 3:659–674.
3. Glassman AJ, Kantor SJ, Shostak M: Depression, delusions, and drug response. *Am J Psychiatry* 1975; 132:716–719.
4. Scovern AW, Kilmann PR: Status of ECT: A review of the outcome literature. *Psychol Bull* 1980; 87:260–303.
5. Minter RE, Mandel MR: The treatment of psychotic major depressive disorder with drugs and electroconvulsive therapy. *J Nerv Ment Dis* 1979; 167:726–733.
6. Abrams R, Taylor MA: Catatonia: A prospective clinical study. *Arch Gen Psychiatry* 1976; 33:579–581.
7. Salzman C: The use of ECT in the treatment of schizophrenia. *Am J Psychiatry* 1980; 137:1032–1041.
8. McCabe MS: ECT in the treatment of mania: A controlled study. *Am J Psychiatry* 1976; 133:688–691.
9. Heshe J, Roeder E: Electroconvulsive therapy in Denmark. *Br J Psychiatry* 1976; 128:241–245.
10. Regestein QR, Reich P: Electroconvulsive therapy in patients at high risk for physical complications. *Convulsive Ther* 1985; 1:101–114.
11. Dec GW, Stern TA, Welch C: The effects of electroconvulsive therapy on serial electrocardiograms and serum cardiac enzyme values. *JAMA* 1985; 253:2525–2529.
12. Abrams J, Roberts R: First North American conference on nitroglycerine therapy. *Am J Med* 1983; 74:1–66.
13. Flaherty JT: Comparison of intravenous nitroglycerine and sodium nitroprusside in acute myocardial infarction. *Am J Med* 1983; 74:53–60.
14. Price TRP: Short- and long-term cognitive effects of ECT: Part 1—Effects on memory. *Psychopharmacol Bull* 1982; 18:81–91.
15. Welch C: The relative efficacy of unilateral non-dominant and bilateral stimulation. *Psychopharmacol Bull* 1982; 18:68–70.
16. Horne RL, Pettinati HM, Sugarman AA, et al: Comparing bilateral to unilateral electroconvulsive therapy in a randomized trial with EEG monitoring. *Arch Gen Psychiatry* 1985; 42:1087–1092.
17. Price TRP: Unilateral electroconvulsive therapy for depression. *N Engl J Med* 1981; 304:53.
18. Daniel WF, Weiner RD, Crovitz, HF: Autobiographical amnesia with ECT: An analysis of the roles of stimulus waveform, electrode placement, stimulus energy, and seizure length. *Biol Psychiatry* 1983; 18:121–126.
19. Ottoson JO: Experimental studies on the mode of action of electroconvulsive therapy. *Acta Psychiatr Neurol Scand* 1960; 35 (suppl 145):1–141.
20. Fink M: *Convulsive Therapy: Theory and Practice.* New York, Raven Press, 1979.

21. Weiner RD: Does electroconvulsive therapy cause brain damage? *Behav Brain Sci* 1984; 7:1–54.
22. Squire LR, Slater PC: Electroconvulsive therapy and complaints of memory dysfunction: A prospective three-year follow-up study. *Br J Psychiatry* 1983; 142:1–8.
23. Zis AP, Grof P, Webster MA, et al: Prediction of relapse in recurrent affective disorder. *Psychopharmacol Bull* 1980; 16:47–49.

14

Suicide and Other Disruptive States

THOMAS P. HACKETT and THEODORE A. STERN

A number of emotionally charged situations occur regularly in a general hospital. Although they often defy standard diagnostic classification, they usually become the responsibility of the psychiatrist. Many of these situations are dealt with in individual chapters, but a mixed bag remains. Those here described by no means constitute the complete repertoire, but they do represent the more commonly encountered disruptive states.

THE SUICIDAL PATIENT

Within the confines of the general hospital, psychiatrists are generally called upon to evaluate and treat patients who have contemplated, threatened, or attempted suicide. These assessments may occur either in the emergency room (ER) or on general medical or surgical floors.

Suicide is common, and attempts to commit suicide are even more common. Currently suicide is the tenth leading cause of death in this country and one of the leading causes of death among younger age groups, accounting for approximately 25,000 deaths per year.[1] Moreover, a dramatic increase in the suicide rate among adolescents and young adults has been detected,[2-4] making suicide a major public health problem. This situation is particularly tragic because suicide is in large measure preventable. It is also important to remember that the person who either attempts or commits suicide is not the only victim. After a suicide, family members and friends must deal with their doubts, anger, and guilt as well as their loss.

Among those who attempt suicide, drug overdose is the most common method, especially by the young. More violent means are also used (eg, shooting, slashing, hanging, and jumping from a height), usually, but not exclusively, by males. When self-mutilation is involved, the underlying psychiatric illness is usually severe, and staff reactions toward these individuals are generally intense.[5]

Overall factors that predispose to suicide include depression, alcoholism, personality disorders, addiction, and schizophrenia.[1,6–9] In addition, a host of demographic risk factors exist: (1) the psychiatric disorders listed above, (2) a history of suicide attempts and/or threats of suicide, (3) male sex, (4) advanced age, (5) a recent loss, (6) being unskilled or unemployed, (7) being single or widowed, (8) being psychotic, (9) having a chronic illness and/or pain, and (10) feeling hopeless. The evaluation of the suicidal patient must not, however, be restricted to a search for these factors. The clinician's task is too assess the severity and/or risk of an attempt and predict the likelihood of its occurrence in the future. Unfortunately, there are no absolute predictive tests or criteria that establish who will, or who will not, commit suicide. suicide.

The goal of a suicide evaluation is to elicit the true feelings and thoughts of an individual and place them in the context of the aforementioned demographic and social risk factors so that appropriate treatment may be undertaken. An example of this is as follows:

> Ms R., a 25-year-old white, single hospital employee was admitted to the medical intensive care unit (ICU) in coma, requiring assisted ventilation, following an intentional overdose with amitriptyline hydrochloride, fluphenazine, and flurazepam hydrochloride.
>
> Twenty-four hours after admission she awoke and was extubated. Ms R. was an attractive, slender woman lying in bed in four-point leather restraints; nonetheless, she was polite and cooperative. She was drowsy and spoke in a slow, soft whisper.
>
> Her past psychiatric history was notable for a chronic state of depression and a borderline personality disorder. She had attempted suicide via drug overdose on three prior occasions and had been hospitalized twice. She reported that this attempt was made during her psychiatrist's vacation after feelings of loneliness increased. She had not informed others of her intent and was surprised to learn that she had been found. Her mood was depressed and lonely; she thought that nothing had been changed by her survival. Ms R. was cognitively intact, not psychotic, and still wanted to be dead.
>
> Two days later, after an uneventful recovery, she was transferred to a private psychiatric hospital under the care of her psychiatrist, who had returned from vacation. In the interim, despite an endearing quality that led staff to feel sorry for her, Ms R. was maintained on suicide precautions (with one-to-one supervision and/or leather restraints, as dictated by staff comfort and availability) so that neither self-harm nor premature discharge would occur.

As a general rule, the emergency evaluation of a suicidal patient should proceed in a fashion similar to the direct, medically oriented approach that one uses in any emergency. A rapid assessment is required so that triage can be carried out expeditiously. However, one should always err on the side of conservatism so that needless fatalities do not result. The thought that "those who talk about suicide don't do it" is a myth; all potentially fatal threats, gestures, and attempts should be taken seriously.

Every patient who has survived a suicide attempt should be seen by a psychiatrist. A suicide evaluation should also be done on all patients who complain of suicidal thoughts and on those who admit to suicidal ideation upon questioning. In addition, all patients whose actions suggest suicidal intent or potential, despite their protests to the contrary, should be screened for suicidal risk.

Unless one entertains the possibility that a patient may be suicidal, the diagnosis will be missed. Patients must be asked about suicidal thoughts, ideas, wishes, motives, intent, and plans; asking these questions will not plant the idea in their minds. In fact, most patients are grateful for the chance to discuss this issue.

When confronted with a patient who has made a suicide attempt, it is essential to ensure his physical safety. This includes prompt attention to any medical complications that have either occurred or may develop. Subsequent to this, the severity of an attempt can be assessed. The determination of the relative risk of an attempt (lethality of method) versus the likelihood for rescue after the attempt helps to establish the seriousness of the attempt.[10] It is also useful to know if the patient believed his method would lead to his death and if survival was a disappointment. For most patients the question of "why now?" is crucial. If a precipitant or crisis led to anger, helplessness, depression and/or suicidal ideation, it is essential to determine if that situation has resolved. If the situation and social framework are unchanged, it is likely that a subsequent attempt will take place.

Since affective illness commonly leads to suicide, physicians who perform suicide evaluations must always screen for the presence of depression. Criteria for the diagnosis of depression are presented in chapter 12. In addition, when psychosis (especially when manifested by command hallucinations) and suicidal ideation coexist, a deadly combination is present and protection of the patient is mandated until the psychosis and suicidality resolve.

Suicide attempts commonly lead to ER assessment. At the Massachusetts General Hospital (MGH), 1% to 2% of all ER visits[11] or 5% of all admissions to a medical ICU[12] are a direct result of drug overdose, the most common method of attempted suicide. After evaluating patients for suicide in the ER, the psychiatrist has several options available. The patient can be sent home with a recommendation for outpatient follow-up; the patient can be admitted to a general hospital unit for medical treatment where psychiatric care is available; the patient can be voluntarily admitted to a psychiatric unit; or the patient can be involuntarily admitted to a psychiatric facility. These decisions are based upon clinical judgment. If one is confident that the patient is not psychotic, significantly depressed, or intoxicated; that the crisis leading to an impulsive attempt has resolved, and that reasonable follow-up can be assured, then discharge can generally be arranged. However, if one is unsure about the ongoing safety of a patient (by virtue of ongoing depression or psychosis), the patient should be admitted for further psychiatric evaluation and treatment. In a recent study at MGH (TAS, unpublished data, 1985) 47% of all patients evaluated in the ER for a drug overdose required inpatient treatment on a medical, surgical, or psychiatric unit. As a rule, it is better to hospitalize a patient, even involuntarily, if doubt exists about suicidality. In this age of litigation it is well to remember that being sued for battery (as would be the case for mandatory commitment) is far easier to defend than the charge of negligence.

Throughout the evaluation period and until transfer to a secure facility is achieved, the suicidal patient must be protected from harm. Protection of the patient has traditionally been referred to as taking suicide precautions. These precautions prevent the patient from eloping from the hospital or from self-injury. Depending on the nature, severity, urgency, and intent of the patient's plans to hurt himself, a number of maneuvers can be employed. These range from constant, one-to-one supervision with nurses, aides, and security personnel, to tranquilization with or without physical restraint. One always tries to use the least restrictive treatment available to assure the ultimate safety of the patient. Frequently this involves the use of locked leather restraints until the clinical situation has been clarified and the intent of the patient re-evaluated. In addition, potentially dangerous objects should be removed from contact with the suicidal patient, including access to an intravenous (IV) bottle which can be broken and used for cutting.

The clinical impressions and disposition plan based upon the evaluation should be clearly documented in the medical record. Once the patient has been transferred to a medical or surgical unit for complications of a suicide attempt, the patient's mental status should be reassessed at least daily by the psychiatric consultant.

Many patients, despite having taken serious drug overdoses that result in coma, respiratory arrest, and admission to an ICU, deny suicidal intent.[13] In rare cases, this may be true. For example:

> A psychiatrist was asked to see Mr Z., a 22-year-old white, single male, for an evaluation of suicidal risk following his admission in a comatose state to the medical ICU from a polydrug overdose (secobarbital, glutethimide, acetaminophen, and codeine).
>
> The patient had a long-standing addiction to several drugs, especially barbiturates, with several episodes of barbiturate withdrawal seizures. Hospitalization had been required several times for treatment of substance abuse. His disorder met criteria for borderline personality organization. In addition, he had been recently diagnosed as having hepatitis.
>
> Upon examination, Mr Z. was noted to be a well-muscled young man, lying in bed in four-point restraints, screaming and cursing at staff to have him unchained. After being told by the psychiatrist that the restraints would not be removed prior to his interview, Mr Z. calmed down. He reported that his overdose was a result of a vigorous celebration on the birth of a friend's child. Although he was annoyed at himself for having underestimated the effects of the drugs he had taken, he was neither depressed nor suicidal. There was no evidence of psychosis, and he was cognitively intact.
>
> The psychiatrist's impression was that he was not suicidal, and suicide precautions were discontinued. Mr Z. was advised that it would be to his benefit to re-enter a therapeutic relationship where he could learn to decrease his impulsivity and drug abuse.

In one recent study of ICU patients who survived drug overdose[13] only 39% of patients reported feeling depressed or hopeless at the time of their overdose, and only 45% admitted to suicidal intent. A majority of these overdose patients had received psychiatric treatment and had made previous suicide attempts. Moreover, although a formal diagnosis was not given to all of them, character pathology replete with impulsivity and a history of drug and alcohol abuse was common.

An alliance with the suicidal patient should be established during evaluation and disposition. This is often difficult to achieve because of the patient's negativity, hostility, and rage at having survived. By the time the psychiatrist is called to see the patient, the staff may be highly polarized against his continued care. Not uncommonly, the staff expresses the wish that the patient had died. It is the psychiatrist's task to diffuse these charged situations. Despite the potential countertransference problems that may arise in dealing with these patients, concern should be demonstrated.[14] Furthermore, the psychiatric consultant should hold group meetings with the personnel involved in their care to make sure that the caretakers are aware of their own negative feelings for these patients. Anger, when unrecognized, may endanger the patient through mismanagement and premature discharge. Often the examiner needs to take an active role in order to elicit information and to emphasize options the patient has for the future. For many individuals, suicide occurs only when they perceive no other option except death. Social supports often provide a source of alternatives which should be assessed and used.

What about the patient who recovers from a suicide attempt and is admitted to a medical or surgical ward? The suicide risk must be constantly estimated in these patients. Antidepressant medication or treatment should be started if this is appropriate, and constant vigilance must be maintained to prevent a recurrence of suicide. It is unusual for the suicidal patient to make a further attempt while confined to a medical or surgical ward. This may be due to the care and attention he receives from the medical caretakers. He may also experience a resurgence of care and attention from his family. There may be a cathartic effect from the suicide attempt. Despite this low incidence of recurrent suicide attempts, constant vigilance must be maintained.

Reich and Kelly[15] have written a study on 17 attempts by medical and surgical patients to commit suicide in a general hospital. These were impulsive and in no case was the immediate suicide risk predicted or even suspected by the staff. However, the study disclosed that in each case there had been either a rising tide of anger or agitation, sudden mood change, or a psychotic episode. In 15 of these cases, there was a disruption in a medical relationship. The principal ingredient in these suicide attempts was the presence of a mental disorder in 15 out of the 17 cases. In those two who had no antecedent psychopathology the attempt occurred when the staff became discouraged about treatment outcome.

Another study has shown that cardiorespiratory patients are more apt to commit suicide when compared to a matched control population.[16] Factors that distinguished potential suicide candidates were: (1) excessive emotional stress over the disease, (2) low tolerance for pain and discomfort, (3) need for attention and reassurance with demanding behavior, (4) need to control the treatment, (5) high degree of alertness and good orientation, (6) exhaustion and lack of support from the family and the hospital, and (7) prior or present suicidal threats.

Attention has been called by some to the importance of organic brain syndromes in in-hospital suicidality. This may particularly be true in patients fearing Alzheimer's disease. There is a high incidence of suicide of patients on renal dialysis. They are reported to have a suicide rate 400 times that of the general population.[17]

THE PATIENT WHO THREATENS TO SIGN OUT AGAINST MEDICAL ADVICE

Each year on the consultation service at MGH there are five to ten occasions when the issues of signing out against medical advice (AMA) pose a serious, life-threatening problem to a patient. At such a time, the confidence of the primary physician is shaken and the hospital's reputation endangered. These situations reach the psychiatric consultant at the eleventh hour. In fact, only about 5% of sign-outs are seen by a psychiatrist. For each serious threat there are perhaps 20 manipulative threats that fall short of emergencies.

A careful study of the premature sign-out process over a recent 3-year period revealed that it is, in nearly all instances, a two-way transaction. The patient threatens to sign out because in his eyes he has been mistreated, misunderstood, misinformed, or in some way mismanaged. While this is not always an accurate observation, since the misunderstanding may well be the fault of the patient, it is crucial to realize that the serious threat to leave the hospital is rarely a sudden act of rash bravado. Most often it is the result of a series of transactions between patient and staff that progressively set the points of the patient's compass toward the front door. Discharges against medical advice accounted for less than 1% of hospital discharges at another local general hospital,[18,19] and addiction to drugs or alcohol was present in 22% and 42%, respectively.[18] A majority of those discharges occurred in the first five days after admission, and almost all the patients maintained some contact with the hospital after their departure.[19] A history of previous sign-outs is always a danger signal and should alert the admitting physician or the ward physician of the possibility of a forthcoming sign-out. Similarly, alcohol and drug abuse are linked with sign-outs. In fact, Jankowsky and Drum[18] believe that the differential diagnosis of any general hospital patient who signs out against advice should prioritize alcoholism or drug addiction until proved otherwise. Impulsivity, however, is more likely to pre-empt the importance of the diagnosis in signing out. Sign-outs against medical advice are not related to specific diagnostic categories. Schizophrenia, affective disorders, personality disorders, and organic mental illness are all represented in the list of sign-out diagnoses.

It is interesting that most of the literature on sign-out from psychiatric hospitals agree that the single most important feature that leads the patient to thinking about leaving is inadequate preparation of the patient and the family by the staff. Patients enter the hospital thinking that they will be there for a brief stay and then are surprised that it will be ten days, 2 weeks, or more. Most of the patients who sign out in the first five days do so because they have not been adequately prepared.

Whether the setting is a general or a psychiatric hospital, a disturbance in the doctor-patient relationship is without question one of the most frequent causes for sign-out. The doctor gets angry at the patient. There is a misunderstanding between them and the patient thinks that he has been misinformed or gulled into expecting a shorter stay when in fact a longer stay was anticipated. All of these things make for difficult doctor-patient interrelations which can result in sign-out.

Schlauch et al[19] found that the largest number of sign-outs were on the ward service. The patients were young and none was critically ill. Much of what they say centers around the feeling of helplessness. Anger and anxiety are disguises for a sense of helplessness which is sometimes augmented by the patient's low socioeconomic status. This makes patients feel defensive and may cause them to misinterpret feelings from the staff as prejudicial, arrogant, or dismissive.

There may be a conspiracy on the part of the caretakers, based upon unconsciously hostile wishes, to get the patient out. Medication can be changed without warning; the patient can be moved without preparation. All kinds of things can be done to antagonize the patient and to intensify whatever underlying anger he may have, which results in the sign-out. Most of the sign-out patients feel as though they have been wronged.

Albert and Kornfeld[20] repeat a theme emphasized by Schlauch et al.[19] There are three basic factors behind the majority of sign-outs: (1) fear of what is going to happen; (2) anger at fate, at the medical establishment, at the caretakers, or all three; and (3) psychotic reactions and/or depression. These authors point out that the premonitory signs in addition to anger are insomnia, daytime crying, boredom, voicing the complaint of boredom, and anger at the staff. Sometimes it might be important when these premonitory signs are present to ask the person "Do you feel like signing out?" And when they say they do, say, "Let's sit down and talk it over."

There are two statements of Albert and Kornfeld[20] which we think are worth remembering: "The threat to sign out is the last desperate act of a patient to whom no other solution seems available to deal with intense emotional distress." Rather than take the sign-out threat personally, which so many physicians do, one should realize that the patient is leaving because he is feeling driven out and can do nothing else but go. The second memorable quote is: "It is when we are too proud as physicians or frightened to admit an error that the patient may escalate his feelings to threats of leaving or litigation." Don't let pride get in the way of admitting you are wrong if indeed you are.

The first tack any consultant should take when faced with a patient about to sign out is to ally himself with that patient. "What's wrong? What can I do to help? What have people done to you? Is there something that I can negotiate to make you stay? Is there some wrong that can be put right?" One can assume that a mistake or misunderstanding has occurred. Whether it stems from an act by the hospital personnel or by the patient is less important than getting the aggrieved parties together for a reconciliation. It is also important to let the patient know he has the freedom to leave. Assuming that the patient's judgment is sound and that he is not taking his life in his hands by departing, point out that he is free to go and indicate that the door is always open for return. It is always wrong to issue an ultimatum. Most patients who sign out tend to keep contact through the outpatient department; a number of them come back to the hospital the next day. Approximately 94% return to the hospital. If you leave the door open, they are apt to return.

Once the patient feels he has an ally, he is usually willing to delay his sign-out long enough to have the problem aired to the concerned parties. This generally effects a resolution. Patients are usually relieved at the chance to remain—especially if a concession is made to them. As mentioned above, the sign-out, for most patients, is a desperate act, one they are forced into by what they believe is an immutable pattern of behavior on the part of the staff.

There are exceptions to this rule. Perhaps the most common is the individual with organic brain disease. His difficulty with memory and orientation and his low tolerance for anxiety leave him ill-equipped to cope with the strangeness of the hospital setting and primed for panic. An impatient nurse or an abrupt physician may induce an alarm response and a threatened sign-out. Careful explanations, round-the-clock visitation by trusted family members, and patience are usually the answer to such problems.

Although psychotropic medications are useful with psychotic patients who threaten to sign out as a result of delusions or hallucinations, the last thing one should do in facing the nonpsychotic patient who threatens to sign out is to "snow" him with drugs. Such an attempt is often regarded as the "last straw." It may well confirm the patient's fear of coercive betrayal.

As a final strategy, it often helps to suggest that the patient leave the hospital on an overnight pass if this is compatible with good medical management. A sense of autonomy is restored by giving him the option of leaving the hospital with the understanding that he can return. So often it is the unfortunate decision, wrought in anger, usually by a young staff physician or house officer, that the patient who leaves is no longer entitled to return. In the opinion of Albert and Kornfeld, this attitude "rarely dissuades the patient from leaving, but it may make continuing outpatient treatment less likely."[20]

> M.P. was a friendly, 72-year-old pharmacist who had undergone an open heart procedure 5 years earlier. He had unpleasant memories of the postoperative period when he had been delirious for five successive days. It had been a frightening time, and he held his surgeon accountable for not providing proper medication for sleep. The only hypnotic in which the patient had any faith was phenobarbital. His surgeon had given him one of the newer sedatives and it hadn't worked. This time he wanted to make certain he would get phenobarbital for sleep. Everyone assured him that he would. He was amiable and good-natured and did not strongly press this demand. As a consequence, his request was forgotten until after his subtotal gastrectomy. On his first postoperative day he moaned incessantly, asking for phenobarbital. Instead he was given small doses of diazepam (Valium). Throughout the night he continued to whine and moan piteously, reminding everyone that he had been promised a barbiturate. The recovery room people who were now responsible for his care had never met him before and knew nothing about promised medication. The following day he howled in a loud voice that unless he saw his physician by midday and was given something to help him sleep he was going to remove his tubes and walk out. Although his physician did his best to meet the deadline, he was late by ten minutes, during which time the patient had removed a catheter and an IV line. The physician immediately ordered phenobarbital and the patient went into a relaxed sleep. This medication was continued until the patient's discharge.

The smoke signals in this case were the patient's reasonable request for a specific hypnotic and his past history of postoperative delirium. His easygoing manner and confidence that his request would be carried out worked against him. Furthermore, he had no idea that barbiturates are thought by some to contribute to the incidence of postoperative delirium and therefore are seldom used. Requests for specific medication should always be heeded, especially when they come from people with a medical background. A promise made to use a drug should certainly be carried out or a reasonable explanation for the drug's omission or substitution must be given.

> Mr J. was a valued hospital employee who worked in the engineering shop for 20 years. He was admitted to the coronary care unit (CCU) with

an acute myocardial infarction. Popular with the nurses, he was usually gregarious, but after 3 days he became visibly apprehensive. A snowstorm had moved in and winds from the Atlantic had whipped the snow into blinding flurries that rendered driving hazardous from Maine to New Jersey. The patient's frequent requests to use the telephone meant moving it into his room and then returning it to its stand. No one had time to wonder why Mr J. needed to make these calls. At midday two persons were admitted and the patient's request for the telephone could not be honored for about three hours. When the nurse finally agreed to bring him the phone, she did so with a trace of anger. In the interval of delay between the promise to bring the phone and her actual arrival, the patient had removed his monitoring leads, taken out his IV tubing, and was in the midst of putting on his clothes. The nurse was stunned by this unexpected spectacle and angry at herself for being the probable cause. He refused to speak, just shook his head sadly, and continued tying his shoestring. The house officer on duty approached the patient quietly and gently inquired what we had done to make him want to leave. Mr J. continued to shake his head and tie his shoestring. Finally, in response to the repeated urgings of the house officer, Mr J. said that his son was driving up from New Jersey and that he had been calling hourly to make sure everything was all right. The telephone was his lifeline. Without it he felt powerless. Leaving the hospital seemed his only alternative. The house officer immediately apologized for the lack of a telephone and instantly called the patient's home to check on his son. He then got a telephone from another floor for the patient. Mr J. agreed to return to bed as long as he could keep the phone in his room. This request was immediately granted.

In retrospect it is easy to see that someone should have asked Mr J. why he needed the telephone so frequently and so urgently. However, the lesson of this case is taught by the intern. His immediate response was not to blame the patient for acting foolishly, but to assume that the unit was at fault. This is an ideal tactic when the physician faces a prospective sign-out patient whose motive is not immediately discernible. It allows the patient a chance to explain without being defensive. With or without cause, the patient usually feels aggrieved and angry. The medical caregiver should be prepared to be scapegoated either directly or symbolically. If an error has been made, it is imperative that the individual involved acknowledge the mistake.

THE SEDUCTIVE FEMALE

When a male physician thinks of a sexually provocative patient, the usual image brought to mind is that of a young, partially clad, attractive woman whose working diagnosis is hysteria. The scenario would then call for a young, earnest, but inexperienced physician to take charge of the patient and be seduced into making a fool of himself. This seldom occurs. Physicians are possibly less sexually naive than was the case a decade ago. They seem less susceptible to coercion through overt seduction. However, a more subtle type of seduction sometimes occurs, usually directed by an attractive woman who is not necessarily hysterical. She finds in the physician someone who is patient, kind, and, perhaps, aware of her charms. Generally a marital problem is part of her clinical picture. She has a husband who, for one reason or another, does not understand her. During a period of turning to the physician for comfort, she develops a warm, compassionate, platonically romantic attachment to him. A relationship then develops that sometimes leads the physician to make serious errors in judgement without ever realizing the impropriety of his action. More often than not, the physician is unaware of the romantic fantasies of the patient.

Mrs C.L. was an attractive brunette who, at age 38, looked 10 years younger and had a good sense of humor. She was married to a physician who spent most of his time attending to his practice. They had been married for almost 20 years and over the last 15 years he had been slowly losing interest in her. Nonetheless, he was a loyal husband who had developed no liaisons and was essentially married to her for life.

The patient developed a low back pain syndrome. The neurosurgeon who attended her was married and well respected by his colleagues. He kept his patient in the hospital for 2 months, during which time he saw her daily. In the course of his visits the patient told him how she had been maritally neglected for years. She made much of her husband's drinking and claimed that his partners were fed up with him because of it. A psychiatric consultant was called in to advise the patient about her husband's alleged alcoholism. When the psychiatrist asked the neurosurgeon if he had spoken to the patient's husband, he found that no contact had been made. The psychiatrist pointed out that the neurosurgeon had in fact accused a colleague on circumstantial evidence and had entered this in the patient's chart without ever having confirmed the story. The surgeon quickly saw the need to see his patient's husband, but was unwilling to do so himself. An interview between the husband and the psychiatrist and phone calls to medical colleagues of the husband revealed that the problem was in the marriage and not in alcohol.

The referring neurosurgeon was infuriated with himself, but quickly turned this anger toward the patient. The psychiatric consultant pointed out that both patient and surgeon were culpable and encouraged him to discuss the situation with his patient. The woman felt betrayed and forsaken by her physician. Her marriage ultimately ended also. Much, if not all, of this unpleasantness could have been averted if the neurosurgeon had been less naive.

When sex is used, either actually or symbolically, between patient and doctor in a manipulative way, look for a mantrap. The entrapment may not be deliberate, but the net result is the same. The storm warning should be out when one senses a seduction. It might also be valuable to warn one's colleagues when one sees it.

THE MALE SEXUAL PROVOCATEUR

The male sexual provocateur has an altogether different approach, and his disruptive effect is far more immediate and intense. There are roughly three varieties of male sexual disturbance commonly seen in a general hospital. They represent degrees on a sliding scale of indiscretion. The mildest indiscretion is the flirt. He is constantly making excessive references to the physical attributes of those who care for him, using pet names, and sometimes suggesting sexual activities, but rarely offering a serious proposition. Generally, he embarrasses the nursing personnel more than he angers or frightens them. Next is the obscene seducer. His idea of seduction is to tell dirty jokes or make lewd comments about the anatomical parts of the nurses. His coarseness and vulgarity are offensive and sometimes he does make serious advances. The obscene seducer usually induces reactions of revulsion and anger from the nursing staff. The most indiscreet is the exhibitionist who exposes himself either passively by letting the sheet fall away from his genitals or actively by openly masturbating in the presence of the nurse. The exhibitionist causes the same response as the obscene seducer, but combined with a fear that something is so unbalanced in the patient that a more serious assault might occur.

To understand these three degrees of maladaptive behavior, one must recognize that serious illness, such as myocardial infarction, even when its full impact is denied, is a major threat to the masculine ego. The fear of functional castration is apt to be more pronounced in individuals who value their sexual ability above other personal attributes. It is also found in individuals who have had problems with sexual adequacy before their illness. In any event, attempting to arouse a show of interest from the nurses by flirting is often no more than a man's harmless method of testing sexual viability. Engaging in sexual banter with nurses may also be an attempt to prove potency by evoking an erection. Usually the perpetrator is unaware of his motive, just as he is blind to the impact of his behavior on others.

> C.G. was a 42-year-old maritime pilot whose myocardial infarction occurred 3 months after his wife divorced him. He was tall, thin, somber, and solemn. The second day in the unit he began addressing the nurses as "gorgeous," "hot lips," "luscious," and "sex pot." He also managed to pat the posterior of the charge nurse and tried to kiss

another when she was taking his temperature. It was done in a humorless and mechanical way as though he were a wind-up doll programmed to make advances. By the third day his advances increased in frequency. Any dialogue with a nurse was embellished with amorous epithets and archly suggestive allusions.

A psychiatric consultant was asked to speak to the patient. During this conversation the patient appeared likable but quite despondent about his recent divorce. His wife was the only woman he had ever known well. He had spent most of his life on the oceans of the world and had had such little contact with women that he behaved toward them in a stereotyped way. He said that he had always called women "dear" or "sweetie" instead of using proper names. When confronted with the fact that he had tried to kiss one of the nurses and given another a friendly pat, he said that he thought this would make them like him more and it would give them "encouragement." "I lost one wife because I wasn't a ladies' man. Now with my ticker on the fritz I'm even less a ladies' man." The psychiatrist suggested he stop trying to give the girls "encouragement" and try to treat them like shipmates. (He got along very well with men.) The nurses warmed up to him as soon as the phony flirting stopped. Their changed attitude reinforced his altered patterns of behavior, and by the time he left the hospital he was communicating with women more naturally.

It was apparent that this man was quite innocent in his attempts at flirting. He had no idea that his efforts were clumsy and awkward. His self-esteem with regard to women had always been low and assumed a new depth now that his "ticker was on the fritz." The term "encouragement" seemed a projection of his own need. When the psychiatrist told him literally how to behave, he did so and received immediate and genuine encouragement. The nurses, had they been advised, might have done the same for him from the start.

Q.B., a paunchy, 62-year-old educator with thickset facial features cast in a dour expression, was admitted with his second myocardial infarction in 7 years. His cardiac condition had stabilized by the second day. While bathing the patient that morning, the nurse observed him fondling his penis into semierection. Every time she drew the sheet over his hips, he removed it. She left the room. When she returned, he had finished bathing and said nothing to her. Throughout the rest of the day the nurses noted that he lay in bed fully exposed. This was disconcerting to them. With considerable tact the head nurse confronted him about his exhibitionism. Contending that his sheet had merely slipped down, Q.B. denied intent. The next day another nurse who bathed him had the same experience. His physician was asked to help him curb his exposing, but the patient simply assumed an air of injured innocence. At this point the psychiatrist was called. The patient again denied any wrongdoing just as he did not acknowledge any fear of impaired sexuality. His mental status was quite normal. He showed no evidence of psychosis and was not delirious. Because no individual had been able to halt this man's denial, a more imposing confrontation was thought to be called for.

After consulting his physician and gaining permission, the nursing staff of the afternoon and evening shifts, accompanied by the psychiatrist, entered the patient's room. The chief nurse took on the role of spokesperson. Pleasantly, with even-toned assurance, she told the patient that his behavior had worried all of the nurses. They wondered whether or not he knew what he was doing and, more importantly, the effect that it was having on them. She assured him that the staff liked him and regretted his misfortune. However, they were sufficiently distressed by his behavior that some were reluctant to help him bathe. She went on to explain that they had come in a group to make sure he knew that they all felt the same way. Surveying them with a visage that displayed neither alarm nor embarrassment, he denied any notion of what they were talking about. The nurses responded almost in chorus that they knew he did. They expressed a desire to help him. He made no effort to respond. The meeting ended, and the nurses felt even more frustrated and powerless. However, at the next bath he behaved in a sullen but modest manner, a pattern that continued throughout his hospitalization.

It is difficult to imagine what went on in this man's mind to change his behavior. There had been no threat offered, nor had there been any display of vindictive animosity. The reason may have been the size of the assemblage and their unity in expressing opposition. This type of confrontation has been successful in similar cases. It is harsh treatment and requires the presence of a psychiatrist skilled in group techniques to ensure that the situation does not get out of hand. There is always the danger that the stress incurred may adversely affect the patient's heart, but this must be weighed against the toll such behavior takes from the nursing staff.

THE MALINGERER

Malingering (V65.20 DSM III) is the conscious simulation of an illness or symptom. Illness is feigned by the patient in order to accomplish a particular goal. This goal may be a financial reward, the avoidance of an unpopular duty, or the creation of guilt in the minds of involved friends or family. Whatever the motive, the modus operandi is the same: faking for gain. Hypochondriasis, compensation neurosis, and Munchausen's syndrome are sometimes confused with malingering.[21-23] Because it is difficult to spot the malingerer, we should keep him in mind when dealing with the symptoms where elements of secondary gain are prominent. Usually malingerers are found in armed services medical facilities or Veteran's Administration hospitals rather than in general hospitals. Aside from the prominence of secondary gain, they usually have a past history of malingering, or "goldbricking," that can be unearthed from old records. An important characteristic of the malingerer is that he often has a record of antisocial acts. Although he manages to avoid jail he may have a bad conduct discharge from the armed forces and a history of being expelled from school and fired from jobs. The tracks of his misbehavior meander back through early adolescence. The most dramatic of the malingerers to have come our way was a prototypical charlatan.

Some years ago a young man from the Himalayas came to MGH for an examination of his blindness. He was well over 6 ft tall and had the finely chiseled handsomeness of a mountain prince. He wore a turban and long white cape. Allegedly he had been kicked by a horse. Although his face bore no scars and his eyes were the best feature of his impressive face, he nonetheless had radiologic evidence of an old fracture over the occipital area. In his country, due to political connections and personal magnetism, he had formed a school for the blind and infirm. In order to subsidize it he took lecture tours around the world. That was his reason for being in the United States. He spoke excellent English. His tour through the United States had been very successful and was ending in New England. It was because he had attracted so much attention and won so many friends that he found himself on the neurologic service of MGH. His friends had literally forced him to become a patient in order to afford him the best appraisal modern medicine could offer on the faint chance that something could be done to help his blindness.

It soon became apparent by all tests that he had excellent visual acuity. Although he was highly skilled in behaving as a totally sightless person, he was unable to outwit the various neuro-opthhalmologic tests. After these tests had demonstrated the soundness of his optic system, we were faced with the dilemma of having to deal with a fraud who was in the United States at the invitation of our government. In addition, he enjoyed the friendship of many individuals in high places, including benefactors of the hospital.

It was decided to give him the opportunity to bow out gracefully. He would be told that all of the tests had been performed and the results were excellent. His prognosis was far better than anyone could have imagined at the time of his admission. He had a type of blindness that could be cured. A treatment had recently been devised at the hospital wherein, employing a combination of eyewashings and certain injections, he would begin to regain light perception within as little time as a day. He was then instructed in the following manner: "When you begin to see light, as we know you will, the following will happen. You will begin to feel much better by the third treatment. The following day you will begin to see forms and movement. This will improve your mood to the point of happiness. The following morning you will begin to see faces, and by that afternoon you will be able to perceive the visual world as you did before the horse kicked you. One of your first acts after full restoration of your vision will be to obtain air transportation to your homeland. With that accomplished, your case will be closed at the hospital, and no follow-up will be done. However, if you fail for some reason to depart the country and return to your sanitorium, where you are badly needed, additional follow-up investigations might have to be done and disclosures of a painful nature made." He was quick to get the point, smiled faintly as the instructions were given him, nodded his head, and said, "I understand and I thank you." He performed his part of the bargain, and we kept our word.

The malingerer is often a charming person. Unlike the hypochondriac, he is not querulous and demanding. While willing to have some diagnostic tests, he is unlikely to submit to painful procedures or surgery that patients with Munchausen's syndrome commonly undergo. The review of symptoms and past history is atypical for somatoform disorder, and generally he does not have a lawyer or the history of litigation with industrial accident boards, which is the case with the compensation neurotic. According to DSM-III, the criteria by which the diagnosis can be made are: (1) ruling out the other diagnoses already mentioned, (2) noting a large element of secondary gain with a discrepancy between the disability and objective findings, (3) finding a past history of antisocial personality disorder, (4) noting lack of cooperation with diagnostic evaluation and treatment regimen, and (5) observing a medicolegal context of presentation.

MUNCHAUSEN'S SYNDROME

Munchausen's syndrome has been called by DSM-III *factitious disorder with either psychological* (300.16) or *physical* (301.51) *symptoms*. It is defined on the basis of three principle features: (1) psychological and/or physical symptoms are produced that are apparently under the individual's voluntary control, (2) the symptoms that are produced are not explained by any other mental or physical disorder (although they may be superimposed on one), (3) the individual's goal is apparently to assume the "patient role" and is not otherwise understandable in light of the individual's environmental circumstance (as is the case in malingering).

Individuals with Munchausen's syndrome plagued physicians even before Asher gave this syndrome of factitious illness its name in 1951.[24] Uniformly, patients with this disorder wreak havoc once they have been admitted to a hospital. Yet only 50% of them are ever seen by psychiatric consultants.[25] When they are seen, recommendations for psychiatric follow-up care are invariably rejected. Successful treatment for this disorder is rare, and clear management strategies for dealing with these patients during their hospital stay are lacking.

Early efforts in managing the Munchausen patient were directed toward saving physicians from being duped, rather than toward treatment. To this end the methods suggested included the creation of blacklists and a central registry with photographs and fingerprints of these patients. Although Asher first wondered what the psychological kink might be to cause these individuals to act as they did, it was not until years later that others postulated dynamic hypotheses to account for the patient's impostureship, pseudologia phantastica, itinerant lives, absence of close relationships, and masochistic acceptance of painful procedures.[21,26] Along these lines a wide range of psychiatric diagnoses have been recorded for these patients: hysterical, psychopathic, masochistic, and borderline personalities; schizophrenia; and malingering. Prior to the creation of the DSM-III diagnosis of chronic factitious disorder with physical symptoms, alternative labels for Munchausen patients included hospital hoboes, Kopenicades, peregrinating problem patients, hospital addicts, and sufferers of the Ahasuerus syndrome.

The following case of a young woman with Munchausen's syndrome illustrates the value of psychiatric consultation in preventing needless surgical interventions and decreasing the countertransference hatred of the hospital staff.

> Ms L.C., a 27-year-old, widowed, full-blooded Navajo Indian was admitted to MGH with a chief complaint of abdominal pain, nausea, vomiting, and watery diarrhea.
>
> Her past medical history included childhood asthma, and rheumatic fever at age 7 years, an appendectomy at age 20, and an emergency cholecystectomy following a car accident in Colorado. She could not recall the name of the Colorado hospital. At ages 21 and 27 she underwent caesarian sections at a New York hospital.
>
> Ms C. said she was raised in Brooklyn. Her father died when she was 4 years old. She had five brothers, one of whom she said lived in the Boston area. Her husband was killed in a motor vehicle accident during her second pregnancy. She reported coming to Boston 6 weeks prior to admission to find work and start college. Her two children remained in New York City under the care of her mother. Since her arrival in Boston she had become engaged to a truck driver, who at the time of her admission was in North Dakota.
>
> On physical examination Ms C. was a thin, white female in considerable abdominal distress. Temperature was 102°F orally, pulse was 104 beats/min, blood pressure was 160/70 mmHg, and respirations were 20/min. Her abdominal examination was notable for multiple midline scars and for moderate tenderness with guarding over the right

upper rectus abdominus muscle. The remainder of her examination was entirely normal.

Ms C. was taken to the operating room for exploratory laparotomy which, except for numerous adhesions, was normal. Postoperatively, she complained of continued right upper quadrant abdominal pain. She had severe tenderness to mild palpation, diffuse guarding, but no rebound. Beginning on the second postoperative day she spiked nightly fevers, all greater than 103°F. On the third hospital day a *Klebsiella* infection in the urine was identified and successfully treated with antibiotics; however, the spiking fevers and abdominal pain persisted. For this pain, Ms C. required intramuscular (IM) injections of meperidine hydrochloride. A kidneys, ureter, bladder (KUB) examination, upright abdominal plain film, ultrasound of the abdomen and pelvis, and computed tomography (CT) scan of her abdomen were all normal. Intravenous pyelography was planned, but she refused, stating a similar test several years earlier had nearly killed her. Instead, an ultrasound record of the kidneys was obtained and was normal. On the ninth hospital day she underwent cystoscopy with bilateral retrograde ureterograms which were also normal.

Infectious disease consultants were called in to evaluate Ms C's nightly fevers. Ten blood cultures were negative, as were cultures of the stool, urine, and sputum. Results of a lumbar puncture were also normal. Her WBC at all times remained between 6000 and 10,000 cells/cm^3 with a normal differential. Multiple cultures of sputum and urine were negative for tuberculosis, and an apical lordotic view of the chest was normal.

On the 18th hospital day psychiatric consultation was requested since no clear organic cause could be detected for the patient's continuing fevers and abdominal pain. Ms C. was noted by the psychiatrist to be alert, oriented, and without either a formal thought disorder or depression. However, she appeared distant and indifferent to questions or events. She answered questions slowly and occasionally grabbed her right side and moaned, "Oh, the pain."

The psychiatrist thought that the patient's presentation was consistent with Munchausen's syndrome. Her account was replete with impostureship and pseudologia phantastica (ie, telephone numbers she gave were false, she had no knowledge of Navaho customs, her work and school history were not verifiable, and the hospitals she claimed to have had surgery in had no record of her). She displayed an equanimity to invasive procedures and a medical sophistication by virtue of previous job experience in medical laboratories. In addition, there was evidence of drug abuse, a poor interpersonal style (she had no visitors and received no phone calls), and threats to sign out AMA unless her pain medications were increased. Moreover, a review of her behavior within the hospital revealed her to be demanding, evasive, and frequently noncompliant with hospital rules. She would, for example, page the intern from the hall telephone to demand treatments or would call the senior resident at home to arrange medications. Elements of her history were also consistent with a diagnosis of Munchausen's syndrome: an acute, but not entirely convincing presentation, a childhood history of deprivation and rejection, a history of illness as a child, and frequent travel. The psychiatric consultant planned to administer psychologic tests. He informed the staff about the need to set limits on her demands and to supervise temperature taking (to eliminate the possibility of factitious fevers) and warned the staff about the likelihood of her signing out AMA. Ms C. refused psychologic testing.

Over the next three days the psychiatrist did not challenge her complaint of pain but confronted her with the staff's impression that her pain had no medical basis. During this time she had been afebrile. Ms C. insisted that her care be transferred to a senior attending surgeon so that she might get a more "experienced work-up." However, she did not deny that she was either misrepresenting or fabricating her pain or fevers.

The senior surgeon was consulted and agreed with the need for further psychiatric treatment (including possible in-patient care) and out-patient medical follow-up. That night her unsupervised temperature was 103°F but was 98°F when supervised, and she was noted to be scratching at her surgical scars.

Since she had no hospital insurance, no financial support, and no verifiable address, transfer to a local state psychiatric facility was considered. When Ms C. was asked if she desired in-patient psychiatric care at the state hospital or, out-patient follow-up, she stated she planned to stay in MGH, despite the fact that the surgeon clearly stated this was not indicated. Discharge was then urged so that Ms C. would not further harm herself and require a longer hospitalization. Ms C. was escorted out of the hospital by security personnel.

The above case presents essentially all of the features generally associated with Munchausen's syndrome. Despite the anger of staff toward Ms C., psychiatric consultation was delayed until the 18th hospital day. Once the possibility of Munchausen's syndrome was raised, detective work carried out, and the dynamics discussed with staff, unproductive struggles with the patient decreased. The patient's discomfort could be addressed and she could be confronted in a supportive context. Although Ms C. failed to take advantage of psychiatric follow-up, further invasive treatments were prevented. Without an awareness of the diagnosis and of the physician's countertransference feelings, the percentage of successful psychiatric referrals will be low and the patient will continue to be at risk from her illness.

THE DEMANDING PATIENT

The demanding patient is a person who requests more service than the staff believes he is entitled to. There are, however, wide variations in the tolerance of individual caregivers. What is demanding to one nurse or physician may not be to another. Also, there are levels of subtlety in the way demands are voiced such that some caregivers, rather than feeling used, are only aware of a growing antagonism toward a patient.

Consultation psychiatrists are perhaps overly sensitive to the demanding patient. Oftentimes they misconstrue perfectly legitimate requests as evidence of demanding behavior. For example, someone immobilized by a cast often asks a visitor to perform such tasks as lighting a cigarette, handing water cups, or elevating the bed. Frequently a rash of these requests will be made as soon as the physician enters the room. This may be less the sign of a demanding nature than evidence of an overburdened nursing staff. It is important that a diagnosis of demanding behavior be based not on one but many such instances. There are a number of types of demanding behavior, some examples of which are the following.

The Perfectionist

Perfectionism is perhaps the most frequently encountered type of demanding behavior. The perfectionist is usually obsessive-compulsive by nature. He knows the room rate and his rights. Punctuality is expected. Meals are to be given at a certain time, pills and shots at another. Complaints are issued when service lags. When criticism is accompanied by a sense of humor, little difficulty arises, but the same complaint offered sullenly will earn short shrift for the patient. The perfectionist is not so apt to ask for special favors as he is to insist on being given what is due him at the time it is due. Individuals of this sort are seldom referred to a psychiatrist unless they are in the hospital for a period of weeks. If this happens, their sense of entitlement may gnaw away at staff patience and alienate nurses and physicians to the point where they insist something must be done.

The most effective type of intervention for perfectionism is confrontation. One may begin by agreeing that the patient has certain rights as a paying guest at a medical hostelry. However, because it is medical, there are apt to be emergencies and unforeseen incidences that make it impossible for the staff to serve patients in a fashion they might expect aboard a luxury liner. Perfectionists, the patient can be told, unless they are critically ill, tend to be served last. Sometimes this message is written in a letter and handed out like a business card to appropriate patients. The staff often has its own way of reacting to the person who demands too much.

The Reactive Demander

Demandingness of the reactive type is a form of hospital regressive behavior. The hospital environment tends to favor regressive behavior and the more severe or chronic the illness, the more regressed the individual can become. Demandingness of this type is apt to occur in compensation for the sense of impairment or helplessness that a patient feels. One phase of the adaptation to quadriplegia is demandingness. As a phase, it eventually passes. Similarly, patients with severe burns, multiple fractures, or any other injury or surgical illness that necessitates long hospitalization and dependency, will demonstrate demanding behavior.

A 32-year-old woman was hospitalized to have an ileostomy for severe ulcerative colitis. She had had many previous hospitalizations, all in an effort to avoid the ileostomy, but now her condition necessitated surgery. After the ileostomy she refused to take care of the stoma. She only halfheartedly cooperated with those who taught her how to adjust the bag. Before long, a series of stomal abscesses formed. These were suppurative, ugly, and malodorous. Feces stained her fingers and her bed. She began to talk in a lispy, whiny tone and to request all types of service, from having her hands and face washed to back rubs at all hours. Nurses began to avoid her room and refer to her as "psychotic." Her physician had lost patience with her when she refused to cooperate with the nurse who taught stomal care. He rarely visited her for more than two minutes at a time and the floor nurses could not depend on him to establish any discipline with the patient. With reluctance he agreed to make a request for a psychiatric consultation.

The psychiatrist was appalled by the condition of the room and the patient. The patient's first comment was, "I want the nurse and my cigarettes." Although she answered questions in monosyllables, she paid little attention to the examiner and seemed entirely unaware of her unwholesome surroundings. While there was no evidence of psychosis, it was clear that she was living in a world whose unnaturalness verged on the insane.

After a consultation with the nurses and her physician about his strategy, the psychiatrist again approached the patient. She was told that one reason the nurses and her physician did not visit her was the stench—for which she seemed to accept no responsibility. Like a child, she had turned over her personal hygiene to others. She broke into tears and replied, "Well, how do you think I feel?" The consultant acknowledged that she must feel dreadful, but also explained that if she continued to let herself go, the result could be serious and possibly fatal. To assist her in mending her relationship with her caregivers, a list of rules was prescribed including cooperation with the nurse who taught her stomal care, improved personal hygiene, friendliness to the nursing staff, and ambulation. In return she would be moved to a new room with a much better view (the current room faced an air shaft), be provided with a new television set, and receive daily visits from the psychiatrist. The alternative would mean continued poor nursing care, loneliness, and eventually transfer to a psychiatric facility.

The psychiatrist knew that the patient was depressed. She had told him so. Her situation was evidence of passive neglect by the medical community, an unconscious or indeliberate manifestation of their anger. The anger of the psychiatric consultant at this demanding infantile patient, though felt, was not expressed until he had spoken with the nurses and had examined the patient to reassure himself that she was not psychotic. He then used his anger to call the patient's attention vividly to the circumstances of her condition. "Your room stinks and so do you!," he said. Next came the setting of limits, followed by the alternative rewards or punishments. This program could only be carried out with the understanding, agreement, and cooperation of the nurses.

This case points out three principles for management of the demanding patient:

1. *Self-awareness.* Be aware of the response the patient arouses in you. If it is anger, acknowledge it as such. Some individuals act out their anger covertly by avoiding the person who causes it. Avoidance had been one of the major responses to this patient. Anger at someone who is desperately ill is hard to countenance, yet it is human and must be contended with.

2. *Limit-setting.* It is important to list the things one wants to accomplish. Talk them over with the patient, see what is reasonable and what is not until both parties—caregiver and patient—can arrive at a suitable compromise. The rewards and punishments of the system should be made clear.

3. *Confrontation.* It is always better to confront patients with their demanding behavior rather than to let the demands continue uncontested. The confrontation should be made before the staff has become so angry that the message contains unnecessary belligerence. The confrontation should be firm but gentle; for example, "Do you realize that you are only commenting on things we do wrong? You never say a word when we do something right. You comment when the pill is five minutes late, the same way you do when it is half an hour late. You leave us no latitude."

The Demanding Hypomanic Patient

Many patients are not so demanding as they are hyperactive. These are people who resist being sick because they cannot stand to be inactive. The tendency to activity stands them in good stead if they are undergoing a course of rehabilitation that requires full cooperation. However, it is apt to become a problem when they are forced into the passive role. In this situation the hospital staff must realize how inflexible hospital routines are apt to be. Sometimes the answer is to loosen these routines if it can be done with no inconvenience to other patients and no harm to the hyperactive patient.

Mr A.J., a 49-year-old silk importer, was basically well-intentioned and courteous, but he was accustomed to giving orders like a drill instructor. As soon as the nursing staff reminded him that this was not Parris Island, he apologized and phrased his requests more politely. The main problem, however, was not the manner of his requests, but the content. He insisted on having two telephones—one line directly to his office, the other for outside calls. He also wanted a small bar in his room for the business meetings that he began scheduling. He had just entered the CCU with what appeared to be a septal infarction. At first the nurses thought his requests were the result of morphine-induced euphoria. As a consequence morphine was withheld and the patient experienced a return of chest pain. This was enough to quiet him for a while. He was given a large oral dose of a hypnotic for sleep, which carried him through the night.

The next day he awoke pain-free and in excellent spirits. His energy had returned and he was about to leave his room when he was halted by a team of nurses who rushed in because his actions had dislodged one of the monitoring electrodes and set off an alarm. He returned to bed without protest, but once again asked for telephones and a bar. On morning rounds, his physician told him that alcohol in any form was prohibited in the hospital. This he accepted gracefully, but he told the physician that the telephones were a necessity. The physician said that he would consider it, but increased his dosage of tranquilizer instead. This produced an outburst of anger from Mr A.J. He felt "patronized" and "ignored." He declared, "My doctor gave me the medicinal brush-off." He once again left his bed and paced the floor, tripping the alarm and triggering a series of premature ventricular contractions. His physician was summoned and spent 20 minutes talking with him about the need for absolute bed rest and avoidance of excitement. The patient pointed out that he could not control his nerves, that he was used to being active during the day, that several things were happening to his business requiring his immediate attention, and that no amount of sedation was going to soothe his nerves while his business was about to be dismantled in his absence.

He was a man who had never been ill before in his life. He had made no provision for illness, never having even considered the possibility. He still refused to admit that he was as sick as his ECGs and enzymes indicated. Part of his desire for telephone contact with the outside world was interpreted by the physician as an attempt to deny the seriousness of his plight. This was pointed out to him, but had no effect whatsoever. As midafternoon approached, his agitation seemed to mount and he refused to take any more tranquilizers. He was so restless in bed that his nurse made the comment, "If anybody could pace the floor while remaining in bed, Mr A.J. would be the man to do it." By late afternoon his physician thought it wise to meet him halfway by putting in one telephone that he could use without restrictions.

The result was immediate. The patient called his secretary and began lining up telephone calls and scheduling activities. There was an immediate change in his manner. He became much more himself and had a notable decrease in ventricular irritability in the next 48 hours. An agreement was reached with the physician that there would be no business meetings until he left the CCU, but that two telephones would be installed as long as his secretary could help him with business. Although the telephones were in constant use from dawn until dusk, he did agree to take three one-hour rest periods during the day, at which time the phones were unplugged. The remainder of his stay in the CCU was altogether uncomplicated. When Mr A.J. left the unit, his physician allowed him to have daily business meetings. He was monitored for the first two days, but the meetings were quiet and produced no disturbance in mood or myocardium.

Clearly in this instance, physical and mental inactivity were more stressful than "business as usual." Medical caregivers must be prepared to recognize individuals whose mental well-being depends on activity and to shape their therapeutic program to reduce emotional wear. Although some activities may violate the policy of a unit, enough latitude should be available to accommodate the exceptional person. Furthermore, in an instance such as the one described, the patient was under constant monitoring. If conducting business increased myocardial irritability, an alternative activity could be found. Bargains can always be made with the movers and shakers. They are usually practical individuals, more inclined toward self-preservation than reckless misbehavior. If a program of physical conditioning is available in the hospital, these individuals are likely to enjoy participating since it gives them something to do. Also, having a business partner visit a patient regularly can be of value.

The Passive-Aggressive Patient with Demanding Behavior

There are a number of patients whose demands are a form of hostility. At times of stress this tendency may be more apparent. Usually these individuals have a long history of personality malfunction studded with incidents in which they have alienated people or caused rows of various sorts. Often they can be immediately identified by a sense of entitlement so ingrained that they feel no need to acknowledge a service rendered. The pleasantry "thank you" may not be in their vocabulary.

Mr G., a 57-year-old accountant, occupied a bed on the convalescence floor of a CCU where he had gained the title, "Mr Coffee Nerves." Every time one of his fellow patients turned a radio up, "Mr Coffee Nerves" would shout across, "Turn that god-damn thing down!" Whenever the nurse was delayed in bringing a medication he would shout at her, "Get your sweet little ass over here, honey!" On rounds he would address the medical students and interns as "boy." "Boy, hand me that paper before you leave" was said to an intern on rounds; or, "Sonny, you come back when I'm feeling better before you listen to my chest. I'm tired of being a pincushion for you kids." The second week he insisted on smoking on the ward, which was against rules, and threatened to sign out unless they allowed him this privilege. The resident in charge said he would not allow him to smoke and if he wanted to sign out against advice he not only would allow him to do so, but would open the door for him. This in fact is what happened. The patient walked out, went home, and shortly afterward died.

It is difficult to know how this individual could have been managed to everyone's satisfaction. The likelihood is that any attempt to do so would have been met with a hostile, negative rebuff. However, a psychiatrist should have been called in as was agreed on during the postmortem discussion. Confrontation and limit-setting also ought to have been the order of the day as soon as the early signs of this type of behavior began to occur.

THE ASSAULTIVE PATIENT

Patients who are physically combative or dangerously assaultive are rarely encountered by psychiatrists on general medical or surgical floors. Far more common is the disruptive, disoriented, delirious individual, someone with strength enough to harm himself, but with neither the intention nor the wherewithal for injuring another. However, occasionally delirious patients, such as individuals in withdrawal states, can pose a problem on the ward as can the psychotic in catatonic furor or the epileptic in epileptic furor. Prevention is the best type of management. Individuals with a potential for dangerous assault who can be identified by virtue of their previous performance or past history elsewhere should be covered with an appropriate medication. In addition, a special attendant should be available along with a trusted friend or relative. The latter are often the most effective instruments available to avert violence. Room confinement or body restraint is at times necessary. It must be cautioned, however, that physical restraint in the odd case can serve as a precipitant to increased truculence rather than to submissiveness.

When a patient becomes unexpectedly obstreperous, seeks exit from the ward, and threatens to dispose of anybody who obstructs his way, quick action is called for. Most often the psychiatrist is the one who is expected to interpose some form of barricade between the patient and the door. Most psychiatrists have enough sense to resist the role of David without a sling. A very quick survey of the situation is usually enough to determine whether or not the patient is amenable to conversation. Is the patient, for example, willing to accept medication as long as he is not asked to return to bed? Before an interview is conducted, however, the psychiatrist should make sure that the security forces are alerted and several male attendants are on their way to the location where they should remain out of sight unless needed. If the individual will take medication, it should be given. The security force should remain in the area until the patient is fully sedated. An effective dose is one that leaves the individual asleep or semistuporous.

If, on the other hand, the individual is not amenable to conversation (generally they are not because persuasive methods have been attempted long before the psychiatrist is called), then the psychiatrist should follow one cardinal rule of conduct: Never move in on a violent assaultive patient without at least four assistants. The rule of thumb is one helper for each extremity, and, optimally, an extra person for holding the head. The bigger the assistants, the better. It is better to have ten than five, and the progression is linear in direct proportion to the patient's size and pugilistic talent. A show of force of this kind is often enough in itself to stop the individual from acting out. A smaller number might serve as a challenge to the patient's sense of machismo or the patient might have sufficient martial skills to believe that he can handle himself against anything but a mob.

During the service of one of us (TPH) as a Public Health Service officer at a federal reformatory, an experience occurred that serves as a model for handling a violent patient.

A 6 ft, 7 in., 260-lb inmate was admitted to the reformatory hospital on his way to the federal hospital at Springfield, Mo. He was diagnosed as having paranoid schizophrenia. The prison attendants had never seen a larger or more heavily muscled man. After being unshackled he was placed in a security room within the neuropsychiatric section of the hospital. Shortly thereafter, for reasons that are unknown, he tore the iron gate from the wall of his cell and within minutes dislodged the entire cell door. Using this as a flail, he was terrifying the other inmates, who screamed for help. When the psychiatrist arrived, he foolishly walked toward the patient and asked him to sit down and talk. Instead he flung the door at the doctor, a distance of some 20 feet. Fortunately, he missed.

The doctor realized that if he tried to subdue the patient with the five or six orderlies on duty a massacre would result. He evacuated the ward of everyone but the patient and asked the warden to send over the riot squad along with a riot truck. The warden questioned his judgment, but was eventually persuaded. With a squadron of 30 guards at his back and a riot truck bearing tear gas canisters and a riot hose positioned at a window facing him, the doctor advanced with a syringe containing a sedative. The inmate was told that he could have it his way or our way, but in any event he was going to be sedated. One way he would get hurt, as would we; the other way, no one would be harmed. For a moment he paused, looking at the phalanx in a menacing way, and then simply said, "Aw, shit, go ahead," dropped his pants, and turned around so that the doctor had easy access to an injection site in his buttock.

This case report illustrates the principle of force. The greater the force, the less apt there is to be bloodshed or fracture.

The intervention strategies in the case reports mainly demonstrate the practice of common sense. Interwoven with common sense are a few psychological principles that are important. It is the authors' hope that the case examples are vivid enough to serve as a hook for memory.

REFERENCES

1. Miles CP: Conditions predisposing to suicide: A review. *J Nerv Ment Dis* 1977; 164:231–246.
2. Crumley FE: Adolescent suicide attempts. *JAMA* 1979; 241:2404–2407.
3. Holinger CP: Adolescent suicide: An epidemiological study of recent trends. *Am J Psychiatry* 1978; 135:754–756.
4. Hellon CP, Solomon MI: Suicide and age in Alberta, Canada, 1951–1977: The changing profile. *Arch Gen Psychiatry* 1980; 37:505–510.
5. Greilsheimer H, Groves JE: Male genital self-mutilation. *Arch Gen Psychiatry* 1979; 36:441–446.
6. Murphy GE: The physician's responsibility for suicide: II. Errors of omission. *Ann Intern Med* 1975; 82:305–309.
7. Tsuang MT: Suicide in schizophrenics, manics, depressives, and surgical controls: A comparison with general population suicide mortality. *Arch Gen Psychiatry* 1978; 35:153–155.
8. Roy A: Risk factors for suicide in psychiatric patients. *Arch Gen Psychiatry* 1982; 39:1089–1095.
9. Barraclough B, Bunch J, Nelson E, et al: A hundred cases of suicide: Clinical aspects. *Br J Psychiatry* 1974; 125:355–373.
10. Weisman AD, Worden JW: Risk-rescue rating in suicide assessment. *Arch Gen Psychiatry* 1972; 26:553–560.
11. O'Brien JP: Increases in suicide attempts by drug ingestion: The Boston experience; 1964–1974. *Arch Gen Psychiatry* 1977; 34:1165–1169.
12. Thibault GE, Mulley AG, Barnett GO, et al: Medical intensive care: Indications, interventions, and outcomes. *N Engl J Med* 1980; 302:938–942.
13. Stern TA, Mulley AG, Thibault GE: Life-threatening drug overdose: Precipitants and prognosis. *JAMA* 1984; 257:1983–1985.

14. Maltsberger JT, Buie DH: Countertransference hate in the treatment of suicidal patients. *Arch Gen Psychiatry* 1974; 30:625–633.
15. Reich P, Kelly MJ: Suicide attempts by hospitalized medical and surgical patients. *N Eng J Med* 1976; 294:298–301.
16. Farberow NL, McKelligott JW, Cohen S, Darbonne A: Suicide among patients with cardiorespiratory illness. *JAMA* 1966; 195:422–428.
17. Abram HS, Moore GL, Westervelt FB Jr: Suicidal behavior in chronic dialysis patients. *Am J Psychiatry* 1971; 127:1199–1204.
18. Jankowski CB, Drum DE: Diagnostic correlates of discharge against medical advice. *Arch Gen Psychiatry* 1977; 34:153–155.
19. Schlauch RK, Reich P, Kelly MD: Leaving the hospital against medical advice. *N Engl J Med* 1979; 300:22–24.
20. Albert HD, Kornfeld DS: The threat to sign out against medical advice. *Ann Intern Med* 1973; 79:888–891.
21. Cramer B, Gershberg MR, Stern M: Munchausen syndrome: its relationship to malingering, hysteria, and the physician-patient relationship. *Arch Gen Psychiatry* 1971; 24:573–578.
22. Hackett TP, Weisman AD: Psychiatric management of operative syndromes I. *Psychosom Med* 1960; 22:267.
23. Hackett TP, Weisman AD: Psychiatric management of operative syndromes II. *Psychosom Med* 1960; 22:356.
24. Asher R: Munchausen's syndrome. *Lancet* 1951; 1:339–341.
25. Stern TA: Munchausen's syndrome revisited. *Psychosomatics* 1980; 21:329–336.
26. Ford CV: The Munchausen syndrome: A report of four new cases and a review of psychodynamic considerations. *Psychiatry Med* 1973; 4:31–45.

15

Coping with Illness

AVERY D. WEISMAN

Coping with illness is a problem for both patient and physician. Indeed, anyone engaged in the management of illness or involved in its psychosocial complications is required to cope and understand how others cope. For the patient and physician, however, coping together may be a mutually constructive or a depleting job, since the coping strategies used by one participant are likely to be the mirror image of strategies used by the other.

In general, *coping* is best defined as problem solving behavior designed to bring about relief, reward, quiescence, and equilibrium. There is nothing in this definition that promises permanent resolution of problems. It does imply, however, that effective problem solving behavior must be preceded by adequate appraisal of the significant issues.

In ordinary language and usage, asking how one coped refers to the outcome, not to the intermediary processes of appraisal and performance that problem solving requires. In the sense of this discussion, coping is an extensive, recursive process of self-exploration, self-instruction, self-correction, self-rehearsal, and self-assessment, combined with other functions such as cognition, memory, judgment, reflection, and so forth, taken from that factory of functions called ego/personality.

Coping with illness is an inescapable part of medical practice, although hospital psychiatrists are apt to see more clearly how being sick entails a variety of psychosocial problems that may require the intervention of other specialists.

Most psychosocial problems go beyond the narrow limits of physical symptoms and disabilities. The issues involve complex interaction of a person within the social groupings that characterize the range of individual life. That one copes with nondisease factors cannot be doubted. Only a narrow-visioned superspecialist immersed in technology would claim that every patient undergoes similar risks and problems, corresponding to standard treatment, and that psychosocial issues are irrelevant.

297

How one copes depends on the nature of a problem as well as on the mental, emotional, and physical equipment one has to cope with. The hospital psychiatrist or anyone qualified to make a psychosocial assessment is in an advantageous position to integrate and evaluate how physical illness interferes with the conduct of life, and how psychosocial issues infringe upon the course of illness and recovery. The psychiatrist's principal job is to understand which psychosocial problems are pertinent, which physical problems are distressing, which interpersonal relations support or undermine coping. The psychiatrist must also assume that current coping is inimical or inadequate to the best possible resolution related to physical recovery.

In restricting assessment to the here-and-now, the hospital psychiatrist will be concerned with details of previous problems only insofar as they illuminate the present predicament. Long-range forays into past history will, as a rule, be neither practical nor useful.

WHO ARE GOOD COPERS?

There are few paragons who cope exceedingly well with every problem likely to occur. If such people exist, the psychiatrist would be unlikely to see or be one. For everyone else, psychiatrists included, sickness imposes a personal and social burden, threat, and risk which are seldom precisely proportional to the actual dangers of the primary disease. Therefore, the good copers may be regarded as individuals with a special skill or with personal traits that enable them to master many difficulties. What characterizes good copers?

1. They are optimistic about mastering problems, and despite setbacks, generally maintain a high level of morale.
2. They tend to be practical in emphasizing immediate problems, issues, and obstacles which must be conquered before even visualizing a remote or ideal resolution.
3. By selecting from a wide range of potential strategies and tactics, their policy is not to be at a loss for fallback methods. In this respect, they are resourceful.
4. In heeding various possible outcomes, they improve coping by being aware of consequences.
5. They are generally flexible in being open to suggestions, without losing the final say in decisions.
6. They are quite composed though vigilant in avoiding emotional extremes that could impair judgment.

These are collective tendencies, seldom typifying any specific individual, except the very heroic or idealized. No one copes superlatively at all times, especially with problems that impose a risk and might well be overwhelming. Notably, however, the really good copers seem able to choose the kind of situation they are most effective in. Unless a particular plight is thrust upon them, good copers have enough confidence to feel resourceful enough to survive intact. I also have the impression that good copers do not pretend to knowledge they do not have, and therefore feel comfortable about turning to experts in whom they trust.

The clinical importance of this characterization is that it can help assess how patients cope by pinpointing what trait they seem to lack.

WHO ARE BAD COPERS?

Bad copers are not necessarily bad people, nor even incorrigibly ineffective people. It is too schematic merely to indicate that bad copers have the opposite characteristics of good copers. Bad copers are those who have more problems in coping with unusual, intense, and unexpected difficulties because of the following traits:

1. They tend to be excessive in self-expectation, rigid in outlook, inflexible in standards, and reluctant to compromise or ask for help.
2. Their opinion of how people should behave is narrow and absolute, allowing very little room for tolerance.
3. While prone to firm adherence to preconceptions, bad copers may show unexpected compliance or be very suggestible on specious grounds, with little cause.
4. They are inclined to excessive denial, elaborate rationalization, and the inability to focus on salient problems.
5. Because they find it difficult to weigh feasible alternatives, bad copers may be more passive than usual, and fail to initiate action on their own behalf.
6. Occasionally, the rigidity lapses, and bad copers will subject themselves to impulsive judgments or atypical behavior which fails to be effective.

THE MEDICAL PREDICAMENT

Coping refers to a patient's response within the total complex of factors related to illness: disease, sickness, and vulnerability. Assessing how patients cope will be diffuse impressionism unless the psychiatrist can focus, without distraction, on the immediate illness and its surrounding circumstances, social and emotional. For example, a key question is, Why now? Has the patient's clinical plight become too difficult? Or does the request for help reflect the attending physician's exasperation or sense of futility? How have present difficulties come about to the present time?

Disease is assuredly not the same as being sick, because patients with the same diagnosis can be sick in wholly different ways. Cancer patients, for example, are sick in different ways, from one diagnosis to the next, from one phase and stage, depending upon a host of physical and personality issues. Cancer certainly differs from heart disease, and most other diseases, not just in the organs involved, but in symptoms and social expectations. Most prominently, diseases differ also in their sense of threat and risk. The medical predicament is also influenced by a set of expectations generated by rules and principles that direct how physicians, patients, and supportive others should behave. The cultural match between professional staff and social grouping may also be a factor in generating specific problems that both must cope with.

The psychiatrist will also try to compare how a patient deals with outside problems when assessing the difficulty that the patient encounters within the institutional setting, with its regulated expectations. There is always an implicit social code that patients either comply with or violate.

If there is any doubt about how staff and patients differ in social expectations and cultural bias, listen to the conversation at the bedside. Words have different meanings, and messages are usually garbled. It is often a wonder that we understand each other as well as we do. The semantics of clinical discussion may have a distinct influence on the outcome of how patients are expected to cope. While the importance of a good doctor-patient relationship has never been minimized, its exact constituents must include a degree of mutual communication. This in turn makes for more effective, better understood coping. Therefore, when assessing how any patient copes, it is essential to examine how that patient communicates and fails to communicate with the staff, and the reverse, at key moments. When communication breaks down, previous agreement is lost. The result may be negativism, denial, antagonism, and unexpected, unwarranted, unacceptable behavior. Coping well involves a kind of social compact that insists upon certain values and appropriate behavior. It also defines potential threats and implied risks.

How to cope is inescapably tied to how one is expected to cope in order to be judged. Not all of this is explicit, since communication is often more effective when words are few than when much talk goes on. Some things are far too important to be put into words. A good psychiatrist appreciates the autonomy of good coping, and knows that people can talk incessantly without coming to terms about the best way to handle problems. When the staff becomes an adversary, problems change, and the original difficulty may become even more problematic.

The psychiatrist is not the only professional concerned about coping with illness. In fact, psychiatrists are seldom called upon to be asked about rehabilitation and recovery. There are trained specialists who direct and instruct and give much support and information about issues that interfere with recovery. For example, there are experts in nutrition, dialysis, colostomy care, chemotherapy, physical rehabilitation, social work, hospice services, and pain control, to mention only a few who are actively engaged in helping patients cope better by correcting problems and deficiencies.

Long-term illness obviously has a profound effect on self-image, self-expectation, and social function. Its effect on significant others is almost immeasurable. Complications can snowball, leading to progressive impairment of coping. Moreover, however adept these trained "para-professionals" (paraprofessional to whom?), few can adequately cope with the existential issues underlying much chronic disease. Death, transience, disability, alienation, and so forth are drawn inconspicuously into the clinical scene.

It is wise to remember that psychiatry does not arbitrarily introduce existential issues into the appraisal. If a patient is found to have an unspoken but vivid fear of death, that fear is already there, and not an artifact of the evaluation process.

Being sick is, of course, somewhat easier for some patients than others, and for certain patients it is much preferred over trying to make it in the outside world. There is much anxiety and inadequacy, failure and frustration, in holding one's own in a job or family. At key moments of life, being sick may be a better solution than continuing to struggle and fail. Although healthy people are expected to withstand defeat, others legitimize their disappointment in and through illness. A passive-dependent person may tenaciously hang onto the face saving of disabling symptoms long after other patients are back working again. Such patients not only tend to thrive in a complaining atmosphere but even blame their physicians. Demands are almost triumphant since the patient, sooner or later, wants to share failure with the doctor.

Hospital psychiatrists readily observe how chronic invalidism may become a perverse form of success representing retaliation against those who cope very well, namely, members of the professional community. Denial and hypochrondriacal elaboration underscore the essential failure of coping.

Every patient needs a measure of support, sustenance, security, and self-esteem, even if they are not patients at all. No one gets very far, or feels very well, for very long, without drawing on someone or something from the outside that provides these four factors that are necessary for coping well. Patients pointing toward recovery simply need more.

In assessing how patients cope, their needs with respect to support, sustenance, security, and self-esteem can be determined by identifying *potential pressure point problems* in the following areas:

1. Health and well-being
2. Family and marital responsibility
3. Marital and sexual roles
4. Vocational and economic solvency
5. Social and community expectations
6. Religious and cultural demands
7. Self-image problems
8. Existential concerns

What this means from a practical viewpoint is that if special pressure point problems can be singled out, it is possible then to identify problems pertaining to support, sustenance, security, and self-esteem with which the patient is trying to cope.

COURAGE AND VULNERABILITY

Most psychiatric assessments emphasize shortcomings, deficiencies, defects, and aberrant symptoms. Seldom does the examiner pay enough attention to a patient's strengths or positive attributes. This is unfortunate because strengths can counterbalance many inimical forces. Examiners overlook hope, confidence, intelligence, loyalty, and many other so-called virtues, as if they were simply pathologic manifestations of something else. A conspicuous example of a praiseworthy trait is courage.

Clinical courage in this sense should not be confused with "bravery under fire." The derring-do of heroic exploits is seldom found among ordinary people, but courage is more common than realized. Everyone, at some time, is obliged to take steps to deal with a serious threat. Such threats occur on several levels, ranging from actual injury and death, to failure, disgrace, humiliation, and so forth. The courage to cope is generally found in a wish to perform competently and responsibly despite barriers. This is what is meant by "moral courage."

If an examiner were to include assessments of positive attributes in evaluating the capacity to cope well, a patient's overall coping might be understood better. If a patient indicates that in the past he had failed over and over because of shortcomings in himself, not necessarily because of external circumstances, the psychosocial assessment would show that bad coping needed to be supplemented. Courage would also require bolstering, because hope, confidence, and morale join together in the cause of coping well. Patients who cannot perform competently or who never live up to their standards are more than the familiar "inadequate" personalities; they will certainly need help in containing distress and contending with potential obstacles. Naturally, few people readily admit their tendency to fail or to behave in unworthy ways. A skillful interview, however, can get behind the denial, rationalization, and externalizations to form a better picture of what the patient is like.

Courage requires an awareness of risk. Without a substantial sense of anxiety, fear, tension, and worry about being able to manage and withstand pressure, courage cannot exist. In a word, courage is always accompanied by vulnerability.

Like courage, vulnerability is present in us all. It shows up at times of stress, crisis, calamity, risk, or profound threat to well-being and identity. Actually, vulnerability has a double meaning: (1) the disposi-

Table 15-1. Vulnerability

Hopelessness: Patient believes that all is lost; effort is futile; no chance at all; passive surrender to the inevitable

Turmoil/Perturbation: Patient is tense, agitated, restless, hyperalert to all potential risk, real and imagined

Frustration: Patient is angry about inability to progress, recover, get satisfactory answers, or to get relief

Despondency/Depression: Patient is dejected, withdrawn, apathetic, tearful, often inaccessible to verbal interaction

Helplessness/Powerlessness: Patient complains of being too weak to struggle any more; cannot initiate action or make decisions that stick

Anxiety/Fear: Patient feels on the edge of dissolution, with dread and specific fears about impending doom and disaster

Exhaustion/Apathy: Patient feels too worn out and depleted to care; more indifference than sadness

Worthlessness/Self-rebuke: Patient feels persistent self-blame, no good, finding numerous causes for weakness, failure, incompetence

Painful isolation/Abandonment: Patient is lonely, feeling ignored and alienated from significant others

Denial/Avoidance: Patient speaks or acts as if threatening aspects of illness are minimal, almost showing a jolly interpretation of related events, or else a serious disinclination to examine potential problems

Truculence/Annoyance: Patient is embittered, not openly angry, but feeling mistreated, victimized, duped by forces or people

Repudiation of Significant Others: Patient rejects or antagonizes significant others, including family, friends, professional sources of support

Closed Time Perspective: Patient may show any or all of the above, but in addition foresees an exceedingly limited future

---

tion or potential for suffering in various ways, and (2) the dysphoric experience of distress.

In order to find out, for example, how a patient facing a serious operation will cope, ask that patient how he or she imagines or visualizes each step of the procedure leading up to the feared event. Which step was most difficult? Prediagnosis? Relation to the doctor? Family issues? Going under anesthesia? Possible postoperative pain?

Coping and vulnerability have a loose kind of reciprocal relationship. The better one copes, as a rule, the less distress. Conversely, much distress often means ineffective coping with a current problem. This does not mean that those who deny even mild problems, or disavow any emotional concern, are therefore really good copers. Courage requires substantial anxiety, or concern, which is reflected in measurable distress, not in stolid unresponsiveness.

Tables 15-1 and 15-2 labelled Vulnerability and Cope, respectively, show 13 common types of distress, and 15 different coping strategies.

Table 15-2. Cope (To Find out How a Patient Copes)

Problem: In your opinion, what has been most difficult for you since your illness started? How has it troubled you?
Strategy: What did you do (or are doing) about the problem?
01. Get more information (rational/intellectual approach)
02. Talk it over with others to relieve distress (share concern)
03. Try to laugh it off; make light of it (reverse affect)
04. Put it out of mind; try to forget (suppression/denial)
05. Distract myself by doing other things (displacement/dissipation)
06. Take positive step based on present understanding (confrontation)
07. Accept, but change the meaning to something easier to deal with (redefinition)
08. Submit, yield, surrender to the inevitable (passivity/fatalism)
09. Do something, anything, reckless or impractical (acting out)
10. Look for feasible alternatives to negotiate (if *x*, then *y*)
11. Drink, eat, take drugs, etc to reduce tension (tension reduction)
12. Withdraw, get away, seek isolation (stimulus reduction)
13. Blame someone or something (projection/disowning/externalization)
14. Go along with directives from authority (compliance)
15. Blame yourself for faults; sacrifice or atone (undoing/self-pity)
Resolution: How has it worked out so far?
01. Not at all
02. Doubtful relief
03. Limited relief but better
04. Much better; actual resolution

Adapted with permission from Weisman AD: *The Realization of Death: A Guide for the Psychological Autopsy*. New York, Jason Aronson, Inc, 1974, pp 172–173.

While few strategies occur in unamalgamated form, unmixed with others, it is a useful exercise to carry out the appraisal recommended in Table 15-2, and to identify specific kinds of dysphoria defined in Table 15-1. One should always compare the characteristics of good copers with his patient's report. Whenever a problem is identified, find out whether the risk visualized is related to threat of death, the risk of not performing well in front of others, being thought cowardly, etc.

Questionnaires have limited value. Careful interviewing asking only pertinent and precise questions about what a patient did or tried to do, together with what actually happened, will be more helpful than giving formal tests.

Examiners should realize in assessing how patients cope with illness that the moment of consultation or even a short period of illness itself may not be typical of how a patient handles problems. The consultation itself may be a sign that the staff or primary physician feels very vulnerable in dealing with a particular clinical issue. Therefore the physician may seek help, more information, or just want to share his concern. Among various forms of dysphoria, the most common is depression, with its associated signs, such as dejection, exhaustion, guilt, and so forth. Anger, of course, is easiest to diagnose because its target tends to be easily identified. Anxiety is very prevalent but often under-diagnosed. Other forms of vulnerability are seldom recognized at all.

HOW TO FIND OUT MORE ABOUT COPING

Thus far, I have pointed out (1) characteristics of good copers and bad copers, and suggested that deficits in patients who are thus identified should direct the clinician how to strengthen coping in specific ways, (2) potential pressure point problems that will alert clinicians to different kinds of psychosocial difficulties, (3) types of emotional vulnerability, and (4) a format for listing different coping strategies, along with questions about resolution.

The assessment and identification of ways in which a patient copes or fails to cope with specific problems requires both description by the patient and interpretation by the psychiatrist. Even so, this may not be enough. Details of descriptive importance may not be explicit. The clinician is then required to pursue relentlessly. If not, the result is only a soft approximation that generalizes where it should be specific. By "pursue relentlessly," I mean that the clinician should ask again and again about a topic that is unclear, rephrasing, without yielding to clichés and general impressions. The examiner can also inquire, "How satisfied were you with what you tried to do?"

Psychiatrists have been imbued with the value of so-called empathy and intuition. While immediate insights and inferences can be very pleasing to the examiner, sometimes these conclusions can be misleading and totally wrong. It is far more empathic to respect each patient's individuality and unique slant on the world by making sure that the examiner accurately describes in detail how problems are confronted. To draw a quick inference without being sure about a highly private state of mind is distinctly unempathic. Like most of us, patients give themselves the benefit of the doubt, and claim to resolve problems in a socially desirable and potentially effective way. It takes little experience to realize that disavowal of any problem through pleasant distortions is itself a coping strategy, not necessarily an accurate description of how one coped.

Simple and straightforward problems are usually someone else's problems. It is difficult to translate complex events into understandable language without sounding pedantic or glossing over ambiguities. Good coping usually means less distress and very little dysphoria, so it is hard to identify what patients do when coping is successful. Consequently, relentless pursuit will be guided by the spoor of painful affect. Is the patient able to indicate *any* problem or does he immediately set up a granitic denial? It is here that an examiner asks, "What if. . ." questions, such as "What if someone like you had a boss (or wife or husband) who was never satisfied and always picked you apart, how should that person handle it?"

Good copers are not only flexible, resourceful, optimistic, and practical, but good at indicating pressure points and problem areas, and instructing themselves what to do. On the other hand, there are two groups of patients who are bad copers. One group adamantly denies any difficulty of any description. The second group floods the interview with details of how badly the world and its occupants have treated them. In the first group, militant denial is the major strategy. In the second, the chief strategy is to put off the interviewer by appealing for pity and rescue. By seeking credit for having suffered so much, such patients reject any implication that they might have prevented or deflected or corrected what has befallen them. Their coping is covered by strategies 13 and 15 in Table 15-2.

Suppression, isolation, and projection are common defenses. This makes it difficult to evaluate the scope of denial and to credit the reports that many patients give. To believe or not to believe is always an open question. But good copers do seem to pinpoint problems clearly, while bad copers, as well as those with strong defenses, seem only to seek relief from further questions, without attempting anything suggesting reflective analysis.

In learning how anyone copes, a measure of authentic skepticism is always appropriate, but combined with a willingness to correction later on. The balance between denial and affirmation is always uncertain. The key is to focus on points of ambiguity, anxiety, and ambivalence while tactfully preserving a patient's self-esteem. A tactful examiner might say, for example, "I'm really not clear about what exactly bothered you, and what you really did...."

The purpose of focusing is to avoid premature formulations that gloss over points of ambiguity. An overly rigid format in approaching any evaluation risks overlooking individual tactics that deny, avoid, dissemble, and blame others for difficulties. Patients, too, can be very rigid, discouraging alliance, rebuffing collaboration, and preventing an effective doctor-patient relationship.

HOW TO BE A BETTER COPER

Coping with illness is only one special area of human behavior. It is important to recognize that in evaluating how patients cope, we, as examiners, should learn our own coping styles, and in effect, learn from patients. Knowledge of medication, psychodynamic theory, and descriptive psychiatry have less to do with the outcome of psychotherapeutic intervention than the doctor's integrity and informed compassion. Credentials, of course, are important, but we are seldom sure which credentials are essential. But clearly it is not enough to mean well, have a warm heart, or a head filled with scientific information. Coping well requires open-ended communication and self-awareness. No technique for coping is applicable to one and all. In fact, the very concept of technique may be antithetical to true understanding. A false objectivity obstructs appraisal; an exaggerated subjectivity only confuses what is being said about whom.

Psychiatrists and patients, indeed almost anyone, can become a better coper by cultivating characteristics of good copers. Coping is, after all, a skill that is useful in a variety of situations, although many modifications of basic principles are called for. Confidence in being able to cope can only be enhanced through self-appraisal, self-instruction, and self-correction over and over. Coping well with illness, and with any other problem, does not predict invariable success, but it does provide a foundation for becoming a better coper.

SUGGESTED READING

Bird B: *Talking with Patients*, ed 2. Philadelphia, JB Lippincott Co, 1973.

Coelho G, Hamburg D, Adams J (eds): *Coping and Adaptation*. New York, Basic Books, Inc, 1974.

Jackson E: *Coping with the Crises in Your Life*. New York, Hawthorn Books, Inc, 1974.

Moos R (ed): *Human Adaptation: Coping with Life Crises*. Lexington, Mass, DC Heath & Co, 1976.

Murphy L, Moriarty A: *Vulnerability, Coping and Growth*. New Haven, Yale University Press, 1976.

Weisman A: *The Coping Capacity: On the Nature of Being Mortal*. New York, Human Sciences Press, 1984.

16

Brief Psychotherapy

JAMES E. GROVES and ANASTASIA KUCHARSKI

"The tranquilizers can only do so much. I wish somebody
would *talk* to me about this cancer thing...."

Surgical patient to consultant.

Tranquilizers can only do so much for the medical or surgical patient
coping with psychological stresses imposed by illness and hospitalization. The hospital staff can do only so much reassuring, explaining, and
talking to the patient. In fact, staff members had spent hours talking
with the patient quoted in the epigraph, yet the patient felt no one
"talked" about the "cancer thing." What patients in this situation
usually mean by "talking" is a specialized kind of listening by the
caregiver—listening and responding based on an understanding of what
the illness or surgery means to patients, to their self-image and to their
lives, careers, and families. This specialized kind of listening, psychotherapy, is a complicated intellectual and empathic relationship
between the patient and the physician.

"Psychotherapy" can refer to transactions continuing for months or
years, but it can also refer to interactions of a few minutes in which only
a few sentences are exchanged—provided they are the right sentences.
Brief psychotherapy on the medical or surgical ward deserves consideration in consultation psychiatry because psychiatrists must combine a
knowledge of medicine and surgery with an understanding of stress
response syndromes. Psychiatrists should know how to listen and to
respond on three levels—medical, social, and psychological—simultaneously. The role of the consultant who comes to the stressed patient is
mainly that of fostering optimal adaptation to painful reality. How well
the consultant succeeds in a small number of interviews depends on the
ability to understand how personality interacts with illness to produce
stress responses. Such work begins with the consultant's understanding
why psychiatric consultation is requested.

WHY CONSULTATION IS REQUESTED

Cassem and Hackett[1] found that the three most common reasons for consultation requests to see myocardial infarction patients in a coronary care unit (CCU) are patient anxiety (32%), depression (30%), and problem behavior (20%). Other reasons include the patient's hostility, delirium, depression, psychosis, delayed recovery, predilection to death, family problems, and sleep disturbance.[2,3] Also, the physician may seek medication advice. Behavior problems seem to stem from excessive denial of illness, euphoria, inappropriate sexual behavior, or hostile-dependent conflicts with the staff. Interventions by the consultant include medication, explanation and reassurance, changes in the patient's immediate environment, confrontation of disruptive behavior, and hypnosis.

Based on these and several other studies,[4-8] there are three broad categories of indications for psychotherapy in the general hospital:

1. Problems with *cognition*—delirium, psychosis, excessive denial, and other states in which the patient is not processing information the way caregivers think the patient should
2. Problems with *affect*—anxiety, depression, apathy, hostility, euphoria
3. Problems with *behavior*—dependency, expression of hostility, noncompliance, manipulativeness, withdrawal, flight

Clearly, these categories overlap; they are all found in responses to stress. In the following sections we will attempt to discuss stress responses under the category that is most relevant to the consultation.

Therapy for Disturbances of Cognition

By "cognition" we mean the complicated mechanisms by which human beings process information: they attend (focus information-gathering apparatuses), they perceive (take in information), they register (encode new information), they recall (retrieve previously stored information that is relevant), they understand (integrate new information with previously stored and processed information), and they plan responses (anticipate consequences of the product of new with old information). Disorders of consciousness impair attention and perception; disorders of memory impair registry and recall; disorders of intellect impair understanding and planning. Medical and surgical illnesses typically engender more than one of these deficits. Delirium, for instance, especially affects the ability to attend and register; dementia affects the recall and integration of previously stored information. *Therapy for a disturbance of cognition consists mainly of recognizing the nature of the impairment and, as much as possible, helping the patient compensate for it.*

> The consultant was called to see an 80-year-old widow who had been hospitalized for treatment of viral pneumonia. Consultation was sought because the patient frequently awoke confused, dressed, packed, and tried to leave. When she was prevented from leaving, she always wept piteously. The consultee thought she might be depressed.
> When examined, the patient was fully oriented and seemed not to recall her nocturnal adventures. Her memory of recent events was impaired, but she was a storehouse of information about World War I when she was a nurse in France. She was optimistic about her improvement. She was dismayed by the quality of hospital food, especially since her appetite was returning. She especially missed the photographs of her husband and her children. These mementos had been left behind in confusion the day she was rushed by ambulance to the hospital.
> The consultant recommended that she be given 1 mg of haloperidol at bedtime as a sedative. Also, it was recommended that her mementos be brought from home, prominently displayed by her bedside, and brightly lit throughout the night.

Simple orienting objects such as clocks, calendars, and familiar possessions frequently suffice to correct cognitive disturbances such as those associated with senile dementia and "sundowning" in the aged. More severe disturbances, such as those accompanying toxic or metabolic encephalopathies, require environmental adjustment of a more restrictive sort (such as restraints) along with correction of the underlying cause of the organic dysfunction.

Another sort of disordered cognition arises when the patient is ignorant of certain aspects of the illness or medical procedure, or when there is misperception or miscommunication between physician and patient.

> A beefy, middle-aged longshoreman was convalescing unremarkably following a myocardial infarction until suddenly one afternoon he threw a glass across his room and roared out his intention to leave the hospital immediately. He refused to speak with his physician or with the psychiatric consultant who had been called soon after the incident started. When they pleaded with the patient to say what had upset him, he muttered that he knew "what fibrillation means," but would say no more. With the intern and the consultant half-blocking the door to the patient's room, the consultant asked the physician to describe the clinical course of the patient during hospitalization. The patient had electrocardiographic and enzyme evidence of a recent myocardial infarction and tracings indicating a previous myocardial infarction (MI). He

had also had episodes of atrial fibrillation which had responded to digitalization.

With the words "fibrillation that had responded" the patient sat heavily down and began to sob—as he later explained—with relief.

Late that afternoon when the patient was again settled in bed, he explained to the consultant the series of events that had led to his outburst. The previous day he had been told that he had had an earlier MI that left a scar on his heart. This scar he visualized as an ominously fragile, thin lesion in his heart wall similar to the "scars of tuberculosis that killed my dad." He had worried about the scar through the night and then on the morning of the incident heard the team talking at the foot of his bed about "fibrillation." Fibrillation, he said, filled him with dread because it ". . . is what the patient on the hospital shows on television always gets just before he dies."

The patient was an intelligent and keenly interested man who derived much satisfaction from following his own course and much comfort from learning some details of cardiology—such as the difference between atrial and ventricular fibrillation. He did well until his MI extended and he died suddenly the day before he was to go home.

In this example the patient required additional information in order to avoid flight. In the following, the patient appeared to flee from more information than he could tolerate.

> A successful young businessman and father of three small children was hospitalized for treatment of fulminant acute myelogenous leukemia that had failed to respond to a succession of chemotherapeutic agents. He was dying and arrangements were being made to place him in a terminal care facility. Consultation was sought at the urgent request of his wife because the patient stoutly denied he was more than mildly ill. The wife knew the patient was dying. She explained to the consultant that although she hoped no one would think her mercenary, she was frantic because the patient had no life insurance. Also, he was a member in a limited partnership of a small electronics firm, and she believed the contract specified that if a partner died intestate, all interest reverted to the firm. The consultant understood her desire to provide for herself and the children, and suggested that she find an estate attorney while the consultant spoke with the patient.
>
> The consultant found the patient to be an emaciated man who was slightly euphoric. Although he identified his illness as leukemia, he said firmly, "It's not going to kill me. I can assure you of that." The patient's history included extreme childhood poverty, an absent father, and a depressed, hypochondriacal mother who "was constantly dying."
>
> The consultant briefly explained that leukemia is usually considered to be fatal, but that progress has been made in its treatment. The consultant also stated a belief that persons who were able to put the illness out of their mind or to fight it, as this patient was doing, were those who survived longest. After a period of silence, the consultant told

the patient of his wife's concerns and asked why the patient had deferred making a will. The patient replied that his "one superstition" was that to make a will was to "invite trouble."

The consultant gently confronted this notion reminding the patient how hard he was "fighting it" and how that helped the prognosis. With these going for him, he had no need for such superstitions—especially when his wife was so distraught. For his wife's peace of mind, would the patient please make a will? The patient agreed to do so.

In this example, the patient's stalwart refusal to process information about his dying was responsible for maladaptive behavior. The consultant saw no harm in the patient's denial except that it prevented him from providing for his family. A direct assault on the denial of impending death would not have changed cognition but, rather, would only have alienated the patient and rigidified the behavior. The consultant supported the denial, strengthened it, and then confronted the behavior and unhooked it from the denial.

Therapy for Disturbances of Affect

Affects—even negative affects such as anxiety, depression, anger—are not inimical to health and adaptation in the human organism. Perhaps they even facilitate growth by motivating change in cognition and behavior. Affects become a problem on the medical or surgical ward when they are (1) inappropriate, (2) too intense, or (3) autonomous—beyond the power of the individual or the environment to change them. They also tend to become a problem when they are based on inaccurate cognition or when they give rise to maladaptive behavior. *Therapy for disturbance of affect in a stressed patient consists mainly of recognizing the causes of disturbance and restoring appropriate affect and control over its intensity and expression.*

Anxiety, depression, and hostility that stem from a psychotic or depressive disorder presumably with a biochemical substrate seem to be autonomous, having "a life of their own" and existing apart from any ability of the individual or of the environment to change them. Psychological or environmental factors may obscure the evidence of biological illness.

A 50-year-old, single, female, classical languages professor whose mother had died a month before was brought to the hospital in a diabetic coma. After the correction of her metabolic imbalance, she refused further treatment saying, "Let me die. It's my right to die and I choose to do so." She also refused to be examined by a psychiatrist until the consultant haltingly interviewed her in Latin. Haughty and contemptuous of the consultant's grammar, she nonetheless consented to be interviewed in Latin and eventually agreed to use English. The consultant found that the patient had suffered from early morning awakening and severe weight loss during the past year, starting some months before her mother became ill. Her mother had had two postpartum depressions and her father had died of alcoholic cirrhosis. The patient also displayed a paranoid delusion in which her academic rivals gave her diabetes by wireless devices in order to sabotage her work. She also had a plan to commit suicide at home.

Working with the hospital lawyer, the consultant obtained a court order that mandated treatment of both her depression and her diabetes. After eight unilateral electroconvulsive treatments her psychotic depression responded and she was given follow-up care by an internist and a psychiatrist after her discharge home.

In addition to being aware of the possibility of a functional psychosis, the consultant should be aware of the possibility that the illness or the medical regimen itself could be the cause of inappropriate, too intense, or autonomous affects.

Another middle-aged woman was hospitalized for regulation of her diabetic regimen. Because she was anxious and sleepless and had had an idiosyncratic reaction to sedative-hypnotics, she was given haloperidol in small doses as a sedative. After a few days in the hospital she became panicky, impulsive, uncooperative, and hostile. Her condition only worsened with an increased dose of her tranquilizing medication.

The psychiatric consultant believed that the patient had akathisia. Indeed, she improved within half an hour after being given intramuscular (IM) benztropine mesylate.

While disturbances of affect are occasionally caused by undiagnosed schizophrenia, manic-depressive illness, medication side effects, or metabolic disturbances related to the medical illness, more often disturbances of affect encountered by the consultant are psychological or psychosocial reactions to the illness or surgery and require a psychodynamic formulation and psychotherapeutic intervention.

A 60-year-old truck farmer was hospitalized for radiation therapy for cancer of the larynx that was too extensive for surgery. The patient also had severe psoriasis, the history of which began in his childhood. Psychiatric consultation was sought because of the patient's severe depression, because of his extreme anxiety—extending as it did even to the most innocent and routine medical procedures, to which he attached dire significance—and because of a hostile dependent attitude. The patient had been given large doses of a tricyclic antidepressant for several weeks but this seemed to help little.

The patient was very eager to consult the psychiatrist. He seemed anxious to go into great detail about his lifelong struggle with psoriasis.

When he spoke of his skin, his voice rose and he assumed a declamatory, vibrant posture. He was the youngest of seven children of a hard-working widowed seamstress. He gave particular emphasis to an incident that had occurred when he was 6 years old. He was returning home from Sunday school with his entire family who boarded the trolley car. Because of crowds the patient had been sent to sit away from his mother at the other end of the car. He felt humiliated, he recalled, and sat feeling defective and ugly because his skin was "all broken out" that day. As he sat his rage grew until suddenly he jumped up and ran to his mother. "You treat me like a leper!" he accused her, pleased with the stares of the other passengers. "You treat me like a leper!" After a momentary pause, his mother picked him up, hugged him, and held him in her lap all the way home. Ever since then he had believed that he was his mother's favorite and, in fact, he had been her sole heir. With the inheritance money he bought his farm. "From that day on," he said, "I been a loudmouth and that's what I'll always be."

The consultant now understood that the patient valued most his ability to speak out and was depressed by the possibility that his most valued possession—his voice—would be taken away. The consultant recommended to the staff that they compliment the patient's loudness and forcefulness. Over a period of time the consultant reassured the patient that no one would take his voice away. He died several months later, after a discharge and subsequent readmission, shouting to the end.

For many patients, it is easier to be angry than to be sad. Sometimes culture, sometimes notions of gender-appropriate behavior, and sometimes simply aloneness prohibit the patient from being sad about losses and give rise to depression accompanied by hostility or uncooperativeness. "Nobody to cry with," one patient said.

A roisterous, elderly ex-convict delighted in shattering the surgical ward with the most vile, obscene, vituperative cussing that any staff member could ever recall. Patently sociopathic, he had "gotten by" until a dissecting aneurysm of the aorta had necessitated a Teflon graft. His postoperative course was punctuated by life-threatening crises. Hypotension, cardiac arrhythmias, septic emboli, a succession of febrile episodes, anemia, renal failure, stress ulcers, and more, all seemed destined, as he put it, "to do me in." Finally, the disruption of the ward became so intense one day when the patient had (1) stolen another patient's wallet, (2) kicked in a television set, and (3) grabbed three nurses that a psychiatric consultation was sought to find appropriate medication for the patient.

The consultant, tired at the end of a long day, sat down with the patient. A chain smoker, the consultant managed somehow to get smoke in the eyes and tears began to stream out. "I know how you feel, Doc," the patient exclaimed. "It's not dying I mind—it's this rot, rot, rot all day long—and nobody to cry with that I mind." After that, the consultant made it a point to go at the end of a day to have a cigarette with the patient so they could be sad together. The patient's behavior improved—not a lot—but a little.

Losses stir up feelings of hopelessness and depression that—until there is time and opportunity for the patient to understand the possibility for repair—seem beyond the reach of any human help.

> A young Vietnam combat veteran had lost a leg because of a shrapnel injury. In the hospital for revision of his below-the-knee amputation, he became increasingly despondent. The psychiatric consultant was called to evaluate his deteriorating psychological status. It was a bad war, a foolish war, the patient ruminated, a war that shouldn't have been fought. What possible sense did it make, and for what possible reason had the leg been lost? The consultant conceded the futility of the war and after a period of silence asked the patient what came to mind. "My son, my 3-year-old," the patient replied. "He's big into guns now. Bang! bang! bang! All the time. At times," he confided, "I hate him...hate his stupid playing." "Perhaps he only wants to be brave like you," the consultant offered. The veteran grimaced and said nothing. "Perhaps he sees you as a hero and wants to be a hero too."
> The patient seemed to reject his idea but said he'd like to have the consultant come again. Through the many hours they sat together, the idea of the war came up again and again, often associated in the veteran's mind with his son. Eventually the consultant began to see that the son represented to the father a part of himself, albeit a stupid, immature, aggressive part. "You love that kid, I can tell. But he reminds you of yourself, going blindly off to the war—and you hate it, you just hate it. Maybe that's what you can use your lost leg for—to understand him and teach him about that part of all of us that has such a romantic fascination for violence." The veteran said nothing, but the staff later reported that the patient seemed gradually to have lost some of his despair and seemed to have some new motivation, some purpose.

While depression, sadness, and apathy are affective states, with which the consultant has time and some leverage to work, there are emotions such as panic that require an emergency response not based on a leisurely examination and a stately approach to treatment.

> A 36-year-old single man was hospitalized for revision of a colostomy for ulcerative colitis. Consultation was sought because the patient became anxious, hostile, paranoid, and completely noncompliant with staff during the evening shift.
> The consultant found that the patient, a night watchman, was a self-described "loner" with no family or friends. He lived a simple, isolated existence most of his life in fantasy punctuated by occasional visits to pornographic films. The consultant believed that the patient had a stable schizoid or paranoid character structure that was threatened by

the forced intimacies of the hospital situation. The consultant gingerly asked him why he became upset in the evening. "It's that faggot nurse Eddie!" the patient exclaimed and proceeded to aim a deluge of paranoid vituperation at the male licensed practical nurse on the ward, growing increasingly hostile by the second and developing loose associations.

The consultant was fearful and immediately told the patient that the hospital was aware of the "situation" with Eddie and that the consultant would "take steps" to ensure that the patient would be safe from Eddie. "Masculine men like yourself are often put off by people like Eddie, but I think you'll relax about it if you stop a second to realize that you're strong enough to protect yourself from anybody, including Eddie, and, besides, you don't go to sleep until 11:00 PM anyway, and by that time, Eddie's long gone." Immediately the patient calmed down. He showed no further panic during his hospitalization after the consultant recommended that only female nurses be assigned to work with the patient.

In each of the preceding examples, the consultant moved to restore appropriateness of affect and to give the patient control of its intensity and expression. Such interventions are based on an assessment of whether the affect is autonomous, that is, governed by metabolic or biochemical substrates, or whether it is amenable to psychodynamic formulation and explanation. When explanation is possible, its form depends on the personality and capacity of the patient to understand.

Therapy for Disturbances of Behavior

Disturbances of behavior arise from some sort of disordered information-processing—cognition—or from some inappropriate, uncontrollable, or autonomous affect. *Therapy with a stressed patient having a disturbance of behavior consists mainly of understanding the behavior as it relates to the affects associated with it and cognition—the patient's picture of the self with an illness.* As shown by the examples already given, disruptive behavior results from affects of anger or depression based on cognitions that embody hopelessness or frustration of goals for successful adaptation. Noncompliance and therapeutic negativism are variations of these behaviors. Withdrawal and flight are maladaptive responses to the hospital environment mediated by incorrect cognitions and governed by fearful affects. Behaviors of hopelessness and their accompanying affects are related to incomplete perceptions of options for better adaptation.

Inappropriate sexual behavior by the medical or surgical patient usually represents an attempt to repair some real or imagined loss of masculine or feminine appeal rather than truly erotic aims. When the behavior is viewed in its proper perspective and "unlinked" by the consultant from guilt-inducing cognitions in the staff,[9] patients who display inappropriate sexual behavior respond dramatically to limits on inappropriate behavior coupled with reassurance that they are still attractive men or women.

> A middle-aged married male shop owner was hospitalized for treatment of a myocardial infarction. During his convalescence consultation was sought because the patient constantly fondled or pinched the female nurses who were caring for him. When examined the patient appeared quite anxious and concerned about his cardiac condition and asked many questions about how much it would impair his ability to "exercise." The consultant responded to these concerns and gradually brought up the subject of sexual functioning as an example of exercise. The patient was told how soon he could return to full sexual activity. "A lot of people are afraid that when they have a heart attack their sex life is over, but that's simply not true." After this interview the patient's anxiety was considerably lower and his inappropriate sexual overtures to the nurses ceased.

Such behavior is a good example of how disordered cognition ("I am sexually defective because of my heart attack") leads to intense and ungovernable affects (here, anxiety and despair), which, in turn, lead to a maladaptive attempt to repair the damage through undoing and acting out.

Far more difficult are those consultations involving pathologic dependency and its manifestations. Pathologic dependency in the hospitalized medical or surgical patient presents as (1) intense, implacable, clinging behavior and constant requests for reassurance and attention, (2) constant requests for anxiolytic or pain medication, (3) manipulative and contradictory demands for emotional supplies, and (4) chaotic, destructive, hostile-dependent or passive-aggressive behavior that makes the staff furious or frustrated and that makes every encounter with the patient a ghastly chore. While mild or moderate forms of clinging and demanding behavior are often seen in emotionally healthy individuals who have regressed to an infantile dependence under the multiple stresses of hospitalization and illness, pathologic dependency in its full-blown form typically occurs in persons with long-standing character pathology. Such persons usually feel empty and worthless even without a physical illness and have an intense desire for closeness but a simultaneous fear of intimacy. This pervasive fear of what they most long for leads them to thrash about emotionally, simultaneously demanding and rejecting help and then destroying whatever help is given. A conviction of interior emptiness and worthlessness, along with hurricanes of affect—rage, despair, terror, hate—are important in the genesis of pathologically dependent behaviors. Also important is the fact that while self-defeating and contradictory demands are obvious to the caregivers, such patients typically lack the ability to step aside and observe the nature and consequences of their own behavior. For this reason and because such individuals do not make good alliances with caregivers, interpretation of the self-defeating nature of the character pathology does not work; interpretations such as, "You are so hungry for care that you drive others away, fearful of your devouring needs," are either heard as sadistic or not heard at all. Such techniques simply do not succeed in the short-term treatment of such patients. They feel entitled to all they demand; but this feeling of entitlement is a fragile, primitive thing at best. Any interpretation that challenges the entitlement makes such a patient prey to intense despair and rage.

Psychotherapy with patients displaying pathologically dependent behaviors on the medical or surgical ward requires (1) clear communication among the staff and with the patient, (2) not challenging entitlement and needed defenses, (3) constant personnel and support but without too close a stance that threatens the patient's need for privacy and distance, (4) liberal use of major tranquilizers when indicated to help calm the hurricanes of affect, and (5) most importantly, firm, consistent, repeated limit setting on demanding and self-destructive behaviors. This limit setting reassures such patients that they cannot destroy the caregiving system, however much they may wish or fear it.

The behavior of such patients under stress stirs up sadistic feelings in caregivers, who, in turn, may flinch from necessary firm limits because such drastic control may somehow seem sadistic.

> An 18-year-old man, self-described as a "speed freak," terrorized the orthopedic floor where he was in traction following multiple long bone fractures received in a motorcycle accident. He demanded excessive doses of narcotics, ripped out intravenous lines, threatened extortion and litigation if he were not given his way, threw food, shouted, and was menacing toward the staff. The consultant recommended a treatment plan based on clear communication; constant personnel; firm, consistent, noninterpretive limits; and 25 to 50 mg of chlorpromazine given IM or orally every two to eight hours as needed. With the consultant present, the orthopedist informed the patient that his narcotics would be tapered very gradually but that any threatening or acting-out behavior would immediately result in the patient being restrained even more than he already was. Ten minutes later, the patient broke a drinking glass and inflicted superficial lacerations on his wrist. He was placed in four-point restraints and given chlorpromazine until heavily sedated.
>
> Throughout his course, this regimen was followed. Any acting-out

behavior immediately resulted in restraint and sedation. While this regimen did little to control verbal assaults and demanding behavior, it drastically reduced his physical destructiveness.

This is a behavioral response to stress occurring in a man with an obviously abnormal personality.

STRESS RESPONSES, PERSONALITY, AND DEFENSES

With an understanding of cognition, affects, and behavior the consultant can proceed to the four major features of the psychiatric consultation:

1. Rapid evaluation of the most pressing psychiatric problems
2. Explicit psychodynamic formulation of predominant conflicts
3. Proposal of a practical program of management
4. Active participation by the psychiatrist

But psychodynamic formulation presupposes an understanding of the personality and defenses as they relate to stress:

A 37-year-old married mother of two school-aged children was also a successful attorney. She had coped well with the multiple demands of home and career until she underwent a radical mastectomy for carcinoma of the breast. After the surgery she seemed to do well for a time but then developed anxiety, severe depression, insomnia, weeping spells, and angry outbursts which responded only partly to sedatives. Her surgeon had carefully explained the procedure and had discussed with her its impact on her self-image and sexual functioning, but she felt little better and eventually requested a psychiatric consultation.

"It's like a traffic accident!" the patient exclaimed. "I can't stand to look—but I can't look away either." On initial examination, the consultant found nothing that the surgeon had not already noted and it was not until the following day that an explanation became apparent. The patient reported a dream. "I am in court and trying the case of someone accused of larceny. My client is clearly guilty and the judge is overruling me time after time. It's an all-male jury and they go out to deliberate before I can even make my summation." Asked for her associations to the dream she promptly told the consultant that she felt that she had not really deserved to go to law school, even though she had graduated near the top of her class. She felt, she said, that her classmates had secretly suspected her of being a lesbian because she had been so orderly and logical. She became silent. After a long pause the consultant suggested that perhaps it was really she who was on trial for larceny. Perhaps her crime had been to succeed in a man's world and perhaps the punishment was to be made into a man.

"It's true, you know," she replied, "I guess I always expected that eventually I'd have to pay for becoming a lawyer. Did I tell you? My father is a lawyer."

The next day the patient told the consultant that she had had her first night of sound sleep in the hospital. She felt "at peace for some reason" and a few days later went home to convalesce uneventfully from both her surgery and her stress reaction.

There have been numerous descriptions of the personality and its cognitive, affective, and behavioral phases of response to a crisis. Cannon,[10] Lindemann,[11] Anna Freud,[12] Menninger,[13] and Caplan,[14] among others, have worked on various aspects of what Horowitz synthesizes as typical phases of response to a stressful event[15] (see Figure 16-1). When confronted with a catastrophic event, the individual typically responds with outcry ("Oh God! Oh God! Oh God!"), denial ("It isn't true! You're joking! It's not true!"), or affective numbing and repetitive thoughts about the event. Not uncommonly the individual, like the patient with the mastectomy, will vacillate among these first three phases. As noted by Caplan[14] and Lindemann,[11] these initial reactions to catastrophe are reflexive and probably serve some adaptive

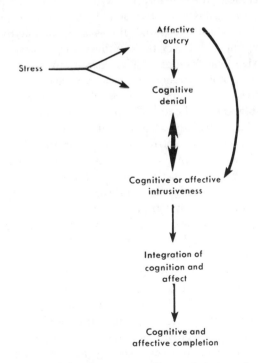

Figure 16-1. Phases of response after a stressful event (adapted with permission from Horowitz[15]).

function. Outcry is accompanied by an autonomic discharge like the flight-fight response described by Cannon,[10] and denial has a resemblance to dissociative mechanisms of ego defense.[12] Caplan traces the sequence of responses from the dazed impact or flight-fight response to affective flooding that, in turn, is followed by coping efforts.

The unwanted intrusion of thoughts and feelings about the stress event and the inability either to look or to look away probably represent an unstable equilibrium between the need to come to cognitive and affective completion in service of adaptation and the need to defend against affects that are painful. The need to process information about a crisis seems to be innate, and phenomena noted by Zeigarnik,[16] Festinger,[17] and Piaget[18] show that the human being remembers uncompleted tasks, experiences discomfort from doubt and dissonance, and generally moves in the direction of cognitive completion when possible in order to adapt to the environment. But the need to defend against painful feelings associated with a crisis is also adaptive. The consultant ought not to come to the consultation with a bias toward affective outpouring and a bias against cognitive denial. Hackett and coworkers[19-21] found that patients facing terminal illness who are able to defend well (major deniers) not only lower their anxiety and raise their hopes, but also survive significantly longer. The consultant should not confuse neurotic denial in nonemergency situations with "denial in service of the need to survive,"[22] nor apply concepts about long-term growth in the ability to master painful affects[23] to denial in the acute stress response.

The phase of cognitive and affective integration is best examined by referring to the model of the ego described by Hartmann[24] as that central, creative part of the personality that synthesizes, rationalizes, and makes do with whatever tools it has in order to bring to the individual the greatest possible peace and function during deviations from the "average expectable environment" that trauma violates. Integration is accomplished when the individual optimally balances mechanisms of defense[12] with the capacity for the tolerance of negative affects[23] and emerges with flexible yet realistic plans for dealing with trauma in the present and anticipating problems that may emerge in the future.[15]

Integration depends at least partially on the stressed individual's ability to shoulder what Lindemann aptly terms "grief work."[11] Grief work is the process of experiencing the painful affects associated with mourning in order to gain emancipation from bondage to the lost object. For Lindemann, the major obstacle to doing grief work is the individual's unwillingness to suffer the pain of mourning. He noted that the psychotherapist's task in such work is evocative (vivifying the trauma), hortatory (encouraging grief), and supportive (being with the grieving individual).

While Lindemann focused on the affective response to trauma, Horowitz[15] explored the cognitive aspects of integration. A series of theoretically ideal steps emerge that can be applied, for example, to the cancer patient who had a mastectomy:

First, she should perceive the event correctly ("A total mastectomy has taken my breast, leaving me mutilated.")

Next, she should translate this perception into meaningful ideas about the world. ("By allowing myself to be mutilated, I have probably been cured of cancer.")

Next, she should relate these meanings to her attitudes about the world and her place in it. ("It is better to be mutilated than to die.")

Next, she should plan responses to the event appropriate to this idea of her place in the world. ("With a prosthesis and new wardrobe I will hide my mutilation. When I can't, as with my husband, I will work out new techniques to minimize the impact of this mutilation on him and me.")

Then, she should revise her habitual attitudes so that her plans are not sabotaged. ("It is not necessarily true of my body and relationships, as I had previously thought, that anything less than perfect is grotesque.")

And, finally, she should not ward off the full implications of the event, lest denial of some important aspect of reality impair her ability to work through the steps of information processing. ("I can't kid myself. This looks awful—awful enough to cause me to give up or to pull away in shame, which I must not do.")

In real life, the patient said that she could neither look nor look away. She needed to look because the trauma contained information essential for coping with reality. She needed to look away because it hurt. She was in the unstable equilibrium represented by the two-headed arrow in Figure 16-1. Her paralysis was exacerbated by an unconscious, painful assumption or syllogism in addition to the terribly painful fact of the loss of her breast. The unconscious meaning of the loss was that it represented a punishment for something "bad" she had done—that is, she succeeded by "unfeminine" means. Her dream illustrated the unconscious idea that the "punishment" fits the "crime." Her associations to the dream revealed the basis of her guilt, an ambivalent identification with her father. By using the consultant's interpretation, she was able to unlink the loss of her breast from her neurotic syllogism and habitual information-processing about herself and subtract the unconscious painful affect of guilt from the total suffering she was experiencing. Thus, she could move the equilibrium forward into affective and cognitive integration.

It is when the patient is in this unstable equilibrium between intrusiveness and denial that the consultant is often called. Sometimes there is an unconscious conflict underlying the maladaptive paralysis; sometimes there is not. But in each consultation the psychiatrist must understand the patient's habitual ways of processing information and defending against negative affects.

Shapiro's[25] descriptions of neurotic styles of personality and the discussion by Bibring and Kahana[26] of personalities encountered in the general hospital provide details of the leading traits and defenses of various personality types, their typical reactions to the stress of illness, and strategies of therapy for each. These styles are summarized in Table 16-1.

The patient who had the mastectomy had a mixture of styles:

> I guess the main thing my father taught me is to do one thing at a time, to make lists of priorities...hierarchies, you know. And then to work through them in a logical way—playing advocate to first one and then another idea before coming up with a judgment or decision. On the other hand...on the other hand I guess I also owe a lot to my mother because I inherited her "woman's intuition" as it's stupidly called. Sometimes I just *know* things. Sometimes I just get the big picture and make a snap decision and it's right! Call it a hunch or whatever, but I still do it and it pays off.

She processes information in at least two ways—one, orderly and sequential—the other, intuitive, holistic, gestalt-oriented.

Horowitz[15] chooses three personality styles, their information processing and problem-solving habits, and their defenses to illustrate the interplay between stress and personality. The histrionic personality has as a perceptual mode a global, holistic intake of information without much attention to detail. Information processing is impressionistic and affect-oriented rather than sequential, with a limited translation of images into words. Such a style is vulnerable to stereotyping and conclusion jumping, and therefore problem solving is rapid but prone to error and sometimes marred by avoidance or wishful thinking. The obsessive personality has as a typical perceptual mode a preoccupation with detail at the expense of gestalten. Information processing is orderly but often neglects the importance of affects and fails to make meaningful connections between ideas and their emotional impact. Problem solving may be active but it is slowed by prolonged reasoning back and forth, so that affective and cognitive integration is tediously late in coming. The

Table 16-1. Personality Types in the General Hospital

"Name"/Leading Traits	Reaction to Illness	Suggested Management
"Histrionic"/ dramatic, vivid, likable, anxious, involved	As if illness were a punishment for or an attack on masculinity or femininity	Appreciation of attractiveness/courage; ventilation of fears; supportive but not detailed explanations
"Obsessive"/ orderly, dull, likable, anxious, involved	As if illness were a punishment for letting things get out of control	Detailed "scientific" explanations, intellectualizations, and making the patient a partner in therapeutic decisions
*"Narcissistic"/*self-involved, controlling, angry, independent, perfectionistic	As if illness were an attack on autonomy and perfection of the self; the leading fear (and wish) is of being taken care of	Supporting strength and integrity of the self by making patient equal, independent partner in own care
*"Oral"/*clinging, demanding, attention-seeking	As if illness posed the threat of abandonment	Warm support but firm limits on undue neediness and manipulativeness
*"Masochistic"/*long-suffering, depressed, help-rejecting	As if illness were a deserved, expected punishment for worthlessness	Appreciation of courage in suffering without undue reassurance or optimism; appeal to altruism
*"Schizoid"/*remote, unsociable, uninvolved	As if illness threatened a dangerous invasion of privacy	Muted interest in patient but respect for need for privacy and distance
*"Paranoid"/*wary, suspicious, aggrieved, querulous, blaming, hypersensitive	As if illness were an annihilating assault coming from everywhere outside the self	Honest, simple, full, repeated explanations; accusations neither disputed nor confirmed but explained as coming from illness rather than from someone trying to injure patient

Based on Bibring and Kahana,[26] and adapted from an unpublished summary by TF Dwyer.

narcissistic personality (resembling also depressive-masochistic, paranoid, and borderline personalities, some of which are included in Table 16-1) has as a perceptual mode a search from the environment for data that protect the self or blame others, as if the self were desperately fragile. Information processing may be either too impressionistic or too detailed, but its aim is to hide damaging implications from the individual. Thus problem-solving behavior is poor and sometimes self-destructive since it is based on too few accurate cues from the environment and the emotions.

Therapy with the histrionic patient involves controlling affects and slowing down information processing to include sequence and logic. Therapy with the obsessive personality involves eliciting overall views and blending in affects as tolerated. Therapy with the narcissistic patient involves shoring up primitive defenses, controlling affects, and lending reality testing and logic—all within a firm, noninterpretive supportive relationship. The patient who had the mastectomy used very little narcissistic information processing and her mixture of histrionic and obsessive styles actually helped each other once the neurotic assumption was interpreted away. Therapy with any patient involves helping the patient combine as many cognitive facts as are needed for adaptation with as much of their associated affects as the patient can stand—all without assaulting needed defenses.

To clarify the psychoanalytic concepts of ego defense mechanisms, Vaillant[27,28] proposes a theoretical hierarchy of defenses and ways of coping. Some defenses are associated with psychological health; some are less effective for adaptation than others. But *all* of them help the individual cope with painful affects. Table 16-2 presents this hierarchy.

Vaillant believes that narcissistic defenses are less effective and more costly than immature defenses, which are less adaptive, in turn, than neurotic defenses, and so on. In this schema defenses are not drawn up in a single line against a threat but rather form concentric walls about the vulnerable core person; the closer to the center, the more archaic the wall. Vaillant provides a pivotal clarification by subtracting from this hierarchy of defenses the mechanism of regression, which he chooses to see as reflecting shifts in levels of defenses toward the vulnerable center rather than a mechanism of defense per se. This crucial point implies that all defenses at all levels are to be respected. Depending on their capacity, individuals may be able to use only primitive defenses in the service of adaptation. Psychologically less healthy individuals such as paranoid and schizoid personalities typically use narcissistic defenses. Masochistic, oral, and narcissistic individuals (see Table 16-1) tend to use immature defenses. Histrionic, obsessive, and mixed personalities use neurotic and mature defenses. Stressors such as illness and surgery are associated with a regressive shift to lower levels of defenses. But environmental manipulation and therapeutic interpersonal intervention can facilitate shifts to higher levels (outer walls) of defenses—progression.

Table 16-2. Theoretical Hierarchy of Adaptive Ego Defenses

"Narcissistic" defenses are common in "healthy" individuals before age 5 years and in adult dreams and fantasy; such mechanisms alter reality for the user but to the beholder they appear "crazy"; they tend to be refractory to change by conventional psychotherapeutic interpretation but are altered by change in reality (eg, antipsychotic medication, removal of stressor); in therapy they can be given up temporarily by interpersonal support combined with direct confrontation with ignored reality.

1. *Delusional projection*—paranoid attribution of internal feelings as coming from outside "reality"
2. *Psychotic denial*—unshakably ignoring some aspect of external reality
3. *Distortion*—gross reshaping of external reality to suit inner needs

"Immature" defenses are common in "healthy" individuals between ages 3 and 16 years, in "character" and affective disorders, and in individuals in psychotherapy; such mechanisms mitigate the "dangers" of interpersonal intimacy for the user but to the beholder they appear socially undesirable and self-defeating; they may be altered by prolonged relationships with intuitive, mature individuals.

1. *Projection*—attribution of one's own undesirable, unaccepted, unacknowledged feelings to others
2. *Schizoid fantasy*—retreat into autistic daydreams for the purpose of conflict resolution and gratification
3. *Hypochondriasis*—transformation of reproach toward the self or others into somatic symptoms
4. *Passive aggression*—overt compliance but covertly hostile behavior designed to punsh others
5. *Acting out*—direct behavioral expression of unconscious conflict in order to avoid consciousness of the affect that accompanies the conflict

"Neurotic" defenses are common in "healthy" adults with neurotic disorders and in mastering acute adult distress; such mechanisms alter private feelings or instinctual expression (sexual or aggressive) for the user but to the beholder appear as quirks or "hang-ups;" often they can be dramatically changed by conventional brief psychotherapeutic clarification of unconscious wishes or fears.

1. *Intellectualization*—subtraction of affective implication from reality with simultaneous overattention to detail
2. *Repression*—forgetting some aspect of reality often accompanied by highly symbolic behavior that suggests that the repressed idea is not really forgotten
3. *Displacement*—redirection of conflicted feelings toward a relatively less-cared-for object than the person or situation arousing the feelings (eg, jokes, phobias, hysterical conversion reactions)
4. *Reaction formation*—affect or behavior opposite to an unconscious, unwanted sexual or aggressive wish
5. *Dissociation*—temporary but drastic modification of character or of the sense of personal identity to avoid emotional distress (eg, amnesia)

"Mature" defenses are common in "healthy" adults during optimal functioning; they are often regarded as so adaptive and conscious as to be not defenses but rather "coping mechanisms;" for the user these mechanisms integrate conscience, reality, interpersonal relationships, and private feelings; to the beholder they appear as convenient virtues; under increasing stress they may change to less mature mechanisms.

1. *Altruism*—vicarious but constructive and gratifying service to others
2. *Humor*—overt expression of feelings without discomfort or immobilization and without unpleasant effects on others; it releases tension and is gratifying both for the user and for the beholder
3. *Suppression*—conscious decision to postpone paying attention to a feeling or fact and, indeed, later attending to and integrating the conflict
4. *Anticipation*—realistic planning for and experiencing future discomfort
5. *Sublimation*—indirect or partial expression of sexual and aggressive needs without either adverse consequences or loss of pleasure

Regression and progression—not defenses but, rather, reflected by shifts in levels of defenses.

Adapted with permission from Vaillant.[27]

Both clinical and experimental evidence exists to support the concept of a hierarchy of defenses or responses to stress ranging from maladaptive to adaptive. The clinical work of Hackett and coworkers[19-21] concerning the responses of patients faced with life-threatening illness, such as myocardial infarction or cancer, parallels the experimental work of Funkenstein et al[29] in which normal subjects were stressed in a laboratory situation. These experimental subjects appeared to respond in three ways to unexpected situations that required the mastery of stress in task-performance:

1. They did not notice the stress and remained "un-anxious" from start to finish, carrying out tasks smoothly throughout.
2. They mastered the stressful situation with some anxiety or were dysfunctional at first but went on to master the anxiety and successfully carry out tasks.
3. They were anxious from the outset and deteriorated in performance as the experiment progressed.

Those rarer individuals who either did not notice the stress or who noticed it too much represented extremes, whereas those numerous individuals who noticed stress but eventually overcame it represented the mean. Thus, to notice stress and be bothered by it, but then eventually to master it, seems normal.

Hackett and coworkers[19-21] find a similar set of phenomena in individuals who suffer life-threatening illness: "major deniers" tend not to notice the illness, to brush off its implications, to pooh-pooh the necessary medical regimen for its care. The average patient tends to be anxious and compliant with a medical regimen, but to go on to adjust to the illness. The "ontological denier" may resemble the major denier in avoiding compliance with the medical regimen, but this type of patient is angry, difficult to deal with, and displays to the observer—if not to the self—evidence of severe and dysfunctional anxiety. Weisman and Hackett[21] note that "bullies, braggarts and bigots are specialists in ontological denial: they attempt to destroy another person's autonomy simply because they feel challenged by his dissenting version of reality."

The consultant is called frequently for major deniers and ontological deniers because they stand out from the average patient who gets along. The major denier coolly refuses to process threatening information; the ontological denier hotly attacks the staff members as if they and not the illness were the threat. But although the noncompliance with a regimen may be similar, the prognosis is not. Major deniers who can get to the hospital in time and who can be persuaded to follow enough of their regimen survive longer than normal persons. Thus, although it is abnormal not to notice the threat of an illness, it does have adaptive value in major deniers; they illustrate the paradox that it can be healthier to be abnormal.

Ontological deniers are another story altogether: they resemble the less adaptive personality types, paranoid and schizoid, described in Table 16-1, and they utilize narcissistic and immature defenses. Unlike major deniers who settle comfortably into cognitive denial (see Figure 16-1), the ontological deniers vacillate between denial and cognitive or affective intrusion (the two-headed arrow) and never seem able to arrive at a stage of cognitive and affective equilibrium.

The vignettes of the noncompliant night watchman in the homosexual panic and the "speed freak" who had the motorcycle accident provide examples of ontological denial. The man with leukemia who almost died without writing a will is a classic example of a major denier. The woman with the mastectomy falls into the large group of patients who at first experience dysfunctional anxiety but go on to master it—with or without the help of a psychiatrist. Under the stress of an illness and mutilation she had regressed from mature to neurotic defenses. By partially interpreting her sexual-aggressive confusion, the consultant helped her move from behavior that seemed to reflect oral and masochistic personality traits to her customary histrionic and obsessive traits. This the consultant knew how to do by using the traditional clinical tools, the history and mental status examination, and by formulating her conflict in terms of (1) the stage of stress response—stuck between intrusiveness and denial, (2) personality style—mixed histrionic and obsessive, and (3) defenses—habitually mature or neurotic but now regressed. This patient occupies a central place in our discussion because she represents both a norm and an extreme—the norm, in that she is highly adaptive—the extreme, in that the consultant is rarely called to see such a healthy patient. In comparison to that of the major deniers, her denial is the flexible sort based on the defense of repression. Her affects, unlike those of the ontological denier, are tolerated over time, are governable, and eventually submit to cognition.

CONCLUSION

The psychiatric consultant summoned to evaluate medical or surgical patients in the general hospital should be prepared to encounter a stress response in some phase of its evolution, manifesting problems in information processing (cognition), feelings (affects), or behavior (the product of cognition and affect). The consultant should be prepared to encounter patients with distinctive personality styles, encompassing the capacity—or lack of it—to tolerate and master affects by utilizing a hierarchy of defenses. These patients will in all likelihood be in some state of regression from their customary levels of defenses. But whatever the state of the patients' defenses, the consultant's most intelligent and most appropriate strategy is to recognize that such defenses as they are *now* are the best available for the moment and not to be assaulted. Rather, they are to be strengthened and worked with in order to return the patients to their previous level of functioning. Meanwhile, the patients' cognitions of self and illness are assessed in order to help patients integrate, so far as personality and defenses permit, both painful affects and facts necessary for optimal adaptation.

REFERENCES

1. Cassem NH, Hackett TP: Psychiatric consultations in a coronary care unit. *Ann Intern Med* 1971; 75:9–14.
2. Hackett TP, Weisman AD: Psychiatric management of operative syndromes. I. The therapeutic consultation and the effect of noninterpretive intervention. *Psychosom Med* 1960; 22:267–282.
3. Hackett TP, Weisman AD: Psychiatric management of operative syndromes. II. Psychodynamic factors in formulation and management. *Psychosom Med* 1960; 22:356–372.
4. Meyer E, Mendelson M: Psychiatric consultations with patients on medical and surgical wards: patterns and processes. *Psychiatry* 1961; 24:197–220.
5. Lipowski ZJ: Review of consultation psychiatry and psychosomatic medicine. I. General principles. *Psychosom Med* 1967; 29:153–171.
6. Lipowski ZJ: Review of consultation psychiatry and psychosomatic medicine. II. Clinical aspects. *Psychosom Med* 1967; 29:201–224.

7. Lipowski ZJ: Review of consultation psychiatry and psychosomatic medicine. III. Theoretical issues. *Psychosom Med* 1968; 30:395–422.
8. Lipowski ZJ: Consultation-liaison psychiatry: an overview. *Am J Psychiatry* 1974; 131:623–630.
9. Kucharski A, Groves JE: The so-called "inappropriate" psychiatric consultation request on a medical or surgical ward. *Int J Psychiatry Med* 1976–1977; 7:209–220.
10. Cannon WB: *The Wisdom of the Body.* New York, WW Norton & Co Inc, 1932.
11. Lindemann E: Symptomatology and management of acute grief. *Am J Psychiatry* 1944; 101:141–149.
12. Freud A: *The Ego and the Mechanisms of Defense.* New York, International Universities Press, 1946.
13. Menninger KA: *The Vital Balance.* New York, Viking Press Inc, 1963.
14. Caplan G: *Principles of Preventive Psychiatry.* New York, Basic Books, Inc, 1964.
15. Horowitz MJ: *Stress Response Syndromes.* New York, Jason Aronson, Inc, 1976.
16. Zeigarnik BW: Über das Behalten von erledigter und unerledigter Handlungen. *Psychol Forsch* 1927; 9:1–85.
17. Festinger L: *A Theory of Cognitive Dissonance.* New York, Row, Peterson, 1957.
18. Piaget J: *The Construction of Reality in the Child.* New York, Basic Books, Inc, 1954.
19. Hackett TP, Weisman AD: Denial as a factor in patients with heart disease and cancer. *Ann NY Acad Sci* 1969; 164:802–817.
20. Hackett TP, Cassem NH: Psychological reactions to the life-threatening illness, in Abram H (ed): *Psychological Aspects of Stress.* Springfield, Ill, Charles C Thomas Publisher, 1970.
21. Weisman AD, Hackett TP: Denial as a social act, in Levin S, Kahana R (eds): *Creativity, Reminiscing and Dying.* New York, International Universities Press, 1966.
22. Geleerd ER: Two kinds of denial: neurotic denial and denial in service of the need to survive, in Schur M (ed): *Drives, Affects, Behavior.* New York, International Universities Press, 1965, vol 2.
23. Zetzel ER: *The Capacity for Emotional Growth.* New York, International Universities Press, 1970.
24. Hartmann H: *Ego Psychology and the Problem of Adaptation.* New York, International Universities Press, 1958.
25. Shapiro D: *Neurotic Styles.* New York, Basic Books, Inc, 1965.
26. Bibring GL, Kahana RJ: *Lectures in Medical Psychology: An Introduction to the Care of Patients.* New York, International Universities Press, 1968.
27. Vaillant GE: Theoretical hierarchy of adaptive ego mechanisms. *Arch Gen Psychiatry* 1971; 24:107–118.
28. Vaillant GE: Natural history of male psychological health. *Arch Gen Psychiatry* 1976; 33:535–545.
29. Funkenstein DH, King SH, Drolette ME: *Mastery of Stress.* Cambridge, Harvard University Press, 1957.

17

The Dying Patient

NED H. CASSEM

Oncologists, cardiologists, and nephrologists, long accustomed to caring for the whole person, typify experienced physicians faced with the management of the dying patient. These individuals have seen every variety of emotional reaction, so that the request for psychiatric consultation usually comes for a patient with the most difficult problems. The commonest of these turn out to be major depression with hopelessness, withdrawal, and the wish to be dead (but rarely suicidal); delirium and organic brain syndromes with or without cerebral metastases or known metabolic (eg, hypercalcemia) or paraneoplastic disorders; personality disorders—splitting, hostility, treatment rejection, litigation threats, substance abuse, outrage at having the illness; treatment-resistant continuous pain syndromes; and despondencies—grief, giving up long before the illness seems terminal, having life plans shattered. Also found are denial, the inability to accept diagnosis or treatment, unrealistic hopes for miracles, or persistent questions as why there is no improvement; anxiety, often extreme, with near panic and unspecifiable fears about dying; ambivalence and guilt, such as the ambivalence of the daughter with vaginal cancer on learning that the diethylstilbestrol her mother took during pregnancy is implicated and the guilt felt by her mother; and unrelated bad news, for example, whether a dying person should be told of a relative's death when ability to tolerate another trauma is seriously questioned. The physician requesting the consultation may or may not be able to specify the disorder. An occasional request may read: "Very difficult situation for unfortunate 32-year-old father of two with widely metastatic adenocarcinoma of unknown origin; please evaluate. Any suggestions appreciated."

The family of the dying person may be included in or made the specific subject of the consultation. A family member may be the first to notice a difficulty (like a personality change) or may be having more difficulty coping with the illness than the patient. This can irritate caregivers, isolate the patient (visits are made so as to avoid the family), and seriously jeopardize treatment.

Nurses make routine observations about the patient, family, and visitors and their interactions. This information can provide an invaluable perspective on any patient or family problem.

Although some of the histrionic and prurient interests in "death and dying" of the 1970's have subsided, that element of the cult still lives which assigns major blame to physicians for absence of the guarantee that death will come to all with peace, grace, comfort, and cosmetic dignity. The quest of the scapegoater for an object is made easier by the contemporary stereotype of the physician as cold, uncaring, mechanical, and mercenary. The psychiatric consultant who believes that psychiatry is that specialty of medicine with a unique claim on humanitarian perspective, compassion, and ethical principles is headed for deserved trouble.

Referring physicians, on the other hand, may retain a certain distorted view of psychiatry as a discipline of good bedside manner and interpersonal relations. In such a case, consultation may represent a sense of guilt over failure to meet the responsibilities of the primary-care physician, a deficiency which the consultant will "see" and possibly rebuke after evaluating the patient. Sensitivity to these pressures on the referring physician will strengthen the relationship with the patient, a factor essential to the patient's continued well-being.

Confronted by this array of clinical and sociocultural pressures, the consultant can take consolation from knowing that the job is no different with the terminally ill than with any other patient: diagnosis and treatment. We neither work miracles nor have answers for all questions. No matter how tragic and devastating the fatally ill person's predicament, we are always willing to see him so that we may do what we do for other patients—diagnose their conditions and prescribe appropriate treatments. Using the cancer patient as a type of person with a terminal illness, Table 17-1 outlines an approach to diagnosis and treatment, listing four common problems encountered in these patients.

ANXIETY IN TERMINAL ILLNESS

Impending death can generate severe anxiety in the patients facing it, in their families and their friends, and in those who take care of them. When panic, phobia, generalized anxiety, and the other conditions listed in the differential diagnostic outline of chapter 9 have been sought by the consultant and not found, the four commonest fears associated with death are: (1) helplessness or loss of control, (2) being bad (guilt and punishment), (3) physical injury or symbolic injury (castration), and (4) abandonment.[2,3]

In the clinical examination, the patient is not likely to easily find what

Table 17-1. Problems Encountered in Consultation to the Cancer Patient

Depression
   Incidence: 20% with major depression
      Not greater than in other medical illness
      Not greater in mastectomy than in surgery for other tumors
      Not related to physical performance status
      Not related to nearness to death
   Suicide: small increase in risk over normal rate, possibly in men only
   Diagnosis: made as described, chapter 12
   Drugs implicated
      Procarbazine hydrochloride
      L-Asparaginase
      Methotrexate, high IV dose
      Steroids
      5-Azacytadine
      Cytarabine hydrochloride
      Vincristine sulfate, vinblastine sulfate
      Hormones
         Aminoglutethimide
         Tamoxifen citrate
         Testosterone (mainly irritability in breast cancer patients)

Delirium
   Second commonest consultation problem
   Often mislabeled depression
   Diagnosis: made as described, chapter 6
   Drugs implicated: essentially same as above
   Treatment: in accord with diagnosis of etiology (see chapter 18)

Weakness
   Differential diagnosis
      Illness itself
      Major depression (see chapter 12)
   Drugs implicated (see also above)
      Vincristine: neuropathy
      Steroids: myopathy
      Combined chemo- and radiation therapy
      Bed rest itself (see chapter 12)
   Treatment
      Specific to diagnosis: antidepressants; stopping a drug; if bed rest,
         physical therapy and/or physical exercise
      Psychotherapy: clarify weakness *not* due to progressing cancer

Treatment-Resistant Pain
   See chapter 4

Anticipatory Nausea
   Incidence: about 50% of chemotherapy patients with GI toxicity
      Typically occurs after fourth or fifth treatment, quickly escalates

Table 17-1. Problems Encountered in Consultation to the Cancer
Patient—continued

Best predictor of severity: severity of vomiting induced by prior
   treatments
Diagnosis: conditioned aversive response (of GI toxicity to stimuli
   such as those listed below)
Precipitating stimuli
   Thought/sight of hospital/clinic
   Thought of chemotherapy
   Smell of hospital/clinic setting, alcohol wipe
   Sight of red fluid (doxorubicin hydrochloride), syringe
Treatment
   Systematic desensitization
   Hypnosis, relaxation techniques
   Benzodiazepines: alprazolam and others for anticipatory anxiety

---

Reproduced with permission from Greenberg et al.[1]

it is about death which is so frightening, unless, of course, the anxiety is
mild. In the latter case, memories of someone who died of the same
illness or associations to the illness will produce specific material (it will
be painful, disfiguring, etc). Truly disruptive anxiety states are usually
related to the patient's developmental history: defective ability to trust
or unresolved dependency conflicts, for example, the fear of helplessness,
and loss of control. Conflicts over guilt and castration will be lifelong.
The worst anxiety encountered may be that associated with defective
maternal bonding, where abandonment appears to be the object of fear.
Characteristic would be the dying daughter, now overwhelmed by
anxiety she cannot pinpoint or understand, for whom separation from
mother had always been a major unresolved issue. Where the mother is
available and willing, therapy of both simultaneously can be helpful, but
since death's separation seems so irreversibly final, considerable discomfort may remain throughout the time left for treatment.

Clinical research provides additional information useful in the treatment of terminally ill persons. This will include what is known about
dying as a psychophysiologic process, the goals of treatment, management recommendations, breaking the bad news, truth-telling, the
function of religious faith and value systems, and the emotional
problems of physicians and nurses who care for the dying.

PSYCHOPHYSIOLOGIC PROCESS OF DYING

Dying is a process that keeps the body near the forefront of the mind.
Having contracted a disease that may eventually cut him down (like
heart disease) or devour him (like cancer), the patient interprets or even

anticipates bodily changes as ominous. When present, symptoms are likely to produce fear, but fear is often present long before their arrival. The body, once regarded as a friend, may seem more like a dormant adversary, programmed for betrayal. Dying persons, even before disintegration begins, fear many things. Loss of autonomy, disfigurement, being a burden, becoming physically repulsive, letting the family down, facing the unknown, and many other concerns are commonly expressed. When all fears were compared for frequency in one sample of cancer patients,[4] the three that occurred most often were abandonment by others, pain, and shortness of breath. These fears were expressed before the patients were symptomatic. Patients thought that as their illness progressed family and hospital staff would gradually avoid them, their condition would become increasingly more painful, or the illness would encroach on their breathing capacity and suffocate them.

Because physicians and families also worry about what will happen to the dying person, it is helpful to know which difficulties are, in fact, the most distressing when the patient is terminally ill. Saunders[4] documented the exact incidence of practical problems in terminal cancer at St Joseph's Hospital in London. She found that the three most common complaints were (1) nausea and vomiting, (2) shortness of breath, and (3) dysphagia. Largely because of her efforts, avoidance of dying patients was not a problem at St Joseph's Hospital, but one would expect to find it in many hospitals or nursing homes with chronically ill patients. It was striking that pain did not appear high on the problem list. Nausea and dyspnea are miserable psychophysiologic states. Relief of these and other troublesome symptoms helps restore peace of mind.

In a work which evoked worldwide interest in dying persons, Kubler-Ross[5] presented a framework of five stages according to which dying persons reacted to the threat of death: (1) shock and denial, (2) anger, (3) bargaining, (4) depression, and (5) acceptance. Fear and anxiety are not represented. The concept of stages of adaptation is by no means new and is not restricted to dying. As a dynamic process, dying is a special case of loss and the stages represent a dynamic model of emotional adaptation to any physical or emotional loss. A common misdirection in caring for dying patients is the attempt to help an individual through the stages one after the other. It is more accurate and therapeutically more practical to regard the stages as normal reactions to any loss. They may be present simultaneously, disappear and reappear, or occur in any order.

Resort to Quackery

Even well-educated persons with potentially fatal illnesses will seek out unorthodox or even potentially harmful treatments in hope they will cure or alleviate their disease. Cassileth et al[6] interviewed 304 cancer center inpatients and 356 patients under the care of unorthodox practitioners. Although they found only 8% of patients had had no conventional treatment, 54% had combined unorthodox with conventional treatment, and 40% had abandoned conventional care entirely after beginning unorthodox treatment. Moreover, 60% of the unorthodox practitioners were physicians. Patients that resorted to unorthodox therapies, either exclusively or in part, were significantly more likely to be white and better educated than patients who used conventional therapy only. The nonconventional therapies included, in descending order of frequency, metabolic therapy, diet therapies, megavitamins, mental imagery for antitumor effect, spiritual or faith healing, and "immune" therapy. These data were gathered after the laetrile hoax was put to rest, although laetrile had been shown to cause agranulocytosis, congenital malformations, and death from cyanide poisoning before the US Supreme Court finally undid lower court mischief and, in Curran's words "stop[ped] the nonsense."[7] Useful, informative summaries[8,9] are sober testimony to how far desperate persons will go for cure and how lenient society may become out of compassion for them, even to the point of endangering them further.

Of the unconventional therapies mentioned in the study of Cassileth et al,[6] two have been publically censured by the American Cancer Society (ACS) for their misleading and unproven claims: the metabolic therapy of Harold Manner featuring pretreatment hair or blood analysis, "detoxification" with a daily coffee enema, digestive and "antineoplastic" enzymes, vitamins, counseling, and an announced "success rate of 68 per cent in the treatment of cancer,"[10] and mental imagery, most notably that proposed by O. Carl Simonton.[11] "Basically a self-help program," Simonton's center uses relaxation and mental imagery, emphasizing the role of the mind and of stress in the development of cancer.[12] The main objection of the ACS is that there is no evidence to support this supposition, which could be interpreted by patients as blaming them for having the disease and for being unable to cure it themselves.

Patients resort to unproven treatment methods for many reasons. Holland noted that an estimated $2 billion are spent annually on worthless tests and treatments.[13] Fear of and refusal to accept death, struggling for a way to "do something" positive, family and social pressures "to leave no stone unturned," the simplicity and harmlessness of many of the treatments, and the basic appeal of "natural" methods are the chief reasons patients seek unorthodox therapies. The methodologies also capitalize on individuals' narcissism, that foundation stone of so many of the "holistic" health movements. The basic attitude stresses the ignorance of orthodox physicians (basically antiauthoritarianism) and the expertise of minimally trained therapists and their patients, ever ready to capitalize on any outrage against organized medicine. For many patients, vitamins, laughter, relaxation, and Tibetan gong therapy are less threatening than chemotherapy with its many distressing side effects. An honest disapprobation by the physician, an article to read, or referral to the American Cancer Society may help patients evaluate an unorthodox treatment. The responsibility of the physician is to prescribe what is considered reasonable and helpful and to encourage compliance, but noncomplying patients are the rule, not the exception. Even when noncompliance undermines a course of treatment, the patient can still be offered whatever remains available, to the extent that he can accept it.

CARE AND MANAGEMENT OF THE DYING

In addition to the specifics of psychiatric diagnosis and treatment mentioned above, several practical considerations for management are added to support the goals of treatment.

Goals of Treatment

Deutsch[3] observed from his clinical sample of dying patients that the decline in vital processes is accompanied by a parallel decline in the intensity of instinctual aggressive and erotic drives. With the reduction of these drives, fear of dying is also reduced. The illness could be viewed by the patient as a hostile attack by an outside enemy such as God or fate, or as a punishment for being bad. Since patients could complicate their conditions by reacting with increasing hostility toward outside objects or with self-punitive actions to offset guilt, Deutsch's therapeutic objective is a "settlement of differences." The ideal stage is reached when all guilt and aggression are dissipated.

For Eissler,[14] therapeutic success depends on the psychiatrist's ability to share the patient's basic beliefs in immortality and indestructibility. The main forces in the psychiatrist's supportive relationship with the patient are his ability to share the patients' defenses and to develop a strong admiration for their patients' inner strength, beauty, intelligence, courage, and honesty. Kubler-Ross[5] described the unfinished business of the dying—reconciliations, resolution of conflicts, and pursuit of specific remaining hopes. Saunders[15] has stated that the aim is to keep patients feeling like themselves as long as possible. For her, dying is also a "coming together time" when patient, family, and staff help one another share the burden of saying appropriate goodbyes. The LeShans[16,17] have deliberately chosen not to focus on dying (the minor problem), but to search aggressively with patients for what they wish to accomplish in living (the major problem). Weisman and Hackett[18] have coined the term "appropriate death." To achieve this patients should (1) be relatively pain-free, (2) operate on as effective a level as possible within the limits of their disability, (3) recognize and resolve residual conflicts, (4) satisfy those remaining wishes that are consistent with their conditions and ego ideals, and (5) be able to yield control to others in whom they have confidence.

Perhaps more important than any other principle is that the treatment be individualized. This can be accomplished only by getting to know the patient, responding to his needs and interests, proceeding at his pace, and allowing him to shape the manner in which those in attendance behave. There is no one "best" way to die.

Treatment Recommendations

Much of the psychosocial information about dying persons comes from them and their families. In the area of experiential reality the patients are the teachers, while those who care for them always have something further to learn. Over the years, observations made by patients on various aspects of their management have helped in the formulation of nine essential features in the care and management of the dying patient.[19]

Competence. In an era where some discussions of the dying patient seem to suggest that love covers a multitude of sins, it would be unfortunate to encourage the misconception that competence in physicians and nurses is of secondary importance to dying patients. Competence is reassuring, and when one's life or comfort depends on it, personality considerations become secondary. Being good at what one does brings emotional as well as scientific benefits to the patient. For example, no matter how charming physicians, nurses, or technicians may be, the person who is most skillful at venipuncture brings the greatest relief to a patient who is anxious about having his blood withdrawn.

Concern. Of all attributes in physicians and nurses none is more highly valued by terminal patients than compassion. Although they may never convey it precisely by words, some physicians and nurses are able to tell the patient that they are genuinely touched by his or her predicament. A striking example came from a mother's description of her dying son's pediatrician: "You know, that doctor loves Michael."

Compassion cannot be feigned. Although universally praised as a quality for a health professional, compassion exacts a cost usually overlooked in professional training. This price of compassion is conveyed by the two Latin roots, *com-*, "with," and *passio* ("suffering"), from *pati*, "to suffer," which together mean "to suffer *with*" another person. One must be touched by the tragedy of the patient in a literal way, a process that occurs through experiential identification with the dying person. The process of empathy, when evoked by a person facing death or tragic disability, ordinarily produces uncomfortable, burdensome feelings to which internal resistance can arise defensively. Who can bear the thought of dying at age 20? It is not perverse but natural for us to discourage discussion of such a topic by the individual facing it. Also, students are sometimes advised to guard against involvement with a patient. When a patient becomes upset, hasty exits or avoidance are likely.

Few things infuriate patients more than contrived involvement. For this reason, the patient may excuse even an inability to answer direct questions when the inability stems from genuine discomfort on the physician's part. One woman preferred to ask her physician as few questions as possible, even though she wanted more information about how much longer she could expect to survive with stage IV Hodgkin's disease. "Whenever I try to ask him about this, he looks very pained and becomes very hesitant. I don't want to rub it in. After all, he really likes me."

Involvement—real involvement—is not only unavoidable, but necessary in the therapeutic encounter. Patients recognize it instantly. As a hematologist percussed the right side of his 29-year-old patient's chest, his discovery of pleural effusion brought the realization that a remission had abruptly ended. "Oh shit!" he muttered. Then, realizing what he had said, he added hastily, "Oh, excuse me, Bill." "That's all right," the young man replied. "It's nice to know that you care."

Comfort. With the terminally ill patient, comfort has a technology all its own. "Comfort measures" never indicate that less attention should be paid to the patient's needs. In fact, ensuring the comfort of a terminally ill person requires meticulous devotion to myriad details, great practical knowledge, and continual exercise of creative ingenuity.

Freedom from pain is basic to every care plan, and should be achievable in 90% of cases. Pain control for the cancer patient is described in detail in chapter 4. Table 17-2 presents a list of the practical problems commonly found in the care of the terminally ill. This subject is covered in detail by Billings.[20] If one claims to be committed to keeping the

Table 17-2. Symptom Control in Terminal Illness

Pain control
Nausea and vomiting
Hiccoughs
Anorexia and nutritional care
Constipation, diarrhea, GI problems
   Incontinence
   Obstruction
   Hepatic encephalopathy
Mouth problems, dysphagia
Dyspnea, cough, respiratory symptoms
   "Death rattle"
Urinary tract symptoms
   Incontinence
   Indwelling catheters
   Renal failure, obstruction
Skin problems
   Pruritus
   Pressure sores
   Fungating tumors, ulcerating wounds
     Odor
     Bleeding
     Drainage, fistulas
Fluid accumulation
   Edema
   Ascites
   Pleural/pericardial effusions
Dehydration
Neuropsychiatric symptoms, brain tumors
Weakness, fatigue
   Spinal cord compression
   Spasticity
Infections, fevers, sweats
Anemia and transfusions
Emergencies
   Superior vena cava syndrome
   Pathologic fractures

Adapted with permission from Billings.[20]

terminally ill person comfortable until death comes, one must be prepared, at the very least, to manage the difficulties listed in Table 17-2.

Communication. Talking with the dying is a paradoxical skill. The wish to find the right thing to say is a well-meaning but misguided hope among persons who work with terminally ill patients. Practically every empirical study has emphasized the ability to listen over the ability to say something. Saunders summarizes it best when she says, "The real question is not, 'What do you tell your patients?' but rather, 'What do you let your patients tell you?'"[15] Most people have a strong inner resistance to letting dying patients say what is on their minds. If a patient presumed to be 3 months from death says, "My plan was to buy a new car in 6 months, but I guess I won't have to worry about that now," a poor listener would say nothing or, "Right. Don't worry about it." A better listener might say, "Why do you say that?" or, "What do you mean?"

Communication is, however, more than listening. Getting to know the patient as a person is essential. Learning about significant areas of the patient's life—such as family, work, or school—and chatting about common interests are the most natural if not the only way the patient has of coming to feel known. After a 79-year-old man of keen intellect and wit had been interviewed before a group of hospital staff members, one of the staff said, "Before the interview tonight I just thought of him on the ward as another old man in pain." It is not necessary to talk about esoteric things to a dying person. Like anybody else these individuals get self-respect from a sense that others value them for what they have done and for their personal qualities. Allowing dying persons to tell their own stories helps to build a balanced relationship. The effort spent getting to know them does them more psychological good than trying to guess how they will cope with death.

The physician can help dissolve communication barriers for staff members by showing them the uniqueness of each patient. Comments such as "She has 34 grandchildren," or "This woman was an Olympic sprinter" (both were actual patients), convey information that helps the staff find something to talk about with the patients. Awkwardness subsides when a patient seems like a real person and not merely "a breast cancer." This rescue from anonymity is essential to prevent a sense of isolation.

Communication is more than verbal. A pat on the arm, a wave, a wink, or a grin communicate important reassurances, as do careful back rubs and physical examinations.

Patients occasionally complain about professionals and visitors who regard them as "the dying patient," not as a unique individual. A wise precaution is to take conversational cues from the patient whenever possible.

> A woman in her early fifties with breast cancer that had metastasized to bone, brain, lungs, and liver entered the hospital for a course of chemotherapy. During her entire 6-week stay she was irascible,

argumentative, and even abusive to the staff members. To their surprise, she got a good response with a substantial remission and left the hospital. She later told her oncologist, apologizing for her behavior: "I know that I was impossible. But every single nurse who came into my room wanted to talk to me about death. I came there to get help, not to die, and it drove me up a wall."

Had staff members tuned in to this patient as an individual with a courageous attitude toward her illness instead of treating her as "a dying patient," their efforts to comfort would not have backfired.

Children. All investigators have learned that the visits of children are as likely to bring consolation and relief to the terminally ill patient as any other intervention. A useful rule of thumb in determining whether a particular child should visit a dying patient is to ask the child whether he or she wants to visit. No better criterion has been found.

Family cohesion and integration. A burden shared is a burden made lighter. Family members must be helped to support one another, although this requires that the physician get to know each member of the family as well as the patient. Conversely, when patients are permitted to give support to their families, the feeling of being a burden is mitigated.

The often difficult work of bringing the family together for support, reconciliation, or improved relations can prevent disruption when death of the patient begins the work of bereavement. The opportunity to be present at death should be offered to family members, as well as the alternative of being informed about it while waiting for the news at home. Flexibility is the rule, and the wishes of the family and patient are paramount. After the patient has died, family members who wish to should be offered a chance to see the body before it is taken to the morgue. Parkes[21] has documented the critical importance to grief work of seeing the body of the dead person.

Lest one get the idea that simple common sense gives predictive power, recent intensive studies of families of chronically ill dialysis patients gave evidence that patients of families that appeared to have the stronger bonds died significantly sooner than those in apparently "weaker" families.[22]

Cheerfulness. Dying persons have no more relish for sour and somber faces than anybody else. The possessor of a gentle and appropriate sense of humor can bring relief to all parties involved. "What do they think this is?" said one patient of his visitors. "They file past here with flowers and long faces like they were coming to my wake." Patients with a good sense of humor do not enjoy dead audiences either. Their wit softens many a difficult incident. After an embarrassing loss of sphincter control, one elderly man with a tremor said, "This is enough to give anybody Parkinson's disease!"

Wit is not an end in itself. As in all forms of conversation, the listener should take his cue from the patient. Forced or inappropriate mirth with a sick person can increase feelings of distance and isolation.

Consistency and perseverance. Progressive isolation is a realistic fear of the dying patient. A physician or nurse who regularly visits the sickroom provides tangible proof of continued support and concern. Saunders has emphasized that the quality of time is far more important than the quantity.[15] A brief visit is far better than no visit at all and the patient may not be able to tolerate a prolonged visit in any case. Patients are quick to identify those who show interest at first but gradually disappear from the scene. Staying power requires hearing complaints.

> Praising one of her nurses, a 69-year-old woman with advanced cancer said, "She takes all my guff, and I give her plenty. Most people just pass my room, but if she has even a couple of minutes she'll stop and actually listen to what I have to say. Some days I couldn't get through without her."

Equanimity. The capacity to be comfortable with a dying person is another valued quality.

> A 68-year-old woman with two primary pulmonary malignancies fought, as did her physicians, a steadily losing battle against shortness of breath. She often complained that death would be preferable. Nevertheless, she also worried that her criticisms and unanswerable questions placed an unfair burden on her physicians. After making this observation to one of her physicians, she suddenly fixed her piercing blue eyes on him and said, "You know, you're just like an old shoe—comfortable."

Equally prized by the physician, equanimity not only greatly contributes to but is produced by enriching encounters with the terminally ill.

Breaking the Bad News

Because so many reactions to the news of diagnosis are possible, it is helpful to have some plan of action in mind ahead of time that will permit the greatest variation and freedom of response. When the diagnosis is made and it is time to inform the patient, it is best to begin by sitting down with the patient in a private place. Standing while conveying bad news is regarded by patients as unkind and expressive of wanting to leave as quickly as possible. The patient should be informed that when all the tests are completed, the physician will sit down with him again. Spouse and family can be included in the discussion of the findings and treatment. As that day approaches, the patient should be warned again. This permits those patients who wish no or minimal information to say so.

If the findings are unpleasant, for example, a biopsy positive for malignancy, how can it best be conveyed? A good opening statement is one that is (1) rehearsed so that it can be delivered calmly, (2) brief (three sentences or less), (3) designed to encourage further dialogue, and (4) reassuring of continued attention and care. A typical delivery might go as follows: "The tests confirmed that your tumor is malignant (the bad news). I have therefore asked the surgeon (radiotherapist, oncologist) to come by to speak with you, examine you, and make his recommendations for treatment (we will do something about it). As things proceed, I will be by to discuss them with you and how we should proceed (I will stand by you)." Silence and quiet observation for a few moments will yield valuable information about the patient, his emotional reactions, how he deals with it from the start. While observing one can decide on how best to continue with the discussion, but sitting with the patient for a period of time is an essential part of this initial encounter with a grim reality that both patient and physician will continue to confront together, possibly for a very long time.

Telling the Truth

Without honesty, human relationships are destined for shipwreck. If truthfulness and trust are so obviously interdependent, how can there be so much conspiracy to avoid truth with the dying? The paradoxical fact is that for terminally ill patients the need for both honesty and the avoidance of the truth can be intense. Sir William Osler is reputed to have said, "A patient has no more right to all the facts in my head than he does to all the medications in my bag." A routine blood smear has just revealed that a 25-year-old man has acute myelogenous leukemia. If he were married and the father of two small children, should he be told the diagnosis? Is the answer obvious? What if he had had two prior psychotic breaks with less serious illnesses? What if his wife says he once said he never wanted to know if he had a malignancy?

Most empirical studies in which patients were asked whether or not they wanted to be told the truth about malignancy overwhelmingly indicated desire for the truth. When 740 patients in a cancer detection clinic were asked prior to diagnosis if they wanted to be told their diagnosis, 99% said they did.[23] Another group in this same clinic was asked after the diagnosis was established and 89% of them replied affirmatively, as did 82% of another group who had been examined and found to be free of malignancy. Gilbertsen and Wangensteen[24] asked the same questions of 298 survivors of surgery for gastric, colonic, and rectal cancers and found 82% wanted to be told the truth. The same investigators questioned 92 patients who had advanced cancer and were judged by their physicians to be preterminal and found that 73 (79%) of the patients thought they should be informed of their diagnosis.

How many patients do not want to know the truth or regard it as harmful? The effects of blunt truth telling have been studied empirically in both England and the United States. Aitken-Swan and Easson[25] were told by 7% of 231 patients who were explicitly informed of their diagnosis that the frankness of the consultant was resented. Gilbertsen and Wangensteen[24] observed that 4% of a sample of surgical patients became emotionally upset at the time they were told and appeared to remain so throughout the course of their illness. Gerlé et al[26] studied 101 patients that were divided into two groups. Members of one group were told, along with their families, the frank truth of their diagnoses. In the other group, an effort was made to maintain a conspiracy of silence with family and physician excluding the patient from discussion of the diagnosis. At first, greater emotional upset appeared in the group where patient and family were informed together, but the investigators observed in follow-up that the emotional difficulties of the families of those patients shielded from the truth far outweighed those of the patients and families that were told the diagnosis simultaneously. In general, empirical studies support the idea that truth is desired by terminally ill patients and does not harm those to whom it is given. Honesty sustains the relationship with a dying person rather than retarding it.

> Dr. Hackett saw in consultation a 57-year-old housewife with metastatic breast cancer, now far advanced. She reported a persistent headache, which she attributed to nervous tension and asked why she should be nervous. Turning the question back to her, he was told, "I am nervous because I have lost 60 pounds in a year. The priest comes to see me twice a week, which he never did before, and my mother-in-law is nicer to me even though I am meaner to her. Wouldn't this make you nervous?"...[He] said to her, "You mean you think you're dying." "That's right, I do," she replied. He paused and said quietly, "You are." She smiled and said, "Well, I've finally broken the sound barrier; someone's finally told me the truth."[27]

Not all patients can be dealt with so directly. A nuclear physicist greeted his surgeon on the day following exploratory laparotomy with the words, "Lie to me, Steve." Individual variations in willingness to hear the initial diagnosis are extreme, and diagnosis is entirely different from prognosis. Many patients have said they were grateful to their physician for telling them they had a malignancy. Very few, however, reacted positively to being told they are dying. In my experience, "Do I have cancer?" is a common question, while "Am I dying?" is a rare one. The question about dying is more commonly heard from patients who are dying rapidly, such as those in cardiogenic shock.

Physicians today generally prefer to tell cancer patients their diagnoses. Okin's study of 1961 documented that 90% of responding physicians preferred not to tell patients the diagnosis.[28] When Novack et al repeated this questionnaire in 1979, 97% of responding physicians indicated a preference for telling the cancer patient the diagnosis.[29] One hundred percent of the physicians said that patients had a right to know.

Honest communication of the diagnosis (or of any truth) by no means precludes later avoidance or even denial of the truth. In two studies patients who had been explicitly told their diagnosis (using the words "cancer" or "malignancy") were asked 3 weeks later what they had been told. Nineteen percent of one sample[25] and 20% of the other[24] denied that their condition was cancerous or malignant. Likewise, Croog et al[30] interviewed 345 men 3 weeks after myocardial infarction and were told by 20% of them that they had not had a heart attack. All had been explicitly told their diagnosis. For a person to function effectively truth's piercing voice must occasionally be muted or even excluded from awareness. On four consecutive days I spoke with a man who had a widely spread bone cancer. On the first day he said he didn't know what he had and didn't like to ask questions. The second day he said he was "riddled with cancer." On the third day he didn't really know what ailed him. The fourth day he said that even though nobody likes to die that was now his lot.

Truth-telling is no panacea. Communicating a diagnosis honestly, though difficult, is easier than the labors that lie ahead. Telling the truth is merely a way to begin; but since it is an open and honest way, it provides a firm basis on which to build a relationship of trust.

Role of Religious Faith and Value Systems

Investigation of the relationship between religious faith and attitudes toward death has been hampered by differences in methodology. Lester[31] and Feifel[32] have reviewed much of the conflicting literature on the relationship between religious faith and fear of death. Other research has tried to clarify the way belief systems function within the individual.

Allport[33] contrasted an extrinsic religious orientation in which religion is mainly a means to social status, security, or relief from guilt, with an intrinsic religious orientation, in which the values appear to be internalized and subscribed to as ends in themselves. Feagin[34] provided a useful 21 item questionnaire for distinguishing the two types of believers. Experimental work[35] and clinical experience indicate that an extrinsic value system, without internalization, seems to offer no assistance in coping with a fatal illness. A religious commitment that is intrinsic, on the other hand, appears to offer considerable stability and strength to those who possess it.

Many patients are grateful for the chance to express their own thoughts about their faith. For assessing religious faith a useful question that can be asked during discussion of the illness is, "Where do you think God stands in all this?" This question leads to others. "Do you see your illness as imposed on you by God? Why? What sort of a being do you picture God to be?" Answers can be scrutinized for feelings of guilt and for the quality of relationship the individual describes as having with God. Belief in an afterlife is another useful area for questioning and helps to assess tolerance of doubt, an important quality of mature belief. In general, those persons who possess a sense of the personal presence of God, of being cared for or watched over, are more likely to manifest tranquility in their struggle with terminal illness. The presence of firm religious convictions indicates that consultation of the chaplain (or the patient's own minister or rabbi) is important. He or she will usually provide many valuable facts and insights about the patient and family that can smooth the patient's overall course.

DIFFICULTIES OF THOSE WHO CARE FOR THE DYING

A dying person poses a threat to the professional's own human attachments. First of all, the physician is reminded that death means loss of the relationship with the patient and all the investment and caring that has gone into it. Second, imminent loss of a patient reminds professionals of their own losses and of threatened losses. Caring for a dying woman, for example, can remind physicians of the past or feared death of their own mother, sister, or spouse. The wounds of an incompletely grieved loss are reopened. Losses in life are not discreet; they are cumulative. Those who care for the dying sustain repeated bereavement.

Because of the repeated stresses posed by these threats, professionals develop defenses. One course is to avoid involvement with patients in order to minimize personal loss or discomfort. This is one of the causes of adoption of fixed styles of relating to patients. Physicians who follow the initial communication of the diagnosis to the patient with a standardized, nonstop monologue detailing diagnosis, treatment, and course of the disease are not trying to baffle, overwhelm, or lose the patient altogether, but rather are trying to minimize their own anxiety by handling every initial bad news session the same way. Some professionals say the patient "can't take it," which is often a projection of their own fear onto the patient. The point is that the physician's discomfort and avoidance of the patient arise mainly from instincts of self-defense rather than any desire to alienate or harm the patient.

Criticism of physicians tends to be widespread and can generate unfortunate hostilities. Common accusations are that physicians are more afraid of death than other people and that this fear prompted them to enter the medical field in the first place. Sophisticated critics refer to Feifel's[36] study of physicians' attitudes toward death which showed that physicians spent significantly less time in conscious thought about death than did two control groups of professionals. Feifel et al[37] also found more fear of death in medical students than in two control samples. Dissatisfaction with physicians' communication patterns, avoidance of patients, and their manner in the sickroom compounds the alienation.

Although everyone is fascinated with death, physicians grapple with it more frequently than others and are sought out by those who wish to prevent or postpone it. Conflict or discomfort in the presence of death is intensified by the combination of two factors: frequent exposure and high responsibility. The findings of Feifel et al[37] may also be accounted for by the increased exposure of medical students to death and to the widespread belief of the population that the physician is the last barrier against it. Natural disappointment that a terminally ill person cannot be saved can lead to resentment. As one who could not reverse the illness, the physician may become the object of some or all of the family's resentment and blame. Finally, those who accuse physicians of inability to communicate with the dying patient seem to forget that everyone has this difficulty, including members of the patient's family.

Hospice Care of the Terminally Ill

Dame Cicely Saunders traces the notion of hospice therapeutics back to a treatise entitled "The Care of the Aged, the Dying and the Dead," written by a family physician for Harvard Medical School students.[38] Using the work in pain control at St Luke's Hospital in London, St Joseph's Hospice continued development of the hospice concept. St

Christopher's opened in 1967 with Dr Saunders as medical director, dedicated to enabling a patient, in her words, "to live to the limit of his or her potential in physical strength, mental and emotional capacity, and social relationships.... It is the alternative to the negative and socially dangerous suggestion that a patient with an incurable disease likely to cause suffering should have the legal option of actively hastened death, i.e., euthanasia."[38]

St Christopher's exported their expertise to this country with Dr Sylvia Lack, medical director of the New Haven Hospice.[39] The proliferation of hospices has been remarkable. By 1984 the National Hospice Organization (NHO) cited 1345 hospice programs in the United States.[38] The types of hospice available include those which provide home care only, independent inpatient units, and units based within a hospital, either as a separate unit or as a number of beds scattered throughout the hospital.

The NHO definition of hospice is:

> ...a medically directed, nurse coordinated program providing a continuum of home and inpatient care for the terminally ill patient and family. It employs an interdisciplinary team acting under the direction of an autonomous hospice administration. The program provides palliative and supportive care to meet the special needs arising out of the physical, emotional, spiritual, social and economic stresses which are experienced during the final stages of illness and during dying and bereavement.[38]

The special features of hospice care are:
Home care
Symptom control
Physician-directed, nurse-coordinated services
Interdisciplinary team—provided care
Twenty-four hours-per-day, 7-days-per-week coverage
Patient and family as the unit of care
Bereavement follow-up
Volunteers as an integral part of the interdisciplinary team
Structured support of personnel and communication system
Patients taken on basis of need, not on ability to pay

The essential features of hospice care are described in a number of outstanding works.[20,38,40] Whenever there is a hospice care team available to the terminally ill patient, referral can provide unique care for the individual and family.

REFERENCES

1. Greenberg DB, Abrams HE, Cassem EH: Psychologic and family complications of cancer, in *Cancer Manual* (7th ed). Boston, American Cancer Society, 1986, pp 400–413.
2. Freud S: The ego and the id, originally published in 1923. In *Standard Edition*, Strachey J (trans-ed). London, Hogarth Press, 1961, vol 19.
3. Deutsch F: Euthanasia, a clinical study. *Psychoanal Q* 1933; 5:347–368.
4. Saunders C: Care of the dying. *Nursing Times*, Oct 9–Nov 13, 1959.
5. Kubler-Ross E: *On Death and Dying*. New York, Macmillan, Inc, 1969.
6. Cassileth BR, Lusk EJ, Strouse TB, et al: Contemporary unorthodox treatments in cancer medicine. *Ann Intern Med* 1984; 101:105–112.
7. Curran WJ: Laetrile for the terminally ill: Supreme Court stops the nonsense. *N Engl J Med* 1980; 302:619–621.
8. Relman AS: Closing the books on laetrile. *N Engl J Med* 1982; 306:236.
9. Lerner IJ: Laetrile: A lesson in cancer quackery. *CA* 1981; 31:91–95.
10. Unproven methods of cancer management: The metabolic cancer therapy of Harold W. Manner, Ph.D. *CA* 1986; 36:185–189.
11. Unproven methods of cancer management: O Carl Simonton, MD. *CA* 1982; 32:58–61.
12. Simonton OC, Matthews-Simonton S, Creighton JL: *Getting Well Again*. New York, Bantam Books, 1981.
13. Holland JC. Why patients seek unproven cancer remedies: A psychological perspective. *CA* 1982; 32:10–14.
14. Eissler K: *The Psychiatrist and the Dying Patient*. New York, International Universities Press, 1955.
15. Saunders C: The moment of truth: Care of the dying person, in Pearson L (ed): *Death and Dying*. Cleveland, Case Western Reserve University Press, 1969, pp 49–78.
16. LeShan L, LeShan E: Psychotherapy and the patient with a limited life span. *Psychiatry* 1961; 24:318–323.
17. LeShan L: Psychotherapy and the dying patient, in Pearson L (ed): *Death and Dying*. Cleveland, Case Western Reserve University Press, 1969, pp 28–48.
18. Weisman AD, Hackett TP: Predilection to death: Death and dying as a psychiatric problem. *Psychosom Med* 1961; 23:232–256.
19. Cassem NH, Stewart RS: Management and care of the dying patient. *Int J Psychiatry Med* 1975; 6:293–304.
20. Billings JA: *Outpatient Management of Advanced Cancer*. Philadelphia, JB Lippincott Co, 1985.
21. Parkes CM: Bereavement: Studies of grief in adult life. New York, International Universities Press, 1972.
22. Reiss D, Gonzalez S, Kramer N: Family process, chronic illness, and death. *Arch Gen Psychiatry* 1986; 43:795–804.
23. Kelly WD, Friesen SR: Do cancer patients want to be told? *Surgery* 1950; 27:822–826.
24. Gilbertsen VA, Wangensteen OH: Should the doctor tell the patient that the disease is cancer? Surgeon's recommendation, in American Cancer Society: *The Physician and the Total Care of the Cancer Patient*. New York, American Cancer Society, 1962, pp 80–85.

25. Aitken-Swan J, Easson EC: Reactions of cancer patients on being told their diagnosis. *Br Med J* 1959; 1:779–783.
26. Gerlé B, Lunden G, Sandblom P: The patient with inoperable cancer from the psychiatric and social standpoints. *Cancer* 1960; 13:1206–1217.
27. Hackett TP, Weisman AD: The treatment of the dying. *Curr Psychiatr Ther* 1962; 2:121–126.
28. Oken D: What to tell cancer patients: A study of medical attitudes. *JAMA* 1961; 175:1120–1128.
29. Novack DH, Plumer R, Smith RL, et al: Changes in physicians' attitudes toward telling the cancer patient. *JAMA* 1979; 241:897–900.
30. Croog SH, Shapiro SD, Levine S: Denial among male heart patients. *Psychosom Med* 1971; 33:385–397.
31. Lester D: Religious behaviors and attitudes toward death, in Godin A (ed): *Death and Presence.* Brussels, Lumen Vitae, 1972, pp 107–124.
32. Feifel H: Religious conviction and fear of death among the healthy and the terminally ill. *J Sci Study Religion* 1974; 13:353–360.
33. Allport C: *The Nature of Prejudice.* New York, Doubleday & Co, Inc, 1958.
34. Feagin JR: Prejudice and religious types: Focused study, Southern Fundamentalists. *J Sci Study Religion* 1964; 4:3–13.
35. Magni KG: The fear of death, in Godin A (ed): *Death and Presence.* Brussels, Lumen Vitae, 1972, pp 125–138.
36. Feifel H: The function of attitudes toward death, in Group for the Advancement of Psychiatry: *Death and Dying: Attitudes of Patient and Doctor, Symposium 11.* 1965, vol 5, pp 633–641.
37. Feifel H, et al: Physicians consider death. Proceedings of 75th Annual Convention of American Psychological Association, Washington, D.C. 1967, vol 2, pp 201–202.
38. Zimmerman JM: *Hospice: Complete Care for the Terminally Ill.* Baltimore, Urban & Schwarzenberg, 1986, pp xi, xii, 17.
39. Lack SA, Buckingham RW: *First American Hospice: Three Years of Home Care.* New Haven, Hospice, Inc, 1978.
40. Saunders C (ed): *The Management of Terminal Illness.* Chicago, Yearbook Medical Publishers, 1978.

18

The Setting of Intensive Care

NED H. CASSEM and THOMAS P. HACKETT

Constant attendance of the critically ill or the dying began with the deathwatch. By the 1980s, computer-assisted technology had replaced and refined human vigilance in monitoring vital functions of the critically ill patient. Along with it has come a new cadre of medical caregivers, physicians, and nurses especially trained to reverse life-threatening cardiac and respiratory problems; secure the results of heroic surgery; heal and graft burns; and sustain a transplanted kidney, liver, pancreas, heart and/or lungs. Severity of illness and readiness of the staff to launch dramatic lifesaving interventions combine to lend a unique air of danger, urgency, and heroism to these settings. So new was it all 20 years ago that the phenomenon was called an "intensive care syndrome" by McKegney, who discussed a new "disease of medical progress."[1]

Practical issues and consultation problems in the intensive care setting are discussed first according to the setting and the natural course of critical illness. Then the management of each specific problem is discussed in turn.[2]

CONSULTATIONS FROM INTENSIVE CARE SETTINGS

Consultations from intensive care settings, when diagnosed, are very similar to the consultations that arise in other parts of the hospital. The frequencies of any one category of consultation from a particular unit is often determined by the illnesses which brought the patient to the unit. Table 18-1 displays the reasons for psychiatric consultation requests in four different intensive care settings at the Massachusetts General Hospital (MGH). It can be seen, for example, that delirium is far less common in the coronary care unit (CCU) than it is in the surgical intensive care unit (ICU) (this surgical ICU is primarily reserved for patients who have undergone cardiac surgery). In general, the more severe the systemic illness of the patient, the more likely the patient is to have delirium. Early consultations from the burn unit, for example, almost invariably are requests for the management of a delirious patient.

Table 18-1. Reasons for Psychiatric Consult Requests in Various Intensive Care Settings Listed in Order of Decreasing Frequency

Coronary Care Unit	*Surgical ICU*
1. Anxiety	1. Delirium
2. Depression	2. Depression
3. Management of behavior (sign-out, dependency)	3. Anxiety weaning from respirator
4. Hostility	
5. Delirium/psychosis	
Respiratory ICU	*Medical ICU*
1. Depression	1. Suicide attempt, overdose
2. Anxiety weaning from respirator	2. Depression
3. Management (drug dependency, dependency)	3. Character disorder
	4. Delirium
	5. Drug and/or alcohol abuse
	6. Anxiety

When original research was done on consultations coming from the CCU in 1970,[3] delirium represented a consultation request in only 11% of the cases. As technology advanced and interventions became more heroic, more and more patients with acute life-threatening problems were transferred to the unit and the number of consultation requests to manage delirious patients rose steadily. In the medical ICU, suicide attempt by overdose ranks second in frequency of admitting diagnosis, second only to cardiovascular disease. Discussion of the management of these cases is presented in chapter 14.

Reactions to myocardial infarction can serve as a model for the type and pattern of emotional reactions of a patient in a critical care setting (Figure 18-1). Typically, the patient who has had a myocardial infarction exhibits fear and anxiety during and immediately after admission. As symptoms stabilize or subside, some patients may decide that the symptoms, though abated, are so ominous that they must insist on signing out of the hospital and going home. After diagnostic tests confirm the presence of myocardial infarction, feelings of demoralization begin. As the hospitalization progresses, personality problems such as passive-aggressive behavior may complicate interactions between the patient and the hospital personnel and lead to a psychiatric consultation.

This conceptualization can at times be of practical assistance in caring for patients in a critical care setting. For example, if a patient seems impossible to deal with on the day of admission to an ICU, the reason is

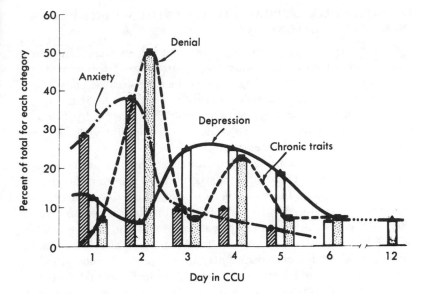

Figure 18-1. Hypothetical sequence of emotional and behavioral reactions of a coronary care unit (CCU) patient, derived from the frequency of psychiatric consultation for each category of reaction.

probably underlying fright. Nothing interferes with interpersonal behavior quite like panic. Staff members are likely to comment three or four days later that this patient seems like a completely different person. On the other hand, when a patient becomes impossible to deal with only after four or five days in the unit, and there has been no new or frightening symptom or complication, his behavior probably reflects a lifelong style or even a personality disorder. In contrast to the patients who are frightened when admitted, those who demonstrate personality problems later (like the dependent patient who has the call light on constantly) are not likely to become favorites of the staff, no matter how long they stay in the unit. By nature they have typically handled threats to their self-esteem either by whining dependency or hostile machismo intimidation, and they can be expected to continue to do so in the critical care setting. The delay in emergence of these character-related interpersonal problems is intriguing but not explained. It is possible that the patient suspends regressive or manipulative interpersonal dealings while his life hangs in the balance, since the threat of death is more immediate and serious than the fear of something else, like dependency.

CONSULTATION APPROACH TO THE CRITICALLY ILL PATIENT: DIFFERENTIAL DIAGNOSIS

Derangements of emotion, cognition, and behavior are common in critical care settings and require prompt attention. No treatment can proceed without a careful diagnostic evaluation. Because consulting a psychiatrist may mean that the consultee believes there is no organic cause for the abnormality, a psychiatric diagnosis must begin by excluding organic factors which could cause symptoms in the realm of thought, emotion, and/or behavior.

The many causes of these psychiatric derangements can be grouped into four categories. First, the abnormality may arise from the effect of the patient's medical illness or its treatment on the CNS, for example, abnormalities produced by hypoxia. Second, the abnormality may be the effect of the medical illness on the patient's mind (the subjective CNS), as with the patient who thinks he is "washed up" after a myocardial infarction. Third, the disturbance may arise from the "mind" primarily, as in a conversion or factitious symptom. A patient may malinger about pain in order to get more narcotics. Finally, the abnormality may be the result of interactions between the sick person and his environment or family, for example, the patient who has no complaints until his family arrives, at which time he promptly acts helpless and complains continuously. For these reasons the consultant must start by becoming acquainted with the disease of the individual patient and, like the renal or infectious disease consultant, review the chart completely. This includes the old chart, no matter how thick. Some patients have had prior psychiatric consultations and have presented similar difficulties on earlier admissions. Other patients have had no psychiatric consultations, but have caused considerable trouble for their caregivers on prior admissions, much of which may be extensively documented.

Throughout the evaluation, it is helpful to have in mind a systematic schema for the exclusion of organic disorders. There is a simple schema which is useful when the intervention for the organic disease needs to be especially prompt, that is, in those cases where prolonged failure to make the diagnosis may result in permanent CNS damage. These conditions are (1) Wernicke's disease, (2) hypoxia, (3) hypoglycemia, (4) hypertensive encephalopathy, (5) intracerebral or subarachnoid hemorrhage, meningitis-encephalitis, and poisoning, whether exogenous or iatrogenic. The consultant working in the emergency room, for example, would find this short list even more useful than would the consultant working in the acute care hospital. When there is a bit more leisure in making the diagnosis, an excellent comprehensive differential diagnostic list, compiled by Ludwig,[4] has been slightly expanded for use (Table 18-2). This 13-category differential diagnostic list goes by the mnemonic "vindictive mad" although it is easier to put it on a 3 × 5 card and carry it on one's person. Since a psychiatric consultant is, to some extent, the last court of appeal for making an organic diagnosis, a systematic approach is warranted. A quick review of this list is recommended even when the consultant is relatively sure of the patient's diagnosis.

Table 18-2. Differential Diagnosis of Brain Dysfunction in Critical Care Patients

General Etiology	Specific Etiologies
Vascular	Hypertensive encephalopathy; cerebral arteriosclerosis; intracranial hemorrhage or thromboses; circulatory collapse (shock); systemic lupus erythematosus; polyarteritis nodosa; thrombotic thrombocytopenic purpura
Infectious	Encephalitis; meningitis; general paresis
Neoplastic	Space-occupying lesions such as gliomas, meningiomas, abscesses
Degenerative	Senile and presenile dementias such as Alzheimer's or Pick's dementia, Huntington's chorea
Intoxication	Chronic intoxication or withdrawal effect of sedative-hypnotic drugs such as bromides, opiates, tranquilizers, anticholinergics, dissociative anesthetics; anticonvulsants
Congenital	Epilepsy; postictal states; aneurysm
Traumatic	Subdural and epidural hematomas; contusion; laceration; postoperative trauma; heat stroke
Intraventricular	Normal pressure hydrocephalus
Vitamin	Deficiencies of thiamine (Wernicke-Korsakoff), niacin (pellagra), B_{12} (pernicious anemia)
Endocrine-Metabolic	Diabetic coma and shock; uremia; myxedema, hyperthyroidism, parathyroid dysfunction; hypoglycemia; hepatic failure; porphyria; severe electrolyte or acid-base disturbances; remote side effect of carcinoma; Cushing's syndrome
Metals	Heavy metals (lead, manganese, mercury); carbon monoxide; toxins
Anoxia	Hypoxia and anoxia secondary to pulmonary or cardiac failure, anesthesia, anemia
Depression-Other	Depressive pseudodementia; hysteria; catatonia

From Ludwig's differential diagnosis of the confusion-delirium-dementia-coma complex.[4]

ICU Psychosis

The term "ICU psychosis" is a popular diagnosis that is often applied to patients exhibiting abnormal behavior in a critical care setting. In fact, the occurrence of acute psychosis in the critical care setting is rare. The term is invoked to imply that the environmental features of critical care settings are themselves capable of inducing psychosis. The rationale given for this is usually either sensory deprivation or monotony. In point of fact, the use of this diagnosis usually means that the etiology of a delirium is simply unknown. There would be more justification for ascribing acute agitation to psychosis if, for example, it were established that the patient's father died at the same age of the same disease in the same hospital during the same month. When used as a convenient diagnostic catchall term, however, "ICU psychosis" has more risks than benefits because it tends to discourage a thorough differential diagnosis.

Drugs Which Can Produce Psychiatric Abnormalities

Of all organic causes of altered mental status in intensive care settings, drugs are probably the most common. Some, like lidocaine, are predictable in their ability to cause an encephalopathic state, and the relationship is clearly dose-related. Others, like the antibiotics, are much rarer causes of delirium and usually occur only in someone whose brain is already vulnerable, as in a patient with a low seizure threshold. Table 18-3 lists some drugs in clinical use that have been associated with delirium.

The number of drugs than can be involved either in direct toxic actions or in toxic effects because of drug interactions are numerous, potentially bewildering, and constantly changing (see chapter 27). Certain sources provide regular reviews of published summaries and updates.[5]

The usual treatment is to stop or reduce the drug. Sometimes this is not possible. For example, in a patient with life-threatening ventricular irritability for whom a high rate of infusion of lidocaine seems essential, there may be no way that one can immediately reduce the dosage even though the etiologic connection with agitation is clear. In that case, treatment of nonspecific delirium, specifically with intravenous (IV) haloperidol, can proceed while the lidocaine is being given. However, the CNS derangement does not cease until the drug is reduced to a nontoxic level or withdrawn. Once a florid delirium with lidocaine begins, reduction of the dosage to a prior level that was not toxic may not eliminate the delirium. The drug often has to be stopped.

Elderly patients are more susceptible to the toxic action of many of

Table 18-3. Drugs in Clinical Use That Have Been Associated with Delirium

β-Adrenergic blockers
  Propranolol hydrochloride
  Timolol maleate
γ-Aminobutyric acid (GABA) agonists
  Baclofen
  Benzodiazepines
Antiarrhythmics
  Diisopropamide
  Lidocaine hydrochloride
  Mexiletine hydrochloride
  Procainamide hydrochloride
  Quinidine
  Tocainide hydrochloride
Antibacterials
  Aminoglycosides
  Amodioquine hydrochloride
  Amphotericin B
  Cephalosporins
  Chloramphenicol
  Chloroquine
  Colistin sulfate
  Ethambutol hydrochloride
  Gentamicin sulfate
  Isoniazid
  Metronidazole
  Rifampin
  Sulfonamides
  Tetracyclines
  Ticarcillin
  Vancomycin hydrochloride
Anticholinergics
  Atropine
  Benztropine mesylate
  Diphenhydramine hydrochloride
  Eye and nose drops
  Scopolamine
  Thioridazine
  Trihexyphenidyl hydrochloride
Anticonvulsants
  Phenytoin
Antihypertensives
  Captopril
  Clonidine hydrochloride
  Methyldopa
  Reserpine

Anti-inflammatory drugs, nonsteroidal
  Ibuprofen
  Indomethacin
  Naprosyn
  Sulindac
Antiviral agents
  Acyclovir
  Interferon
Barbiturates
Digitalis preparations
Disulfiram
Dopamine agonists (central)
  Amantadine hydrochloride
  Bromocriptine mesylate
  Levodopa
Ergotamine tartrate
Histamine H_2 antagonists
  Cimetidine
  Ranitidine hydrochloride
Immunosuppressives
  Aminoglutethamide
  L-Asparaginase
  5-Azacytadine
  Cytarabine hydrochloride (high-dose)
  Dacarbazine
  5-Fluorouracil
  Methenamine
  Methotrexate (high-dose)
  Procarbazine hydrochloride
  Tamoxifen citrate
  Vinblastine sulfate
  Vincristine sulfate
Lithium
Metrizamide
Monoamine oxidase inhibitors
  Isoniazid
  Phenelzine sulfate
  Procarbazine hydrochloride
Narcotic analgesics
  Meperidine hydrochloride (normeperidine)
  Pentazocine lactate
Podophyllum resin (topical)
Steroids
  ACTH
Sympathomimetics
  Aminophylline
  Amphetamines
  Cocaine

Table 18-3. Drugs in Clinical Use That Have Been Associated with Delirium—continued

Ephedrine
Phenylephrine hydrochloride
Phenylpropanolamine hydrochloride
Theophylline
Tricyclic antidepressants
  Amitriptyline hydrochloride
  Desipramine hydrochloride
  Imipramine hydrochloride
  Maprotiline
  Nortriptyline hydrochloride
  Protriptyline hydrochloride
  Trimipramine

these drugs, and some of the agents listed in Table 18-3 have been reported to cause delirium only in elderly patients, for example, nonsteroidal anti-inflammatory drugs and eye and nose drop preparations.

An anticholinergic psychosis can be reversed by IV physostigmine in doses of 0.5 to 2.0 mg administered parenterally. Caution is essential for patients in critical care settings, however, because their autonomic nervous systems are generally less stable than those of patients who have developed an anticholinergic psychosis after a voluntary overdose. Moreover, if there is a reasonably high amount of anticholinergic drug in the system (as in a patient with renal failure on dialysis who has excessive scopolamine on board), the therapeutic effect of physostigmine, although sometimes dramatic, is usually short-lived. The cholinergic reaction to IV physostigmine can cause profound bradycardia and hypotension, thereby multiplying the complications instead of reducing them. It should also be noted, on the other hand, that a continuous IV infusion of physostigmine has been successfully used to manage a case of anticholinergic poisoning.[6] Because of the diagnostic value of physostigmine, one may wish to use it even though its effects may not be permanently therapeutic. If one were to use an IV injection of 1 mg of physostigmine, protection against excessive cholinergic reaction can be provided by preceding this injection with an IV injection of 0.2 mg of glycopyrrolate. This anticholinergic agent does not cross the blood-brain barrier and should protect the patient from the peripheral cholinergic actions of physostigmine.

Figure 18-2 presents a decision tree or quasi-algorithm, according to which the diagnosis and treatment of specific abnormalities in ICU

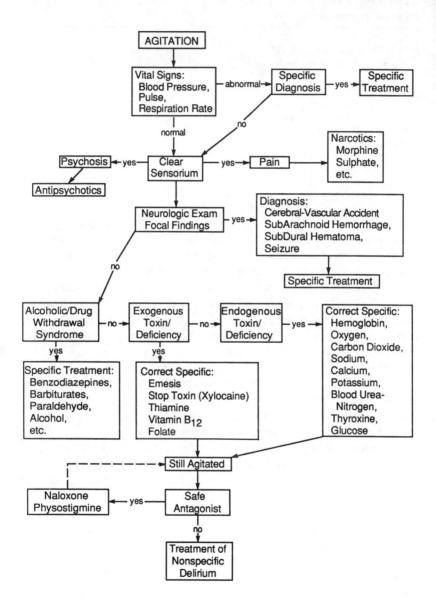

Figure 18-2. Decision tree for diagnosis and treatment of abnormalities in ICU setting.

settings could proceed. Usually the diagnostic and therapeutic considerations contained in this summary algorithm have already been considered by the physicians in the critical care unit prior to the arrival of the psychiatric consultant. It is the obligation of the consultant, however, to reconsider all organic possibilities that may have caused the psychiatric symptomatology of the patient. Sometimes the psychiatric symptomatology is so bizarre or so offensive that prior diagnostic efforts were disrupted and incomplete.

It is idealistic to expect that every psychiatric abnormality in the critically ill patient can be traced to one or more of the specific causes outlined in this differential diagnostic survey. Most of the time there are many known factors that could impair CNS function, but their exact contributions are not clear, some of their elements are beyond correction, and efforts to correct other abnormalities have not resulted in any clear therapeutic response. Nonetheless, having made the best diagnosis possible under the circumstances, the consultant then proceeds to treat the difficulty in accord with that diagnosis.

MANAGEMENT OF SPECIFIC PROBLEMS
Fear and Anxiety

Admission to an intensive care setting is invariably associated with a life-threatening disease. Even after the fear of death has ceased to haunt their consciousness, patients may fear that they will be maimed by the illness or by its treatments. This fear may assume many guises: verbosity, outbursts of anger, paranoia, and silent withdrawal are all behaviors typically produced by fear.

Fear is treated by medication and by quiet reassurance. Unless panic has begun to encroach on rationality, the drugs of choice are the benzodiazepines (Table 18-4). If the patient's condition is one in which autonomic lability may be a hazard (eg, myocardial infarction), routine prescription of one of these agents is recommended whether or not the patient looks anxious. Even when autonomic lability is not a hazard, the anxiety that accompanies severe acute medical illness is the most common indication for the prescription of benzodiazepines.

Of the benzodiazepines available, diazepam probably produces a high blood level most rapidly and is of particular value for the patient who needs to feel tranquilization quickly. If tranquilizers are given routinely to all patients, about 8% of them will complain of feeling sedated. Some of these patients may be reacting to a drug's rapid absorption and would better tolerate the slow, steady accumulation of one of the less lipid-soluble benzodiazepines, such as oxazepam or prazepam.

Table 18-4. Benzodiazepines: Characterization by Half-Life and Metabolism.

	Half-Life (h)	Metabolized to
Short-acting agents		
Oxazepam (Serax)	5–15	
Lorazepam (Ativan)	10–20	
Temazepam (Restoril)	9–12	
Alprazolam (Xanax)	12–15	Three (half-life)
Triazolam (Halcion)	2–3	Two (half-life)
Moderately long-acting agents		
Diazepam (Valium)	26–53	N-Desmethyldiazepam
Chlordiazepoxide hydrochloride		
(Librium)	8–28	Desmethylchlordiazepoxide
		Demoxepam
		N-Desmethyldiazepam
Halazepam (Paxipam)	14	N-Desmethyldiazepam
Long-acting agents		
Clorazepate dipotassium (Tranxene)	30–200	N-Desmethyldiazepam
Prazepam (Centrax)	30–200	N-Desmethyldiazepam
Very long-acting agents		
Flurazepam (Dalmane)	>96	N-Desalkylflurazepam

Clorazepate and prazepam are two long-acting benzodiazepines that are not active in their original form. They both have the same metabolite, N-desmethyldiazepam, which is the only metabolite that produces psychotropic effects. However, clorazepate produces high blood levels within the first hour, whereas prazepam enters the system slowly. By four hours, the concentration of desmethyldiazepam is essentially the same for both of these agents.[7] According to this rationale a clinician would choose diazepam, clorazepate, lorazepam or alprazolam if the patient wanted to experience tranquilization quickly. Oxazepam, prazepam, and temazepam are better for the patient who prefers to get the benefit slowly and imperceptibly.

When using longer-acting agents such as diazepam, whose half-life varies between 20 and 60 hours, the physician can assume that saturation has been attained after two or three days and administer only a bedtime or twice-daily dose thereafter. However, if the patient's anxiety responds best to the impacts of repeated dosing, three or four divided doses a day may remain clinically preferable. In fact, the latter is the most common way of prescribing the agent for both inpatients and outpatients. Parenteral forms of chlordiazepoxide and diazepam are available, but intramuscular (IM) absorption of these two agents is erratic and less complete than absorption of oral doses. For this reason oral or cautious IV administration is recommended. Chlordiazepoxide and diazepam can, on rare occasions, produce paradoxical rage or hostility. The shorter-acting drugs appear to do this far less often and are therefore more appropriate if the patient already seems hostile. Among the short-acting benzodiazepines—oxazepam, lorazepam, and temazepam—lorazepam is the only short-acting drug currently available for parenteral use and, for that reason, has special value in critical care units. Otherwise, the major advantage of these agents is that they have no active metabolite and therefore do not accumulate in blood.

A general rule is to prescribe the simplest and shortest-acting effective drug, for example, 15 mg of oxazepam given three or four times per day. With the physician's permission, the nurse can hold this if it seems excessive or report if the patient seems undermedicated. One of the most sensitive measures of the dose's adequacy is the perception of the critical care nurse. The nurse, who attends the patient for an entire eight-hour shift, is generally able to see whether the patient appears to be growing more anxious or has begun to sleep all the time and is becoming harder to arouse and engage.

Slow accumulation of metabolites is a problem worth worrying about. It is especially likely with flurazepam, diazepam, and all agents in which desmethyldiazepam is a metabolite. In addition, since the metabolism of these agents requires oxidative processes, patients with hepatic impairment are even more likely to accumulate excessive doses. Another major advantage of the three short-acting benzodiazepines is that they require only glucuronide conjugation by the liver to be inactivated. Even in patients with advanced cirrhosis, this metabolic step is achieved simply, and the half-lives of these agents in patients with liver failure remain essentially the same as in patients with normal hepatic function. Accumulation is another problem common to geriatric patients. Long-acting agents are more likely to accumulate and produce toxic effects in the elderly and are better avoided where possible.

There are those patients who maintain that flurazepam, long half-life or not, is the most effective sleeping medication available to them. This claim appears to be correct in many cases, but one must still worry about the dangers of accumulation.

If the patient's fear is sufficiently intense to impair reason, or if the patient appears to be in a state of panic or (transient) psychosis, a *neuroleptic* agent is the drug of choice. Panicked individuals are barely in control, and the benzodiazepines can sometimes further compromise an already diminished ability to cope. The preferred neuroleptic is haloperidol, which can be administered in oral or parenteral form.

Clarification, explanation, and *reassurance* can also have soothing effects on anxious patients, particularly when fear stems from threatening or erroneous misconceptions of disease. Questions such as "Have you ever known anyone with these symptoms?" or "What is your idea of a heart attack?" can be used to uncover misconceptions. When a family member has died of the same condition, his or her age at death may figure heavily in the patient's fear; often the patient expects that fate will take him at the same age.

After false ideas have been corrected, it is important to mention positive aspects of the treatment plan. For example, the cardiac patient might be assured that myocardial healing is complete in 5 to 6 weeks, and that normal activities will be resumed along with an exercise program. Even when the prognosis is grave, as in lung cancer, a calm statement of the treatments planned to counteract and contain the malignant disease is of value to the anxious patient. The more ominous the prognosis, the more important it is to encourage the patient to specify the fear, so that specific and *valid* reassurances (eg, that medication can control pain) can be given. False reassurances are not recommended because they rob the physician of credibility and therefore of the ability to reassure the patient later in the illness. Equanimity has perhaps the most soothing effect on the patient. Anxious patients have a way of making people who take care of them anxious, and a vicious circle may develop. A calm person can break that deleterious interaction.

Denial and the Threat to Sign Out

Denial allows an acutely ill person to avoid panic by minimizing or excluding the threatening implications of his disease.[8] If panic sets in, a patient may get the urge to flee; threatening to sign out is therefore a special case of fear and anxiety (see chapter 14). Although the threat to sign out can mean that the individual does not take the illness seriously, it should be assumed to be a manifestation of panic unless proved otherwise.

Because such persons are desperate and often irrational, antagonism flares when efforts are made to detain them. The patient should not be threatened or given the idea that he is being cornered. Sitting on a chair so that one is physically lower than the patient, speaking in a gentle and quiet voice, and emphasizing the positive aspects of the proposed treatment are likely to be most effective. A gentle approach is essential. For example, the physician might begin by saying, "I am not here to force you to do anything; what I ask is that you let me know your point of view and then let me know that you understand mine."

Seriously ill patients need to hear the truth in direct but quiet, calm terms. They must understand that their illness is manageable if they stay in the hospital: "Your heart is damaged and needs to be carefully monitored to avoid further damage and risk, but it's much like the process of cement setting. At first it's fragile when freshly poured, but if given the chance to firm up, it can hold up a building. The same can be true of your heart muscle if you give it a chance to repair itself." As the patient calms down, he may respond to questions on the source of his fear.

Before talking to the patient who signs out, the physician should ask that the family be mobilized immediately. Their appearance and pleading with the patient, even when hysterical, may induce him to stay. Even if the patient becomes calm, he should be medicated promptly, most often with a neuroleptic such as haloperidol.

Most of these patients (at least the ones who would be able to leave the hospital under their own power) are not mentally incompetent, but requesting a formal psychiatric evaluation is appropriate. Having the patient sign out against medical advice is usually unnecessary if the conversation and circumstances are carefully documented in the chart; furthermore it is of no value as a punitive measure. Even if the patient leaves, he should be told that he is welcome to the appropriate treatment whenever he changes his mind and chooses to return. The emphasis is always on *what is best for the patient*—both in one's conversation with the patient and in making practical judgments about how to handle the sign-out. This can help to undercut the accusation made by some of these patients that the physician is interested only in winning a power struggle.

Delirium

Acute delirium is one of the most common psychiatric problems of critical care. Fifteen years ago it was routine to administer atropine to newly admitted CCU patients who developed bradycardia. Some of these patients, particularly older ones with some pre-existing organic brain disease, developed acute delirium. For such patients, parenteral propantheline bromide (Pro-Banthine), a quarternary ammonium compound that does not cross the blood-brain barrier and is equally effective in treating bradycardia, was substituted. This can still be done, but problems are seldom so simple. Often, the drugs that may be causing the delirium, such as lidocaine or cimetidine, cannot be changed without possible detriment to the patient. Alternatively, pain may be the cause of agitation in a delirious patient. Morphine sulfate can relieve pain, but may be contraindicated by an associated decrease in blood pressure or respiratory rate.

Psychosocial measures are not effective in treating a bona fide delirium of uncertain or unknown etiology. In these cases, treatment options include administration of neuroleptics or paralytics and/or the use of physical restraints. However, restraints are likely to be in place already, particularly if critical lines have been jeopardized by agitation. Moreover, paralytic drugs such as pancuronium bromide require use of mechanical ventilation, which increases the risk of respiratory complications in postoperative patients. Delirium is therefore usually treated with haloperidol or another neuroleptic.

Treatment of delirium with haloperidol. Because an agitated critical care patient may harm himself by pulling out pacemaker wires, pumps, sutures, endotracheal tube, and other therapeutic life lines, the decrease of agitation is the treatment goal against which haloperidol's effects are titrated. Its effects on blood pressure, pulmonary artery pressure, heart rate, and respiration are milder than those of the benzodiazepines, making it an excellent agent for severely ill patients with impaired cardiorespiratory status.[2,9,10] Although haloperidol can be administered orally or parenterally, acute delirium with extreme agitation requires parenteral medication. Intravenous administration is preferable to IM administration for the following reasons: (1) Drug absorption may be poor in distal muscles if a patient's delirium is associated with circulatory compromise or borderline shock; the deltoid is probably better than the gluteus muscle for IM injection, but neither is as reliable as the IV route. (2) The agitated patient is commonly paranoid, and repeated painful IM injections may increase his sense of being attacked by enemy forces. (3) Intramuscular injections can complicate interpretations of muscle enzyme studies if enzyme fractionation is not available. (4) Finally, and most important, IV haloperidol is less likely to produce extrapyramidal side effects.

In contrast to the immediately observable sedation produced by IV diazepam, IV haloperidol has a mean distribution time of 11 minutes in normal volunteers; this may be even longer in critically ill patients. The mean half-life of IV haloperidol's subsequent, slower phase is 14 hours. This is still a more rapid metabolic rate than the overall mean half-lives of 21 and 24 hours for the IM and oral doses, respectively. The oral dose has about half the potency of the parenteral dose, so that 10 mg of haloperidol by mouth corresponds to 5 mg IV or IM.

Haloperidol has not been approved by the Food and Drug Administration for IV administration. Any drug can be used for a patient when justified as "innovative therapy." For critical care units desirous of using IV haloperidol, one approach would be to present this to the hospital's human studies committee with a request to use the drug with careful monitoring of results, based on the fact that it is the drug of choice for the patient's welfare, is the safest drug, and is justifiable as innovative therapy. After a period of monitoring, the committee may choose to use this drug routinely.

In Europe IV haloperidol has been used to treat delirium tremens and acute psychosis and to premedicate patients scheduled for electroconvulsive therapy (ECT). Its use has been associated with few side effects on blood pressure, heart rate, respiratory rate, or urine output and with minimal extrapyramidal side effects. The reason for the last-named is not known. Studies of the use of IV haloperidol in psychiatric patients have not shown that the side effects were fewer. Their less frequent appearance after IV administration in medically ill patients may be due to the fact that many of the medically ill patients are receiving other medications that are protective, especially the benzodiazepines and β-blockers, or that patients with psychiatric disorder, especially schizophrenia, are more susceptible to extrapyramidal side effects.

Before IV haloperidol is administered, the IV line should be flushed with 2 mL of normal saline. Phenytoin precipitates haloperidol, and mixing the two in the same line must be avoided. Rarely, haloperidol may precipitate with heparin sodium, and since all lines in critical care units are usually heparinized, the 2-mL flush is advised. The initial bolus dose of haloperidol varies from 0.5 to 20.0 mg: 2 mg for mild agitation, 5 mg for moderate, and 10 mg for severe. The only time a consultant would use a higher initial dose is when the patient has already been treated with reasonable doses of haloperidol unsuccessfully. To allow for haloperidol's delayed onset, doses are usually staggered by at least a 30-minute interval. If a 5-mg dose does not calm an agitated patient after 30 minutes, 10 mg should be administered. Partial control of agitation usually is not adequate and only prolongs the delirium. Therefore it is recommended that haloperidol be given every 30 minutes until the patient is calm.

After calm is achieved, agitation should be the sign for a repeat dose. Ideally, the total dose of haloperidol on the second day should be a fraction of that on day 1. After complete lucidity has been achieved, the patient needs to be protected from delirium only at night, by small doses of haloperidol (0.5 to 3.0 mg), which can be given orally. This is seldom necessary for more than two or three days. As in the treatment of delirium tremens, the consultant is advised to stop the agitation quickly and completely at the outset rather than barely keeping up with it over several days. The maximum total dose of IV haloperidol to be used as an upper limit has not been established, although IV single-bolus doses of 150 mg have been administered in our institution, and as much as 945 mg total dose has been used in a 24-hour period.[11]

Hypotensive episodes following the administration of IV haloperidol are rare and almost invariably are caused by hypovolemia. Ordinarily this is easily checked in ICU patients who have indwelling pulmonary artery catheters, but since agitation is likely to return, volume replacement is necessary before administering further doses. There are no local caustic effects on veins. Intravenous haloperidol is generally safe for epileptics and patients with head trauma. Although IV haloperidol may be used without mishap an patients receiving epinephrine drips, after very large doses of haloperidol a pressor other than epinephrine, such as norepinephrine, should be used to avoid unopposed β-adrenergic activity.

Intravenous haloperidol does not block the dopamine-mediated increase in renal blood flow. It also appears to be the safest agent for patients with chronic obstructive pulmonary disease.

Combining haloperidol with a benzodiazepine in the treatment of a nonspecific delirium may at times be quite helpful. When repeated doses of haloperidol have failed to give a therapeutic response, another agent, either lorazepam or diazepam, can be tried. Adams has recommended a regular treatment regimen with alternating doses of haloperidol (10 mg) and lorazepam (1 mg) for the treatment of nonspecific delirium.[12]

An alternative agent to haloperidol is IV droperidol, an agent already approved for IV administration by the FDA. This agent, however, is a far more potent α-adrenergic antagonist and is far more likely to lead to difficulties with hypotension, particularly when it is combined with other agents. One such reaction occurred at this hospital when droperidol was used as an IV antiemetic for cancer patients simultaneously receiving oral tetrahydrocannabinol. Intravenous diazepam is used routinely to treat agitated states, particularly delirium tremens, as are IV chlordiazepoxide and lorazepam. Any one of these IV benzodiazepines may be a useful adjunct in the treatment of acute nonspecific delirium. Intravenous alcohol is also extremely effective in the treatment of alcohol withdrawal states. Its disadvantage is that it is toxic in itself to both liver and brain, although its use can be safe if these organs do not already show extensive damage (and sometimes safe even when they do). A 5% solution of alcohol mixed with 5% dextrose in water, run at 1 mL/min, brings a calming effect amazingly quickly. Other parenteral neuroleptic drugs for treatment of agitation are thiothixene, trifluoperazine hydrochloride, fluphenazine, and chlorpromazine. Chlorpromazine is extremely effective, but its potent α-blocking properties can be exceedingly dangerous for critically ill patients. When administered IV or IM, it can abruptly decrease total peripheral resistance and cause a precipitous fall in blood pressure.

Midazolam maleate became available on the US market in mid-1986. Promoted for IV sedation for short diagnostic or endoscopic procedures and preanesthetic medication, midazolam acts even faster than diazepam and is three to four times as potent. Its rapid onset, short elimination half-life from one to four hours, and its amnestic potency make it an ideal short-term sedative. Clinical experience with this agent is not sufficient to evaluate its usefulness for the treatment of acute delirium. Respiratory depression and hypotension have both been reported with midazolam, the latter being particularly severe when the drug is combined with large doses of fentanyl citrate.

Major Depression and Despondency

Consultation to critical care settings results in many discoveries of despondency and major depression. The diagnosis and treatment of these conditions is fully discussed in chapter 13. Intensive care settings demand rapid answers to clinical questions. For example, if the patient's inability to recover seems due to depression, the use of a psychostimulant, as described in chapter 12, makes eminent sense. Many patients in critical care units are not taking anything by the oral route. In the treatment of depression this limits the choice of agents considerably. One alternative in the use of stimulants is to request from the hospital pharmacy a stimulant in suppository form. Theoretically, almost any agent can be given in suppository form, even though this can be a time-consuming task for the pharmacist.

For the depressed patient who requires parenteral drug administration, IV amitriptyline may provide excellent relief.[13] The regimen described is as follows: Amitriptyline, 10 mg in 200 mL of 5% dextrose in water (or half-normal saline) is allowed to infuse over a two-hour period, with vital signs taken every 15 minutes during the first session. If no untoward effects occur with the first administration, one need not expect them later unless the dose is raised. This dosage is repeated at bedtime every night. If the patient shows no immediate response (eg, a better night's sleep), then the dose can be increased by 10 mg per night until some response occurs. Most of the patients responded to a 10-mg dose. In one patient 200 mg was tolerated over a several-week period.[13] Occurrence of dry mouth, tachycardia, and urinary retention was rare. This may be because of the small doses involved.

Anxiety That Inhibits Weaning from the Ventilator

The multimodal treatment of anxiety that inhibits weaning from the ventilator often begins with a benzodiazepine such as lorazepam administered prior to weaning periods or a neuroleptic such as haloperidol if the patient appears to be in a near-panic state. Again, if haloperidol is used, the IV route is recommended.

Persons who suffer acute and chronic respiratory failure and therefore require prolonged mechanical ventilation may become so anxious when the weaning process begins that psychiatric assistance is requested. Even though the patient is physically ready for weaning, anxiety can transiently increase metabolic demands and cardiac work until further weaning becomes impossible.

The consulting psychiatrist who faces the request to help an anxious patient wean will profit from reading Feeley's[14] description of how a respiratory physician determines a patient's readiness for weaning. Basically, Feeley states that six criteria must be met before a patient is considered ready for weaning.

1. The patient must have a vital capacity of at least 10 mL to 15 mL/kg body weight.
2. The maximum inspiratory force exerted by a patient with totally occluded tracheostomy tube should be greater than -2 cm of water. (This does not require the cooperation of the patient.)
3. The oxygen gradient, $AaDO_2^{1.0}$ should be less than 300–350 mmHg.
4. The ratio of dead space to tidal volume V_D/V_T should be less than 0.6.
5. Cardiovascular stability is a must.
6. Metabolic balance must be present.

When these six criteria are met, the patient is hooked up to a T-piece or Brigg's attachment with a heated nebulizer, the inspired oxygen concentration is raised 10% higher than is required for controlled ventilation, and weaning begins. It is quite systematic and logical. Vital signs are taken every five minutes and after 20 minutes arterial blood gases are drawn. If the arterial oxygen pressure is less than 70 mmHg or the pH is less than 7.25, the patient is put back on the ventilator. If not, weaning continues.

Failure to wean may be due to hypoxia or hypercapnia. Arterial blood gases can change, and the consultant who fails to check them is doing both the patient and the consulting physician a disservice. If the arterial oxygen tension has not changed, the physician can quickly check the pH to make sure it is not less than 7.25. Common causes for onset of hypercapnia might be an increase in the dead space, poor muscular function due to weakness or starvation, lack of coordination between the muscles of the diaphragm and the intercostal muscles, bronchospasm, tumor, tracheal stenosis, or a tracheostomy tube that is too narrow.[14]

Most behavioral exercises for relaxation encourage the subject to take slow, deep, easy breaths. This is one of the quickest and surest ways of inducing relaxation for most people, but it is precisely what patients with respiratory problems cannot do and precisely what makes them so anxious. The multimodal treatment of this difficulty often begins with a benzodiazepine administered prior to weaning periods, or a neuroleptic such as haloperidol if the patient appears to be excessively fearful. The patient himself can indicate whether a drug is effective and which drug is most helpful. In some cases it may be possible to use a mixture of nitrous oxide if the respiratory specialist or anesthesiologist is present to administer it. Hypnosis or relaxation techniques are often helpful in distracting the patient from the weaning process. When these are used, the instruction to breathe easily is best omitted from the hypnotic suggestion; the patient should be encouraged to concentrate either on a tranquil scene such as a beach or on a single concept (mantra).[15]

Finally, the patient may be helped by the explanation that the weaning process itself can be expected to produce anxiety. Despondency and major depression, as well as anxiety, can impede weaning so that the treatments of depression listed in the foregoing section may apply here as well.

Cardiac Arrest

The ultimate complication, cardiac arrest, leaves distinctive marks on the minds of patients and staff. After cardiac arrest, the survivor almost invariably shows some natural increase in apprehension, even though it may not be verbalized. Most are amnesic for the arrest episode itself, but manifestations of emotional turmoil, such as nightmares, are common.[16,17] This turmoil is usually transient; the overall capacity of the survivor to adjust is high.[8] Those who adjust poorly usually have prior histories of emotional disturbance.[17] Cardiac arrest does not necessarily justify concomitant pessimism. Lemire and Johnson reviewed the course of 1204 patients resuscitated in a general hospital, of whom 230 (19.1%) survived to discharge.[18] Regardless of the underlying disease, the survival rates of these patients discharged were 74% surviving for 1 year, 59% for 2 years, 51% for 3 years. A study of randomly chosen survivors showed that their functional capacity before and after resuscitation was unchanged. In general, the literature supports the emotional adaptability of survivors of cardiac arrest.[19–21] The consultant armed with these facts is likely to communicate more subjective, tranquil optimism in assisting the patient who is recovering from cardiac arrest. After cardiac arrest the patient's fear of recurrence often takes the form of anxiety about being left alone. Then, emphasis on the watchdog value of the monitor is helpful along with reminders from the staff that the nurses should never be far from the patient.

Survivors of cardiac arrest frequently go on to electrophysiology (EP) studies in an effort to determine whether the antiarrhythmic agents used can prevent a recurrence of the potentially fatal arrhythmia. This necessitates the effort to induce ventricular tachycardia by electrical stimulation. Patients who return to the catheterization laboratory for this test are commonly frightened, come to dread the experience, or even view it as a re-enactment of their prior close call with death. Since countershock may be necessary to halt ventricular tachycardia or fibrillation, and since adequate anesthesia may not always be feasible for this procedure, anticipation of the next EP study may become increasingly negative. Evaluation of such a patient proceeds along the same lines as analysis for the anxious patient. By and large, most of the EP patients do well, but most of them do better with some pharmacotherapy, usually a benzodiazepine. Alprazolam 0.5 to 1.5 mg three times a day along with psychotherapy has been helpful. Psychiatric consultation in patients with cardiac disease, particularly those with sudden arrhythmias, is solidly founded on the premier regulatory role of the CNS on the heart. Cardiac arrhythmias, focal cardiac lesions, pulmonary edema, and sudden death as well as the mediation of environmental stress can be explained by the connections between CNS structure and the heart. Natelson[22] and Samuels[23] have given excellent reviews.

How can psychiatric treatment reduce the incidence of heart disease? It has been mentioned above that for patients with acute stress or acute coronary disease, standing doses of benzodiazepines may to some extent reduce sympathetic arousal and thereby protect the patient from sudden cardiac arrhythmias. β-Adrenergic blockers have been shown to prolong survival in myocardial infarction patients, but these probably work by countering the peripheral activity of the sympathetic nervous system. One of the most important interventions shown to reduce the incidence of initial or recurrent myocardial infarction is the reduction of type A behavior. Friedman describes coronary-prone (type A) behavior as:

> . . . a characteristic action-emotion complex which is exhibited by those individuals who are engaged in a relatively *chronic struggle* to

obtain an *unlimited* number of *poorly defined* things from their environment in the *shortest period of time* and, if necessary, against the opposing efforts of other things or persons in this same environment.[24]

A review panel convened at the request of the National Heart, Lung, and Blood Institute concluded, after review of the studies, that type A behavior was an independent coronary risk factor of the same order of pathogenetic magnitude as that of blood cholesterol, hypertension, or smoking.[25] Since that time, two studies have demonstrated that reducing type A behavior reduced cardiac recurrences in postmyocardial infarction patients and significantly lowered serum cholesterol in a group of healthy middle-aged American military officers.[26,27] The time-urgent and hostile patterns involved in the behavior known as type A are the primary targets of group therapy, which has been described in detail.[28]

Treatment is no simple affair. Groups of approximately 12 patients meet twice a month for 3 months, monthly for 3 months, and every 2 months thereafter. In general, the participants are taught to identify the array of overt manifestations of the type A behavior pattern—for example, reliving anger about the past, arguing tenaciously about minor issues, polyphasic activity, interrupting others, and hypersensitivity to criticism, first from others, then from themselves. Patients' beliefs about themselves—for example, unrealistic appraisals of personal qualities; overemphasis on achievement as a measure of self-worth; hostile, suspicious, vindictive, and competitive attitudes toward others, and their attitudes toward life in general—were topics introduced later in treatment. There is no proof thus far that myocardial infarction patients with type A behavior can sustain their improved health without some form of continued group therapy. Consultants who familiarize themselves with the type A behavior pattern can identify patients who will be suitable for group therapy. We argue that group therapy of this type should be part of an overall cardiac rehabilitation program for cardiac patients.

In his book, *Life After Life*, Moody has stirred tremendous interest in the death experience with reports by survivors of near-death experiences like cardiac arrest and their accounts of "out of body" experiences.[29] Based on the reports of these individuals, Moody has listed the following 15 characteristic aspects described by such survivors: participating in an ineffable and indescribable experience; hearing bystanders pronounce them dead; feeling peaceful and quiet; hearing an unusual noise of some sort such as a buzzing, whistling, or windy sound; traveling through a dark space such as a tunnel; being out of the body; meeting with significant others such as family, God, or the saints, who are often viewed as spiritual rather than physical beings; encountering a very bright light; watching one's life pass in review before the mind's eye; approaching a border such as a fence, shore, or line; feeling a need to "come back" (often with regret); being reluctant to tell others despite their conviction of reality; feeling a dramatic change in their lives; having a new and fearless view of death; and being assured that elements of the story, such as words actually uttered by bystanders, can be corroborated.

We have spoken with a number of MGH patients who have had experiences such as those described by Moody. The actual incidence of these experiences in all survivors of cardiac arrest is not known, but we estimate it at about 2%. It would also be inaccurate to give the impression that these out of body experiences are all pleasant. Moody describes survivors of attempted suicide who awaken with guilt and remorse after having been transported to a frightening place. We have not interviewed any of these individuals, but two patients who had altered mental states during cardiac arrest reported unpleasant experiences.

One woman described seeing all the dead members of her family awaiting her on the other side of a fence. She had no desire whatsoever to join them and resisted desperately their efforts to pull her through the fence. She "came back" with considerable relief.

A 32-year-old psychologist who had a cardiac arrest in the emergency ward experienced himself as a piece of meat in a supermarket being carried along a conveyor belt to the check-out counter. He found himself shouting that he would not be "checked out" and re-entered consciousness in the emergency ward to the sight of several physicians and nurses dressed in white. "Jesus, there are a lot of people in this supermarket!" he exclaimed, a remark that mystified the medical team until he explained it.

The Difficult Patient

By "difficult patient" is meant the patient with a personality disorder. The most difficult are those with narcissistic and borderline personalities. The principles of their treatment in the ICU are no different from those articulated in chapter 10.

Rites of Passage: Transfer out of a Critical Care Setting

Coronary patients experience a dramatic rise in catecholamine excretion on the day of transfer out of the CCU.[30] Transfer from an ICU to a general ward is generally both bad and good news for the patient—bad because it means reduced coverage and observation, good because it means that his condition has improved. Ideally, the discharge date should be made definite at least 24 hours in advance, if possible. Explicit warnings about less frequent checks and fewer nurses should be accompanied by the assurance that intensive care is no longer necessary. In essence, increased independence should be represented as a reward rather than a hazard.

Recommendations for Maintaining ICU Morale

The following practical recommendations for the maintenance of unit morale round out the important work done in these units.

1. Intensive care functions better with a strong medical director who can work in close conjunction with a head nurse. It is impossible to overemphasize the truth of Safer's insight that ICU personnel are happier under a benevolent dictator than they are under a disorganized or passive democracy.[31] This physician-leader must have special competence in critical care and the strengths to keep ICU staff from being caught between physicians of various disciplines who may be feuding over the care of a patient.

2. A quiet, reasonably secluded place with a coffee pot is helpful to unit morale.

3. A psychiatric nurse-clinician can teach the staff about difficulties with specific patients as well as ways in which the group as a unit can deal with crisis and stress.

4. The steps required for successful group resolution of conflict could be summarized as: (a) identification and acknowledgment of feelings, (b) sharing of and reaction to these feelings by the group, (c) review of the experience with criticism, support, and praise, and (d) integration of what is learned with application to future experience.

5. Families should be allies wherever possible, so as to reduce their potential as distractions or obstacles to care. They should be allowed to share in the realities of the patient's illness, whether the prospects be optimistic or tragic.

Intensive care settings reveal humanity at its best and at its worst. This is as true for the staff as it is for the patients. Those who serve in intensive care settings in a true sense risk their own lives, their own feelings, their own self-esteem, and their own self-respect. Those who face these risks receive opportunities to mature. The unit that faces these responsibilities together does best. The responsibility of the psychiatric consultant is to see the patient, make a diagnosis, and prescribe appropriate treatment. The therapeutic approach is multimodal and closely integrated with the rest of the patient's critical care.

REFERENCES

1. McKegney FP: Intensive care syndrome: definition, treatment and prevention of new "disease of medical progress." *Conn Med* 1966; 30:633–636.
2. Cassem NH: Critical care psychiatry, in Shoemaker WC, Thompson WL, Holbrook PR (eds): *Textbook of Critical Care*. Philadelphia, WB Saunders Co, 1984, pp 981–989.
3. Cassem NH, Hackett TP: Psychiatric consultation in a coronary care unit. *Ann Intern Med* 1971; 75:9–14.
4. Ludwig AM: *Principles of Clinical Psychiatry*. New York, The Free Press, 1980, p 234.
5. Drugs that cause psychiatric symptoms. *Med Lett Drugs Ther* 1981; 23:9.
6. Stern TA: Continuous infusion of physostigmine in anticholinergic delirium: case report. *J Clin Psychiatry* 1983; 44:463–464.
7. Greenblatt DJ: Pharmacokinetic comparisons. *Psychosomatics* 1980; 21 (suppl):9–14.
8. Hackett TP, Cassem NH, Wishnie HA: The coronary care unit: an appraisal of its psychological hazards. *N Engl J Med* 1968; 279:1365–1370.
9. Sos J, Cassem NH: Managing postoperative agitation. *Drug Ther* 1980; 10:103–106.
10. Ayd FJ: Intravenous haloperidol therapy. *Int Drug Ther Newsletter* 1978; 13:20–23.
11. Tesar GE, Murray GB, Cassem NH: Use of high-dose intravenous haloperidol in the treatment of agitated cardiac patients. *J Clin Psychopharmacol* 1985; 5:344–347.
12. Adams F, Fernandez F, Andersson BS: Emergency pharmacotherapy of delirium in the critically ill cancer patient. *Psychosomatics* 1986; 27(suppl): 33–37.
13. Adams F: Cardiovascular effects of phenelzine and amitriptyline. *J Clin Psychiatry* 1982; 43:472.
14. Feeley TW: Problems in weaning patients from ventilators. *Resident Staff Physician* 1976; 22:51–55.
15. Benson HA: *The Relaxation Response*. New York, William Morrow & Co, Inc, 1975.
16. Druss RG, Kornfeld DS: The survivors of cardiac arrest. *JAMA* 1967; 201:291–296.
17. Dlin BM, Stern A, Poliakoff SJ: Survivors of cardiac arrest. *Psychosomatics* 1974; 15:61–67.
18. Lemire JG, Johnson AL: Is cardiac resuscitation worthwhile? *N Engl J Med* 1972; 286:970–972.
19. Minuck M, Perkins R: Long-term study of patients successfully resuscitated following cardiac arrest. *Anesth Analg* 1970; 49:115–118.
20. White RL, Liddon SC. Ten survivors of cardiac arrest. *Psychiatr Med* 1972; 3:219–225.
21. Hackett TP: The Lazarus complex revisited. *Ann Intern Med* 1972; 76:135–136.
22. Netelson BH: Neurocardiology: an interdisciplinary area for the 80's. *Arch Neurol* 1985; 42:178–184.
23. Samuels M: Electrocardiographic manifestations of neurologic disease.

Semin Neurol 1984; 4:453–461.

24. Friedman M: *Pathogenesis of Coronary Artery Disease.* New York, McGraw-Hill Book Co, 1969.

25. The Review Panel on Coronary-Prone Behavior and Coronary Heart Disease: Coronary-Prone Behavior and Coronary Heart Disease. A critical review. *Circulation* 1981; 63:1199–1215.

26. Friedman M, Thoresen CE, Gill JJ, et al: Alteration of type A behavior and its effect on cardiac recurrences in post myocardial infarction patients: Summary results of the recurrent coronary prevention project. *Am Heart J* 1986; 112:653–665.

27. Gill JJ, Price VA, Friedman M, et al: Reduction in type A behavior in healthy middle-aged American military officers. *Am Heart J* 1985; 110:503–514.

28. Powell LH, Friedman M, Thoresen CE, et al: Can type A behavior pattern be altered after myocardial infarction? A second-year report from the recurrent coronary prevention project. *Psychosom Med* 1984; 46:293–313.

29. Moody RA Jr: *Life after Life.* Atlanta, Mockingbird Books, 1975.

30. Klein RF, et al: Transfer from a coronary care unit: some adverse responses. *Arch Intern Med* 1968; 122:104–108.

31. Safer P, quoted in *Hospital Tribune*, March 17, 1975, p 20.

19

Hemodialysis and Renal Transplantation

OWEN S. SURMAN

Once accessible to only a few, treatment of end-stage renal disease (ESRD) is now a multibillion dollar health care specialty available by law to the 60 to 90 new uremics per million population diagnosed each year in the United States. This chapter addresses the psychological management of dialysis patients and transplant recipients.

THE HEMODIALYSIS PATIENT

Refinements in hemodialysis and peritoneal dialysis have provided a practical alternative utilized by 90% of patients with ESRD. The overall mortality of patients receiving this mode of treatment continues to be approximately 10% per year. But many dialysis patients are able to pursue a satisfying level of work, recreational activity, and family life. One source gives 20% as the rate of total rehabilitation among dialysis patients.[1] More recent data by Evans et al show 45% to 59% of patients functioning with almost normal activity, depending on the type of dialysis.[2] Contributing to the overall adjustment to hemodialysis are the disease variables, treatment aspects, and psychosocial factors.[3]

Disease Variables

Initial experience with hemodialysis is influenced by severity and chronicity of illness, as well as by patient expectation and technical factors. For sicker patients, the relief following initiation of dialysis allows for a so-called honeymoon period. Those with slowly progressive chronic illness may dread the loss of autonomy associated with "the machine." Some may attempt to circumvent the procedure by opting for early transplantation. That may be a practical alternative, at times, but subsequent fears of rejection are potentially compounded when the patient has no prior successful mastery of the dialysis setting.

Those with systemic diseases such as diabetis mellitus, lupus, and hypertension tend to tolerate dialysis less well than patients with primary disease of the kidney. Most vulnerable is the juvenile diabetic patient whose distress is often compounded by fear of retinal hemorrhage in the setting of pre-existent retinopathy. Diabetics do best with sensitive, consistent support by a physician familiar with the special needs of this population. An example is the case of one young diabetic woman with failing vision who left her family home in the Middle West and came to Boston to undergo renal transplantation. While initiating dialysis she simultaneously began a self-managed business venture. Fear of further visual loss and of graft rejection were a source of considerable anxiety best managed with meticulous teaching and care from a nephrologist who provided continuity throughout the patient's course of treatment.

Genetic versus acquired disease may also influence adjustment. Patients with heredofamilial disease may identify with the adverse experience or mortality of their forebearers. Those with children may bear a sense of genetic guilt for their offspring. Awareness may be at a preconscious level for these patients and some may profit from brief psychotherapy.

Central nervous system abnormalities are frequent among dialysis patients. No one toxic metabolic factor is preeminent. Contributing factors are anemia, endocrinopathy, hypertension, and cardiovascular disease. While organicity may be evident in routine mental status examination, an acute change or progression of such deficit should lead to excluding cerebral hemorrhage, seizure disorder, dialysis dysequilibrium, or dialysis dementia. Seizure disorders are especially frequent in this patient population. In the presence of psychotic disturbance or recurrent unexplained lability of affect it is important to be aware that complex partial seizure disorders may be responsible. Even catatonia may present in this fashion.[4] Effective seizure control is often readily obtained with phenytoin or carbamazepine. Patients with this degree of complexity will generally have an array of needs: supportive psychotherapy, family and social intervention, and support of medical and nursing personnel.

Treatment Variables

Hemodialysis is accomplished in a variety of settings. Most familiar to the general hospital physician is the acute care unit where treatment is characteristically initiated. Here the intensity of physician and nursing support are at a maximum. But, for the new dialysand, anxiety may be increased in the presence of a relatively sick patient population. Satellite units provide facilities for chronic care. Patients often describe them as impersonal. But presence of a stable population of chronic dialysis patients offers an intrinsic support. Some who have made a difficult start in the acute setting will improve noticeably once transfer to the satellite unit has been completed. Home dialysis, the third available option, accounts for 16% of worldwide dialysis treatment; it is less costly and affords the greatest degree of autonomy, albeit sometimes at the expense of harmonious family relations. The dialysand's family role may be displaced as he or she takes on the role of patient while the spouse becomes a surrogate nurse. For one couple, an independent entrepreneurial dialysand wife found herself in increasing conflict with a husband who thrived in the role of caregiver. Awareness of the potential for conflict between intelligent assertive individuals placed in this type of setting allows for effective brief psychotherapeutic intervention in which the dynamics may be productively explored. Part-time involvement of a paid dialysis technician may also be beneficial in such situations.

The question of autonomy with hemodialysis is a significant existential issue. Self-care is available to a degree in a number of chronic dialysis units. Many patients are capable of dialyzing themselves with relatively minimal supervision. Since ten to 15 hours per week of dialysis time is required for most patients, scheduling is an added concern. Those desirous of traveling may arrange for a temporary dialysis slot in a distant city. Dialysis cruises have been made available by enterprising individuals.

The central principle of dialysis is exchange of waste for replacement of fluid and solutes across a semipermeable membrane. There are variations in dialysis equipment and variable characteristics of individual adaptiveness.[5,6] Overly vigorous correction of azotemia may be associated with osmotic imbalance and rapid shifts in pH leading to dialysis disequilibrium, a transient disorder varying from headache, nausea, and irritability to seizure and psychosis. Reversible CNS lesions may also be caused by ischemia.[7] Some patients may poorly metabolize acetate, an ingredient of dialysis fluid. These individuals often improve when dialyzed with a bicarbonate bath. For others dietary excess may result in dangerously high potassium levels between treatment. This may be associated with cardiac arrhythmia and death.

Dialysis dementia.   Dialysis dementia is a rare, fatal, complication of hemodialysis thought to be related to excessive exposure to aluminum salts. The symptoms consist of speech abnormality, myoclonus, increasing encephalopathy, seizures, and characteristic EEG findings.[8-10] Timely renal transplantation has on occasion led to significant improvement in this otherwise progressive disorder.

The attitude and rapport of the dialysis staff is of great significance. Invariably, dialysis demands considerable dependence on medical personnel. The associations between patient and physician, patient and dialysis nurse are dynamic, colored by personal style and social setting. Kaplan De-Nour has studied the adverse impact of excessive physician denial on patient adjustment.[11] Physician bias for or against hemodialysis versus alternative uremia therapy is also of importance in patient acceptance.[12] The challenge to the nephrologist is to adapt the treatment of end-stage renal disease to the profile of each individual patient.

Psychosocial Factors

The cost of ESRD management brings attention to the psychological adjustment of patients in this group. Frequent reference is found to the occurrence of depression and its contribution to morbidity and mortality among dialysands.[13,14] Estimates of the suicide rate in the dialysis population vary widely.[14] Neu and Kjellstrand[15] report a 15-fold increase in the rate of suicide among dialysis patients as compared to the general population. The authors differentiate between suicide and a 9% incidence of discontinued dialysis among 1766 patients studied at the Regional Kidney Disease Center, Hennepin County Medical Center, Minnesota. Brain disease and acute catastrophic illness were the most frequent complications, and age and diabetes the strongest risk factors leading to withdrawal from dialysis. Among those who withdrew from treatment, half were competent. Thirty-nine percent of those who were competent had no new medical illness preceding the decision to discontinue dialysis.[15]

Many dialysis patients, even among those interviewed for pretransplant screening, are coping relatively well. One instructive study by Cassileth et al[16] compared 758 patients in six chronic illness categories with measures of psychological status. The cohort included 60 ESRD patients, half of whom were receiving hemodialysis and half chronic abdominal peritoneal dialysis. Other categories of illness were: arthritis, diabetis, cancer, dermatologic illness, and depression. Psychological status did not differ among the groups of somatically impaired patients who appeared to be coping well relative to the general population. But all were significantly better adapted than the patients under treatment for depression.[16]

Sexual dysfunction is common in the dialysis population.[13,17] Women tend to experience altered menstrual function and, often, diminished libido. Pregnancy has been reported but infertility is the rule. Among males there is a reduction of testosterone, and decreased spermatogenesis. For both males and females there is inadequate hypothalamic-pituitary response to gonadal function.[18,19] Endocrine change, antihypertensive medication, general health impairment, altered social roles, and depression contribute to impaired sexual function. Levy used a nationwide questionnaire and reported partial or complete impotence in 56% of dialysis patients and 43% of transplant patients.[20] Generally, transplantation has been associated with improvement in sexual experience.[21,22] Salvatierra et al reported pre-illness levels of sexual function in 27 (84%) of 32 patients with a functioning transplant for 3 or more years.[23] Sexual counseling supports couples in optimizing interaction and maintaining intimacy. Some males with persisting potency impairment may be candidates for a penile prosthesis.

Personality variables are of consequence in all chronic disease. In the case of hemodialysis this is dramatized by the nature of the technology. For some, the dependence on such close medical supervision is painful indeed. One young woman ultimately resolved the issue by learning home dialysis and taking over her entire self-care when a trained partner became unavailable. Some, as previously discussed, have opted out of treatment or discontinued dialysis, a situation somewhat analogous to that presented by the cancer patient who chooses not to undergo chemotherapy. This can be exceedingly stressful for both family and medical staff. But the competent patient has a necessary right to choose between treatment and no treatment.

Some approach hemodialysis with stoic determination, while for others it looms as a formidable barrier. Kaplan De-Nour and Czaczkes studied 136 dialysis patients and found the most successful adaptation to be among those who rejected dependency and who effectively handled anger.[23] Denial is an important defense which allows the dialysand to selectively attend to areas of intact function.

For the overly anxious patient with chronic renal failure the dialysis unit and staff are best introduced several weeks ahead of time. Patients beginning dialysis may benefit from self-help groups such as the National Association of Patients on Hemodialysis and Transplantation (NAPHT) and the Kidney Transplant Dialysis Association (KTDA). Psychotherapy, when introduced in the dialysis setting, is necessarily brief, ego-supportive, and pragmatic in focus. For some patients hypnotherapy has been a useful technique for anxiety reduction and development of psychotherapeutic rapport. Hypnosis is especially suited to the patient whose fears are pain-related, or to the self-care–oriented patient desirous of enhanced control.[24]

Depression is most commonly seen in those of advancing age, with severe illness, and without sufficient family and financial supports. Their special needs highlight the importance of a resourceful, compassionate social worker as a member of the dialysis team. Also at risk for depression are those with personal and family histories of affective disorder and alcohol abuse. When clinical depression is evident, a trial of **antidepressant medication should be entertained. Where sleep disorder is** marked, doxepin hydrochloride and trazodone hydrochloride have frequently been helpful. When depression is combined with panic-type anxiety, imipramine hydrochloride or desipramine hydrochloride may be used alone or in combination with alprazolam. While these drugs are hepatically metabolized, lower doses are more often used than among otherwise healthy depressed psychiatric patients. Maintenance doses for some commonly encountered psychotropic agents have been tabulated by Bennett et al[25] (Table 19-1). One may choose to either increase dosage intervals or to administer smaller doses in keeping with changes in biological half-life as renal function declines.[25] When prescribing trycyclic antidepressants it is convenient to begin empirically with 25 mg of desipramine, or the equivalent dose of another compound, and to titrate the dosage upward in 25-mg increments on successive dialysis days, after observing carefully for anticholinergic effects, orthostatic hypotension, and other side effects. The rate of increase should be further individualized for patients of advanced age or with additional organic dysfunction. In severe, life-threatening depression electroconvulsive therapy (ECT) should be considered, as would be the case in standard psychiatric care.

Ethical Issues in Hemodialysis

Patients with uremia are a singular group for whom catastrophic illness is covered by federal law. Nonetheless Relman and Drummond have observed that utilization of hemodialysis and transplantation varies as widely among the states as it does among nations.[26] The authors aptly conclude that some patients are not being treated who could benefit and some are being treated "who cannot benefit." Regional attitudes tend to vary. As Levy[18] points out, many nephrologists favor the approach most familiar to them. The relationship between a nephrologist and the regional centers of transplantation is also important. And "selfish economic factors" may at times influence the decision to continue a patient on an established treatment program as opposed to losing that patient to a surgical center.[18]

Many clinicians are concerned about the possibility of future health care rationing in the United States. At the same time, there are genuine

Table 19-1. Psychotropic Medication in Renal Failure

| Drug | Route of Excretion | Normal Half-Life (h) | Maintenance Dose Intervals | | | | Significant Dialysis of Drug | Toxic Effects *Remarks |
| | | | Normal | Renal Failure | | | | |
				Mild	Moderate	Severe		
Barbiturates*								*For drugs in this subgroup, hemodialysis at least two times more effective than peritoneal dialysis
Amobarbital (Amytal)	Hepatic	0.6 (part)‡ 15.8–21 (part)	IM or IV bolus	Unchanged	Unchanged	Unchanged	No (HP)*	†Group toxicity; *Subgroup remarks; hemodialysis may be useful in poisoning; ‡Biexponential pharmacokinetics
Phenobarbital	Hepatic (Renal: 30%)	37–96	q 8 h	q 8 h	q 8 h	q 8–16 h (×2)	Yes (HP)*	†Group toxicity; *Subgroup remarks
Secobarbital (Seconal)	Hepatic	?	q h s	Unchanged	Unchanged	Unchanged	No (HP)	†Group toxicity; *Subgroup remarks; hemodialysis may be useful in poisoning
Benzodiazepines Chlordiazepoxide (Librium)	Hepatic	22–24	q 8 h	q 8 h	q 8–12 h (×1.5)	q 12–24 h (×1.5–3)	No (H)	†Group toxicity
Diazepam (Valium)	Hepatic	2–10 (part)‡ 48–192 (part)	q 8 h	Unchanged	Unchanged	Unchanged	No (H)*	Group toxicity; *May need supplemental dose if used as an anticonvulsant; ‡Complex biexponential pharmacokinetics

Drug	Route	Half-life (h)	Normal	Mild	Moderate	Severe	Dialysis	Comments
Ethchlorvynol (Placidyl)	? Hepatic (Renal)	?21–105	q h s	Unchanged	Unchanged	Unchanged	Yes [HP]	†Group toxicity ? Nephrotoxic
Glutethimide (Doriden)	Hepatic	?10–45‡	q h s	q h s	q h s	Avoid	No (HP)	†Group toxicity *Half-life increase with dose and hypotension
Lithium carbonate	Renal	24–48	q 8 h	q 8 h	Avoid	Avoid	Yes [HP]	†Group toxicity Nephrogenic diabetes insipidus; toxic effects increased by sodium depletion
Meprobamate (Miltown, Equanil)	Hepatic (Renal: 10%)**	8	q 6 h	q 6 h	q 9–12 h (×1.5–2)	q 12–18 h (×2–3)	Yes [HP]*	†Group toxicity *H is two times more effective than P †May be increased by saline diuresis
Methaqualone (Quaalude, Mandrax)	Nonrenal	2.6	q 8 h	Unchanged	Unchanged	Unchanged	Yes [H]	†Group toxicity; contaminant (orthotolidine) may cause hemorrhagic cystitis
Phenothiazines*	Hepatic		q 6 h	q 6 h	q 9–12 h (×1.5–2)	q 12–18 h (×2–3)	No (HP)	†Group toxicity; anticholinergic; may cause urinary retention, pigmentation, lactation *Prototype: chlorpromazine
Tricyclic antidepressants*								*All agents in this subgroup anticholinergic; may cause urinary retention; may decrease hypotensive effects of guanidinium drugs; increased excretion in acid urine (total excretion remains **small**)

Table 19-1. Psychotropic Medication in Renal Failure—continued

Amitriptyline hydrochloride (Elavil)	? Hepatic[+]	41–45	q 8 h	Unchanged	Unchanged	Unchanged	? Yes (P) No (H)	[+]Group toxicity •Subgroup remarks [‡]Metabolized to nortriptyline
Desipramine hydrochloride (Norpramin)	? Hepatic (Renal: <5%)	4–35[‡]	q 8 h	Unchanged	Unchanged	Unchanged	?	[+]Group toxicity •Subgroup remarks [‡]Genetic variation in metabolism
Imipramine hydrochloride (Tofranil)	? Hepatic[+] (? Renal)	3.5	q 8 h	Unchanged	Unchanged	Unchanged	? Yes (P) No (H)	[+]Group toxicity •Subgroup remarks ? Nephrotoxic [‡]Metabolized to desmethylimipramine
Nortriptyline hydrochloride (Aventyl)	? Hepatic (Renal: <5%)	18.1–38[‡]	q 8 h	Unchanged	Unchanged	Unchanged	? Yes (P) No (H)	[+]Group toxicity •Subgroup remarks [‡]Genetic variation in metabolism

Reproduced with permission from Bennett et al.[25]
H = hemodialysis, P = peritoneal dialysis.
[+]All agents in this group may cause excessive sedation.

concerns about overly aggressive medical care for those who are unable themselves to opt out.

Continuous Abdominal Peritoneal Dialysis

Continuous abdominal peritoneal dialysis (CAPD) is a technique which has evolved over the past decade for dialysis between peritoneal fluid and plasma in ambulatory patients. A permanent indwelling catheter is used for exchanges performed by the patient for approximately two hours daily. Advantages include increased patient autonomy and dietary freedom, reduced cardiovascular stress, diminished blood loss, avoidance of anticoagulation with heparin sodium, lack of necessity for vascular access, and diminished blood loss. The method is particularly advantageous for those with severely impaired cardiac function and for stabilization of vision in type 1 diabetic patients. Patients must be well motivated, intelligent, adequately trained, and possess sufficient manual dexterity and special sensory function to follow strict sterile technique. Peritonitis is the main disadvantage and is typically signaled by changes in the color of peritoneal fluid which are readily evident to patients capable of careful self-observation. Additional disadvantages include excessive weight gain, body image distortion, nutritional impairment, and absence of social interactions of the dialysis center. Those most likely to fail at CAPD are the elderly, the intellectually impaired, and patients with poor motivation or inadequate social support.[27,28]

There is some evidence for comparable life styles among CAPD patients and in-center dialysis patients. Direct measurement of adjustment to CAPD versus hemodialysis requires large prospective studies of patients with similar medical findings and psychosocial features.[2] Analysis of CAPD registry data indicates that over a 2-year period there is increasing transfer from CAPD to hemodialysis. Transfer is related to repeated episodes of peritonitis or other medical complications, to patient noncompliance, or to patient and family preference.[28-30]

THE RENAL TRANSPLANT PATIENT

At the forefront of renal transplantation are concerns about delivery of care. Renal tranplantation enjoys full government support but accounts for only 10% of ESRD management. Some blame medical economics, and especially the for-profit dialysis centers for the discrepancy in incidence of prescribed therapy with hemodialysis versus transplantation. Most evident is the relative shortage of donor organs and the growing lists of immunologically sensitized individuals awaiting grafts. Currently there are two sources of transplantable organs: living donors and cadaveric donors. A third approach, xenografts from other species, may someday be a source of treatment and of controversy.[31]

Transplant Donors

Since the first successful renal transplant between human twins, medical and legal opinion in the United States has supported living related organ donation, not only from healthy adults capable of informed consent, but in selected instances from assenting minors and, at least in one case, from a retarded donor.[32] In support of this approach is the significant likelihood of success for the recipient, a low complication rate for the donor, and a conviction that the living related donor will be disadvantaged by the death or continuing illness of the recipient. For a brief time pioneering efforts in transplantation allowed for participation by prisoner volunteers. The latter practice ended once ethical constraints were evident.

Early psychological observation led to inquiry into the validity of donor altruism. Depression noted among some donors following surgery was explainable by separation in hospital from the supportive influence of the transplant unit staff and the allograft recipient. Another concern was family coercion, particularly in instances where a "black sheep" donor sought improved recognition within the family system. Fellner and Marshall demonstrated that the decision to be a donor was frequently a spontaneous act of giving.[33] Others, especially Simmons et al, confirmed the long-term psychological benefits of organ donorship.[21]

The concept of living related organ donation has not received worldwide acceptance. Serious postoperative complications are uncommon.[34] Death following kidney donation is rare but documented. (The risk of death for donors is thought equivalent to the risk for urban commuters driving 16 miles daily.) A growing success rate with cadaveric organ transplants is an added factor in the desirability of this approach.[35] Brain death following catastrophic accidents is the source of cadaver kidneys. The possibility of transplantation provides hope to the ESRD patient and meaning to the bereaved family of the donor. But despite the utilitarian value of cadaveric transplant surgery, the availability of organs is inadequate. Several countries have addressed this problem with laws of presumed consent. These so-called opting-out laws provide availability of transplantable organs unless informed family members choose actively against organ donation. While it remains to be established that this approach would or would not be acceptable to the American public, some in the United States are concerned about backlash with this type of legislation. Caplan[36] has suggested "required consent" by hospital authorities from the relatives of brain-dead individuals.[31] The impact of organ retrieval on hospital personnel and families has been discussed by Youngner et al.[37]

Advantages of living related donor participation include: availability and improved condition of retrieved organs, and the opportunity for donor-specific pretransplantation transfusion. Transfusion, a topic of current controversy, may be associated with improved outcome for allograft recipients, possibly because immunologic suppressor systems are activated.[38] And there are psychologic benefits for the recipient who can be spared the uncertain timing of cadaveric transplantation. These advantages have led some to consider the ethics of living nonrelatives as candidates for organ donorship.[39] Some centers, notably the University of Minnesota, have experience in work with spousal donors and distant relatives.[40]

Donor Selection

The selection of organ donors requires an evaluating physician who can act as health care advocate for the donor. And there must be available psychiatric consultation. Generally, those potential donors with major active psychiatric disorders are screened out by the recipient, the family, the primary care health provider, or the evaluating nephrologist. The transplant unit at Massachusetts General Hospital (MGH) provides for weekly "family meetings" which allow for mutual assessment and development of rapport between patients and the surgical team. Present at these meetings are the recipient, potential donors, immediate family (or close friends), staff nephrologist, staff surgeon, unit social worker, and consulting psychiatrist. The central topic is informed consent. The team provides factual data about transplant surgery while respectfully acknowledging the deliberative process and stresses experienced by the family. Specific psychiatric evaluation is provided in the event of ambivalence, untoward anxiety, depression, or disconcerting behavior on the part of the recipient or donor.

The anxious donor presents a challenge similar to the anxious patient encountering elective surgery. A cognitive behavioral approach is appropriate for desensitization of mild phobic symptoms in a donor who has made a clear choice. The ambivalent donor often resolves the conundrum in a passive way by choosing to avoid the necessary steps (eg, tissue typing) for transplant. Alternatively, a brief series of visits with the psychiatrist allows the ambivalent donor to approach the pros and cons of further involvement in a setting where factual feedback and acceptance are both at hand. Four donors in the past few years have given preoperative evidence of alcohol abuse. The first three were encouraged to become abstinent prior to surgery but were involved in no formal rehabilitation program. Surgery proved psychologically uneventful in only one of these three cases.[3] Although the three recipients had prolonged allograft survival it seemed prudent when the fourth alcoholic donor presented to mandate an alcohol rehabilitation program. In this instance, the HLA (the major histocompatibility gene complex)-identical donor brother indicated a strong willingness to pursue surgery and entered a previously encountered alcohol rehabilitation program. His sobriety lasted less than a month and he was engaged in no further discussion of organ donorship with the family or transplant staff. The intended recipient was placed on the cadaveric donor list.

At times there is an unusual element of human drama associated with organ donation. In one instance a hospital employee offered to donate a kidney to anyone in need. This type of offer is not unknown and is appropriately met with appreciation and a gentle no. In another case an adopted patient in his early twenties met his biological mother for the first time and was the recipient of a kidney. The allograft did not survive but their new relationship prospered. Complications may occur unexpectedly when the donor work-up yields evidence of differing parentage among siblings. And there are cases where an able donor withdraws because of financial concerns or pressure brought to bear by an unwilling spouse. In one recent case an intended donor came to psychiatric consultation with his wife who had avoided meeting with our transplant team. This young woman proved knowledgeable about the risks and benefits of her husband's planned organ donation; but she came from a broken, alcohol-impaired, family setting and the remote possibility of sustaining a further loss had precipitated a depression. Once able to understand the basis of his wife's distress, the donor withdrew from the planned procedure and another member of his family of origin proceeded with a donor work-up.

One requirement in organ donation is that the donor not profit monetarily. The ethics are clear enough. But donors do at times undergo legitimate hardship from loss of work or travel expense. Some form of government-approved compensation for these losses seems appropriate to this author.[31] A more pressing current issue is the need for vigilance for fictitious relatives pressed into service by affluent individuals from other lands.

Four factors interact to determine the outcome of renal transplantation: (1) the rejection reaction, (2) the side effects of immunosuppressive medication, (3) the pathophysiology of underlying disease, and (4) the psychosocial setting.

Graft Survival

Absence of a rejection reaction to the renal allograft is an uncommon event.[41] Only identical twins have identical immunologic characteristics. Currently, living related donor (LRD) transplants at MGH have an 80% to 90% 1-year survival rate. Cadaveric transplants (CD) are viable at 1 year approximately 80% of the time. Current figures for 3-year renal allograft survival are: living related kidneys, 80%; cadaveric kidneys, 55%. Recent improvements at 1 year suggest that 3-year statistics will also improve. The overall 1-year mortality rate after renal transplantation at MGH is less than 5%; the rate declines progressively with each succeeding year of allograft survival (Cosimi AB, personal communication, November, 1986). Evans et al studied 859 ESRD patients and found that 79% of transplant recipients (half having received LRD, and half CD transplants) were functioning at "nearly normal" levels.[2]

Immunosuppressant Side Effects

Techniques for controlling rejection include immunosuppressant drugs, graft radiation, and total lymphatic irradiation (TLI). Most important among the immunosuppressant drugs are prednisone, azathioprine, antithymocyte globulin, anti-T cell subtype monoclonal antibodies, and cyclosporine.

The side effects of prednisone are well known. Most noteworthy from a psychiatric perspective are altered mood states which we observe in approximately 15% of transplant recipients. Most infrequent is the full-blown syndrome of steroid psychosis which presents characteristically as an affective psychosis with mixed manic and depressive features. More often one encounters volatility of mood, as well as restlessness and irritability which is often more evident to family members and coworkers than to the patient. One possibility is that some of these phenomena might represent a complex partial seizure event.[4]

Reactions to steroid medication and other chemotherapeutic agents is most intense in the early transplant period. By 3 to 6 months a majority of patients are experiencing stable allograft function and a concomitant reduction in the need for these medications. For some, a frank cushingoid syndrome develops and persists with associated weakness, centripital obesity, acniform lesions, and other stigmata. Cataracts, diabetes mellitus, and bone abnormalities are among the potential complications of prednisone.

Of greatest concern is the threat of infection to the immunosuppressed transplant recipient. Infection in this setting has a high rate of morbidity and mortality. Infections typically occur with resident organisms of the herpes virus group (especially cytomegalovirus [CMV], herpes simplex virus [HSV], and varicella zoster virus [VZV]). The results are often debilitating with systemic manifestations, pain, and/or reversible cosmetic effects. Of particular interest is the occurrence of depression in these patients.[3] Depressed affect and mood accompanied by social withdrawal, decreased physical activity, impaired vegetative function, and decreased verbal communication occurs frequently with the *CMV mononucleosis syndrome*. The degree of depression in these patients may attract psychiatric consultation before the infectious aspects are clearly documented. Typically, these patients do not express feelings of worthlessness, hopelessness, or suicidal ideation and there is usually no prior history of depressive disorder. Other types of infection may occur with common bacterial agents or more exotic organisms such as *Pneumocystis*, *Legionella*, or fungi: *Aspergillus*, *Candida*, or *Cryptoccocus*. Meningitis and brain abcess of fungal etiology must be considered as a cause of altered cognition, especially when accompanied by headache and febrile illness. These otherwise uncommon maladies become a part of the differential diagnosis in the transplant patient referred for psychiatic evaluation.

The newcomer among immunosuppressive agents is cyclosporine,[1] credited with the recently improved results in organ transplantation. Cyclosporine allows for rapid reduction in prednisone dose and a reduction in steroid-linked morbidity. One patient with a past history of prednisone psychosis prior to transplantation had no untoward psychiatric effects in the first year following transplantation with a protocol of cyclosporine and prednisone. But cyclosporine is a toxic agent with nephrotoxic, hepatotoxic, and neurotoxic properties. Blood pressure elevation and a coarse resting tremor are at times associated with its administration. A further limiting factor and source of psychological stress is the cost of cyclosporine: approximately $5000 per year per patient.[18]

Disease Recurrence and Progression

For some renal transplant candidates there is a possibility of recurrence of the underlying lesion. Some cases of focal sclerosis are examples of this. One of our patients had a marked intolerance for hemodialysis. A series of four transplants ensued, followed in each instance by graft loss. In diabetes mellitus, recurrence of the renal lesion is sufficiently slow to allow for effective long-term renal allograft function. But prednisone undermines established diabetic control. Over the years following transplantation these patients suffer from tragic progression of diabetic morbidity. Recent progress with pancreatic transplants is an exciting development for the future care of these patients. Another experimental effort is injection of pancreatic islet cells to promote endogenous insulin production in an organ system other than the pancreas (Russell PS, personal communication, May, 1985).

Psychological Aspects of Kidney Transplantation

Regardless of the physiologic health of the individual patient and skill of the transplant team, successful organ transplantation can be seriously undermined in an unfavorable psychosocial environment. One adolescent patient would react to his mother's periodic return to a violent love relationship with a male friend by discontinuing medication and forcing hospitalization with graft rejection. A second transplant in the same individual is hostage to his intolerance of prednisone-induced alteration of body image. Another adolescent has a borderline personality and extensive family history of sexual abuse and emotional deprivation. Multiple psychiatric hospitalizations and out-patient psychiatric support were insufficient to prevent repeated immunosuppressant dosing irregularities and graft loss. One adult male has chronic failure of his renal allograft as a result of numerous episodes of alcohol excess and forgotten doses of immunosuppressive agents.

Acute psychological disturbance can seriously undermine the necessary partnership between transplant patient and surgical team. Disruption of medical compliance may occur in the case of acute depression, psychotic disturbances, and CNS disorders which interfere with memory and cognition. In most instances patients are able to draw from family or other environmental supports, rapport with the transplant team, and supportive psychiatric intervention to continue satisfactory medical management despite acute stress or chronic psychological impairment.

Patient Selection

The selection of transplant patients was once a matter for special boards which became known as "God squads." Renal transplantation is now a well-established technique. The mix of patients provides a broad social cross-section with an incidence of major primary psychiatric abnormalities in approximate proportion to the general population. In recent years we have treated four patients with borderline to moderate mental retardation, one with bipolar affective disorder, two with histories of incarceration for antisocial acts, and several with diagnoses of anxiety or depressive disorder, alcoholism, and personality disturbance. One patient has had marked improvement with transplant following a well-established diagnosis of dialysis dementia. Preoperative depression in the ESRD patient is often an incentive to surgery rather than a cause for postponement. Primary depressive disorders are optimally treated prior to transplantation. Age is not an isolated exclusion criterion. One 68-year-old man sought renal transplantation to improve his capacity for physical activity. He wished to build a rock wall and did so following his surgery.

Renal transplantation does not necessitate exclusive psychosocial criteria. Ability to predict long-term graft survival from psychosocial determinants is limited. Any motivated patient who can medically tolerate transplantation and has a reasonable physiologic chance of benefiting is a potential candidate. The likelihood of success is enhanced with mobilization of appropriate social supports for the patient with special needs.

Postoperative Adjustment

Early psychiatric observation of transplant patients focused on psychological incorporation of the new graft.[42] There are isolated accounts of altered identity in transplant patients. Abram wrote of a Ku Klux Klan grand dragon who joined the NAACP upon learning that his renal allograft came from a black donor.[43] Most often patients express a sense of gratitude without guilt about their allograft. For some there may be a special term of endearment applied to the new organ or plans for an anniversary celebration.

The increasingly routine nature of renal transplant mitigates against untoward psychological events. Rarely, a patient experiences guilt related to a contemporary on dialysis who faired less well. Brief psychotherapy is effective in such cases.

Uncertainty is the principal psychological stress for the transplant patient. First there is the wait, at times extensive, for those on cadaveric donor lists. In the immediate period following surgery there may be a time of impaired graft function, from acute tubular injury, for example, which necessitates a brief return to dialysis. Renal allografts often function immediately with rapid reduction of azotemia. Improved strength and a period of understandable euphoria may be followed by the stress of rejection, typically first encountered at seven to ten days. In the presence of rejection there is a reversible depression of mood accompanied by decreased activity and social withdrawal.

For a short period before and after hospital discharge, the transplant recipient may be apprehensive about absence of close daily observation. Such concern recedes as the patient returns to clinic with improved physical repair and function. In the absence of major complications patients return to work at 4 to 6 months, and by 1 year are experiencing increasingly normal function and appearance.

Occasionally one encounters prolonged convalescence. Typically, this occurs with chronically ill individuals in whom the sudden return to health pulls temporarily at established family and social patterns.[3] Some patients develop adjustment disorders with mild anxiety or depression associated with subjective complaints in the absence of identifiable malfunction. It is helpful in such instances to gently discuss potential identification with others who are undergoing active surgical complications.

Generally, as Abram observed, the emotional well-being of transplant patients runs parallel to success of allograft function.[43] With optimal surgical outcome, there is a dramatic reduction of medical dependency.

Psychiatric Intervention

As in the case of the dialysis patient, effective psychiatric consultation utilizes short-term supportive intervention combined with an understanding of psychodynamics. One middle-aged female was seen preoperatively because of untoward anxiety about her forthcoming transplant. Following surgery she experienced a transient steroid-induced mood change and mild encephalopathy. Following a reduction of steroid dosage and return of normal renal function she continued to be mildly anxious and depressed despite excellent participation and encouragement by her husband and daughter. When the patient was an adolescent her mother required dialysis treatment for renal failure secondary to amyloid disease. A period of prolonged coma ensued prior to death. Closeness between mother and daughter made this an especially tragic loss. The patient's subsequent development was satisfactory with the exception of a persisting mild anxiety disorder of the agoraphobic type. Psychiatric intervention prior to surgery proceeded with hypnosis and cognitively oriented behavior therapy. Postoperatively, a careful exploration of unresolved feelings about her mother's death was followed by the suggestion that she recapture the special meaning of their relationship. With the aid of hypnosis she was able to recall a pleasurable childhood scene of playing on a swing with her mother nearby. The patient learned to repeat this exercise on her own and did so with progressive improvement of mood and affect. Following hospital discharge she was seen for three follow-up psychotherapy sessions in which increased social activity was encouraged. The remaining phobic symptoms resolved despite newly acquired information that she too had amyloid pathology. No psychopharmacologic intervention proved necessary.

When brief supportive measures fail to ameliorate anxiety or depressive symptoms, routine pharmacologic intervention with anxiolytic agents and antidepressants is helpful. We have preferred alprazolam, starting with low doses, for the primarily anxious patient. In two instances this approach proved especially effective in weaning patients from respirator care. Treatment with alprazolam must be individualized. Some patients are unusually sensitive and may experience CNS depression or urinary retention. Others, who tolerate the drug well, have required a gradual dose increase to levels that infrequently exceed 4 to 6 mg daily. To begin treatment, a test dose of 0.25 mg may typically be followed by three-to four-times-daily administration. Doxepin has been well tolerated and effective for patients with pain, depression, and insomnia. Trazodone is an alternative if urinary retention or other disadvantageous anticholinergic effects occur. Desipramine hydrochloride, commencing at 25 mg, followed by 25-mg increments, has worked best for depressed patients experiencing lethargy and anxiety in the absence of prominent sleep impairment.

Steroid psychosis is very infrequent and may be treated with low doses of haloperidol or, in our experience, with carbamazepine when symptoms persist.[4] Whether carbamazepine has been effective in these cases because of its anticonvulsant or psychotropic properties is not clear. We also prefer carbamazepine, if well tolerated, for the prospective transplant patient with an established seizure disorder. Phenobarbital and phenytoin appear more likely to precipitate graft rejection by accelerating prednisone metabolism with induction of liver microsomal enzyme systems.

One patient of ours with bipolar affective disorder has been maintained on lithium carbonate 600 mg daily with therapeutic blood levels and prevention of mania. However lithium does have immune stimulant properties[44] and it may be preferable to use carbamazepine as substitute therapy for a manic patient who has not been maintained on lithium prior to surgery.

Transplant recipients often use denial and repression as successful defenses, especially in situations of acute medical stress. But the mobility of the transplant patient and his freedom from the encumbrance of dialysis makes him generally more available for psychotherapy. And for many the ability to speak with a psychiatrist familiar with the potential frustrations of transplantation proves a welcome relief.

Behavioral nursing approaches beneficial to care of the difficult patient may be suggested by the psychiatrist and elucidated by the psychiatric nurse clinician. At other times the psychiatrist, social worker, and psychiatric nurse-clinician interact with complementary supportive intervention in the setting of terminal care. Patient groups have been employed with varying success for transplant recipients or those awaiting surgery.

The preoperative family meeting is especially beneficial for mobilizing relatives who cannot be organ donors but may wish to play a supportive role. It allows a view of the patient's resources and prospective need for special provisions directed to an anxious patient or impaired family member. It is also a good time to address problems related to alcohol and nicotine use and to set the stage for postoperative dietary management for those who later experience prednisone-related eating disorders. The presence of a psychiatrist and social worker at the time of informed consent legitimizes the role of the health care worker and makes an important statement about the team's interest in the patient's quality of life. It is also a time that allows for introduction to the physical plant of the transplant unit and to nursing personnel. This commences an important bonding process between the patient and the transplant health team.

For optimal psychiatric care of the transplant patient the psychiatric consultant should be an identifiable member of the team who shares a common goal for patient care and rehabilitation. As a team member the psychiatrist joins in the process of teaching and learning and develops a working relationship based on understanding and respect for the style of contemporaries from other specialties. This type of association facilitates the referral process and places the psychiatrist in a supportive position relative to the team. This is desirable because of the long-term nature of the surgical team's relationship with each patient and the uncertainty which both patient and clinician encounter. The greatest psychological support to the team comes from knowledge that informed and compassionate help is at hand for emotional disorders which may follow from surgical complication or which may confound effective delivery of care. The transplant team in turn provides an opportunity for the psychiatric specialist to participate with expertise in his discipline at the forward edge of medical research and progress. With able leadership the team becomes a setting for competent health care and scientific inquiry in a spiritually productive network.

REFERENCES

1. Carpenter CB, Lazarus JM: Dialysis and transplantation in the treatment of renal failure, in Petersdorf RG, Adams RD, Braunwald E, et al (eds): *Harrison's Principles of Internal Medicine*, ed 10. New York, McGraw-Hill Book Co,

1983, pp 1619–1627.

2. Evans RW, Manninen DL, Garrison LP, et al: The quality of life of patients with end stage renal disease. *N Engl J Med* 1985; 312:553–559.

3. Surman OS: Psychiatric medicine update, in *Massachusetts General Hospital Reviews for Physicians*. New York, Elsevier Biomedical Press, 1981, pp 155–175.

4. Surman OS, Parker SW: Complex partial seizures and psychiatric disturbance in end-stage renal disease. *Psychosomatics* 1981; 22:134–137.

5. Massry SG, Sellers AL (eds): *Clinical Aspects of Uremia and Dialysis*. Springfield, Ill, Charles C Thomas Publisher, 1976.

6. Friedman EA: *Strategy in Renal Failure*. New York, John Wiley & Sons, Inc, 1978.

7. Meyrier A, Blanc F, Reignier A, et al: Unusual aspects of the dialysis disequilibrium syndrome. *Clin Nephrol* 1976; 6:311–314.

8. Alfrey AC: Dialysis encephalopathy syndrome. *Ann Rev Med* 1978; 29:93–98.

9. McDermott JR, Smith AI, Ward MK, et al: Brain aluminum concentration in dialysis encephalopathy. *Lancet* 1978; 1:901–903.

10. Victor M, Adams RD: Metabolic diseases of the nervous system, in Petersdorf RG, Adams RD, Braunwald E, et al (eds.): *Harrison's Principles of Internal Medicine*, ed 10. New York, McGraw-Hill Book Co, 1983, p 1981.

11. Kaplan De-Nour A: Prediction of adjustment to chronic hemodialysis, in Levy NB (ed.): *Psychonephrology 1 Psychological Factors in Hemodialysis and Transplantation*. New York, Plenum Medical Book Co, 1981, pp 117–133.

12. Blagg CR: Objective quantification of rehabilitation in dialysis and transplantation in Fiedman EA (ed): *Strategy in Renal Failure*. New York, John Wiley & Sons, Inc, 1970, pp 415–435.

13. Levy NB, Wynbrandt GD: The quality of life on maintenance hemodialysis. *Lancet* 1975; 1:1328–1330.

14. Burton HJ, Kline SA, Lindsay RM, et al: The relationship of depression to survival in chronic renal failure. *Psychosom Med* 1986; 48:261–269.

15. Neu S, Kjellstrand CM: Stopping long-term dialysis. *N Engl J Med* 1986; 314:14–20.

16. Cassileth BR, Lusk EJ, Strouse TB, et al: Psychosocial status in chronic illness: A comparative analysis of six diagnostic groups. *N Engl J Med* 1984; 311:506–511.

17. Levy NB: What's new on cause and treatment of sexual dysfunction in end stage renal disease, in Levy NB (ed): *Psychonephrology 1 Psychological Factors in Hemodialysis and Transplantation*. New York, Plenum Medical Book Co, 1981, pp 43–47.

18. Levy NB: Renal transplantation and the new medical era. *Adv Psychosom Med* 1986; 15:167–179.

19. Drueke T: Endocrine disorders in chronic hemodialysis patients (with the exclusion of hypoparathyroidism), in Hamburger J, Crosnier J, Grunfeld J-P, et al (eds): *Advances in Nephrology*. Chicago, Yearbook Medical Publishers Inc, 1981, vol 10, pp 351–382.

20. Levy NB: Sexual adjustment to maintenance hemodialysis and renal transplantation: national survey by questionnaire: preliminary report. *Trans Am Soc Artif Intern Organs* 1973; 19:138–142.

21. Simmons RG, Klein SD, Simmons RC: *Gift of Life: The Social and Psychological Impact of Organ Transplantation.* New York, John Wiley & Sons, Inc, 1977.
22. Salvatierra O, Fortmann JL, Belzer FO: Sexual function in males before and after renal transplantation. *Urology* 1975; 5:64–66.
23. Kaplan De-Nour A, Czaczkes JW: The influence of patient's personality in adjustment to chronic dialysis: A predictive study. *J Nerv Ment Dis* 1976; 2:323–333.
24. Surman OS, Tolkoff-Rubin N: Use of hypnosis in patients receiving hemodialysis for end stage renal disease. *Gen Hosp Psychiatry* 1984; 6:31–35.
25. Bennett WM, Singer I, Coggins CJ: A guide to drug therapy in renal failure. *JAMA* 1974; 230:1544–1553.
26. Relman AS, Drummond RD: Free but not equal. Treatment of end-stage renal disease. *N Engl J Med* 1980; 303:996–998.
27. Vantelon J, Verger C, Glennie N, et al: Pros and cons of continuous ambulatory peritoneal dialysis, in Hamburger J, Crosnier J, Grunfeld J-P (eds): *Advances in Nephrology.* Chicago, Yearbook Medical Publishers, 1982, vol 11, pp 401–424.
28. Fellner S: Continuous ambulatory peritoneal dialysis (CAPD): Update 1986. *AKF Nephrol Lett* 1986; 3:1–8.
29. Nolph KD, Cutler SJ, Steinberg SM, et al: Continuous ambulatory care peritoneal dialysis in the United States: a three year study. *Kidney Int* 1985; 28:198.
30. Steinberg SM, Cutler SJ, Nolph KD, et al: A comprehensive report on the experience of patients on continuous ambulatory peritoneal dialysis for the treatment of end stage renal disease. *Am J Kidney Dis* 1984; 4:233.
31. Surman OS: Toward greater donor organ availability for transplantation, letter. *N Engl J Med* 1985; 312:318.
32. Fabro AJ: Legal aspects of organ transplant, Strunk vs. Strunk. *Conn Med* 1970; 34:583.
33. Fellner CH, Marshall JR: Kidney donors—the myth of informed consent. *Am J Psychiatry* 126:1245–1251.
34. Cosimi AB: The donor and donor nephrectomy, in Morris PJ (ed): *Renal Transplantation—Principle and Practice.* Grune & Stratton, New York, 1979, pp 69–87.
35. Starzyl T: The present state of organ transplantation. Presented at Transplantation and Artificial Organs: Issues Along the Experiment-to-Therapy Spectrum. An Interdisciplinary Conference, sponsored by The Acadia Institute and Public Responsibility in Medicine and Research, The Hyatt Regency Hotel, Cambridge, Mass, Nov 5, 1985.
36. Caplan AL: Ethical and policy issues in the procurement of cadaver organs for transplantation. *N Engl J Med* 1985; 311:981–983.
37. Youngner SJ, Allen M, Bartlett ET, et al: Psychosocial and ethical implications of organ retrieval. *N Engl J Med* 1985; 313:321–323.
38. Opelz G, Terasaki PI: Improvement of kidney-graft survival with increased numbers of blood transfusion. *N Engl J Med* 1978; 299:799–803.
39. Surman OS: Participation of living non related donors in renal transplantation, in Hardy M, Appel G, Kiernan J, et al (eds): *Positive Aspects to Living With End Stage Renal Disease*: Psychosocial and Thanatological Aspects.

Prager, New York, in press.
40. Najarian JS, Van Hook EJ, Simmons RL: Kidney transplant from distant relatives. *Am J Surg* 1978; 135:362–366.
41. Cosimi AB, Russell PS: Tissue and organ transplantation, in Nardi GL, Zuidema GD (eds): *Surgery: A Concise Guide to Clinical Practice*, ed 4. Boston, Little, Brown & Co, 1982, pp 2688–2695.
42. Castelnuovo-Tedesco P: Transplantation: Psychological implications of changes in body image, in Levy NB (ed): *Psychonephrology 1 Psychological Factors in Hemodialysis and Transplantation*. New York, Plenum Medical Book Co, 1981, pp 219–225.
43. Abram HS: Renal transplantation, in Hackett TP, Cassem NH (eds): *Massachusetts General Hospital Handbook of General Hospital Psychiatry*. St Louis, CV Mosby Co, 1978, pp 365–379.
44. Calabrese JR, Gulledge AD, Hahn K, et al: Autoimmune thyroiditis in manic-depressive patients treated with lithium. *Am J Psychiatry* 1985; 142:1318–1321.

20

Accident Proneness and Accident Victims

JERROLD F. ROSENBAUM and JAMES E. GROVES

Despite apparent randomness, accidents often appear clinically to have been partly determined by the victim's recent emotional state and life events. After diligent investigation, or sometimes serendipitously, psychological explanations of these "chance occurrences" frequently and convincingly become accessible to the psychiatric consultant.

The general hospital patient population can be thought of as comprising two categories of individuals—the ill and the injured. While injured patients may be distinguished from ill patients by a number of characteristics such as age (younger) and prior physical condition (healthier), a major distinction is that injured persons or accident victims—formerly whole and healthy—suddenly and unexpectedly change course in their lives because of a traumatizing encounter with the physical environment. In a single moment, unanticipated and unprepared for, accident victims begin a complicated process of injury, coping, and rehabilitation.

Accident victims are found on orthopedic, general, and plastic surgery services, in burn units and intensive care units, and on rehabilitation and physical medicine wards. Accidents are the leading cause of death for individuals under the age of 44 years[1] and are responsible for disabilities accounting for billions of dollars of annual payments through insurance companies and workmen's compensation funds.[2,3] The sum total of pain, suffering, disability, and shattered dreams is not measurable. For all these reasons, the crucial moment of "the accident" clearly deserves scrutiny. Psychological understanding may perhaps prevent some serious accidents and can add to the treatment of the consequences of others.

ACCIDENTS

In *The Psychopathology of Everyday Life*[4] Freud discusses how unconscious motivation, discerned from psychoanalytic observation, appears to play a primary role in ordinary, daily accidents. An accident can be useful in a number of ways: as a self-punishment to alleviate guilt, as an excuse to avoid an unpleasant situation, as a symbolic castration, and so forth.

> What happens is that an impulse to self-punishment, which is constantly on the watch and which normally finds expression in self-reproach or contributes to the formation of a symptom, takes ingenious advantage of an external situation that chance happens to offer, or lends assistance to that situation until the desired injurious effect is brought about.[4]

In considering serious or fatal accidents, Freud invoked the concept of a death instinct. Other analytic writers expanded the notion of man's innate self-destructive forces. Menninger,[5] for instance, cites four examples of individuals killed or maimed by "forgetting" their own burglar traps and walking into them.

Whether life-threatening behavior and subintentional suicide are manifestations of thanatos, the basic death instinct, or, on the other hand, are even adequate explanations for most accidents is controversial. Psychodynamic theory offers self-destructiveness as a plausible component of the moment of self-injury but evidence supporting its primacy as the cause of most accidents is mixed. Sobel and Margolis[6] underscore how repeated accidental poisoning in children reflects family pathology. One study of people who attempted suicide[7] revealed an 81% higher accident rate than the rate for control individuals, and another report on patients with self-destructive tendencies[8] described an accident frequency twice that of the control population. Selzer et al[9] noted an **incidence of history of suicidal proclivity in 21% (compared to 8% of** the matched control group) of 96 drivers involved in fatal accidents. Tabachnick,[10] however, found that self-destructiveness is not a significant cause of accidents, and the recent thorough review of Tsuang et al[11] concluded that suicidal motivation is but a small factor in the production of motor vehicle accidents.

While suicidal and self-destructive drives are not clearly shown to be consistently linked with self-injury, the data for other psychological factors are more impressive. A number of reports suggest the importance of a variety of life changes, vocational and interpersonal stresses, and recent emotional upset in the causation of traffic accidents.[12-14] Using a modified Holmes-Rahe Scale, Selzer and Vinokur[15] emphasize the role of life events and subjective stress as precipitants of accidents. In one study, ten of 15 drivers killed in traffic accidents either had been recently given positions of increased responsibility or had been considering such a change.[16] In another study, 19 (20%) of 96 drivers involved in fatal accidents were noted to have been acutely upset in the six-hour period prior to accident, usually as the result of violent quarrels with wives or girl friends.[9] Alcohol abuse has been repeatedly indicted as a crucial contributing factor to traffic accidents[10,17,18] and is connected with at least half of all motor vehicle fatalities;[11] acute or chronic alcoholism is presumed to be a reflection of acute or chronic emotional stresses and the inability to cope with them.

While the relation of life stress to accidents via alcohol is a major route, the effect of life stress alone may also be important. In one of the two prospective studies of accidents in the literature, Sheehan et al[19] found a statistical correlation between the accident/error rate of 31 student nurses performing normal patient-care tasks on a ward during a week-long study period and their prospectively rated 2-year life-change scale. The amount of adjustment required to cope with those life changes, along with social supports, were the most powerful predictors of mishap rates and together accounted for 70% of the variance, whereas depression and innate coping skills had less predictive power than prior life stress. On the other hand, the recent review by Tsuang et al[11] acknowledged the support of earlier studies for the role of life event stress but concluded that most recent studies find very little evidence for its general importance in traffic accidents.

ACCIDENT PRONENESS

In 1919 the classic paper of Greenwood and Woods[20,21] appeared in England, a study of minor accidents befalling 648 women working in a munitions factory. Inspection of the factory accident records revealed that a minority (10%) of workers had a majority (56%) of accidents in a 13-month period, and 4% of the workers accounted for 28% of all accidents. Similarly, Marbe[22] studied 3000 German commissioned and noncomissioned officers over the period of a decade, comparing mishaps in the first and last 2- and 5-year periods. In all cases, those individuals with the most accidents in the first time periods showed an excess in the second as well. These results were later interpreted as "proving statistically"[23] that there was increased probability for accidents for an individual who had previous accidents, thus demonstrating the existence of an "accident habit."[24] There were, however, major problems with the statistical methodology.[25]

Farmer and Chambers[26–29] coined the term "accident proneness" to denote[28] "a personal idiosyncrasy predisposing the individual who possesses it in a marked degree to a relatively high accident rate." They continued to believe in it as a real thing despite statistical methodologic problems and the failure to show a correlation between proneness to major accidents as judged from minor ones or to show correlations between "proneness" in various categories of accidents, for example, home and workplace.[25] As a real statistical phenomenon, the concept has never been proved to exist,* but it was an idea that continued to appeal to researchers—despite repeated failures to prove it—through the 1950s. In fact, nowadays, researchers regard most victims, even of multiple accidents, as simply unlucky, not "accident prone."[30]

The observation that a small percentage of individuals is responsible for a relatively high percentage of industrial and traffic accidents led Dunbar,[23,31] Alexander,[32,33] and others to posit the existence of accident prone individuals having certain personality traits (such as impulsiveness and resentment against authority) that made them vulnerable to accidents under certain stresses that threaten their sense of independence. The recent literature suggests, however, that accident proneness as a lifelong, permanent condition is not a concept consistent with the data. While a few accident victims may be chronically accident prone, the group of accident repeaters appears to change from one time period to the next: Most accidents seem to reflect a transient accident syndrome, involving a variety of personality traits and recent life stresses, rather than a chronic process.[11,25,34,35] In studies of psychopathology of groups of individuals having a high incidence of accidents, impulsivity, aggressiveness, paranoid traits, unmet dependency needs, and depressive tendencies have been prevalent.[9,16,36,37]

The search for enduring personality traits to predict accident proneness arose from the ashes of the concept of statistical proneness,[25] and its development paralleled that of other aspects of psychosomatic medicine and met the same fate: Personality traits associated with accidents have been unprovable, just as they were not related to asthma

---

* And it probably never will be proved mathematically. The problem lies in getting a sufficiently large sample to discriminate between stochastic phenomena that lend the *illusion* of patterns in natural phenomena on the one hand and patterns that actually reveal causal connections on the other. It may appear that 4% of workers causing 28% of accidents implies statistical significance, but it does not. Most accident repeaters are simply the victims of random events. Furthermore, great trouble arises in the possibility that the occurrence of one accident may affect an individual's "learning" and change the likelihood of the production of a subsequent one (either in the positive or negative direction). Jacobs[30] estimated that empirical testing of plausible mathematical models to 90% confidence limits would require studying more than 500 individuals over a period of time long enough to allow each individual to *average* 12 accidents!

or ulcerative colitis. Now research has withered and interest in this area has waned. Yet some gross association of accident frequency with "immaturity" (either in age or in what is generally considered to be psychophysiologic maturity) continues to suggest itself both intuitively and empirically.

The recent review of Tsuang et al[11] held that persons involved in traffic accidents manifest excessive hostility and dyscontrol of it, less anxiety tolerance, less conformity, more difficulty with authority, more hyperactivity, and a tendency toward risk-taking—all age-related traits associated with psychological "immaturity." They give some weight to the findings of Conger et al[36,38] comparing airmen who had been involved in accidents with those not involved in accidents. Airmen involved in accidents displayed poorer control of hostility, lower tension tolerance, higher separation anxiety, higher dependency needs on interviews and psychological tests (MMPI, Thurstone Temperament Survey, Allport-Vernon-Linsay Study of Values), and psychophysiological measures (coordination and reaction time tests). Interestingly, those who had not been in accidents were more oriented toward religious values and less toward esthetic and theoretical values than men who had been involved in accidents.

Also with airmen, similar data emerged independently. Biesheuvel[39] had utilized a clinical approach to flying accidents in World War II and studied two groups of air force pilots: an accident group of 200 men in training who had been involved in flying accidents at elementary and advanced flying schools in 1941–1944, and a matched control group of 400 pilots who had completed both elementary and advanced training without any accidents. Each group was tested on intelligence, measures of two-hand coordination, steadiness of movement, choice reaction time, and mechanical aptitude, and each group was tested on personality, including suitability to being a pilot based on observational, biographical, and interview data. These researchers found it possible to credit "safety indicators" to each pilot on the basis of those tests found to have discriminating value: (1) two-hand coordination, high in both speed and quality, (2) good mechanical aptitude, (3) appropriate tempo, variability, stimulability, and impulsiveness of behavior, and (4) appropriate activity of drive and persistence in the face of obstacles. Similarly, they debited each pilot with "accident indicators" based on finding that: (1) to a high degree, feeling or emotionality was a "determining factor" in behavior, (2) there was absence of a broad sporting background but excellence in a single sport, (3) a *positive* parental attitude toward the subject's flying, or (4) a history of death of a parent, especially the father.

Using cumulative scores to compute risk scales, these researchers were able prospectively to predict blindly two thirds of the increased-risk pilots who actually later had accidents, a remarkable success considering that the accident cases consisted of pilots who largely (77%) had only one accident. A second validation study on 17 pilots with accidents correctly predicted 77% of the pilots who would go on to have accidents. The "safer" group has a fairly close resemblance to LeShan's "safety prone" individuals,[40,41] those found by the Worthingham Personal History test to be more obsessive and have higher "castration anxiety" than accident prone individuals. The safety prone person had warm relationships with others, high impulse control, vigilance, good space-time location of the self, strong identification with father and father's social class, and lack of rebellion toward authority. LeShan hypothesized that high castration anxiety along with the warm relationships with others both protected against acting out self-destruction and defended against guilt about repressed hostility and sexuality.[40,41]

ACCIDENT "VICTIMS"

While the literature cited above highlights the importance of psychological factors in accident causation, its relevance to the hospitalized accident victim is less clearly evident. These studies do alert clinicians to the role of emotional issues in some accident victims and lend credibility to the pursuit of psychosocial explanations in individual cases. However, the clinical psychiatric approach to the patient in hospital is more problematic. At first sight, most accidents do, indeed, appear to have been just chance events. Even when historical data are readily available indicating recent emotional upset or major life changes, the issue of unconscious causation is often still rather vague; that is, information suggesting psychological stress prior to accident is rarely sufficient evidence to prove a direct causal link to the accident.

Unconscious dynamics that may be implicated as accident precipitants are often only accessible after extended investigation in interview. This investigative interviewing, while often dramatically revealing, is too rarely accomplished. To the consulting psychiatrist, the reasons for doing it are often not clear and to the consultee physician, surgeon, patient, and much of the rest of the world, the rationale for it is obscure: After all, most people do tend to accept "it was just an accident" as a reasonable accounting of causality. However, as Rome has stated:

> Very little in nature is truly capricious, deserving of the designation "accident." For the most part, our use of the term actually means that

the antecedents of the event have not been analyzed in sufficient detail to establish the logical, scientific basis required for a suitably parsimonious explanation of its pathogenesis.[42]

The weight of evidence implicating psychodynamic causes for accidents will often become available through psychological detective work. Alexander[33] emphasized that traditional psychological testing failed to provide the evidence necessary to define the psychological aspects of accident causation. He believed that detailed psychiatric interview provided the most reliable method. Psychiatric consultation in our experience has time and again revealed striking examples of psychological causes for accidents, fractures, burns, and multiple trauma. For the moment, clinical cases remain the best evidence of psychological determinants in the accident process.

If the foregoing comments appear to overstate the importance of psychosocial and psychodynamic issues in accidents, the primary reason is that the error is all too often made in the opposite direction, overlooking unconscious motivations. While there are indeed "true" or "pure" accidents, such as a flowerpot falling off a ledge and striking an unaware pedestrian (assuming the pedestrian had not ignored potential warnings), often the victim is in some way an agent or prime mover for the sequence of events. The accident victims seen on the Massachusetts General Hospital (MGH) Consultation Service show a broad spectrum of ages and injuries. There is some consistency in the affects most keenly experienced prior to the time of the accident, especially anger, guilt, grief, or loneliness. Many accident victims possess personality characteristics related to one or more of the following three categories:
1. Chronic masochistic character traits or transient masochistic defenses with anger leading to guilt and self-punishment
2. Grief, sadness, loneliness, or depression
3. Counterdependent defenses acutely threatened by increased dependent feelings, with predominant themes of overindependence, bravado, impulsiveness, or rebelliousness, coexisting with neediness

Masochism

The use of the term "masochism" in the first of these three accident victim categories refers to the process whereby angry feelings toward important others are intolerable and generate severe guilt feelings that are relieved only by self-punishment, by being hurt. Punishment expiates the guilt these individuals feel at their anger, especially when their anger is directed toward people on whom they are dependent for nurturance.

> A 32-year-old housewife came to the surgical service after accidentally shooting off her right foot with a shotgun. She stated she was routinely putting away the weapon, which her husband used for hunting. The psychiatric interview revealed a history suggestive of masochistic personality traits and physical abuse by her husband, but at the end of the first interview, the psychiatrist did not have evidence of any acute psychological motivation for the accident. On return visit, however, the interviewer learned that just hours before the accident, her husband had pointed the rifle at the patient and threatened to kill her.

The masochistic person often follows a pattern of introjecting other people's anger, taking it in, feeling it is deserved, feeling guilty and worthless. This woman quite concretely directed her husband's rage at herself.

Even when the patient does not have masochistic personality features, a history of rage toward spouse, lover, or parent is often followed by self-injury. Not infrequent are scenarios like the following:

> A 23-year-old woman was admitted for fractures and lacerations from an automobile accident. She had been having an ongoing conflict with her boy friend, and after a particularly violent argument that appeared to end the relationship, she stormed furiously out of his apartment and drove off. Within minutes she had lost control of her car and struck a tree. Noting the anger at her boy friend she said, "Hurting myself was the last thing I wanted to do."

Again, rage toward an emotionally significant person eventuated in self-injury. In the words of another patient, acknowledging that he was angrier than he had admitted, "Of course I'm angry—at myself!"

Depression and Grief

The second category of psychological predisposition to accidental trauma includes depressive affects, sadness, loneliness, and unresolved grief.

> A 78-year-old man was admitted to hospital for treatment of severe chemical esophageal burns. He was living at home alone and had gotten up in the night to take a dose of antacid. Instead, from the medicine chest shelf he got a bottle of liquid drain cleaner and took a swallow before realizing his mistake. He came to the emergency ward immediately. The psychiatrist was suspicious of suicidal intent from the history but, after interview, was satisfied that the patient had no history

of suicidal ideation, intent, or plan. Rather, in the dark of night the patient had made a serious error.

During routine information gathering, however, the interviewer later learned that the date of the ingestion was 5 years to the day since the death of the patient's wife. It was the anniversary of her death.

In addition to sadness and loneliness, guilt feelings are common concomitants of the grieving process. The following case emphasizes this point and also serves as a reminder of how psychological determinants can go undiscovered.

One day on consultation service rounds, the residents presented a case of "an accident that was just an accident"; the psychiatric resident was originally called to see the patient because of a transient delirium.

The patient, an 18-year-old man, who had been visiting friends in an apartment building, was just leaving when the building caught fire. He was trapped by smoke in a stairway leading outside. No one else was injured, but the patient was badly burned and suffered smoke inhalation. To the surprise of the residents, the interview by the staff psychiatrist revealed that at the first sign of fire the patient went back up the stairs, not out of the building. The patient stated that he wanted to rescue others, all of whom had already reached safety.

Psychiatrist: That was a generous act.
Patient: My father would have done the same thing.
Psychiatrist: Your father?
Patient: He was killed in an accident at the shipyard. Two months ago he got caught by a rope and was crushed between a ship and the dock. Nobody was there to help him.

Acute grief and associated guilt feelings played a part in determining this individual's seemingly chance injuries.

Counterdependent Impulsiveness

The third category of psychological predisposition to accidental injury includes individuals, similar to the description of accident prone personalities, who are impulsive and aggressive, or who act independently but have great difficulty with dependent feelings. As noted above, some people manifest these traits for years and have trouble during periods of stress, such as times of separation. Other individuals appear to fit this description only transiently.

A 16-year-old boy was admitted to the burn unit after sustaining multiple burns in a flash fire he touched off climbing a utility pole; he fell to the ground unconscious. That night he had been out drinking with friends, and in a spirit of carousal and daring he climbed the pole (unusual behavior for him). Later, he could not say why he placed himself at such risk. The consultation came as a result of his behavior on the unit. He had periods of anger at the staff for leaving him alone and for hurting him while changing dressings, and this alternated with periods of contrition and remorse in which he begged forgiveness for the anger.

On interview the boy said he was living at home alone for 3 weeks while his parents were in Europe. This was the first time in his life that he had been left alone; his older brother had left for college earlier in the year. After a pause he spontaneously said, "I wasn't angry that my parents were away." Unit staff reported that his first question on regaining consciousness was, "Have my parents started back?"

The patient had only one prior accident in his life. At age 4 years he tripped and fell and lost a finger tip in a lawn mower while running across the yard to greet his parents arriving home from a trip.

This young accident victim had been engaged in an unaccustomed act of bravado and fearlessness at a time when he was feeling most lonely and needy. His behavior on the ward also suggested problems with guilt resulting from angry feelings toward caregivers. Other victims who fit in this category of pseudoindependent behavior have often had an acute falling-out with someone whom they need for support, despite their feelings of angry self-sufficiency. Traffic accident victims in particular seem to fit this category.

These three categories are not exhaustive but represent the most familiar themes elicited on interview with accident patients. Other issues, conflicts, needs, fears, and stresses may be involved as precipitants of accidents. In general, there are a variety of stresses that can render many different individuals accident prone or vulnerable to having an accident at certain periods in their lives.

> A 33-year-old janitor suffered a posterior dislocation of the knee severing the posterior tibial artery when he tripped in a pothole. Formerly in good health, the patient had now been hospitalized three times in 6 months. The first admission was for a circumcision; the second was for concussion suffered in an automobile accident. On psychiatric interview the patient appeared a chronic loner and seemed to have schizoid personality; 6 months earlier, he had married for the first time.

At times an accident appears to be an attempt to resolve a conflict acceptably. In this case a wish to escape from a conflictual situation— closeness with another person—seems to have led the patient to his frequent hospitalizations.

At times there appears to be, in addition to psychological motivation for self-injury, particular significance attached to the nature or site of the injury, much in the same manner attributed to certain conversion symptoms.[43] These may have symbolic meaning, resolve a particular conflict, indicate identification with another injured person, and so forth.

> A 21-year-old woman was admitted to surgery after she severed the distal third of the ring finger of her left hand in an industrial accident. She recalled being angry with her employer that day because he switched her to an unsafe machine that her mother—employed by the same company—used to operate. Later in the interview she also mentioned that the day just before the accident, she had broken off her engagement to her fiancé.
>
> While the injury to her ring finger clearly seemed quite psychologically overdetermined to the psychiatrist, ward staff members were previously quite certain that this was a chance accident.

Hirschfeld and Behan[34,44,45] have reviewed 300 cases of industrial accidents and injuries and emphasize the concept of the accident process. They note that accidents do not just occur but "rather, they are events which are captured by the personality for the purpose of solving the individual's life problem." The process begins with the build-up of conflict and anxiety that are resolved by the accident. Since the accident and resulting injury succeed in resolving the antecedent conflict, the patient becomes a high risk for ongoing disability and for failure to respond to rehabilitation measures or pain relief:

> A 47-year-old father of five was admitted for evaluation of intractable pain. Four years earlier he fell off a loading dock and broke his left ulna and radius. After surgery he complained of constant pain despite apparently normal neurologic findings. He had been receiving disability payments since that time and had a lawsuit pending against his employer.
>
> When interviewed, he described his childhood as "never had one." His father, abusive and alcoholic, abandoned his mother and three sisters when the patient was 11 years old. At age 12 the patient began taking part-time jobs to help support the family and at age 16 he left school to work full time. He had never had a respite. At times he held two jobs to support his own family. Shortly before the accident, he was passed over for promotion to foreman, a position he felt he deserved.

In this case the patient had never had relief from the burden of work and financial pressures. In addition, he was furious with his employer. The accident and subsequent disability provided short- and long-term resolutions to his conflicts about his anger. They also offered him relief from the pressures of providing for others, a relief to which he felt entitled.

THE PSYCHIATRIST'S THERAPEUTIC ROLE

The preceding discussion emphasizes the detective and diagnostic aspects of the evaluation of the accident victim to determine the nature and extent of psychological motivation. While instructive about unconscious processes, the foregoing begs the question of the therapeutic utility of these endeavors. There are, however, clinical reasons for the rigorous psychological evaluation of the accident victim.

The search for the unconscious antecedents of accidents has repeatedly uncovered pre-existing psychopathology that often had been compromising the patient's general functioning—psychopathology such as unresolved grief, depression, or acute situational disturbances. Generally these three conditions offer the psychiatrist opportunities to make dramatic clinical interventions with a variety of short-term therapeutic modalities. Since these states perhaps predisposed the patient to accidental injury, failure to diagnose and treat them might lead to a missed opportunity for preventive medicine and leave the patient vulnerable to future injury in the same way. Since accident repeaters are a changing group, a person injured for the first time may be one of these transiently accident prone individuals, and the acute process may be prevented from progressing to chronic invalidism.

More chronic psychopathology, such as masochistic personality traits, success neurosis, or unresolved dependent feelings, is of course more resistant to treatment. However, some individuals with these conditions will improve their patterns of interpersonal relationships and their response to life change in long-term dynamic or supportive psychotherapy. When, for various reasons, these patients are not candidates for treatment, a very direct explanation of their vulnerability to specific stresses should be offered. Masochistic persons may be spared repeated trauma if instructed about the role of unacceptable anger in their self-injury and if cautioned to be wary of certain situations that bring increased danger. For those who have a success neurosis, who injure themselves at times of moving ahead in life, a warning about times of critical risk may easily be communicated. Such a warning would at least be humane and ethical, if not certainly therapeutic.

Another important therapeutic role for the psychiatrist evolves from the understanding of the accident-process concept. Many persons have a high risk of permanent disability after they have captured the accident moment. As time passes these patients will become increasingly resistant to physical and psychological interventions.[46] Early discovery of the anxieties, stresses, and conflicts involved in the accident process will increase the likelihood that psychiatric treatment can be directed to these underlying factors, possibly avoiding enduring disability. Psychological consultation with those involved in the physical rehabilitation and treatment of these patients can at least increase the effectiveness of their work and minimize the possibility of increasing disability for the patients.[46]

A number of emotional sequelae of accidents may be discovered by the therapist in interviews. Feelings of guilt and responsibility are at times evident, especially if others were injured or killed. Whether or not other people were involved, the patient may have a semiawareness of the role of recent upsets or angry feelings in accident causation and be troubled by this. A chance to talk openly with the psychiatrist is then likely to relieve some of this vague uneasiness and to facilitate coping with hospitalization.

> A surgical ward requested consultation for a 19-year-old man who was very nervous and agitated. He was in the hospital for multiple fractures and lacerations sustained in a motorcycle accident. The nursing staff was frustrated because the patient was "always on the light" (the signal for assistance). When they responded, he would make apparently trivial requests for a Kleenex, a sip of water, fluffing of the pillow, and the like. His behavior generated anger in nursing and house staff although they knew he was anxious. They asked the consultant to suggest an anti-anxiety drug.
>
> The psychiatrist learned that the patient had a young girl as his passenger on the motorcycle; she was killed in the accident, a fact which family and staff knew but not the patient. The staff and family believed the patient had amnesia for the events of the accident day, and had agreed to keep the secret until "he was strong enough to know." The patient told the psychiatrist he thought he was going crazy.
>
> The psychiatrist was convinced that the patient knew more than others suspected, that the secret was the toxin in the environment, and that the patient accepted the conspiracy of silence fearing there was some terrible reason why he was being held in ignorance. Meetings with staff and family ensued and finally the parents agreed to tell the patient. The following morning the patient told the psychiatrist, "My memory came back." He proceeded to tell the psychiatrist about the young girl, and he cried. Then he said, "At least I know that people still love me." His aggravating behavior on the ward ceased immediately.

The time and effort involved in eliciting detailed history from accident victims are more than justified by the pain and cost of their injuries to themselves, to their families, and to society. Accidents are a major public health issue. The more that is known about their causes both at the individual and at the population level, the greater will be the chances for more effective prevention.

A variety of emotional factors and life stresses can be implicated as important causes of many apparently fortuitous accidents. Usually the accident results from the momentary convergence of psychological vulnerability, transient life stresses, and the physical opportunity for the accident at one point in time. A detailed, investigative psychological interview will often elicit evidence indicating the psychological determinants and permit the consideration of various therapeutic options.

REFERENCES

1. Baker SP, O'Neill B, Karpf RS: *The Injury Fact Book.* Lexington, Mass, Lexington Books/DC Heath, 1984.
2. National Academy of Sciences, Division of Medical Sciences, Committee on Trauma, Committee on Shock: *Accidental Death and Disability: The Neglected Disease of Modern Society.* US Dept of Health, Education, and Welfare, 1966.
3. Dickerson OD: *Health Insurance.* Homewood, Ill, Richard D Irwin, Inc, 1963.
4. Freud S: The psychopathology of everyday life, originally published in 1901. In *Standard Edition*, Strachey J (trans-ed). London, Hogarth Press, 1960, vol 6, p 179.
5. Menninger KA: Purposive accidents as an expression of self-destructive tendencies. *Int J Psychoanal* 1936; 17:6–16.
6. Sobel R, Margolis J: Repetitive poisoning in children, a psychological study. *Pediatrics* 1965; 35:641–651.
7. Crancer A Jr, Quiring DL Jr: Driving records of persons hospitalized for suicidal gestures. *Behav Res Highway Safety* 1970; 1:33–43.
8. Selzer ML, Payne CE: Automobile accidents, suicide, and unconscious motivation. *Am J Psychiatry* 1962; 119:237–240.
9. Selzer ML, Rogers JE, Kern S: Fatal accidents: the role of psychopathology, social stress, and acute disturbance. *Am J Psychiatry* 1968; 124:1028–1038.
10. Tabachnick ND (ed): *Accident or Suicide: Destruction by Automobile.* Springfield, Ill, Charles C Thomas Publisher, 1973.
11. Tsuang MT, Boor M, Fleming J: Psychiatric aspects of traffic accidents. *Am J Psychiatry* 1985; 142:538–546.
12. McMurray L: Emotional stress and driving performance: the effect of divorce. *Behav Res Highway Safety* 1970; 1:100–114.
13. McFarland RA, Moseley AL: Human factors in highway transport safety. Cambridge, Mass, Harvard School of Public Health, 1954.
14. Selzer ML, et al: Automobile accidents as an expression of psychopathology in an alcoholic population. *QJ Stud Alcohol* 1967; 28:505–516.
15. Selzer ML, Vinokur A: Life events, subjective stress and traffic accidents. *Am J Psychiatry* 1974; 131:903–906.
16. Tabachnick ND, et al: Comparative psychiatric study of accidental and suicidal death. *Arch Gen Psychiatry* 1966; 14:60–68.
17. Selzer ML: Alcoholism, mental illness, and stress in 96 drivers causing fatal accidents. *Behav Sci* 1969; 14:1–10.
18. Waller JA, Turkel HW: Alcoholism and traffic deaths. *N Engl J Med* 1966; 275:532–536.

19. Sheehan DV, et al: Psychosocial predictors of accident/error rates in nursing students: a prospective study. *Int J Psychiatry Med* 1981–1982; 11:125–136.

20. Greenwood M, Woods HM: The incidence of industrial accidents upon individuals with special reference to multiple accidents. London: Industrial Fatigue Research Board Rep No. 4, 1919.

21. Greenwood M, Woods HM: The incidence of industrial accidents upon individuals with special reference to multiple accidents, in Haddon W, Suchman E, Klein D (eds): *Accident Research*. New York, Harper & Row, 1964, pp 389–397.

22. Marbe K: *Praktische Psychologie der Unfälle und Betrieb-Schäden*. Munich, Springer, 1926.

23. Dunbar F: *Mind and Body*. New York, Random House, 1955.

24. Joseph ED, Schwartz AH: Accident proneness, in Kaplan HI, Freedman AM, Sadock BJ (eds): *Comprehensive Textbook of Psychiatry*, ed 3. Baltimore, Williams & Wilkins Co, 1980, pp 1953–1957.

25. Arbous AG, Kerrick JE: Accident statistics and the concept of accident-proneness. *Biometrics* 1951; 7:340–432.

26. Farmer E, Chambers EG: A psychological study of individual differences in accident rates. London, Industrial Health Research Board Rep No. 38, 1926.

27. Farmer E, Chambers EG: A study of personal qualities in accident proneness and proficiency. London, Industrial Health Research Board Rep No. 55, 1929.

28. Farmer E, Chambers EG: Tests for accident proneness. London, Industrial Health Research Board Rep No. 68, 1933.

29. Farmer E, Chambers EG: A study of accident proneness among motor drivers. London, Industrial Health Research Board Rep No. 84, 1939.

30. Jacobs HH: Conceptual and methodological problems in accident research, in Jacobs HH, et al (eds): *Behavioral Approaches to Accident Research*. New York, Association for the Aid of Crippled Children, 1961, pp 3–25.

31. Dunbar F: *Psychosomatic Diagnosis*. New York, Paul B Hoeber, Inc, 1943.

32. Alexander F: The accident prone individual. *Public Health Rep* 1949; 64:357–362.

33. Alexander F: *Psychosomatic Medicine*. New York, WW Norton & Co, Inc, 1950.

34. Hirshfeld AH, Behan RC: The accident process: I. Etiological considerations of industrial injuries. *JAMA* 1963; 186:193–199.

35. Schulzinger MS: Accident syndrome. *Arch Indust Hyg Occup Med* 1954; 10:426–433.

36. Conger JJ, et al: Psychological and psychophysiological factors in motor vehicle accidents. *JAMA* 1959; 169:1581–1587.

37. Tillman WA, Hobbs GE: The accident-prone automobile driver: a study of the psychiatric and social background. *Am J Psychiatry* 1949; 106:321–331.

38. Conger JJ, et al: Psychological and psychophysiological factors in motor vehicle accidents. *Am J Psychiatry* 1957; 113:1969–1074.

39. Biesheuvel S: The human factor in flying accidents. *S Afr A F J* 1949; 1:25–31.

40. LeShan L: Dynamics in accident prone behavior. *Psychiatry* 1952; 15:73–80.

41. LeShan L: The safety prone, an approach to the accident-free person. *Psychiatry* 1952; 15:465–468.

42. Rome HP: Emotional problems leading to cardiovascular accidents. *Psychiat Ann* 1975; 5:6–14.

43. Engel GL: Conversion symptoms, in MacBryde CM, Blacklow RS (eds): *Signs and Symptoms.* Philadelphia, JB Lippincott Co, 1970, pp 650–668.
44. Behan RC, Hirschfeld AH: The accident process: II. Toward more rational treatment of industrial injuries. *JAMA* 1963; 186:300–306.
45. Hirschfeld AH, Behan RC: The accident process: III. Disability: acceptable and unacceptable. *JAMA* 1966; 197:85–89.
46. Nemiah JC: Psychological complications in industrial injuries. *Arch Environ Health* 1963; 7:481–486.

21

The Emergency Room

WILLIAM H. ANDERSON

"If you can keep your head when all about you are losing theirs
and blaming it on you
If you can trust yourself when all men doubt you, but make
allowance for their doubting, too"

—*Rudyard Kipling*

Psychiatric consultation in the emergency room is a task that differs
from other consultation services in several important ways. The physical
and psychological environment of the emergency ward is unique in the
hospital setting. The time frame, the nature of decision making, and the
expectations of staff and patients all combine to present the psychiatrist
with unusual challenges. In contrast to other patient care areas, the
physical and psychosocial environment is highly unpredictable. There is
no way to know from minute to minute whether the number of patients
will be increased suddenly or whether another arrival will require
redeployment of therapeutic resources. It is a place where unusual and
even unreasonable demands are made frequently. The clinical problems
are full of ambiguity and often without an obvious method of approach.
Often the physicians who work in the emergency service are not based
there primarily and thus are not familiar with the routines of ancillary
services. These factors combine to distract the physician from the
critical decision-making tasks.

Patients whose problems do not fit neatly into the domain of another
specialty are frequently assigned to the psychiatry service. These may
include those who are unable to give a coherent history as well as those
whose demeanor is assertive and obnoxious rather than passive and
obsequious.

The presence of an active psychiatry consultation service in the
emergency room provides a safety net for patients with complaints that
are not identified by other services as treatable conditions. Rather than
tell a patient that his concern is involved or unreal, physicians may

sometimes suggest that a "nervous disturbance" may be at the root of the problem. A psychiatric referral may then follow.

All these conditions suggest that the psychiatric consultant to the emergency service must have a strong background in general medicine. The psychiatrist must think of himself first as a physician who has been asked to take a second look at a puzzling clinical problem. Only after such assessment ought he to think in psychiatric terms.

THE EMERGENCY ROOM MILIEU

Emergency decisions. Decision making in an emergency room is quite different from that which is usually practiced on other services and at other locations. The physician is usually most comfortable when approaching questions of diagnosis and treatment in a systematic way. The emergency department has concerns that come even before diagnosis. The first branch of the decision tree concerns a judgment as to the seriousness of the patient's condition. Those patients perceived to have life-threatening emergencies are, of course, examined first. This judgment may inadvertently be based on nonclinical considerations such as the fanfare with which the patient enters. Next comes the decision to admit the patient or to attempt final diagnosis and treatment in the outpatient service. This decision is also heavily influenced by nonclinical factors such as the availability of beds. Then a decision must be made concerning the service to which the patient should be admitted. When behavioral abnormalities are the presenting symptoms, this decision is not always obvious. Psychiatry, neurology, general medicine, or neurosurgery may be the most appropriate service for definitive management, depending on the circumstances.

Time frame. Among the uppermost considerations in patient evaluation is the passage of time. In contrast to other patient-care environments, the emergency room most frequently has a rigid requirement that patients may not stay beyond a small number of hours. Problems of psychiatric assessment are not always easy to fit into such time restrictions. The psychiatric consultant may not be notified of the patient's needs until much of the available time has expired. Furthermore, the patient may not be able to give a coherent history and may not be cooperative to examination. Nevertheless, the time frame is constrained for generally sound reasons and one must try to work within it. This requires that the consultant be familiar with methods of rapid diagnosis, treatment, and disposition that are not normally required on other clinical services. The consultant should make every effort to have the patient leave the emergency area as soon as possible.

Patients. Patients who appear for psychiatric consultation in emergency services are not always similar to psychiatric patients in outpatient clinics or inpatient services. They may not define their problem as psychiatric, and they may be correct in this. They may be disruptive or violent, or they may be physically restrained prior to or during the consultation examination. If they are self-referred, they see their problem as extremely urgent and expect its early resolution.

Staff. Every consultation is defined by the desires and expectations of the physician who requests it. With inpatient consultation it is clear that the patient remains the responsibility of the original service and may be transferred only after the primary medical or surgical condition is resolved. In an emergency room this convention is less clear. Consultations are centered more on staff and institutional needs than on a patient's condition. Thus the consultant may be asked for advice on diagnosis or treatment, or, even more often, may be asked explicitly to take over all responsibility for the case.

Consultant. One of the primary missions of the psychiatric consultant is to restore peace and order to the emergency room when it is disrupted by the behavioral excess of a patient. This task, of course, is not an end in itself. While administrators, physicians, and nurses may be forgiven for assuming that the purpose of psychiatry is merely deviance control, the psychiatrist must remember that this chore is merely a preliminary to the actual work of identification of the causes of the unusual behavior and the application of appropriate treatment.

It is equally important that the psychiatric consultant be satisfied that no concomitant acute medical or surgical illness exists. Frequently a patient will enter the emergency service with psychosis or other bizarre behavior that is brought about by acute organic brain disease. Because the behavioral manifestations are often much more prominent than other signs of illness and because these behavioral manifestations often compromise such routine measures as checking vital signs, taking a history, and performing a physical examination, the psychiatric consultant must remain alert to the possibility of subtle organic disease. The consultant should never routinely trust another physician's judgment that organic disease has been ruled out.

Medical clearance. This term usually implies the practice of having an internist see every patient prior to psychiatric referral for the purpose of excluding "organic" disease. Often the practical effect is that a patient is given a cursory examination by a medical intern. In any case it is not criticism of the medical service to point out that very frequently such attempts fail to identify significant illness.

Whether the patient has been seen by other services or not, it is imperative that the psychiatric consultant not take for granted that any illness found will be purely "psychiatric." Estimates of prevalence of medical illness in patients thus referred to psychiatry vary from 5% to 30%. Hence it is fair to say that the concept and practice of "medical clearance" should be abandoned.

Restraint.   There are unusual circumstances when a patient must be placed under restraint in order to prevent harm to himself or others, or to prevent premature departure of a psychotic or incompetent patient with life-threatening illness.

A patient who is fully competent and informed of his condition has the right to refuse treatment even if, in the opinion of the medical staff, his life is in danger. On the other hand, a patient has the right to expect that physicians and hospitals will take all necessary measures to protect him from the consequences of serious illness with impaired mental status and judgment. Deciding which of these principles should apply often devolves to the psychiatric consultant.

A patient who arrives in the emergency service either on his own volition or with the help of relatives or police may at first be assumed to have some serious medical concern. If he should then be unable to give a coherent history of antecedent events, or if he refuses examination, the psychiatric consultant is faced with the decision to insist on medical examination or to allow the patient to leave without examination. The former course invites a lawsuit for assault, whereas the latter leaves the consultant vulnerable to negligence charges.

In this situation nothing can take the place of sound judgment, concern for the patient, and common sense. If the evidence, however meager, suggests the possibility of serious psychiatric or medical illness, then the consultant must insist on such examination procedures as may be necessary to exclude them. Courtesy and diplomacy are the best tools. A patient may not be restrained or examined against his will simply because he is obnoxious or insulting. Likewise, obnoxious and insulting behavior may be the result of acute illness. It is usually better to run the risk of an assault charge rather than one of negligence. In doing so the utmost courtesy and gentleness are called for.

Keeping these concerns in mind, a patient may be restrained and examined against his will if the physician has reason to believe that he may be suffering from serious illness and his judgment is impaired. Common examples are psychotic depression, suicidal ideation, or acute delirium. In all cases, of course, the physician's actions must be in compliance with state law.

The general principles of effective emergency room consultation are as follows:

1. The constraints of time must be respected. It is seldom possible to develop a thoroughly satisfactory psychiatric diagnosis of a patient's difficulty in the time and circumstances available in an emergency room. It is therefore necessary that the patient's condition be assessed quickly for any acute occult medical illness, for psychosis or other serious psychiatric illness, and for suicide potential. On the basis of these assessments the decision whether the patient needs inpatient or outpatient care should be clear and, in either case, expeditious.

2. The psychiatrist must have confidence in a method of identifying major organic illnesses that may resemble psychiatric conditions. This requires familiarity with the relevant methods of history taking, physical examination, and laboratory work.

3. Any ambiguity of responsibility must be clarified at once to determine whether the patient may be diagnosed and treated as the psychiatrist sees fit, or whether the psychiatrist's role is the more traditional one of an advising consultant.

4. Clear orders will assure the necessary degree of safety and security for patient and staff. Notes should be short and free of jargon. The psychiatrist must specify how medication is to be given and whether restraints or constant supervision is needed.

PSYCHIATRIC EMERGENCIES
Psychosis: Differential Diagnosis

Psychosis is one of the more frequent emergencies for which psychiatric consultation is requested. Psychosis is a disorder of information processing during which the patient has diminished capacity to receive, retain, process, recall, and act on information in a plausible or culturally acceptable manner. Numerous causes, both identifiable and idiopathic, may be implicated. Physicians unfamiliar with psychosis sometimes assume that any hallucinatory or delusional activity implies a diagnosis of "functional" or, better stated, idiopathic psychosis. There are, of course, cases in which the distinction between organic (identifiable) and idiopathic disease can be difficult and may require expert consultation and extensive laboratory investigation. This is usually not practical in the emergency setting. The emergency room consultant therefore requires a simple method of identifying first those medical and surgical conditions that cause death or irreparable damage in a short time and that may resemble idiopathic psychosis. Fortunately, there are a few general principles that facilitate the recognition of acute identifiable brain disease.

1. In emergency department consultations it is important to retain a high index of suspicion for organic psychosis—to assume that the disordered information processing is a result of organic brain disease until serious medical and surgical conditions are excluded.

2. A psychosis is not idiopathic simply because of a so-called precipitating psychological event. Most illness can be traced to an outside event if the psychiatrist is determined to find one. The "precipitating" event has little value in differential diagnosis.

3. It is dangerous to assume that an illness is idiopathic because of specific mental content. Even the most classical schizophrenic delusions are often seen in identifiable brain disease.

4. The more acute the onset of psychotic illness, the more the psychiatrist must suspect specific causes. Neither schizophrenia nor manic-depressive illness develops in hours or days as a general rule.

5. A first episode of acute psychotic illness in a person over 40 years of age most frequently implies specific cause.

6. A psychosis in a patient who has a previously diagnosed, serious, medical illness is usually a complication of the illness or of its treatment. A major malfunction of the heart, lung, liver, kidney, or endocrine system often announces itself by psychotic decompensation of the mental status. Numerous medications can produce similar changes.

7. Identifiable psychosis is not necessarily excluded by the absence of localized signs. Many such specific psychoses produce such signs late in their course or not at all.

History.   As in all fields of medicine, the history often yields the most diagnostically helpful information. Psychotic patients will often give critical information if examining physicians are patient and tactful in their inquiries. Often the more rewarding inquiries are those about the use of drugs, medications, and alcohol and about any previous metabolic illness. The questioning of relatives and the perusal of medical records are often revealing. Examination of the contents of wallets and pockets is similarly helpful.

Mental status examination.   The mental status examination is also a helpful tool. Most valuable are the evaluation of orientation, memory, and hallucinosis. Failure to identify time or place correctly is evidence for specific brain disease. Difficulty recalling five objects immediately and after five minutes is also an indication of organic disease. Visual or tactile hallucinosis generally suggests organic brain disease of the toxic or metabolic type.

Physical examination. A complete physical examination is always desirable, but not all aspects of it are equally productive of useful information. Checking vital signs, however, including a reliable temperature, is absolutely indispensable. Most of the other important findings are available to careful inspection with a minimum of invasive action. Signs of autonomic dysfunction and abnormal motor activity are especially useful. Examination for head injuries, nystagmus, and pathologic reflexes are often useful.

Laboratory investigation. Laboratory investigation has limited but definite value in otherwise uncertain cases. Among the most useful procedures are electroencephalography and blood tests for such chemical constituents as electrolytes, glucose, BUN, and toxic agents.

Priorities in diagnosis. It is important to recognize that there are clear priorities in diagnosis. In the milieu of the emergency room it is critical to first investigate and confirm or exclude those conditions that are life-threatening.

1. *Meningitis and encephalitis.* Fever, headache, elevated pulse or WBC count, or presence of meningeal signs should suggest this diagnosis.

2. *Adrenergic delirious states.* The patient has tachycardia, hypertension, diaphoresis, and tremor. The pupils are large and reactive. The reflexes are brisk. Common causes include alcohol and sedative withdrawal, hypoglycemia, thyrotoxicosis, and amphetamine or cocaine intoxication.

3. *Hypertensive encephalopathy* and *intracranial hemorrhage.* Headache, stiff neck, elevated blood pressure, and hypertensive retinal changes suggest these emergencies.

4. *Diminished cerebral oxygenation.* Cardiovascular and pulmonary conditions and severe anemia from any cause (including major unrecognized bleeding) may bring about an acute psychotic state. A change in mental status may be the first sign of decompensation of these systems.

5. *Anticholinergic poisonings.* Especially dangerous in overdosage are the tricyclic antidepressants, but phenothiazines, antihistamines and antisecretory agents may be implicated. Clinical signs include dilated fixed pupils, dry mucous membranes, tachycardia, diminished gastrointestinal (GI) motility, difficulty in voiding, choreiform movements, and fever.

6. *Wernicke's encephalopathy.* Although Wernicke's encephalopathy

is not a life-threatening condition, the consequences if untreated are so profound that they must be considered here. Acute confusional states in alcoholic individuals or others who are nutritionally deprived ought to be treated expectantly with parenteral thiamine (50 mg given intravenously (IV) immediately and 50 mg given intramuscularly (IM) daily until normal diet is resumed).

These conditions are medical and surgical emergencies that must be recognized and dealt with at once in order to avoid serious sequelae or death. There are other conditions less critical than those listed that may also appear at first to be acute functional psychosis and that require decisive early action. Among these are: (1) chronic subdural hematoma, (2) subacute bacterial endocarditis, (3) hepatic failure, (4) uremia, and (5) thyroid abnormalities.

Many other conditions may resemble idiopathic psychosis. These are listed in Table 21-1. The recognition of specific brain disease as distinct from idiopathic psychosis continues to be an important function of the consultation psychiatrist. In the setting of an emergency service, this function is especially critical. When the pattern of psychosis is consistent with identifiable brain disease, the first order of business is to make a diagnosis. This usually means hospital admission to whichever service seems most appropriate.

Idiopathic Psychosis

Diagnosis.   After having considered specific causes of psychosis and having rejected organic disease as an hypothesis, the emergency service psychiatric consultant is faced with the differential diagnosis of idiopathic psychosis. The task now is to determine whether the circumstances demand that the patient be admitted to inpatient psychiatric care or whether it is a plausible alternative to consider outpatient treatment as an option.

Disposition.   There are four important questions to answer before determining appropriate disposition for these psychotic patients:

1. Is the illness acute or chronic?
2. Is there suicidal or homicidal danger?
3. Is there viable family or social support?
4. What is the initial response to medication?

Patients in whom psychotic illness is acute should generally be admitted to inpatient status. This provides the necessary degree of stability and allows observation for diagnostic purposes. Early differential diagnosis is aided and treatment with antipsychotics may begin in a controlled environment. In general, "acute" is defined as onset over

Table 21-1. Metabolic and Structural Disorders with Presenting Psychotic Features

---

Space-occupying lesions
Primary tumors
Metastatic carcinoma (lung, breast)
Subdural hematoma
Brain abscess (bacterial, fungal, gumma, cysticercosis)

Cerebral hypoxia
Pulmonary insufficiency
Severe anemia
Diminished cardiac output
Toxic agents such as carbon monoxide

Metabolic and endocrine disorders
Electrolyte imbalance
Calcium metabolism disorders
Thyroid disease (thyrotoxicosis and myxedema)
Pituitary insufficiency
Adrenal disease (Addison's disease, Cushing's disease)
Hypoglycemia
Diabetes
Uremia
Hepatic failure
Porphyria

Exogenous substances
Alcohol (intoxication, withdrawal)
Amphetamines
Antihistamines
Atropine and similar anticholinergic agents
Baclofen
Barbiturates and similar sedatives (intoxication, withdrawal)
Cannabis (marijuana)
Cephalosporins
Chloroquine
Cimetidine
Cocaine
Corticosteroids
Cycloserine
Digitalis
Disopyramide phosphate
Disulfiram
Ephedrine
Heavy metals
Indomethacin
Isoniazid
Levodopa
Methyldopa

Table 21-1. Metabolic and Structural Disorders with Presenting Psychotic Features—continued

Methylphenidate hydrochloride
Phencyclidine hydrochloride
Propoxyphene
Propranolol hydrochloride
Reserpine
Salicylates
Theophylline
Tricyclic antidepressants
Vincristine sulfate

Nutritional deficiencies
Thiamine (Wernicke-Korsakoff syndrome)
Niacin (pellagra)
Cyanocobalamin (vitamin B$_{12}$)
Folic acid

Vascular abnormalities
Intracranial hemorrhage
Lacunar state (hypertension)
Collagen diseases
Aneurysms

Infections
Meningitis (bacterial, fungal, tuberculous)
Encephalitis (viral; eg, herpes), AIDS
Lues
Subacute bacterial endocarditis
Trypanosomiasis
Typhoid
Malaria

Miscellaneous conditions
Normal pressure hydrocephalus
Temporal lobe epilepsy
Huntington chorea
Alzheimer's disease
Remote effects of carcinoma
Wilson's disease
Pancreatitis

previous days or weeks, frequently with perplexity, confusion, or major affect disturbance.

The psychotic patient who has attempted suicide or who has thoughts of self-destruction must be considered to be in extreme danger and in general requires immediate hospital admission, rapid treatment of the psychosis, and close direct observation. For the psychotic patient, suicide is a highly unpredictable consequence. Any hint of impulsive behavior or active bad judgment as to safety should mandate hospitalization. A psychotic patient need not be intentionally suicidal in order to accomplish death. For example, a manic patient may have no intention of harming himself, but his judgment may be so impaired that he will attempt a 30-mile walk in subzero weather.

The next important consideration is the extent and quality of the patient's social support. A psychotic patient who has no available family or friends should be hospitalized. If the patient has a family that is alert, competent, and concerned, and that will provide the patient with environmental protection and will ensure that the patient take medication and continue outpatient visits, hospitalization may sometimes be avoided.

Finally, the response to initial treatment must be considered. Many patients will respond to parenteral antipsychotic medication with a considerable remission of symptoms within several hours. When such a degree of remission occurs, oral medication may be substituted.

Patients whose illness is "chronic" may not require hospitalization. Follow-up examination to detect emerging side effects as well as minor medication adjustments are reasonably done in the outpatient setting. In general, however, when in doubt about any of the aspects of the clinical situation, the best strategy is a brief inpatient stay. This is especially true if less than optimal social supports are available, if response to medication is unclear, or if any hint of self-harming ideation is present.

Method of initial treatment. When the diagnosis of idiopathic psychosis has been made, antipsychotic medicine may be started in the emergency service. Parenteral high-potency drugs are generally preferred. High-potency antipsychotics such as haloperidol or trifluoperazine hydrochloride have relatively little sedative, hypotensive, or anticholinergic effect. The parenteral route is preferred because of more rapid response. Sedation, per se, is often an undesirable side effect for the patient who has acute psychosis. Lower potency drugs that have greater sedative properties, such as chlorpromazine, are less useful in rapid treatment because side effects limit the amount that can be used within a few hours in the emergency setting. A typical regimen might include an initial 5-mg dose of haloperidol that might be repeated hourly with 5-mg or 10-mg doses. Frequent observation is required to determine whether satisfactory improvement occurs or whether side effects will limit further treatment. First-day remission will occur in about half of the cases with doses of IM haloperidol ranging between 15 mg and 45 mg. There is no evidence that higher doses promote further improvement on the first day. The physician should be alert for the development of acute dystonia, which occurs in about a third of the cases so treated.

Dystonia generally appears within the first several days of treatment with a high-potency antipsychotic drug. It is usually characterized by spasm of the muscles of the face, neck, and pharynx. Rarely, the laryngeal muscles may be involved, with compromise of the airway. Dystonia may be intermittent. It is made worse by stress, responds transiently to suggestion or concentration, and so may give every appearance of volitional or "hysterical" movement.

In general, it should be assumed that any involuntary postures, movements, or muscle spasms that occur within hours or days of antipsychotic medicine use are acute dystonias. Their incidence may be markedly decreased by the prophylactic use of benztropine mesylate 1 to 2 mg orally beginning with the first use of antipsychotics. After they occur, dystonias are best treated by the use of diphenhydramine hydrochloride, 25 to 50 mg by slow IV injection.

The use of prophylactic anticholinergics such as benztropine mesylate must be judged in each individual case. Dystonias are more common in young patients, and the anticholinergic side effects are usually not too bothersome. Elderly patients have dystonias less frequently, but are prone to have more serious anticholinergic side effects, such as delirium, tachycardia, or difficulty in voiding. Thus it would seem rational to give prophylactic anticholinergic drugs more liberally in younger patients.

Continued treatment.   Most patients with idiopathic psychosis will experience some improvement with initial treatment as described above, but relatively few will have a response so complete that hospitalization may be avoided. This is due to lack of adequate social support, the presence of suidical ideation, need for observation for diagnosis, and incomplete response to medication. Some patients may be discharged from the emergency room to continue outpatient treatment when diagnostic issues are clear and when the home environment is safe, supportive, and will insure continued medication and maintenance of outpatient visits. Oral medication is substituted for parenteral medication and the dosage adjusted for optimal response.

Suicide

Remarks will be restricted here to the special problems of consultation of a suicidal patient in an emergency department.

Patients who have made suicide attempts or who have suicidal ideation or even depression seem to elicit little sympathetic understanding in the emergency milieu. Physicians and nurses often assume a punitive or derisory attitude that is, to say the least, countertherapeutic. Since the typical emergency department is not always suitable for on-the-spot staff education, often the most prudent choice is to remove the patient to more peaceful and less abrasive surroundings while evaluation takes place. At all times it must be kept in mind that the emergency room is a fertile field for obtaining means of self-harm. Ideally the patient should be kept under constant observation with adequate security measures to prevent further attempts.

Psychiatric consultants must remember that their basic task is to decide whether suicidal or depressed patients require inpatient or outpatient care. All other concerns are secondary, since time is not on the side of adaptive response in most cases.

The time of most critical danger exists when the patient still requires medical assessment or treatment for poisoning or injury. It is important to remember that two suicidal methods may have been used simultaneously. For example, a patient may have taken a lethal dose of barbiturates as well as having lacerated himself. Constant direct supervision is required when the patient is in a medical or surgical area.

Risk factors. Patients who attempt or contemplate suicide by violent means are among the gravest risks in the emergency room situation. Shooting, hanging, and mutilation suggest the more profound disturbances and argue for immediate hospitalization in a secure facility, and expeditious treatment of the underlying disorder. A combination of a highly lethal method and survival only by good fortune should call for constant vigilance and security.

Psychosis with attempted or contemplated suicide is also an indication for the most zealous and watchful care. It is important to remember that manic patients often have the combination of impaired judgment and increased energy that makes a completed suicide or accidental death possible.

Intoxication presents some of the most difficult problems in emergency service psychiatry. Ideally, intoxicated patients should be kept under close observation until they are thoroughly detoxified from the alcohol or other sedative drug. A meaningful evaluation is hardly possible until this has been accomplished. Unfortunately it is not always possible to keep the patient in the emergency department for the length of time required. In such a case the best solution is to admit the patient to a psychiatric facility where adequate medical attention as well as suicide prevention is possible.

Severe depression is another risk factor that makes rapid decision necessary. This is especially true if the depression is mixed with agitation such that ample energy is available for self-harm.

Other conditions which increase the risk of subsequent completed suicide include a history of impaired impulse control, previous suicide attempts, concurrent serious medical illness, social isolation, recent major loss of self-esteem, and a family history of suicide or affect disorder.

Violent and Aggressive Behavior

Violent and aggressive patients are among the most difficult patients the emergency service psychiatrist must face. An emergency service frequently becomes paralyzed when confronted by unrestricted violence. Consultants can find themselves without the accustomed help of colleagues. Three tasks are defined: the situation must be controlled, the presumptive etiology identified, and the patient treated.

It is best to marshal more than sufficient force before the initial confrontation to bring the situation under control so that evaluation can be made. It is worse than useless to attempt to interrupt violence with inadequate or marginal countermeasures. Fewer injuries and less damage will result if the counterforce is overwhelming and rapid. It is best if there is a trained security force to accomplish the task of applying physical restraint.

Once the patient is under control, the task is to identify possible underlying causes of the violence. Violent behavior of organic etiology includes alcohol and sedative intoxication or withdrawal, amphetamine intoxication, thyroid dysfunction, hypoglycemia, and temporal lobe epilepsy. Idiopathic causes include the psychoses with paranoid features, mania, catatonic excitement, impulsive character disorder, and anti-social personality.

Chemotherapy is often necessary even before a diagnosis is made. High-potency antipsychotic drugs in adequate parenteral dosage are the most useful agents. Nonspecific sedatives such as barbiturates or benzodiazepines are likely to make the situation worse by promoting further disinhibition unless the cause of the violence is alcohol or sedative withdrawal.

Every effort must be made to insure a thorough medical and psychiatric evaluation of the violent patient. The social ecology of the emergency ward setting makes this task difficult, since the rules are not designed to cope with deviance control. The most practical solution often is to admit the patient to a medical psychiatry unit where rapid behavioral control may proceed together with efficient diagnostic assessment.

It should be noted that a number of serious or life-threatening illnesses may at first appear as violent behavior. There is, therefore, no substitute for history, physical and neurologic examination, and appropriate laboratory assessment. If the patient must be transferred to another hospital for management, then diagnostic evaluation must be completed in the emergency room.

Alcoholism

Psychiatric consultation in the emergency service is often requested prematurely—that is, before a reasonable medical evaluation for serious concomitant illness has been accomplished. Alcohol abuse is most frequently viewed by emergency staff as a problem in deviance control rather than diagnosis and treatment. Thus the psychiatric consultant may be asked implicitly or explicitly to cause the patient to be removed before adequate assessment is done.

This tendency must be resisted with the utmost vigor. First, we must recognize that no adequate psychiatric evaluation is possible of an intoxicated patient. Second, we must remember that many serious conditions—medical, surgical, and psychiatric—may be masked by alcohol intoxication. It is our task as consultants to see that patients are protected and that provision is made for thorough diagnostic evaluation of these problems.

Frequently it becomes necessary to manage the excesses of a patient who enters the emergency room in an aggressive and boisterous manner, presumably because of alcohol intoxication. Upon the initial presentation a history and physical examination are often not possible. The patient is clearly unable to care for himself, an emergency exists, and therefore protective action is required. The patient should be restrained in a comfortable prone position such that possible subsequent emesis will be less likely to be aspirated. If necessary to produce calming, and so to allow examination, a small dose of high-potency antipsychotic (eg, haloperidol 2–5 mg IM) may be given without producing excessive sedation.

Physical assessment should include whatever history can be obtained for the patient or his relatives. A reliable measurement of vital signs, including temperature, is invaluable. Attention should especially be directed to possible conditions known to be associated with alcoholism. These include GI disturbances such as upper GI bleeding, liver disease, and pancreatitis. Neurologic complications are likewise to be anticipated. Alcoholic patients are vulnerable to subdural hematomas. The early symptoms and signs resemble intoxications. Hypoglycemia and vitamin deficiencies are likely also. A wide variety of other neurologic disorders including withdrawal states, seizure disorders, and degenerative conditions must be considered as well.

In addition to a history and physical examination with special attention to GI and neurologic features, the patient should have a standard profile of laboratory tests, including complete blood count, urinalysis, and glucose, electrolyte, and liver function tests. When the patient has been examined in sufficient depth so as to exclude serious medical and neurologic conditions, and when his intoxication begins to abate, a psychiatric evaluation should be performed with the goal in mind of determining a treatment recommendation. Suicidal and homicidal ideas should be investigated, since many of these events have alcohol as part of the picture. If chronic alcoholism is well established, a recommendation for inpatient care for detoxification and further psychiatric assessment is reasonable. Major affect disorders are frequent concomitants of alcoholism, and the patient should receive treatment for these conditions when they are identified.

Substance Abuse

The task of the psychiatry consultant in the emergency service is to recognize drug intoxication as the cause of aberrant mental status, to identify the offending substance when possible, and to insure that appropriate treatment is initiated. History is of limited value in these clinical matters. Although the patient usually is aware that he has ingested a drug, he is often less than candid, and he may be unaware of the genuine contents and dosage.

Certain clinical factors suggest the likelihood of drug intoxication. Youth is more vulnerable than age. Sudden onset of mental status change in previously lucid patients indicates intoxication. The presence of changes in vital signs and autonomic responses is often helpful in pointing to a particular class of drug.

Heroin and other opiates. Diagnosis of opiate intoxication is indicated by pinpoint pupils, a smiling sleepiness, stupor, and respiratory depression. Visible signs of habitual IV injection, such as venous sclerosis may be seen. (Meperidine hydrochloride does not cause pinpoint pupils.) Such intoxications may be treated with naloxone hydrochloride.

Opiate withdrawal is suggested by a plausible history of discontinuance plus signs of sympathetic overactivity such as diaphoresis, mydriasis, gooseflesh, and hyperreflexia. Withdrawal typically lasts for a few days at most and is not life-threatening unless other complications of drug abuse are present. If a patient is to be admitted to the hospital, he may be made more comfortable by the use of clonidine hydrochloride or small amounts of methadone hydrochloride. It is generally unwise to attempt outpatient controlled withdrawal by prescription of narcotics, however.

Amphetamines and cocaine.   Acute overdosage with these central stimulants may provoke psychosis, often with paranoid features. Sympathetic autonomic activity is usually present, and tachycardia, hypertension, mydriasis, and diaphoresis may be seen, as well as auditory and visual hallucinosis, tremor, and disorientation. A small amount of a high-potency antipsychotic drug such as haloperidol 2 to 5 mg IM usually brings about a rapid remission.

LSD and similar hallucinogens.   Those patients who appear in the emergency service generally experience dysphoria and acute anxiety along with intense visual hallucinosis. This intoxicated state may persist for hours. It may be ameliorated by the use of oral diazepam 5 to 15 mg. Antipsychotics have been reported to exacerbate the condition.

Marijuana.   Serious dysphoric reaction to the cannabis derivatives is unusual, but may occur with strong preparations or inexperienced users. The patient frequently carries the odor of burning rope, and the conjunctivae may be intensely red. There may be tachycardia, disorientation, paranoia, space and time disorientation, and anxiety. Visual hallucinations may also occur. Rest and reassurance is generally all that is required, with recovery in a few hours.

Phencyclidine.   The popular hallucinatory dissociative anesthetic phencyclidine hydrochloride has many pernicious properties. Clinical presentation varies from stupor to extreme agitation and violence. Mental status is highly labile, and a quiet patient is not necessarily reassuring. Other clinical findings include a blank stare, nystagmus, tachycardia, and hypertension. The serum creatine phosphokinase (CPK) may be elevated, reflecting muscular damage by violent physical encounters.

The patient should be placed in a moderately lighted room under close supervision. Restraint may be necessary. Excretion of the drug is facilitated by gastric suction, which is often impractical, or by acidification of the urine with ammonium chloride or ascorbic acid. Care must be taken when there is significant muscle damage, since liberated myoglobin may precipitate in the renal tubules in a highly acid urine. Treatment is symptomatic and may include antipsychotics, benzodiazepines, β-blockers, or a combination of these drugs.

Barbiturates and other sedatives.   These drugs are all cross-tolerant with alcohol and intoxication and withdrawal symptoms bear many similarities to those seen with that most popular drug. Withdrawal may be subtle at first, with an unexplained delirium which increases in intensity until a hyperpyrexia may become life-threatening. Autonomic signs are not always prominent, and a high index of suspicion is indicated. A history of sedative use is helpful, but not always forthcoming. Any delirium which remains unexplained after initial thorough assessment should be presumed to be sedative withdrawal, at least in part, and treatment attempted with cross-tolerant drugs such as benzodiazepines.

Anticholinergic drugs.   Many prescription and over-the-counter drugs have anticholinergic activity. Antipsychotics, antidepressants, antihistamines, antiparkinsonian, and antisecretory preparations are among them. They may be taken with suicidal intent or with recreational intent.

Mental status may show disorientation, memory loss, visual or tactile hallucinations, and panic. Mydriasis, cycloplegia, tachycardia, dry mouth, difficulty in voiding, and absence of bowel sounds may be seen. Physostigmine is a specific antidote, but must be used cautiously to avoid rebound cholinergic overactivity.

Medical complications.   In addition to their toxic effects on mind and behavior, drugs abused by parenteral injection may produce other complications. Hepatitis, AIDS, tetanus, malaria, syphilis, and bacterial endocarditis are possibilities. Venous sclerosis, local abcess, and septic pulmonary embolism may be seen as well.

Anxiety

Patients who enter the emergency service with the complaint of anxiety may suffer from a wide variety of ailments. A careful history with a view toward differential diagnosis is essential. Many acute medical conditions may make a person anxious. It is hazardous to assume that signs and symptoms of adrenergic hyperactivity stem from psychiatric conditions alone.

Medical conditions as the source of anxiety become increasingly likely with increased patient age. An elderly man who is fearful, sweating, and hyperventilating is more likely to be having a heart attack than an acute identity crisis. Similarly, patients with known systemic disease may often show anxiety symptoms as a result of a worsening of the underlying condition.

Anxiety symptoms may come from toxic or metabolic conditions. Use of amphetamines or large amounts of caffeine may be implicated. Hypoglycemia, electrolyte abnormalities, hypocalcemia, hyperthyroidism, pheochromocytoma, Cushing's disease, and idiosyncratic reactions to medicines may also produce anxiety. Complex partial seizures may also first present as paroxysmal anxiety. Occasionally a sudden serious medical event may be heralded by an anxious state. Myocardial infarction, pulmonary embolism, and anaphylaxis are some examples. Finally, alcohol and sedative withdrawal begins with anxiety and may progress to the full picture of delirium tremens, with life-threatening consequences.

When these conditions have been considered for a patient in the emergency service and have been provisionally rejected as unlikely, it is reasonable to consider the differential diagnosis of anxiety which occurs as part of a more traditional psychiatric syndrome. Among these are panic disorders, agoraphobic states, posttraumatic stress, affect disorders, and incipient psychoses. Anxiety is not a disease in itself, but must be further differentiated so as to provide specific treatment. This is best done outside the emergency service. Depending on the severity of the reaction and on the psychosocial environment, definitive diagnosis and treatment may proceed on an outpatient or inpatient basis.

SUGGESTED READINGS

Anderson WH: The physical examination in office practice. *Am J Psychiatry* 1980; 137:1188–1192.

Anderson WH, Kuehnle JC: Diagnosis and early management of acute psychosis. *N Engl J Med* 1981; 305:1128–1130.

Anderson WH: Psychiatric emergencies, in Wilkins EW Jr (ed): *MGH Textbook of Emergency Medicine*. Baltimore, Williams & Wilkins Co, 1983.

Bristol JH, Giller E, Doherty JP: Trends in emergency psychiatry in the last two decades. *Am J Psychiatry* 1981, 138:623–628.

Gerson S, Bassuk E: Psychiatric emergencies—an overview. *Am J Psychiat* 1980; 137:1–11.

Hall RC: Physical illness presenting as psychiatric disease. *Arch Gen Psychiatry* 1978; 35:1315–1320.

Jenicke MA, Anderson WH: Depression—emergency assessment and differential diagnosis, in Manschreck TC, Murray GB (eds): *Psychiatric Medicine Update*. New York, Elsevier Scientific Publishing Co Inc, 1984.

Murray GB: Violent behavior, in Lazare A (ed): *Outpatient Psychiatry—Diagnosis and Treatment*. Baltimore, Williams & Wilkins Co, 1979.

22

Psychiatric Care of the Burn Victim

CHARLES A. WELCH

Working with burn victims probably places more varied and severe demands on the psychiatrist than any other consultation role. The situation generates negative emotional reactions that make it very difficult to be intimate and encouraging. The problems encountered require special expertise on disparate disciplines, including neurophysiology, pharmacokinetics, psychodynamics, developmental psychology, and family intervention. The job usually includes meticulous attention to staff-oriented consultation, particularly to nurses. The ultimate outcome is often tragic at best and the consultant's self-esteem cannot hinge on the result.

Nevertheless, many elements of caring for the burn victim are well understood and this chapter will review the commonly accepted approaches. The problems will be discussed according to the sequence in which they typically occur, starting with the acute phase, progressing to the reconstitutive phase, and concluding with the long-term adjustment phase, although they do not always occur in that sequence.

CHARACTERISTICS OF BURN VICTIMS

While some burn patients are simply victims of circumstance, the majority carry important predisposing factors. In a study of 155 adults, MacArthur and Moore[1] found that 59% of women and 38% of men had such predisposition. Drug and alcohol abuse was the most prevalent factor, affecting 36% of the predisposed group. Twenty-one percent of the predisposed group suffered from senile degeneration and 20% from chronic mental illness such as schizophrenia or manic-depressive disorder. Of the predisposed persons, 76% suffered their burns at home, typically in a fire involving a bed or mattress.

Children from disturbed or disadvantaged families are at an increased risk for burns. Long and Cope[2] found that in 42% of their sample there was an absent parent, a broken home, or serious psychiatric disturbance in one parent. Over half the children in their sample suffered some serious emotional maladjustment prior to injury. Bernstein[3] in a long-term study of children found that 80% came from disturbed homes, and Martin,[4] in a review of 50 cases, found that in 41 cases (82%) the burns occurred at a time of family crisis or emotional stress. During infancy, the majority of burns are by scalding, and most of these are associated with parental neglect.[5] Older children typically incur their injuries while playing with inflammables or explosives.[6]

These findings indicate that the psychiatric consultant usually must deal not only with the patient, but with a family or living situation that is seriously disturbed. A team approach is necessary, providing at-home family intervention, financial support, residential placement, day care facilities, vocational training, or institutional placement. It is important that the consultant understand and expect this at the outset. Most predisposed patients do not articulate their special needs, and unless the staff anticipate and prepare for them these needs will go unmet.[7]

THE ACUTE PHASE

The acute phase of burn care is in many ways the simplest since immediate surgical care of the burn is the primary issue for all concerned. There is usually an initial lucid period of 24 to 72 hours during which the patient may discuss the situation with remarkable clarity in spite of devastating thermal injury. This is a brief opportunity to assess underlying personality and strengths, and to have a frank dialogue about the extent of the injury and the treatment plan.

Between 30% and 70% of patients start to develop delirium about 48 hours after the burn.[8] Although this is a routine feature of the postburn course, its etiology is not understood, although it appears to be related to stress-induced metabolic disturbances. Severity correlates roughly with extent of burn area. During the delirium, patients may be continually hallucinating, often with vivid re-creation of the scene of injury. Agitation is a serious threat to burn care since patients are usually freshly grafted with delicate suspension of extremities.

Either chlorpromazine or haloperidol may be used to treat burn delirium. Chlorpromazine is sedating but may cause an abrupt drop in blood pressure. Although not approved by the Food and Drug Administration for intravenous (IV) use, 100 mg of chlorpromazine may be instilled in 100 mL of normal saline and infused over 15 to 30 minutes.

Intravenous haloperidol has been studied by Cassem and Sos.[9] They administered doses from 1 to 5 mg as a bolus IV, with total doses as high as 185 mg over 24 hours. Injection was followed by a drop in systolic pressure of 3 to 4 mmHg about four minutes after injection. Sedation appeared after ten to 20 minutes had elapsed. No significant changes in arterial pressure, pulse pressure, mean pressure, ECG, pulmonary arterial pressure, pulmonary wedge pressure, cardiac rhythm, or respiratory rate were observed. In half the patients the regimen was judged to be clearly effective and in the other half partially effective.

With either drug, the initial loading dose should be administered at 30-minute intervals until adequate sedation is achieved; then half the total induction dose is administered every 12 hours to maintain sedation.

Schizophrenia presents a special problem because of the large requirements for antipsychotic medication. Schizophrenics tend to attempt suicide during periods of active psychosis, and consequently these patients often present following self-immolation. Their early course in the hospital may be complicated by severe psychosis, and they may require up to 2400 mg of chlorpromazine IV per 24 hours, or its equivalent. Naturally, very close monitoring of blood pressure is necessary at these doses.

While pain thresholds vary from patient to patient, burns are notorious for the intensity of pain which they can generate. Certainly psychological factors are important in determining pain threshold. However, Szyfelbein et al,[10] in a study of 15 children, found that intensity of pain also varied inversely with plasma β-endorphin levels during dressing changes.

Even with large doses of analgesic, many patients still experience severe pain during dressing changes. If the patient expects that analgesics will eradicate pain, there will be inevitable disappointment. The patient should understand that pain can usually only be modulated by medication. On the other hand, medication should not be sparingly used out of fear of addiction. The incidence of addiction is very low, and probably not correlated with dose.[11] When pain medication is withheld following a request, the patient generally feels the staff is being indifferent or even malevolent and an escalating atmosphere of contention and mistrust may develop.[12] Consequently, patients should always have some form of pain medication available.

The most commonly used IV analgesics are morphine, meperidine hydrochloride, methadone hydrochloride, and fentanyl citrate.[13] Morphine is effective, but may induce nausea and hemodynamic changes. Meperidine is metabolized to normeperidine, a CNS irritant, and should be used only with careful attention to mental status. Methadone is similar to morphine but longer acting, especially after several days of therapy. Fentanyl has the advantage of short duration, making it useful when analgesia is only needed for dressing changes. Optimal dosage varies greatly from patient to patient and should be individualized.[14]

Intramuscular (IM) administration of analgesics should be avoided when practical because of variable kinetics.[15] Oral administration also suffers from variable absorption rates, but may still be the most practical route in the later stages of care. Codeine, oxycodone, and methadone are the most commonly used drugs, typically given one hour prior to dressing changes. Diazepam, hydroxyzine, and chlorpromazine are the psychotropics most commonly used to potentiate the effect of analgesics.

Hypnosis has also been widely used in the control of pain,[16] but its efficacy varies widely, and is largely related to the skill of the hypnotist. For some patients the most gratifying effect is the relaxing quality of the induction. In skilled hands, hypnosis may play an important adjunctive role, but for most clinicians it is not advisable to rely on it as a primary method of pain control.

Two psychological issues predominate in the acute phase: denial and the need for explanation. The intensity of denial is highly variable, and subject to sudden fluctuations.[17] The patient who at one moment does not acknowledge injury may shortly thereafter ask very penetrating questions about the degree of disfigurement. The general rule of dealing with denial is to refrain from confrontation, but to respond when the patient asks questions or expresses a wish to ventilate fear or sadness.

The process of explaining to the patient and family the nature of injury and the treatment involved begins at this point and continues throughout the hospitalization. The psychiatric consultant should be available to discuss these matters with the patient and family, since the surgical staff often does not have the time to explore the emotional impact of the injury or its treatment. It is therefore essential that the psychiatrist be up-to-date about the surgical treatment plan and the expected results.

RECONSTITUTIVE PHASE

The second phase of burn care lasts from the end of acute surgical intervention and delirium until the time of discharge and may take from several days to many months. Psychologically, it is the most difficult phase for most patients, since they must face their injury with a clear sensorium and begin to accept their loss. It is also a period of excrutiating dressing changes, arduous physical therapy, discomfort, uncertainty, and loneliness. It is in this phase that the full scope of the disaster finally settles upon the patient.

It is helpful at this point to review the premorbid psychological status. For instance, the quality of prior relationships often predicts the ways the patient will relate to the medical staff. Patients who have in the past used blaming, denial, and impulsive acts to deal with stress tend to do so in the burn unit. Their work history is also a useful predictor, since it gives some indication whether they have the flexibility, pragmatism, perseverance, and ability to cooperate that the coming weeks will require.

It is also useful to identify the patient's sources of self-esteem. Those patients whose self-esteem is based mainly on physical attractiveness, athletic prowess, or social acceptance tend to have a difficult course, while patients whose self-esteem is based on nonphysical traits such as courage, altruism, perseverance, or empathy carry a better prognosis.

In children it is particularly important to evaluate the family, since the preburn problems of the family tend to define the difficulties that will be encountered in the recovery phase.[18,19] The consultant should carefully observe the parents' initial reactions to the injury. For instance, if they are angry and blaming, this is often a sign of broader family disturbance underneath.

The most concrete role of the consultant in this phase is to continue explanation about what is being done and exploration of the emotional consequences. The psychiatric consultant is a form of trouble-shooter, a role enhanced by the fact that he or she is often the *only* member of the staff not in a pain-inflicting role. At this stage of their care, many patients have difficulty framing questions about what is going on and if the consultant can anticipate their concerns, it often saves the patient from suffering in anxious silence.

Grief work and ventilation are also a major part of the psychiatrist's job. In addition to the loss of their own integrity, patients also have often lost a friend or family member in a fire. Patients who are given opportunities to ventilate these concerns have been observed to have a decrease in psychological disturbances at follow-up.[20] The timing of grief work is unpredictable, and patients may ask to talk and cry about their losses at the most unexpected moments. The consultant should make the staff aware of the importance of this part of burn care, so that, in the pressure of a busy day or night, they still make time for it when the need arises. The combination of a busy work schedule and negative counter-transference to sorrow sometimes makes it an act of discipline to stay at the bedside and hear things out.

For most patients this period also involves accepting the fact that they are altered, and renouncing some of their most fundamental feelings and ideas about themselves. The pace with which a patient learns about new deformities and handicaps should be set by his or her own inquisitiveness. Mirrors should not be conspicuously located on the ward but should be available on request, and many weeks may elapse before a patient indicates a readiness to view the deformity.

The goals of wound healing should be kept to small increments, because the expectation of large leaps inevitably leads to disappointment and discouragement. Small, realistic incremental goals provide the satisfaction of visible progress, particularly when the staff has a positive, reinforcing attitude. Group therapy is also helpful in this regard, in that patients can see progress in others more advanced than they are. It is especially helpful to see burn victims who have resumed normal living, as this provides concrete evidence that life goes on.

Finally, the management of regression is intrinsic to this phase. Limited regression is desirable because it allows patients to adapt to a situation of dependency. For some patients it may help to explicitly encourage regression, by reassuring the patient that it is appropriate to have total care under the circumstances. Other patients regress excessively, and become a management problem because of irritability, crying, angry complaining, insatiable demands, accusations, and persistent complaints of unbearable pain in spite of ample analgesia. In this case the staff must communicate the unacceptability of excessive regression and provide the enthusiasm, coping skills, and interest that the patient is unable to generate.

Giving the patient as much of a decision-making role as possible is usually helpful. Every opportunity should be taken to give him or her a voice in the timing of dressing changes, whether or not tube feeding is to be instituted, the timing of physical therapy and the types of activity to be performed. Generally, regression is more profound in single rooms, occasionally progressing to psychosis, whereas in open wards or semiprivate rooms regressive behavior is less of a problem.

During this phase patients who have been fully cooperative sometimes unexpectedly begin behaving in a hostile and irritable manner toward the staff, just when their wounds begin healing well. This generally does not represent regression, but rather the resolution of earlier dependency and passivity as the patients regain some sense of strength. It is important that this be recognized as a good prognostic sign, rather than as an indication of the staff's failure. Patients who fail to show this kind of irritable or contentious behavior at this stage may be more of a problem. They may tend to remain apathetic and inactive even after discharge and are likely to remain passive and dependent on a permanent basis.

LONG-TERM ADJUSTMENT PHASE

There is controversy about the long-term psychiatric course of burn patients after they leave the hospital. Studies of long-term adjustment have reported a satisfactory outcome ranging from 20% to 70%.[21,22] The most consistent finding is that the degree of subsequent social withdrawal correlates closely with the severity of facial deformity and that facial deformity is a more important determinant of outcome than are personal values, interests, and strengths.[23] This is in contrast to most other forms of disfigurement, where premorbid strengths are the most accurate predictors of long-term outcome.

The most revealing study of facial disfigurement was published in 1953 by MacGregor et al, who studied the subjective response of normal volunteers to the sight of the facially disfigured.[24] Most of the respondents perceived these disfigured persons as mentally inferior or defective, criminal, malevolent, or indolent despite the fact that these traits were not characteristic of the subjects. MacGregor et al found that over 80% of the disfigured underwent a major withdrawal from society. Projective testing revealed repressed hostility, a sense of hopeless isolation, and highly conflicted dependency wishes. The subjects acknowledged that when they were in public places they continued to suffer social ostracism, particularly from staring, questions about their disfigurement, or remarks made about it behind their backs. The subjects reported that their most reliable defenses were defiance, avoidance, and jokes about themselves.

The most discouraging outcome studies pertain to children. Woodward[25] studied 198 children 5 years to more after their burns and found that over 80% were emotionally disturbed, with the most common problems being anxiety states and phobic disorders. Large poor families and families who did not visit during hospitalization were associated with a poor outcome. Sawyer et al[26] reported poor outcome associated with facial burns, frequent moves, and emotionally disturbed mothers. Vigliano et al[27] studied burned children and their mothers a year after hospitalization and found that while the children were aloof and denied anxiety or concern about their disfigurement, on psychological testing they showed overwhelming anxiety and a perception of the world as destructive and overpowering. On interview they denied feelings of weakness but their drawings indicated a ubiquitous sense of vulnerability. Furthermore, 80% of the mothers experienced insomnia, anorexia, loss of sexual interest, crying spells, and strong feelings of guilt during the year following the burn, but generally concealed this from the physicians involved in the burn care.

These studies are important not only for their measure of distress, but also for the finding that burn victims and their families fail to communicate this distress. The data bear out the common clinical observation that denial and repression make it difficult to engage a burn victim in exploratory psychotherapy. In working with these patients one encounters these ego defenses on a scale rarely seen in other nonpsychotic disorders.

Children generally have a greater need for psychotherapy than adults because of the developmental progress to be made after their disfigurement. Stoddard,[28] in a penetrating discussion of the problem, points out that personality disorder need not result from disfiguring injuries, provided staff and parents are able to encourage expression of fear, sadness, guilt, and anger. He recommends that pathologic defenses such as distortion, avoidance, isolation, projection, and pathologic rejection be interpreted and that efforts be directed toward gradual acceptance of a new body image. Ultimately children must face adolescence with its overwhelming focus on physical appearance as the source of self-esteem, and most need a great deal of support during this period. Since the child can only deal openly with the disfigurement if the family is able to do so, skilled family intervention is indicated for most families.

Adults may be more resistant to exploratory work, and sometimes derive greater benefit from a more didactic approach. The focus of the therapy is on teaching coping skills. Weisman and Sobel[29] analyzed good coping in cancer patients and proposed the following approach:

1. Identifying the primary feelings about the injury but refraining from making these the focus of the therapy
2. Defining a hierarchy of problems facing the patient
3. Generating a hierarchy of desired goals and solutions
4. Continuing to work with flexibility toward these goals, and avoiding an all-or-nothing position

In the context of this kind of work, the door should always be left open for exploration of underlying affects. Many burn victims go through sudden lapses in their defensive position and abruptly become quite open to exploratory work, or even request it. As always, versatility is an essential feature of management.

The various consulting roles outlined above may occur in different order, and usually several may be necessary at any given time. Each burn patient naturally follows a different emotional trajectory and this discussion should serve mainly as a framework for organizing clinical formulations and treatment plans. The most important point is that good psychiatric care makes a significant difference in the degree of acute suffering experienced by the patient, and in the long-term adjustment. It is a specialized form of psychiatric consultation and should only be embarked upon after a thoughtful reading of the more important literature on the subject.

REFERENCES

1. MacArthur JD, Moore FD: Epidemiology of burns. *JAMA* 1975; 231:259.
2. Long RT, Cope O: Emotional problems of burned children. *N Engl J Med* 1961; 264:1121–1127.
3. Bernstein NR: *Emotional Care of the Facially Burned and Disfigured.* Boston, Little, Brown & Co, 1976.
4. Martin HL: Parents' and children's reactions to burns and scalds in children. *Br J Med Psychol* 1970; 43:183–191.
5. Savage JP, et al: Childhood burns: A sociological survey and inquiry into causation. *Med J Aust* 1972; 1:1337–1342.
6. Schuhl JF: Suicidal burns. *Anesth Analg* 1973; 30:325–336.
7. Goldberg RT: Rehabilitation of the burn patient. *Rehabil Lit* 1974; 35:73–78.
8. Andreasen NJ, Hartford CE, Knott JR, et al: EEG changes associated with burn delirium. *Dis Nerv Syst* 1977; 38:27–31.
9. Cassem EH, Sos J: The intravenous use of haloperidol for acute delirium in intensive care settings, in Speidel H, Rodewald G (eds): *Psychic and Neurological Dysfunctions after Open-Heart Surgery.* Stuttgart, Georg Thieme Verlag, 1980, pp 196–199.
10. Szyfelbein SK, Osgood PF, Carr DB: The assessment of pain and plasma β-endorphin immunoactivity in burned children. *Pain* 1985; 22:173–182.
11. Porter J, Jick H: Addiction is rare in patients treated with narcotics. *N Engl J Med* 1980; 302:123.
12. Marks RM, Sachar EJ: Undertreatment of medical inpatients with narcotic analgesics. *Ann Intern Med* 1973; 78:173–181.
13. Perry S, Heidrich G: Management of pain during debridement: A survey of U.S. burn units. *Pain* 1982; 13:267–280.
14. Jaffe JJ, Martin WR: Narcotic analgesics and antagonists, in Goodman LS, Goodman A (eds): *The Pharmacological Basis of Therapeutics.* Macmillan Publishing Co, 1983.
15. Stanski DR, Greenblatt DJ, Lowenstein E: Kinetics of intravenous and intramuscular morphine. *Clin Pharmacol Ther* 1978; 24:52–59.
16. Shafer DW: Hypnosis use on a burn unit. *Int J Clin Exp Hypn* 1975; 23:1–14.
17. Hamburg DA, et al: Adaptive problems and mechanisms in severely burned patients. *Psychiatry* 1953; 16:1–20.
18. Holter JC, Friedman SB: Etiology and management of severely burned children. *Am J Dis Child* 1969; 118:680–686.
19. Vigliano A, et al: Psychiatric sequelae of old burns in children and their parents. *Am J Orthopsychiatry* 1964; 34:753–761.
20. Andreasen NJ, et al: Long-term adjustment and adaptation mechanisms in severely burned adults. *J Nerv Ment Dis* 1972; 154:352–362.
21. Andreasen NJ, et al: Long-term adjustment and adaptation mechanisms in severely burned adults. *J Nerv Ment Dis* 1972; 154:352–362.
22. Woodward JM: Emotional disturbances of burned children. *Br Med J* 1959; 1:1009–1013.

23. Goldberg RT: Rehabilitation of the burn patient. *Rehabil Lit* 1974; 35:73–78.
24. MacGregor FC, et al: *Facial Deformities and Plastic Surgery: A Psychosocial Study.* Springfield, Ill, Charles C Thomas Publisher, 1953.
25. Woodward JM: Emotional disturbances of burned children. *Br Med J* 1959; 1:1009–1013.
26. Sawyer MG, Minde K, Zuker R: The burned child—scarred for life? A study of the psychosocial impact of a burn injury at different developmental stages. *Burns* 1982–1983; 9:205–213.
27. Vigliano A, et al: Psychiatric sequelae of old burns in children and their parents. *Am J Orthopsychiatry* 1964; 34:753–761.
28. Stoddard FJ: Body image development in the burned child. *J Am Acad Child Psychiatry* 1982; 21:502–507.
29. Weisman AD, Sobel HJ: Coping with cancer through self-instruction: A hypothesis. *Hum Stress* 1979; 5:3–8.

23

The Spinal Cord-Injured Patient

THOMAS D. STEWART

Is there a role for psychiatry with the spinal cord-injured patient? Certainly the depression, denial, anger, and insecurity permeating such patients (and their caregivers) have a reality anchored in actual tragic loss. What could a psychiatrist trained to treat the pathologic distortions of reality associated with neurosis and psychosis possibly offer?

In this chapter the role for the psychiatrist in the initial evaluation, ongoing assessment, and treatment of the spinal cord-injured patient, with particular emphasis on the use of coping behavior is described. Although the observations and conclusions in this chapter are based on spinal cord injuries, much of the content can also be applied to the understanding of a role for the psychiatrist in the broader areas of rehabilitation medicine and acute traumatology.

INITIAL EVALUATION

The initial psychiatric evaluation lays the foundation for subsequent psychiatric involvement should any be necessary. It is done soon after the patient is admitted and involves interviewing someone who is still acutely injured. The focus is on assessing coping strategies that the patient has used to deal with past stresses and the need, if any, for further psychiatric involvement. In addition, this interview establishes the psychiatrist as a member of the medical team and, thus, as less of a stranger should subsequent psychiatric involvement be required.

On account of the physical and emotional impact of the recent trauma, the patient is approached with caution. Initial questioning centers on his physical state. "Are you in pain?" and "How is your sleep?" are questions asked. Pain is, of course, common, as is marked sleep disturbance. The latter is due to frequent turning and to the proprioceptive disruption in quadriplegia.[1] Further questioning is about postinjury body sensation. In the acute phase, patients may have phantom sensations in which they feel as though their extremities are in positions that are patently impossible.[2–4] For example, patients may feel as though they are astride a motorcycle. Patients may experience this perception and be afraid to mention it for fear of being viewed as crazy. Responding to a question about strange feelings, along with the reassurance that such distortions are normal, can provide much relief. The responses to these questions enable the psychiatrist to assess the appropriateness of further questioning. If patients are too distraught, the interview should be postponed. If not, the second stage of the interview should be initiated.

This stage of the interview begins with questions about work history and social relationships. A stable work history is an important indication of an effective adjustment to the injury. Relationships are explored through traditional questioning about the quality of involvement in marriage or dating and other social interactions. Clues gained from this part of the interview can serve as guides for predicting the ease or difficulty with which patients will work with the hospital staff.

One question stands out in its ability to provide helpful data. It involves finding out whether the patient knows anyone else with a spinal cord injury. It is incredible to see how often the answer is yes when one considers that the injury is rare (30 per million people per year). If he does know someone else with this injury, his expectations about his prognosis will be profoundly influenced by this other person's course. Since the acquaintance's injury and personality might be very different from the patient's, his outcome may be different as well. The psychiatrist needs to help the patient recognize the dissimilarities. This need is especially pressing if the other person was eventually able to walk and the patient lacks such good fortune.

COPING STRATEGIES

The assessment of coping strategies is vital. Coping strategies can be viewed as behavior patterns designed to solve problems and/or reduce stress. A thorough discussion of the distinction between coping behavior and defense mechanisms is beyond the scope of this chapter but is well presented by White in *Coping and Adaptation*.[5] For the purposes of this chapter, the difference centers on the fact that defense mechanisms attempt to avoid anxiety and pain that is often related to long-standing instinctual conflicts, whereas coping behavior attempts to maintain a sense of comfort and continuity in the face of drastic changes that defy familiar patterns of behavior. In an article on the coping behavior of the spinal cord-injured patient, the author reviewed the stages of coping with particular emphasis on depression and grieving.[6] Weisman has described a series of coping strategies used by patients with cancer.[7]

These strategies are also applicable to the adjustment to the sudden stresses of spinal cord injury. A list of these strategies can be found in chapter 15.

The determination of the predominant strategies of a particular patient provides the staff with clues for working with that patient. The answers to a few questions can provide a guide to the strategies favored by the patient. The question, "What is the most upsetting thing that ever happened to you before this injury?" is frequently quite productive. Once the patient answers, he is then asked, "What did you do to ease the frustrations it caused?" This answer will usually spell out one or several favored strategies. Sample answers are, "I kept myself busy" (displacement), "I started reading about it" (rational/intellectual), or "I just got away by myself for a while" (avoidance).

This knowledge of the strategies employed by the patient in adjusting to past stresses allows the staff to work in concert with the patient's efforts to cope with the current situation. For example, displacement calls for active, early engagement of occupational and recreational therapy. The patient using rational/intellectual coping should be given especially thorough explanations of the condition and the required procedures along with available written information about the particular injury. The patient who needs to back off from stress may benefit from a corner bed that can be easily closed off with curtains if the patient uses such "getting away" as a springboard for aggressive rehabilitative efforts. Otherwise, such isolation could promote further withdrawal.

The assessment of coping behavior involves more than a few questions. Further observation during the course of hospitalization along with questions about how the patient managed vocational stresses will fill the picture. The protective denial frequently seen in the acute spinal cord-injured person sometimes makes this extended evaluation especially necessary because of the patient's initial refusal to acknowledge the existence of any problems creating stress.

SYNTHESIS

The data from the interview along with information from the psychologist and social worker provide a working set of hypotheses concerning the psychosocial adjustment and potential problems of the patient. This synthesis of data should take into account several issues relating to disability. First, the impact of the injury on the effectiveness of the patient's coping strategies must be considered. For example, the patient who physically acts out to relieve tension is especially vulnerable to the restrictions of life in a wheelchair, particularly if that patient has a cervical injury. The patient's place in the life cycle can also provide clues to his particular vulnerability.[8] Spinal cord injuries to a patient with an established social and vocational identity is a very different matter than a comparable blow to an adolescent for whom the uncertainty created by the injury adds to the turbulence associated with evolving activity/ passivity and sexual identity conflicts. This disability in the young alters the life cycle by bringing the patient into contact with the feelings of loss and deterioration normally associated with aging. This patient must struggle with the sense of integrity versus despair—the issues of Erikson's eighth and final stage.[9] On the other hand, when this injury occurs to an older person the sense of decline present before the injury is intensified. The disabilities of spinal cord injury synergize with the normal infirmities of aging in a manner that compromises both the length and quality of life.[10] This depletion occurs even more drastically for those with nontraumatic spinal cord impairment (metastases, vascular compromise, etc) whose incidence increases with age.

The effect of this injury on the patient's ability to maintain self-esteem is a vital clue to its impact on the patient's life. Bibring's concept of self-esteem, which he saw as consisting of the sense of being strong, loving, and lovable, is a useful frame of reference.[11] The mechanism of depression, according to Bibring, consists of the ego's awareness of its helplessness in regard to what it must do to maintain self-esteem. From this model, two questions evolve: In what ways did this patient maintain his self-esteem? How will the sensorimotor losses he has suffered disrupt those efforts? Concerns about sexual and vocational functioning become especially relevant in this regard. This injury strikes an especially cruel blow to the patient whose coping efforts centered on physical activity to reduce tension and to increase self-esteem.

INDICATIONS FOR PSYCHIATRIC INVOLVEMENT

There are several specific indications for psychiatric involvement during the initial posttrauma admission. Foremost among these is the history of a suicide attempt, even if the injury itself may not appear to reflect suicidal intent. Early regular involvement is important not only for ongoing assessment, but also for the development of rapport that may have future importance should suicidal behavior reassert itself. This psychotherapeutic investment for the future cannot be overemphasized. The injury may serve as temporary expiation for the impetus behind self-destructive forces in the patient. As a result, suicidal preoccupation may not be apparent initially. The relationship developed with the psychiatrist can increase the likelihood that the patient will reestablish contact after discharge from the hospital when feelings of despair and suicidal thinking recur. For this recontact to occur, however, it is critical that the psychiatrist clearly confront the patient with the fact that he is seen as a suicide risk.[12-13] It should never be assumed that patients cannot kill themselves because they are too disabled. Vigilance and appropriate precautions are required regardless of the patient's level of injury. Suicide attempts during the hospitalization immediately after the trauma are always a possibility.[14]

Frequently, recently injured patients, particularly those with cervical injury, will be disoriented, delusional, and incoherent. It is vital for the psychiatrist to assess such patients and reassure the families and staff that this delirious state does not mean that they have lost their minds along with the use of their arms and legs. The reversibility of this state needs to be emphasized before such patients are irreversibly labeled as "mental."

A history of psychotic behavior, alcoholism, or drug abuse remains a traditional indication for psychiatric involvement. Special considerations with regard to medications useful in the management of these patients is presented in this chapter.

RESISTANCE

There are many sources of resistance to psychiatric involvement and history taking. For the individual with acute and severe injury, the mind is the last bastion of intactness in an otherwise disrupted body. The intrusive questions of a psychiatrist can be viewed as efforts that may trouble the waters in this one otherwise unimpaired area of the patient's life. As one patient said, "With quadriplegia I already feel helpless. Talking to a psychiatrist makes me feel even more so." By holding back from the psychiatrist, the patient can thus protect his remaining sense of intactness. The massive denial frequently found in response to acute stress further restricts the availability of affectively charged data. Weiss believes that this denial continues past the acute phase and becomes a feature of the patient's long-term adjustment.[15] He refers to this as "pseudohysteria." The personality style of the patient is often not suitable for verbal psychotherapeutic methods since spinal cord injuries frequently occur to physically active and impulsive young men whose tensions are acted out rather than talked out. Diller has confirmed the limited appeal of psychotherapy in a survey of 100 patients who had acute spinal cord injuries, of whom only ten (10%) showed any interest in psychotherapy.[16]

STAFF GROUPS

Since individual psychotherapy is not acceptable for most patients, what can the psychiatrist do? Group involvement with the staff is an area where the psychiatrist's skills can be brought to bear. Familiarity with group dynamics, coupled with an understanding of the adjustment to traumatic disability, is especially useful. As a rule those with the most impact on the patient's adjustment are those having the most contact with the patient. Thus, groups are especially important for those in nursing and rehabilitation medicine (physical and occupational therapy). The "inversion effect" often applies to personal knowledge of the patient; that is, those with the least formal education often have the greatest exposure to the patient. Thus, it is important to include nursing assistants in group planning.

Several realities make staff group work in a rehabilitation setting necessary. Prolonged contact with shattered people is a depleting experience. The constant exposure to physical disability can challenge and drain the staff member's sense of intactness. The sharing and mutual support in a group can help offset this. Hospitals are hierarchical, quasi-military organizations in which resentments are passed down the chain of command. Patients often bear the brunt of these resentments since they are sometimes at the bottom of the power structure. Thus, patients may pay both the emotional and financial price of hospital administration. These staff resentments are often vented during group sessions. This ventilation may possibly reduce the pressure that might influence the patient-staff interaction. The prolonged patient contact that occurs in a rehabilitation hospital often activates gratifications and conflicts that staff members would experience in any long-term relationship. During group meetings, the staff member is exposed to peer feedback and psychiatric input, both of which can give perspective to the staff member's distortions, which so easily arise in this work.

Recurrent themes have become evident from the group meetings. The most prominent involves the regressed and demanding behavior characteristic of some spinal cord-injured patients. Such patients will badger the staff with repeated requests for medication, food, and television channel changes. Often the staff is asked to do things that patients are able to do for themselves. Anger, often not expressed verbally, rapidly develops toward this type of patient.

During one group session (not at West Roxbury) the nurses were discussing a man who insisted that they stay at his bedside regardless of

other patients' needs. I pointed out that death wishes for such patients
are not uncommon. Some nurses quickly denied this and others were
silent. One nurse then shared her fantasy of pushing Lubefax into his
tracheostomy site after he had been relentless with her. Other nurses
then more openly shared their angry thoughts. The net effect seemed to
be a reduction in the tension generated by this man.

Another common reaction is the feeling of "helplessness in the
helpers," to use a phrase from Adler.[17] There is a deep wish to do more
for the severely disabled than is actually possible. Guilt is a frequent
sequel to this frustrated wish. Anger at other professionals for not doing
more is also common. Some of the tension on a rehabilitation ward,
however, may be unsolvable because such conflict serves the defensive
purpose of distracting the staff members from the frightening human
tragedies that surround them.

PATIENT GROUP

Group sessions for patients were conducted for an 18-month period by
a social worker and myself. One-hour meetings were held weekly. Such
topics as sex, jobs, life in the hospital, and feelings about the injury were
discussed. When attendance was adequate, the group provided several of
the therapeutic functions described by Yalom.[18] One of these was the
imparting of information. As a physician, I was able to provide information about community resources. Altruism was apparent as the patients
sought to help each other. Paraplegics would offer to help quadriplegics
with tasks they could not manage. Older patients would share their
experiences with younger patients. Catharsis was another therapeutic
function provided by the group with food and the staff being frequent
targets. The feeling of universality, as the patients discovered that others
shared some of their anxieties, helped to reduce their sense of aloneness
in their struggle with the injury.

Consistent attendance, however, was a constant problem. Attendance
varied from two to eight patients. Sudden medical problems, inadequate
staffing, and time conflicts with other therapies interfered. Certainly the
previously described resistance to individual therapy would apply to
group efforts as well. Vigorous efforts on the part of the cotherapists did
little to change the situation. A similarly frustrating experience with
group therapy and patients who have spinal cord injuries was reported by
Cimperman and Dunn.[19] Lipp and Malone, however, reported some
success with a group involving acute amputees in a Veteran's Administration hospital.[20] Their success is encouraging and may have been aided
by the fact that the group meeting was essentially a social event and by

the fact that anxiety-provoking techniques such as open-ended questions about the future were avoided. The efforts of Lipp and Malone indicate that group work with spinal cord-injured patients may be plausible if mutual support is encouraged and defenses are not challenged.

THE FAMILY

Severe disability is a blow to the family as well as to the patient. Prolonged absence of a member from the home, role changes, and grief over what has happened contribute to the stress. In my experience anger with the disabled person is one of the most painful and disguised problems faced by the family. Exclamations like, "How can I be so angry with him!" and "Look at all he's lost!" are common. By pointing out that anger over the personal upheaval caused by the injury is a natural reaction, the psychiatrist can help the family members who feel guilty see their feelings in a more compassionate light. The majority of individual and group family work at our hospital has been carried out by social workers with the psychiatrist serving in a supervisory role.

SEX

Questions about postinjury sexual behavior can be handled by the psychiatrist if he or she is properly versed in the neurophysiology of the injury and is a person with whom the patient is comfortable. The psychiatrist's responses can be helpful on several levels. The first of these involves the interwoven themes of affirmation and grieving. The discussion of sexual possibilities with the patients serves to affirm the reality of sexual behavior and feelings after the injury, a reality the patient often doubts. This talking also presents the opportunity to share with the patient his sadness over what he has lost in both the sexual and nonsexual spheres in his life.

The next level involves the provision of specific information about sexual capabilities. While the patient must experiment to discover what he can do, there are generalizations that can help guide his efforts. After injury there are two types of erections—reflexogenic and psychogenic. The reflexogenic erections are mediated by sacral nerves and initiated by physical contact with or without erotic meaning. Insertion of a catheter would be just as likely to cause an erection as the touch of a loving hand. Psychogenic erections, on the other hand, are a result of erotic thought and fantasy and are mediated by sympathetic nerves. Physical contact of which the patient is not aware can cause a reflexogenic, but not a psychogenic, erection. Reflexogenic erections occur in spastic patients and psychogenic erections in those who are

Table 23-1. Probabilities of Erections in Spinal Cord-Injured Patients

	Reflexogenic Erections	Psychogenic Erections
Spastic, complete	93%	0%
Spastic, incomplete	98%	0%
Flaccid, complete	0%	26%
Flaccid, incomplete	0%	83%

Data from Comarr.[21]

flaccid. The probabilities that such erections will occur are given in Table 23-1. The term "incomplete" is used here to mean that the neurologic impairment below the level of injury is not total.

The spinal cord-injured female retains the capacity to have intercourse. Like the male, she suffers a sensory loss and thus may not be able to climax, depending on the extent of her injury. Unlike most spinal cord-injured males, she retains fertility. Furthermore, she can have a vaginal delivery.[22]

The third level of reponse to sex-related questions involves individual and couple counseling. There are several articles in the literature dealing with this topic.[23-25] Such counseling is similar in some aspects to comparable efforts with the nondisabled. For example, issues relating to intimacy, mutuality, and self-esteem require attention. The first of these is the sense of vulnerability to rejection. During sex the disabled person must expose a damaged body over which he has limited control and must express tenderness with it. The potential for embarrassment, such as a bladder accident, serves to exaggerate whatever insecurity the patient has concerning rejection. Discussion of this feeling along with practical suggestions, eg, advising the patient to void before sex, help. Other issues requiring attention include feelings about oral or manual sexual contact and role conflicts should the sexual partner also be involved in intimate nursing care.

Penile prostheses placed in the corpora cavernosa offer an option for those with erectile dysfunction. Several types are available.[26] The most complex is the Scott prosthesis.[27] This is an inflatable device which can be activated by squeezing a bulb in the scrotum which pumps fluid from a resevoir in the abdomen to balloons in the corpora producing an erection. Detumescence is achieved by squeezing a valve, much as a blood pressure cuff is released. Other implants cause permanent semierect states and are made of silastic. Examples include the Small-Carrion implant and the Jonas implant, which has silver braided wire in the core of the silastic to allow positioning of the penis.[28,29] Careful psychological assessment is necessary to increase the likelihood of a favorable outcome.[30] Although many men are pleased with these implants, some are not.[31,32] Complications in the spinal cord injured are common, the foremost among these being extrusion of the rods.[33] Other problems include possible interference with bladder outflow and interference with subsequent cystoscopy. Their benefits extend beyond sexual function, for they can render condom drainage more reliable.[34]

Affirmation, grieving, advice, and counseling offer a wide range of possibilities for psychiatric involvement.[35] In many institutions, however, most of the sex counseling is done by social workers or psychologists.

PSYCHOPHARMACOLOGY

Knowledge of the effects of psychotropic medication in the neurologically injured patient is a specific contribution that the psychiatrist can offer to the spinal cord-injured person. The disabled individual, like anyone else, can suffer from conditions requiring such medications. This fact can easily be lost sight of, since the physical defects seem to serve as such an obvious cause for depression or alcohol abuse. Autonomic side effects of psychotropic medications present a special threat to the spinal cord-injured patient since the paralysis includes the autonomic nervous system. These side effects in the nondisabled patient have been reviewed by Shader and Mascio.[36] The anticholinergic effects of the major tranquilizers and antidepressants can serve to unbalance the already compromised function of the neurogenic bladder in the spinal cord-injured patient. The α-adrenergic blocking properties of these medications can disrupt the tenuous control the quadriplegic has over his blood pressure since his thoracolumbar sympathetic outflow is disrupted. The result could be serious hypotension.

Proper questioning and medication selection can help avoid these pitfalls. Asking about the type of bladder drainage is crucial. The patient with an indwelling catheter, of course, will present no problem with regard to bladder function. It is quite a different matter for patients with condom drainage because the bladder empties by reflex contractions that are easily disrupted by parasympatholytic agents.

If antipsychotic or antidepressant medication is required for patients with condom drainage, it is important to select agents with fewer anticholinergic effects. Haloperidol or piperazine phenothiazines become reasonable choices.[37] This advantage is lost, however, if antiparkinsonian agents must be used in light of their anticholinergic properties. Care in the selection of antidepressants is equally important. Snyder and Yamamura[38] have shown that the monomethylated tricyclic, desipramine hydrochloride, has fewer anticholinergic properties than the dimethylated forms. Of the latter, imipramine hydrochloride has fewer such effects than amitriptyline hydrochloride. Trazodone hydrochloride has little or no anticholinergic activity.[39] It is quite sedating, however, for many people. Thus it could create problems for the spinal cord-injured who must maintain the vigilence necessary to reposition themselves regularly to avoid skin breaks. Furthermore, it has substantial α-blocking properties.

With respect to cardiovascular effects, haloperidol and piperazine phenothiazines are again the choice since they are less apt to cause a hypotensive episode. The antidepressants with the least α-blocking properties are desipramine and nortriptyline hydrochloride.[40,41] The latter should be given at night when the patient, especially the quadriplegic, is supine.

If injection is required, the potent antipsychotic agents should be used because they appear to be less irritating than injectable chlorpromazine.[42] The irritated injection site on a spinal cord-injured person could become the focus for a bedsore.

Alcohol abuse and its management are frequent problems on a spinal cord unit. Disulfiram has a role in the treatment of this problem in spinal cord-injured patients as it does in the normal population. Special attention, however, must be given to the physiology of an adverse disulfiram reaction due to the autonomic paralysis in some spinal cord-injured patients. The patient with an injury at the T-4 level or above has a severely impaired capacity to regulate blood pressure. In fact, the pressure in such a patient is frequently around 90/60 mmHg. It follows that such a patient would be especially vulnerable to the hypotension that occurs in a disulfiram reaction. As a rule, the author does not use this medication in patients with an injury at the T-4 level or higher. For paraplegics with injury levels of T-4 to T-12 the author does not use dosages of more than 250 mg/d due to reduced sympathetic tone in the lower extremites. For the patient with an injury level of T-12 and below, the full dosage can be used since sympathetic vascular control is intact.

Benzodiazepines are commonly used in the spinal cord-injured patient due to their spasmolytic properties. They can be employed for the management of anxiety with little risk. For those with mixed depression and anxiety, alprazolam would be a reasonable choice.[43] It has no autonomic side effects and may provide relief from depression.

CONCLUSION

Spinal cord injury shatters the crystal of human experience in every facet. Social relationships, intrapersonal dynamics, and neurologic control of functions, seen and unseen, are involved. Nothing is spared. A role for psychiatry is obscured by the traditional emphasis on the treatment of emotional illness per se. Clearly, the anxiety and depression secondary to the injury are not an illness. The psychiatrist has a creative role in the growing understanding of coping behavior. The psychiatrist's grasp of individual and group process can help the staff with their efforts to work in this setting.

Treatable psychiatric illness occurs in the disabled person as well as in able-bodied persons. This fact seems obvious, and yet it is not. The bias revealed in the phrase *mens sana in corpore sano* ("a sound mind in a sound body") is all too widespread. The implication is that a damaged body is to be equated with an unsound mind. Therefore, why should the psychiatrist treat this "unsound mind?" Such treatment is necessary and possible and requires a grasp of the side effects of psychotropic medications in the unsound body.

REFERENCES

1. Adey W, Bors E, Porter R: EEG sleep patterns after high cervical lesions. *Arch Neurol* 1968; 19:377–383.
2. Conomy JP: Disorders of body image after spinal cord injury. *Neurology* 1973; 23:842–850.
3. Wachs H, Zaks M: Studies of body image in men with spinal cord injury. *J Nerv Ment Dis* 1960; 131:121–127.
4. Ettlin TM, Seiler W, Kaeser HE: Phantom and amputation illusions in paraplegic patients. *Eur Neurol* 1980; 19:112–119.
5. White RW: Strategies of adaptation: An attempt at systematic description, in Coehlo G, Hamburg D, Adams J (eds): *Coping and Adaptation*. New York Basic Books, Inc, 1974.
6. Stewart TD: Coping behavior and the moratorium following spinal cord injury. *Paraplegia* 1978; 15:338–342.
7. Weisman, AD: *The Realization of Death*. New York, Jason Aronson, Inc, 1974.
8. Stewart TD, Rossier A: Psychological considerations in the adjustment to spinal cord injury. *Rehabil Lit* 1978; 39:75–80.
9. Erikson EH: *Childhood and Society*. New York, WW Norton & Co, Inc, 1963.
10. Rossier A, Bors E: Problems of the aged with spinal cord injuries. *Paraplegia* 1965; 3:34–45.
11. Bibring E: The mechanism of depression, in Greenacre P (ed): *Affective Disorders*. New York, International Universities Press, 1953.
12. Missel JL: Suicide risk in the medical rehabilitation setting. *Arch Phys Med Rehabil* 1978; 59:371–376.

13. Ducharme S, Freed M: The role of self destruction in spinal cord injury mortality. *Spinal Cord Injury Digest* 1980; 2:27–38.
14. Reich P, Kelly M: Suicide attempts by hospitalized medical and surgical patients. *N Engl J Med* 1976; 294:298–301.
15. Weiss AJ: Reluctant patient—Special problems in psychologic treatment of patients with myelopathy. *NY State J Med* 1968; 68:2049–2053.
16. Diller L: Psychological theory in rehabilitation counseling. *J Counsel Psychol* 1959; 6:189–193.
17. Adler G: Helplessness in the helpers. *Br J Med Psychol* 1972; 45:315–326.
18. Yalom I: *The Theory and Practice of Group Psychotherapy.* New York, Basic Books, Inc, 1970.
19. Cimperman A, Dunn M: Group therapy with spinal cord injured patients. *Rehabil Psychol* 1974; 21:44–48.
20. Lipp M, Malone S: Group rehabilitation of vascular surgery patients. *Arch Phys Med Rehabil* 1976; 57:180–183.
21. Comarr AE: Sexual function among patients with spinal cord injury. *Urol Int* 1970; 25:134–168.
22. Comarr A: Observations on menstruation and pregnancy among female spinal cord injury patients. *Paraplegia* 1966; 3:263–272.
23. Eisenberg M, Rustard L: Sex education and counseling on a spinal cord injury service. *Arch Phys Med Rehabil* 1976; 57:135–140.
24. Griffith F, Trieschmann R: Sexual functioning in women with spinal cord injury: a review. *Arch Phys Med Rehabil* 1975; 56:18–21.
25. Romano M, Lassiter R: Sexual counseling with the spinal cord injured. *Arch Phys Med Rehabil* 1972; 53:568–572.
26. Golgi H: Experience with penile prosthesis in spinal cord injury patients. *J Urol* 1979, 121:288–289.
27. Scott F, Byrd B, Karacan I, et al: Erectile impotence treated with an implantable, inflatable prosthesis. *JAMA* 1983; 241:2609–2612.
28. Krane R, Friedberg P, Siroky M: Jones silicone silver penile prosthesis: initial experience in America. *J Urol* 1981; 126:475–476.
29. Small M, Carrion H, Burdon J: Small-Carrion penile prosthesis. *Urology* 1975; 5:479.
30. Stewart T, Gerson S: Penile prosthesis: psychological factors. *Urology* 1978; 7:400–402.
31. Furlow W: Patient partner satisfaction with the inflatable penile prosthesis. *JAMA* 1980; 243:1714.
32. Beaser R, Vander Hoek C, Jacobson A, et al: Experience with penile prosthesis in the diabetic man. *JAMA* 1982; 240:943–948.
33. Rossier A, Fam B: Indication and results of semirigid penile prosthesis in spinal cord injury patients: long-term follow-up. *J Urol* 1984; 131:59–62.
34. Van Arsdalen K, Klein F, Hackler R, et al: Penile implants in spinal cord injury for maintaining external appliances. *J Urol* 1981; 126:331–332.
35. Stewart T: Sex, spinal cord injury, and staff rapport. *Rehabil Lit* 1981; 42:347–350.
36. Shader R, Mascio D: *Psychotropic Drug Side Effects—Clinical and Theoretical Perspective.* Baltimore, Williams & Wilkins Co, 1970.
37. Snyder S, Greenburg D, Yamamura H: Antischizophrenic drugs and brain cholinergic receptors. *Arch Gen Psychiatry* 1974; 31:58–61.

38. Snyder S, Yamamura H: Antidepressants and the muscarinic acetylcholine receptor. *Arch Gen Psychiatry* 1977; 34:236–239.
39. Newton R: The side effect profile of trazodone in comparison to an active control and placebo. *J Clin Psychopharmacol* 1981; 1:89–93.
40. Richelson E: Pharmacology of antidepressants in use in the United States. *J Clin Psychiatry* 1982; 43:4–11.
41. Roose S, Glassman A, Siris S: Comparison of imipramine and nortriptyline induced orthostatic hypotension: a meaningful difference. *J Clin Psychopharmacol* 1981; 1:316–319.
42. Hollister L: *Clinical Use of Psychotherapeutic Agents.* Springfield, Ill, Charles C Thomas Publisher, 1973.
43. Feighner JP: Benzodiazepines as antidepressants, in Ban TA (ed): *Modern Problems of Pharmacopsychiatry.* Basel, Karger, 1982.

24

The Hospitalized Child: General Considerations

MICHAEL S. JELLINEK

The clear priority of the child psychiatric consultant is to evaluate the biological, psychological, and social status of an ill child living in the seemingly hostile environment of a hospital. Although the child psychiatrist's core function remains diagnostic, the context of consultation is changing and becoming more complex.

The nature of pediatric illness has changed over the past 40 years. In the past, infectious disease was the predominant complaint in both outpatient and inpatient settings. With the availability of antibiotics and immunizations, the nature of presenting complaints is changing so that psychosocial disorders are more prominent in outpatient practice and chronic disease more common on inpatient units. Consequently the child psychiatric consultant often faces difficult differential diagnostic decisions between the primary effects of the chronic illness, the side effects of treatments, and depressive symptomatology. In addition, chronic illness can be uniquely stressful to parents and caretakers. Parents often feel helpless and guilty as they see their child suffering and possibly dying over a period of months or years. Primary nurses often become highly invested in these patients and families and thus share a substantial burden. House staff are frustrated by illnesses that do not easily yield to their interventions and often require them to perform painful procedures; in addition, they face the anguish of the family several times a day.

Beyond the increase in admissions for chronic disease, a second complicating issue for the child psychiatrist is the growing use in some geographic areas of the pediatric unit as a psychiatric facility. Given the limited number of child psychiatric beds and thus the severity of disorders on these units, many children with psychosomatic presentations, depression, neuropsychiatric disorders, and suicidal behavior are being hospitalized in pediatric beds. Although there is a proud tradition within pediatrics to use beds as a shelter or "last resort," pediatrics units are not effectively designed to treat psychiatric disorders. Thus there is often pressure on the child psychiatrist to treat quickly despite the lack of facilities or at least "place" children despite the lack of beds in appropriate units.

The final complicating issue facing child psychiatric consultation is the emphasis on a shortened length of stay. Many pediatric services do not have a child psychiatrist immediately available. The consultation often requires meeting with the child and family several times as well as gathering information from the pediatrician and school. The work has to be coordinated with other medical procedures and schedules since, given the pace of the work-up, children are often off the floor or sedated before or after a procedure. Some children are discharged so quickly that a less thorough outpatient evaluation is the only recourse.

Given the increasing complexity, range, and stress associated with pediatric illness the child psychiatric consultant needs to have skills in diagnosis and liaison work among caretakers, as well as serve as a teacher for house staff. This chapter will discuss these skills in a conceptual manner and the following chapter will review their implementation with specific diagnosis.

GENERAL APPROACH TO DIAGNOSIS

The age and developmental level of the child serve as the basic framework for the consultation.[1,2] The consultant generates hypotheses based on his or her experience and expectations for age appropriate behavior and intrapsychic functioning. For example, the consultant brings to a consultation with an 8-year-old boy definite developmental expectations of ego functioning, maturity of defenses, the ability to cope with certain levels of stress and anxiety, and cognitive functioning marked by concrete operations. The consultant also anticipates the presence of a range of probable fantasies, forms of play, social skills, and a hard-to-define, subjective quality of relatedness. The broad set of developmental expectations form the basis for a subset of hypotheses designed to begin to answer the referring pediatrician's question.

Initial hypotheses are modified and refined as more data are gathered and analyzed. The hypotheses generated on the basis of the patient's age, the specific problem that prompted the consultation request, and the patient's history then undergo careful assessment during clinical interviews with parents and child. The consultant must understand the in-hospital "snapshot" evaluation in the context of a longer-term perspective. For example, a child seen in the hospital in a regressed state marked by depression or unusual anxiety and/or some bizarre ideational content may evidence better psychological resources when the consultant reviews recent functioning and behavior. For the 8-year-old such a "behavioral review of systems"[3] would include previous recovery from stressful circumstances, school performance, peer relationships, style of play, mood in more familiar surroundings, and functioning within the family. The recommendations at the end of the consultation process are based on an integration of the in-hospital "state" observations with the child's and family's history. The consultant's diagnostic impression requires the balancing of many current, historical, and interview variables viewed within a developmental context.

AGE-SPECIFIC EFFECTS OF HOSPITALIZATION

The age-specific effects of hospitalization[4-7] parallel the concept of age-appropriate developmental expectations or norms. For the infant, probably soon after birth, but certainly by age 6 to 8 months, the impact of hospitalization is almost entirely the stress of separation from the mother. Despite the best efforts at continuity of care, the infant is handled by numerous different medical and nursing personnel and, unless the mother is available at all times, has to face separations. Bowlby's observations[8] of separation anxiety are clearly seen in infants and elements of his model are evident in the regressed behavior of all preadolescent children. Bowlby described the following three phases of separation:

1. *Protest.* The infant acutely, vigorously, loudly, and thrashingly attempts to prevent departure of the mother or rapidly attempts to recapture her. In the older child this phase may appear as clinging, nagging, or bargaining as a parent is about to leave.
2. *Despair.* The infant is less active, may cry in a monotone with less vigor, begins to withdraw and appear hopeless. Sometimes the withdrawal phase is misleading since caregivers welcome the quiet and project their own hopes that the child is "settling in."
3. *Detachment.* The infant seems more alert and accepting of nursing care. However, these new attachments are superficial and the infant concomitantly shows a loss of affect or positive feeling when the mother appears. In chronic disease requiring numerous prolonged hospitalizations, the infant and child make many episodic inconsistent attachments and suffer numerous losses.[8]

Tronick et al[9] found antecedents of Bowlby's three phases of separation at very early ages and demonstrated on film that the separation process occurs in microcosm over minutes if the mother is unresponsive to the infant's attempts at relating (entrainment). In response to these findings of short-term and potentially long-term consequences of maternal separations, hospitals are increasingly encouraging mothers to stay overnight with their children and nursing departments have instituted a primary nursing model to limit the number of different nurses caring for the child.

Anna Freud's classic work[6] emphasizes regression, especially in the toddler. The normal child between the ages of 2 and 4 years might lose autonomous functioning (bladder and bowel control, body movement, ego autonomy) under the stress of physical illness and under the regressive, passive pull of nursing care. Prugh et al[4] found that a wide variety of reactions is common in hospitalized children. Virtually all children are anxious; some, seriously so. Older children tend to be irritable, restless, and withdrawn.

Children, especially of younger school age, commonly feel that their illness is a punishment for angry thoughts or misbehavior. This sense of guilt stems from the development of a conscience and from an egocentric view of causation. Thus children who are ill feel that they are the likely cause of the illness and that it is the deserved consequence of not following a parental wish or rule.

The school-age child may share some aspects of the infantile separation phases, but in general develops multiple, often magical, fears about the nature of the illness. Children, especially in the initial interview, may be reluctant to verbalize their fears or fantasies. The draw-a-person test is sometimes initially useful in estimating the child's developmental level and anxiety about his illness. Several drawings over time may demonstrate the child's neurologic and psychological recovery from trauma, surgery, or head injury.

The adolescent is also sensitive to hospitalization and is especially concerned about maintaining a recently won sense of autonomy. Because of the adolescent's tentative identity formation and investment in peer acceptance, physical stigmata or limitations in daily activity arouse significant anxiety. Invariably the illness awakens dependency needs that may be defended against by aggressive assertiveness, denial or refusal to follow medical regimens.

The serious or chronic illness in a child is among the most stressful events in a family's life. The parents must cope with uncertainty and a seemingly endless series of highs and lows. Abnormal laboratory results, adverse reactions, life-threatening crises, limitations on the child's future, and death are not uncommon and all too often regularly recurrent realities. Other members of the family such as siblings or grandparents are also involved on a daily basis. Each member of the family may have different styles of coping—withdrawal, anger, depression, anxiety, or denial. Clearly the family's reaction is the critical mirror that serves as the child's most trusted resource. If the illness creates family conflicts, the child may respond by accepting responsibility for keeping the family together. The child's fear of abandonment may well be rooted in reality since severe or chronic illness may lead to temporary or permanent breakdown of the family unit. The stress of the child's illness may well either increase family cohesiveness or exacerbate areas of conflict.

In general, the maturity of a child's defensive style may help in coping with anxiety; however, defensive patterns are complex. The defense of denial, especially with some isolation and intellectualization, may be very successful in modulating anxiety.[10] Denial, particularly in a withdrawn child, can sometimes obscure psychopathology and prevent psychiatric referral.[11] The consultant must use a developmental perspective in understanding the normal range of responses to hospitalization and then use this understanding in the evaluation of a child's behavior, emotional state, and defensive style.

SOME REASONS FOR CONSULTATION REQUESTS

Why are children and their parents referred for psychiatric consultation?[11-16] The criteria will vary depending on the setting and the age of the child.

In the neonatal intensive care unit (ICU) the basis for referral is either the parents' or staffs' reaction to the infant's serious illness. Parents may be overwhelmed at the sight of their newborn lying passively while attached to multiple life-sustaining equipment. Although many parents adjust, some, especially with poor social support, history of psychiatric disorder, or a painful memory of a close relative's hospital course, may need social service or psychiatric intervention. As the technology advances, a greater percentage of babies are raising chronic care issues as they stay dependent on ventilation for months and sometimes years. The stress on the family and the staff who have become surrogate parents can be very severe. Psychiatric consultation can be used to monitor whether this level of stress is resulting in parental discord, depression, or raising interstaff tension. Inevitably some babies die and psychiatric consultation should be available for parents and staff both acutely and over time for those parents at risk for developing clinical depression as part of prolonged grieving.

For infants and young children the consultant is typically asked to evaluate the quality of the mother-child relationship. In the work-up of failure to thrive, the consultant may find that emotional deprivation is a major factor in the etiology of the child's failure to grow, form affective relationships, or achieve cognitive landmarks.

In the pediatric ICU the range of age and diagnosis is broad but the child's condition is critical. Parental and staff tensions are especially volatile whether the child has been hit by a car, has taken an overdose of medication in a serious suicide attempt, or is having a life-threatening crisis in the course of a chronic disease. Parental guilt and depression, marital discord, and staff tension frequently parallel the child's course.

On the less acute wards, consultation requests usually fall into the categories of psychosomatic differential diagnosis, chronic disease management, and disorders that are traditionally more the realm of psychiatry.

Another unfortunately too common consultation request in young children is evaluation of potential physical or sexual abuse or neglect.[17,18] The child psychiatrist may be asked to help in the differential diagnosis of an "accident" or through play techniques elicit a history of sexual abuse. These findings will often influence both criminal and custody proceedings.

In terms of psychosomatic disorders, school-age children may present with symptoms of unknown etiology and the consultant will be called on to help differentiate functional from organic complaints. A classic example is the child who presents with recurrent abdominal pain as a somatic defense against separation from home (school phobia). Other common referrals for children of this age are functional neurologic presentations (seizures, paresis) and hyperactivity.[19,20]

The early adolescent may complain of a variety of symptoms such as severe headache, chest pain, or dysmenorrhea in response to developmental pressures from peers (dating, rejection by group), or from parents (inhibiting autonomy), or on the basis of intrapsychic conflicts (identity).

The psychological management of chronic disease is an increasing basis of psychiatric referral. With certain disorders such as leukemia, bone cancers, or renal transplantation, it is appropriate to develop a protocol requiring psychiatric assessment at the time of diagnosis, building in the potential role and availability of the consultant from the beginning. With other chronic disorders psychiatric intervention may be indicated by symptoms of depression, noncompliance with essential medical regimens, or helping to deal with anger or anxiety which commonly appear when the limitations imposed by illness interfere with early adolescent development. Lastly, as stated previously, chronic disease has an impact on the family and psychiatric consultation may be useful if there is marital discord or concerns about the patient's siblings.

Pediatric units are increasingly asked to serve a more traditionally psychiatric function. With the rising prevalence of substance abuse, suicidal behavior, and anorexia nervosa, pediatric units are requesting suicide evaluations and the multiple-week evaluation–initial treatment of complex neuropsychiatric disorders and eating disorders. It is noteworthy that accidents are by a factor of five to ten the most common cause of death in childhood and merit more psychiatric attention.

The reasons for consultation requests are both subtle and obvious. The consultant is called quickly for a child who attempts suicide or drives the ward crazy with his behavior. Other times the reasons are more subtle and are based on the pediatrician's sense that an illness had a psychiatric component or that someone in the family needs psychiatric evaluation.

INITIAL STEPS IN THE CONSULTATION PROCESS

After the referral is received, the consultant should contact the pediatrician and, if necessary, clarify or explore the question being asked. Some pediatricians are especially sensitive to psychological concerns and have known the patient and family for several years. In university-affiliated hospitals, the consultant often deals with less experienced house staff on monthly rotating schedules and thus discussion with the "referring physician" will be shifted toward teaching. A crucial function of ongoing consultation is the trust relationship that should develop between pediatrician, ward personnel, and consultant.[21] This trust creates an atmosphere in which the psychological needs of children are recognized and the consultant's recommendations are carried through even when these take considerable time and effort.

The next step in the consultation process is a thorough review of the hospital record. The record describes the course of chronic or acute illnesses (past and present), the utilization of medical facilities, the ability of the child and parents to comply with medical regimens, and a report of previous psychological observations in cases where there have been past problems of a similar nature.

The registration for the current admission often contains relevant social and cultural data. The child's address will determine the availability of community resources. The family's socioeconomic status (SES) can be determined from address, parental level of education, and occupation.[22] The SES is one of the most reliable single indicators of general social stress; a low social class rating increases the probability of poor housing conditions, inadequate schools, unstable families, unemployment, and a high rate of mental illness.[23-25] The type of third-party coverage will place limits on available resources. This kind of information is necessary if the consultant's recommendations are to be realistic. Knowledge of race, religion, and cultural heritage can further refine the consultant's hypotheses.

In the current hospital record, the chief complaint and history of present illness require special attention; they describe the type of illness and, by implication, its probable course. Before considering psychological implications and formulations, the consultant should be keenly aware of the possible organic etiologies of psychological presentations. Some organic etiologies are clear. Head trauma may result acutely in a postconcussive confusional state with altered mental status, and chronically with behavior changes secondary to a subdural hematoma. An altered state of consciousness or unusual behavior may be the first sign of a viral encephalitis. Preinduction anesthesia medication or the anesthetic itself may produce an acute delirium. A psychoticlike state can be seen several days after a major burn or surgery[26] or when the child is metabolically unstable. Certain drugs, for example, phenobarbital, can produce a paradoxical reaction resulting in hyperactivity or, when used for seizure prophylaxis, a state of withdrawal if serum levels become toxic. A frequently overlooked organic etiology is the acute or chronic ingestion of lead which may present as irritability, poor school performance, or aggressiveness. Drug abuse is an important consideration for the adolescent. The consultant must also consider the child's metabolic status. Frequently, electrolytes, BUN, and blood glucose are reviewed in the chart; however, less attention is paid to calcium balance, thyroid status, and blood gases. When a child presents as acutely distraught, the consultant's focus on action can block a careful review of organic possibilities.

> A 14-year-old diabetic girl had a history and initial assessment of moderate ketoacidosis. The patient had a history of difficult, uncooperative behavior which at time of admission was marked and virtually prevented intravenous (IV) treatment. One hour after admission the patient was given 10 mg of diazepam IV for relief of anxiety with little effect. Soon thereafter the patient's pH was obtained with a value of 6.9. On recovery the patient had no memory of her admission to the hospital or of her subsequent behavior. Further history revealed that her current episode of ketoacidosis was precipitated by a suicidal ingestion of ethylene glycol which added to the severity of her metabolic acidosis.

Some organic etiologies are much more subtle or rare. Frequently the most important cue is the mother's vague sense that the child "doesn't look or act right."

A 7-year-old boy with a history of hydrocephalus treated successfully 5 years earlier by shunt presented first with altered behavior (stubbornness) and then with a minimal increase in a long-stable ataxia. The shunt was patent and there were no signs of infection. Despite good communication, the pediatrician, neurologist, and psychiatrist were perplexed. Finally the child developed a mildly edematous arm. Careful examination and radiologic confirmation revealed a venous embolus inhibiting drainage from both the arm and head. His behavior, arm, and gait returned to baseline with resolution of the embolus.

Physical illness can have a major impact on a child's development and emotional life. Most children with acute illness, reasonably sensitive treatment, and parental support recover quickly from the stress of hospitalization. However, chronic illness can be especially devastating[27-29] and serves as a prototype for illnesses leading to severe impairment of self-image. A child may have physical signs of abnormality such as cleft lip, or loss of hair secondary to cancer chemotherapy that can result in a poor body image and scapegoating. Heart disease[30] or renal transplant[5,31] may limit physical activity and therefore radically change peer relationships. Chronic bowel disease or diabetes may require careful attention to diet. Such long-term regimens as multiple medications and pulmonary toilet for cystic fibrosis force the child into daily confrontations with his illness and decrease his sense of autonomy. Chronic disease changes the quality of play, of family and peer relationships, of daily activities, and potentially of every meal.

The family and social history will yield valuable information concerning patterns of family behavior. In addition to a history of the marriage and of parental employment, the chart may contain information that other family members have had illnesses similar to that of the child. Not uncommonly psychosomatic symptoms have a multigenerational history so that headaches or gastrointestinal (GI) symptoms may have been present in the parent and grandparent. Psychiatric histories are not well documented in pediatric records but are available in a social service note. Given the recent evidence of social or genetic transmission of depression, alcoholism, attention deficit disorder and schizophrenia, the family's psychiatric history is becoming increasingly valuable.

Families respond to the illness of their child in a variety of ways.[30,32,33] There is an initial very anxious period of uncertainty; then there is shock when the diagnosis is confirmed. Families may begin to gather data and become heavily invested in the medical center staff's ability to manage the illness. At this point some parents do well and work with the child and pediatrician to maximize development. If the child has a more chronic, disabling, or life-threatening disease, less stable families may lose their respect for medical competency, become angry with the hospital staff, and feel guilty either for bringing about or not adequately protecting their child from the illness. As the disease continues or progresses the family may pull together, especially if they were previously cohesive or, on the other hand, long-standing tension may grow worse and result in open conflict and divorce. Such conflict will, of course, make the child anxious, guilty for having the illness, and depressed about the potential loss of parental support. Parents have many questions about the setting of limits on behavior. They may respond to matters of discipline and activity level by becoming either overprotective or indulgent. If the child's illness is life-threatening, parents will wonder what to tell the child. They may withdraw from the child as a result of anticipatory grieving for the child's unrealizable potential or eventual death.[32]

The other children in the family are frequently affected by their brother's or sister's illness. They may respond in a number of ways including attention-seeking behavior such as regressive nagging, withdrawal, poor school performance, or delinquency. Siblings may also harbor angry thoughts about the patient based on the reality of an altered family life style forced to meet the needs of the ill child. This anger may subsequently arouse feelings of guilt and depression. Probably the best predictor of a family's reaction to stress or their longer-term ability to cope is their past response to crisis. The family's pattern may be documented in the record; if not, this history should be elicited early in the consultant's direct interviewing.

In the review of the medical record, the consultant must pay special attention to the notes made in the chart by ward personnel. The pediatric nurse's observations may be the most helpful in a number of areas. The nurse is a surrogate mother and has considerable objective experience with children of the same age and with the same illness. When a child is admitted, the nurse takes a self-care and daily habit history emphasizing the child's healthy routine functioning. The nurse may also make the most careful observations of the child's level of anxiety, state of regression, and temperamental characteristics.[34,35] Because of the nurse's many contacts over days with the child, her impression of the child's quality of relating may be an important adjunct to the consultant's impression that is based on one or two interviews.

The nurse's notes may be supplemented by other observations from additional personnel such as a child life worker.[36,37] The role of the child life worker, trained in child development, is to help children cope with the stress of hospitalization. By organizing group activities in the playroom or by celebrating a birthday on the ward, the child life worker may make significant observations about the child's ability to interact with peers. Child life workers may also have impressions of the child's intrapsychic life based on preoperative play sessions designed to decrease the child's anxiety about impending surgery. Lastly, some inpatient services have a social worker who reviews all admissions; this expanded social history may be very helpful before the consultant meets the family and child.

LIAISON FUNCTIONS

Child psychiatric consultation almost always involves more than the patient and referring physician. Virtually by definition parents give critical information and will need to be actively involved in implementation of recommendations; nurses serve in loco parentis; the ward rather than the child's room is the temporary home, and behavior has an impact on many other patients and staff. Although adult patients elicit staff reaction, children are likely to evoke broader, more intense feelings. Since their personalities are not fully developed, they are frequently completely innocent victims of their illness, and, since their lives have just begun, they lend themselves to hopeful projections. Since many pediatric units encourage parental visitation and even live-in, the potential impact of a distraught or disturbed parent on the entire ward is substantial. Lastly, there are fewer pediatric units than adult units and since they are usually defined by age level a given patient may return to the same floor over a 5- or 10-year period. Thus many children become well known and the depth of the staff's involvement grows over the years.

Child psychiatric consultation includes an essential liaison role that is relevant to patient and family care, interstaff tensions, and individual staff stress.

A key stressor is inherent to primary nursing. Primary nursing encourages continuity of care as one or two nurses are assigned to the child during the hospitalization and often for repeated admissions. Primary nursing is clearly beneficial for the child's sense of trust, makes the nurse's role more personally satisfying, and can add a needed perspective if too many subspecialists forget the whole child's needs. Unavoidably, primary nurses become intensely involved in the child's personal and family life; thus they have critical information and share the stress of the child's illness. The child psychiatrist can provide suggestions and supervision for dealing with difficult families or crisis, review when psychiatric referral is indicated, and help in understanding the painful issues of chronic disease, suicide, and terminal illness.

For house staff a basic stressor is being relatively inexperienced and yet forced to deal with complex medical and psychological circumstances. The source of stress is clearest in the ICU where frustration mounts rapidly as children do not respond to treatment or suffer life-long physical and neurologic damage. The consequences of multiple stresses —frustration with the patient's course, lack of sleep, and feeling incompetent—may lead to depression, substance abuse, or bitter tensions with other house staff or nurses.

Part of the child psychiatrist's liaison function is to attend rounds, be aware of difficult clinical and family situations, get to know nurses and house staff through teaching and informal discussion concerning patients, and be aware of the early signs of behavior destructive to patient care and fellow staff. With sufficient credibility, the child psychiatric consultant can organize patient care, family, or interstaff meetings that will have a beneficial impact on the unit's functioning as well as relieving family or staff suffering.

BROADER CLINICAL AND ETHICAL ISSUES FACING THE CONSULTANT

Psychiatric consultation faces major barriers because of inadequate funding. The consultation itself may take several hours and require repeated visits with the child, the family, and ward staff. However, reimbursement guidelines do not recognize multiple evaluation visits or the time spent gathering data from other sources. The consultant's recommendations may include long-term psychotherapy or special school classes, both of which are expensive. One of the major frustrations in consultation is the lack of financial support for the hours of consultant time or for implementing the consultant's recommendations. The future of inpatient psychiatric consultation to children depends on recognition by third-party payers that this is a necessary service and that it must be supported financially in all its facets.

The consultant faces some difficult clinical and ethical issues. The clinical interview of the family and child may yield very sensitive information. It is not uncommon to hear family secrets that are kept either from the child or from a spouse. In adolescent patients, the consultant frequently hears very private information about such matters as the first sexual contact, the use of birth control, or pregnancy. It is especially important clinically to build a confidential one-to-one therapeutic alliance; however, it may be therapeutically indicated, but quite complex, to negotiate release of information within a family. An additional problem is how much of all information and inference should be shared with the pediatrician, with the ward nurse, or written in the widely read medical record.

Another frustrating issue for the consultant is the lack of empirical basis for the psychiatric consultation process with children. The current state of the art in child psychiatry research has not developed a methodology to define diagnostic entities adequately or to evaluate interventions. There are too many variables, in both history and illness, to allow for accurate measurement or ready application to other consultations. It is apparent clinically that child psychiatric consultation is essential and useful; however, each consultant develops a personal system of evaluation with only limited systematic data or guidelines.

The psychiatric consultant meets the family and the patient after a thorough process of data gathering and analysis. This process recognizes many sources of both historical and observational data and places special emphasis on developmental expectations for assessing the impact of physical illness. Considering each bit of data within a developmental framework allows the consultant to generate and refine hypotheses to answer the referring physician's questions. In chapter 25 the next step in the consultation process—the direct contact between consultant, patient and family—is reviewed, several diagnostic categories are defined, and specific management interventions are discussed.

Child psychiatric diagnosis, the psychiatric aspects of pediatric diagnosis, the psychological management of chronic disease, the need for liaison and teaching efforts will, if anything, increase in the future. What is in more serious doubt is whether there will be enough child psychiatrists to meet these needs and how these services will be supported.[38,39]

REFERENCES

1. Eisenberg L: Normal child development, in Freedman AM, Kaplan HI, Sadock BJ (eds): *The Comprehensive Textbook of Psychiatry*, ed 2. Baltimore, Williams & Wilkins Co, 1975, pp 2036–2058.
2. Harper G, Richmond J: Normal and abnormal development, in Rudolph AM (ed): *Pediatrics*, ed 16. New York, Appleton-Century-Crofts, 1977, pp 61–95.
3. Jellinek M, Evans N, Knight RB: Evaluating the need for psychiatric referral: use of a behavior checklist on a pediatric inpatient unit. *J Pediatr* 1979; 94:156–158.
4. Prugh DG, Staub EM, Sands H, et al: A study of the emotional reactions of children and families to hospitalization and illness. *Am J Orthopsychiatry* 1953; 23:70–106.
5. Sampson TF: The child in renal failure. *J Am Acad Child Psychiatry* 1975;

14:462–476.

6. Freud A: The role of bodily illness in the child. *Psychoanal Study Child* 1969; 7:69–81.

7. Spitz RA: Hospitalism. *Psychoanal Study Child* 1945; 1:53–74.

8. Bowlby J: Separation anxiety. *Int J Psychoanal* 1960; 41:89–113.

9. Tronick E, Als H, Adamson L, et al: The infant's response to entrapment between contradictory messages in face to face interaction. *J Am Acad Child Psychiatry* 1978; 17:1–13.

10. Knight RB: Coping mechanisms used by children hospitalized for elective surgery, dissertation, Yeshiva University, New York, 1977.

11. Awad GA, Pozanski EO: Psychiatric consultation to a pediatric hospital. *Am J Psychiatry* 1975; 132:915–918.

12. Monnelly EP, Ianzito BM, Stewart MA: Psychiatric consultations in a children's hospital. *Am J Psychiatry* 1973; 139:789–790.

13. Looff DH: Psychophysiologic and conversation reactions in children. *J Am Acad Child Psychiatry* 1970; 9:318–331.

14. Bolian GC: Psychiatric consultation within a community of sick children. *J Am Acad Child Psychiatry* 1971; 10:293–307.

15. Stocking M, Rothney W, Grosser G, et al: Psychopathology in a pediatric hospital: implications for the pediatrician. *Psychiatr Med* 1970; 1:329–338.

16. Schowalter JE: The utilization of child psychiatry on a pediatric adolescent ward. *J Am Acad Child Psychiatry* 1971; 10:689–699.

17. Helfer R, Kempe C: *The Battered Child*, ed 2. Chicago, University of Chicago Press, 1974.

18. Lystad MH: Violence at home: a review of the literature. *Am J Orthopsychiatry* 1975; 45:328–345.

19. Millen JS: Hyperactive children. *Pediatrics* 1978; 61:217–222.

20. Eisenberg L: Hyperkinesis revisited. *Pediatrics* 1978; 61:319–321.

21. Geist RA: Consultation to a pediatric surgical ward: creating an empathic climate. *Am J Orthopsychiatry* 1977; 47:432–444.

22. Redlich FC, Hollingshead AB: *Social Class and Mental Illness: A Community Study*. New York, John Wiley & Sons, Inc, 1958.

23. Eisenberg L: Racism, the family, and society: a crisis in values, in Chess S, Thomas A (ed): *Annual Progress in Child Psychiatry and Child Development*. New York, Brunner/Mazel, Inc, 1969, pp 252–264.

24. Birch HG: Health and the education of the socially disadvantaged child, in Chess S, Thomas A (eds): *Annual Progress in Child Psychiatry and Child Development*. New York, Brunner/Mazel, Inc, 1969, pp 265–291.

25. Rodman H: Family and social pathology in the ghetto, in Chess S, Thomas A (eds): *Annual Progress in Child Psychiatry and Child Development*. New York, Brunner/Mazel, Inc, 1969, pp 291–308.

26. Oanilowica DA, Gabriel HP: Postoperative reactions in hospitalized children: normal and abnormal responses after surgery. *Am J Psychiatry* 1971; 128:185–188.

27. Bergman T: *Children in the Hospital*. New York, International Universities Press, 1965.

28. Minuchin S, Baker L, Rosman BL, et al: A conceptual model of psychosomatic illness in children. *Arch Gen Psychiatry* 1975; 32:1031–1038.

29. Pless IB, Roghman KJ: Chronic illness and its consequences. *J Pediatr* 1971;

79:351–359.

30. Glasser HH, Harrison GS, Lynn DB: Emotional implications of congenital heart disease in children. *Pediatrics* 1964; 33:367–379.
31. Bernstein DM: After transplantation—the child's emotional reactions. *Am J Psychiatry* 1971; 127:1189–1193.
32. Friedman SB, Chodoff P, Mason JS, et al: Behavioral observations on parents anticipating the death of a child. *Pediatrics* 1963; 32:610–625.
33. Gladston R: On borrowed time: observations on children with implanted cardiac pacemakers and their families, in Chess S, Thomas A (eds): *Annual Progress in Child Psychiatry and Child Development.* New York, Brunner/Mazel, Inc, 1970, pp 517–523.
34. Graham P, Rutter, M, George S: Temperamental characteristics as predictors of behavior disorders in children. *Am J Orthopsychiatry* 1973; 43:328–339.
35. Thomas A, Chess S: *Temperament and Development.* New York, Brunner/Mazel, Inc, 1976.
36. Plank EN: *Working with Children in Hospitals.* Cleveland, Western Reserve Press, 1962.
37. Vaughan GF: Children in hospital. *Lancet* 1957; 1:1117–1120.
38. Jellinek MS: The present status of child psychiatry in pediatrics. *N Engl J Med* 1982; 306:1227–1230.
39. Philips I (chairperson), Cohen R, Enzer N (co-chairpersons): *Child Psychiatry: A Plan for the Coming Decades.* Washington, American Academy of Child Psychiatry, 1983.
40. Jellinek M: Recognition and management of discord within house staff teams. *JAMA* 1986; 256(6):754–755.

25

Child Psychiatric Consultation

DAVID B. HERZOG and MICHAEL S. JELLINEK

As was noted in the previous chapter, hospitalized children frequently have psychiatric disorders and psychosocial problems, while at the same time the child psychiatry consultation service is underutilized.[1] Mutter and Schliefer[2] studied latency-age children hospitalized with "nonpsychosomatic" illness and compared them to non-ill children. The hospitalized children had more disorganized families and had suffered more frequent and threatening changes in their environment. Stocking et al[3] found that 64% of children on their pediatric wards had emotional problems that warranted psychiatric consultation, even though only 11% were referred for such consultation. In order for hospitalized children to receive adequate care, the Child Psychiatry Consultation Liaison Service (PCLS) and the department of pediatrics must provide the opportunity for the child psychiatrist and pediatrician to learn from each other. This chapter will review the development of the Massachusetts General Hospital's (MGH) child PCLS, techniques of child psychiatric consultation, and the assessment of the specific childhood conditions and their treatments.

MGH CHILD CONSULTATION LIAISON SERVICE

The MGH child PCLS was established in 1979 and is administered through the Child Psychiatry Service with support from the Department of Pediatrics. The service has three basic roles: to consult with pediatric staff in establishing appropriate diagnosis; to ease suffering of ill children in families; and to support the medical and nursing staff as they face the stress of caring for hospitalized children and their families.[4]

The development of a PCLS has striking similarities to starting a business in a distant land.[5] There are language and culture difficulties. The pediatrician understands the language used in pediatric texts while the psychiatrist is fluent in psychiatric terminology. The pediatrician wants to know the etiology and the treatment, and does not focus on the process of the interview. The pediatrician wants to know facts, not theories. The pediatrician is action-oriented and wants more immediate results and the child psychiatrist is often accustomed to a much longer-term view, based on his or her experience on the psychiatric wards. The pediatrician's ambivalence toward a psychiatrist may be derived from a lack of knowledge of psychiatry, previous exposure with a child psychiatrist who had little interest in consultation liaison work, personal problems that are more difficult to repress in the presence of a psychiatrist, competitive issues, or the feeling that the pediatrician is more knowledgeable and able to manage the emotional problems of children than the psychiatric colleague.

During the initial years of a PCLS the consultant often feels frustrated. Consultations are called only on the day of discharge after an extensive medical work-up has been administered and the family is furious, frustrated by the lack of medical findings and answers. Patients clearly in need of consultation are not referred despite requests from nurses, social workers, and even families. Patients or families are not informed about the referral or are not specifically told that a psychiatrist has been consulted. The note requesting consultation will often state "psych referral" without any explanation. The chart will be incomplete, without any developmental or family history. Treatment recommendations, specifically for psychotherapy, will not be supported. What can change all this? (1) A close working relationship between the chiefs of child psychiatry and pediatrics; (2) support from the chief of pediatrics that the understanding and treatment of emotional problems in children are a priority; (3) the hiring of child psychiatry staff who are also board-certified in pediatrics, interested in consultation liaison, and willing to make themselves available for consultation; (4) the placement of consultants in teaching contact with small groups of pediatric residents, such as senior rounds or as the "visit" on the ward; (5) continuity of personnel; (6) a good track record; (7) the development of house staff and nursing groups. The MGH pediatric service has approximately 85 beds. Since we have been using these guidelines during the course of the past 5 years the number of psychiatric consultations has increased from approximately 10 to 130. Consultations are now called routinely on all children admitted to the oncology service.

TECHNIQUES OF CHILD PSYCHIATRIC CONSULTATION

The request for a child psychiatric consultation initiates a process.[5] The origin of the request should be considered. Ideally, it should come from the primary care physician. Frequently, however, the nurse, social worker, or medical student will initiate the referral. The consultant should take the opportunity to discuss the request for the referral with the various staff, although he should not see the patient until the primary physician agrees to write the order. With better informed staff the likelihood of patient compliance with the consultant's recommendations increases substantially. Furthermore, the more communication between the psychiatric consultant and the ward staff the more discerning will be the observations of the nursing, social worker, and recreational therapy staff—data which the consultant will use to arrive at a diagnostic impression.

The child and family should be prepared for the consultation. It is essential that the referring physician discuss the reasons for the referral with both the child and his parents so that the child feels more included and does not feel that information is being withheld. Parents of a preschool and young school-age child (less than 8 years old) should be interviewed by the psychiatric consultant before the child is interviewed.

The interview of the young child requires largely nonverbal means for the expression of feelings and concerns. In the initial interview the psychiatrist needs to create as normal an environment as possible as he begins to get to know the child. The consultant's attitude should be active, interested, and playful. The room should contain familiar items and not the setting associated with the painful procedures. First, an eyeball examination should be done and then a gross developmental assessment. In the child under 3 years of age, observations of the parent-child dyad are crucial. What is the eye contact like between parent and child? Does the parent respond to cues in the child and vice versa? Are the parent and child in sync? What is the child's temperament like, and how does the parent handle frustration, whether it be as a result of the child's inactivity or excessive activity? How do the child and parent handle separation? How does the child respond to strangers? Stranger anxiety in the very young is expected and the lack of any stranger anxiety may be the sign of inadequate parenting.

The psychiatrist needs to be well equipped to perform such an evaluation. The minimal equipment includes a toy doctor kit, puppets, and a doll house. The evaluation of the child under 1-year-old will include items appropriate for that age group such as rattles.

A classic example of the need for consultation in the very young child is the failure-to-thrive infant. An excellent study of this population showed that children with nonorganic failure to thrive have severe attachment disorder problems, manifested by poor eye contact with their caregivers compared to that with strangers.[6] When, after numerous interventions, the eye contact with the caregiver would begin to improve, the child's weight gain would soon follow.

The 3- to 6-year-old child may still require that a parent be present throughout the interview. That request should be respected, although at some point in the interview an attempt should be made to have the parent leave the room. Developmental assesssment, including language, social interaction, and gross and fine motor coordination is a mandatory part of the interview. Drawings become a more important tool for expressing troublesome thoughts and feelings. The psychiatrist should not expect to complete the evaluation in one visit. It may take several sessions and the sessions may be shorter than the usual hour because of the child's fatigue or because other tests have been scheduled.

The latency-age child can be a more verbal participant in the interview. The child should be questioned about current and previous school attendance, school behavior, school performance, after-school activities, friends, health (including mental health) of family members, family problems, and interaction of family members in response to traumatic events. Mental status examination should initially focus on the manner of relating. The child may be active and verbal or shy and inhibited. The consultant's approach should be flexible depending on the child's way of relating. The active verbal child can be approached in the more traditional interview. The shy child may be engaged through drawings or games such as checkers or video arcade games. These activities can prove helpful in facilitating an alliance and in demonstrating organic deficits. Consultation to the 6-year-old with a chronic disease like leukemia will require several sessions before the child can have trust that the psychiatric consultant will not be performing another invasive procedure. The leukemic child may also be extremely uncomfortable from the disease itself or its treatment. The first few sessions may be brief and consist of supportive comments, gross developmental assessment (past and current), assessment of several symptoms, including pain, anorexia, and insomnia, assessment of the usual coping strategies, and suggestions for ways to deal with symptoms and feelings. The role of the psychiatric consultant for these children has many features of a "professional friend" and after a few sessions the consultant may only drop in for several minutes during rounds. Recreational therapy often plays a prominent role for these children. A 6-year-old with a somatizing symptom such as absent spells merits a different approach. A thorough psychiatric assessment of such a child is then mandated, including an individual interview of the child, psychological testing, and a complete family assessment.

Interviewing an adolescent can pose a true challenge. Some adolescents will flatly refuse to talk and others will substantially distort their psychosocial histories. They are often labile and experience emotions intensely. How does the consultant proceed with the silent adolescent? Often the adolescent's initial anxiety and resistance are difficult to surmount. The consultant should not become discouraged and interpret the silence in response to a question as a personal blunder. The adolescent should be given a thorough explanation and reason for the referral. It is often helpful to reassure the adolescent about the consultant's knowledge of the adolescent's physical problems and clinical procedures. The limits and expectations of the interview should be clarified, and the necessary information gathered to better understand what may be bothering the adolescent and how to best approach helping him. The adolescent is told that the interview will be 30 minutes long, and that although it is preferable to talk about feelings, periods of silence are also acceptable. Confidentiality should be assured and interviews should take place in a private setting. In general, the consultant should be patient and easygoing. It may be necessary to initiate the conversation with some safe topic that the adolescent can easily relate to, such as a sporting event, a rock group, or a television program. The consultant should visit the adolescent frequently, if only for brief periods, and inform the adolescent how long he will stay with him. If the patient appears to be taking a paranoid stance he should be given more control. The majority of introductory sessions do go smoothly. Over time, questions about body image, school, family relationships, friendship patterns, goals, and sexuality need to be addressed.

The role of the family interview as the initial interview for the assessment of a child is somewhat controversial. Some clinicians feel that a family evaluation is mandatory to understand the child.[7] We use a family evaluation for certain disorders, specifically psychosomatic disorders (anorexia nervosa, school phobia, recurrent abdominal pain) where family interaction may either precipitate or maintain the symptoms. In the pediatric intensive care unit (PICU), we routinely prescribe family evaluation sessions for families with the following characteristics: when the response to the child's hospitalization is inappropriate (either excessive or severely constricted); when there is a history of psychiatric illness in family members; when there is a question of abuse or neglect; or when there is a question of whether the family is able to adequately comprehend the clinical information.[8] For other families the evaluation sessions are more optional. Families of ill children need to express their feelings about hospitalization and obtain emotional support. Siblings often have distorted concepts of their brother's or sister's illness which need to be corrected. A carefully planned family meeting can clarify distortions, reduce family turmoil, improve coping skills, and dispel conflicts between family and staff. During the meeting the ward staff or the psychiatrist should make an evaluation of the family's psychological state, including coping mechanisms, anxiety level, available support and ability to comprehend information.

PSYCHIATRIC REFERRAL

The types of problems that are referred to the child PCLS include: (1) depression; (2) concerns about the child's reaction to illness and hospitalization; (3) psychosomatic disorders; (4) suicide gestures; (5) familial grief; (6) behavior problems; (7) problems specific to the preschool child; and (8) problems specific to the intensive care unit.

Depression

Depression is a frequent child psychiatric disorder in hospitalized children. It may be secondary adjustment reaction to acute or chronic illness, or be primary and present with psychosomatic symptoms and behavior problems. Until recently, depression was a neglected area in child psychiatry and some still question its existence, particularly in the very young child.

Depression can be a mood, symptom, or a syndrome. As a syndrome, depression in childhood is characterized by a persistent mood disorder, dysfunctional behavior, and in school-age children, self-deprecatory ideation. These symptoms or behaviors should represent a significant change in the child's premorbid functioning and not be a long-standing character trait. The DSM-III[9] criteria for *depression* are the same for adults and children over age 6 years. For those under 6 years of age, the criteria include: (1) dysphoric mood that may have to be inferred from persistent sad facial expressions; and (2) three of the following: (a) poor appetite or failure to gain expected weight; (b) disturbance of sleep, (c) hypoactivity, and (d) loss of interest and indifference to surroundings (apathy).

Kashani et al[10] investigated depression among hospitalized children (age 6 to 12 years) in a pediatric ward and found that 7% (seven out of 100) met the DSM-III criteria for *depression* and an additional 38% exhibited *dysphoric mood*. The loss of a significant adult figure due to death, chronic or disabling illness, or desertion was present in 86% of the latter sample. The depressed children had a significantly higher frequency of headache, abdominal pain, and parental depression than the nondepressed, hospitalized children. The differential diagnosis is lengthy and may include endocrinopathies (hypothyroidism, hyperglycemia), neurologic disorders (eg, brain tumor), hyperactivity with or without an attentional deficit disorder, chronic illness (eg, renal disease, cardiac disease), and illnesses that have both medical and psychiatric components such as ulcerative colitis and anorexia nervosa.

Some investigators have noted that the form in which the depression appears in childhood is a function of the child's developmental level.[11] Most agree that as the child approaches adolescence, the clinical picture takes on the more topical presentation of the adult patient. The following case examples highlight the heterogeneity and developmental specificity of depressive symptoms in children.[11]

> A 6-year-old girl was brought to the emergency ward after putting a knife to her neck and saying she wanted to kill herself. The precipitant of the action was the loss of her dog. She was currently struggling with loss. She asked, "Have you seen my father? He wears a white coat and I think he works here. I am dying to see him." She added that he went away when she was very young; that he calls sometimes but never visits. She did not engage in spontaneous play and appeared pseudomature, too preoccupied with worries for a 6-year-old. She also was preoccupied with morbid events, talked about funeral homes, and asked questions like, "Did you hear about the two children who were killed last weekend?"

> A 16-year-old boy was hospitalized in the ICU after taking an overdose of sleeping pills while under the influence of alcohol. Symptoms of depression during the previous month had included decreased sleep and appetite; feelings of sadness and hopelessness; decreased interest in friends, school, and hobbies; and suicidal ideation. Precipitants to the overdose included a recent rejection by a girl friend, an increase in his father's drinking, and an exacerbation of the boy's ileitis. Notable in the history was the death of the boy's mother when he was 8 years old, an event he had difficulty in recalling.

Physiologic indices such as plasma cortisol and growth hormone hypersecretion[12,13] have been noted in some depressed children but are not generally helpful in making a diagnosis.

Antidepressants used in conjunction with psychotherapy and recreational programs may improve and hasten the relief of symptoms in depressed, school-age children.[14–16] The tricyclic antidepressants (specifically imipramine hydrochloride and amitriptypline hydrochloride) are the most commonly used drugs in the treatment of childhood and adolescent depression. The usual dosage is 2 to 5 mg/kg/d. The medication regimen should be started at a dose of 1.5 mg/kg/d, and slowly increased over a period of 2 weeks, until the serum level is within the therapeutic range. Plasma levels may be important in terms of the clinical response.[17] Response to medication usually takes 3 to 4 weeks. Blood pressure should be monitored because of hypotension and reports of paradoxical hypertension. In the child, a baseline EEG and periodic ECG monitoring are indicated as there are reports of increased heart rate, increased PR and widened QRS intervals and nonspecific T wave changes.[18] These ECG changes, however, have not been associated with clinical symptoms.

Reaction to illness or hospitalization

A substantial number of patients are referred by their primary physician because they respond to illness in ways that interfere with medical treatment or psychosocial development. In our tertiary facility over one third of the children in this group have an invasive malignancy. Differential diagnosis requires a careful assessment of CNS functioning, side effects of medication, the nutritional state, and psychodynamic factors. These children commonly have depressive symptomatology. Chronic illness, like depression, is often manifested by weight loss, insomnia, dysphoric mood, and anhedonia. The psychodynamic issues may include understanding the illness as a punishment or excessive concern about the pain the child is causing the family. Fears of intolerable pain and death are common. These children may substantially distort the surgeries they have had or are about to have. The consultant's role has several functions: to help these children tolerate pain, and thoughts of death; to help them follow their medical regimen (including invasive procedures); and to help them master their appropriate developmental tasks.[3] In almost every case the consultant works with the staff and with the patient's family concerning their feelings of anger, impotence, and helplessness in the face of the relentless course of the child's illness. The consultant helps the child bear the stress of the illness and its impact on the child's life.

A 10-year-old girl, whose parents were divorced, was admitted for chemotherapy after being diagnosed as having acute lymphocytic leukemia. She responded favorably to treatment and was scheduled for repeated hospitalizations in order to maintain her state of remission.

During each of the several-day periods of inpatient chemotherapy, she was whiny, demanding, and inseparable from her mother. She would lie in bed angry and would often complain of pain at the intravenous (IV) site and cry incessantly at any IV reinsertion. Her anger would usually resolve or lessen during visits from her sister and father. In the initial interviews, the patient's overall anger was substantial, although her withdrawal limited expression of her feelings about her illness. She appeared depressed and stated that her illness had dramatically interfered with many of her usual activities. The patient and her mother both had a sense of entitlement that angered and frustrated the medical staff, since nothing they could do was sufficient to please either the patient or her mother. It quickly became apparent that both the patient's and the mother's sense of entitlement were characterologic and in view of the critical condition of the child's health the consultant decided not to explore those issues.

After several interviews, the consultant decided that the staff, the patient's family, and the patient herself had to be approached. First, he met with the medical staff and clarified the relevant sources of the patient's anger and her attitude of entitlement. Her anger was related to the side effects of the medication, to the frequent invasive procedures, and to her mother's inability to care for herself and keep her marriage together. She feared the consultant would abandon her just as she perceived her father had. It gradually became clear that part of the staff's response to her demanding behavior was related to their own feelings of ambivalence toward the girl's life-threatening, chronic disease. Some of the staff would at times articulate their wishes that the patient die soon. Family meetings were then initiated with the unit social worker. The patient and her sister were able to share some of their feelings of anger, and some of the family's concerns and anxieties were openly discussed. The consultant met individually with the patient. Her anger and isolation were directly confronted, specifically in the context of the length of the sessions. The child repeatedly attempted to shorten the time of the session and the consultant refused to permit that. Her response to this perceived "attack," was fury and she said, "You're picking on me. Stop bothering me!" The consultant pointed out that it was not he bothering her, but perhaps others—physicians and her father and mother. The patient's anger subsided and the chemotherapy proceeded without interference. She became less isolated, was able to talk more freely about her feelings, and on follow-up has continued to do well.

Children's reactions to illness and hospitalization vary. The most common reactions are denial, passive-aggressive behavior, and withdrawal. Some denial is healthy (eg, the patient denies the poor prognosis of his tumor) and the consultant only needs to clarify these issues with the staff. When denial is more severe (interferes with the medical care of the child or puts the child at risk of greater injury) the denial should be confronted, but in stages and with caution. The timing and manner of confronting denial depend on how complete the medical and psychiatric picture is, the consultant's preferred style, and the family's need and tolerance.

The passive-aggressive reaction, such as secretive noncompliance with the medical regimen, can be quite serious. The consultant should attempt to make the angry feelings more conscious and available and able to be talked about. The angry reaction may be positive if it does not interfere with medical care. Again, with this kind of reaction the staff may only need increased understanding. The goal is to help the child talk about the anger and not act on it. Other avenues to channel this anger may need to be made available, such as sticking needles in puppets for the younger child or vigorous (violent) video games for the adolescent.

Withdrawal may represent the response to a fear, to actual pain, to depressive thoughts, or to having all control removed. Exploration of these various possibilities is necessary prior to deciding on an intervention. The clinical approach may be giving the child more control, such as the timing of various procedures, or more selection in his diet.

Psychosomatic disorders

Some patients are referred by pediatricians who question whether emotional factors are the cause of the patients' illness. Psychosomatic disorders refer to those illnesses at the interface between the psyche and the soma. They include somatopsychic disorders (eg, diabetes mellitus) in which the primary problem is medical, psychosomatic disorders in which the medical and the psychiatric components are more intertwined (eg, anorexia nervosa), and psychosomatic disorders that are primarily psychiatric.

A hallmark of psychosomatic disorders is the great pressure on the doctor to (1) define the disorder in biomedical terms, and (2) to do so without a total medical evaluation of the child, specifically without exploring the child's emotional or family life.[18] The families are characterized by their inability to speak in psychological terms and their denial of family involvement in the child's symptoms.[18] They prefer to talk about their daughter's amenorrhea and the need for a laparotomy rather than what the daughter was experiencing as a result of poor school performance due to a recently identified learning disability. They deny any possible relationship between the child's symptoms and even the most painful issues in family life, such as threatened parental separation or extramarital affairs. Furthermore, these families pay attention to borderline test findings and the doctor is constantly pressured to attend to these findings. Young clinicians are particularly vulnerable since they are not yet comfortable with assessing and dismissing irrelevant data. These characteristics interfere with the family's ability to trust one physician and these families often see specialist after specialist.

The consultant can intervene with the primary physician, the patient, and the family. Therapeutic intervention with the primary physician may take several forms. The pediatrician may feel pressure to rule out every possible medical basis for the symptoms though such an approach has drawn fresh criticism on both conceptual and cost-effective grounds. The consultant may help the pediatrician to define a rational approach. The rule-out approach in these disorders is problematic because it reinforces the biomedical tunnel vision of the family and delays their obtaining effective help with the denied or ignored psychosocial issues. Furthermore, the consultant can help the primary caregivers attempt the differential diagnosis of the source of anxiety that surrounds these cases. When excessive anxiety is noted in the family's communication about the child's illness, the concept of displacement may be applied as a way of understanding and managing this anxiety for the family.[18] Displacement implies that the manifest anxiety about the vomiting or abdominal pain is magnified by unacknowledged anxiety about something else in the life of the child or family. The primary focus of the anxiety may be an emotionally traumatic issue such as impending divorce, and displacement occurs when the primary focus is too frightening to be acknowledged. The secondary focus for the anxiety—the child's symptoms—come to stand for the primary focus. Some helpful tools for making these diagnoses include[19]:

1. Watchful waiting: It is not necessary to make the whole diagnosis the first day, week or month, despite the wishes of the family.
2. Judicious disregard: Use of restraint in the pursuit of equivocal organic findings.
3. Multiple diagnoses: It is not necessary to reduce the symptoms to one disorder. (A child at the same time may have atypical asthma, family tension, and a depressive disorder.)
4. Diagnosis in context: Children often have shifting levels of functioning in different settings.

Therapeutic interventions for the patient include a medical psychiatric team approach. Such an approach is often directly helpful and at other times, at least initially, serves as a graceful way out of a tense situation. The development of the relationship with the child and family is critical. It is also important to be aware that children with these kinds of symptoms are at risk for medical abandonment, especially after psychiatric referral. Pediatric re-examinations and the inclusion of both pediatrician and consultant in treatment planning conferences and in forming conferences with parents are useful. Since the child's symptoms frequently serve to stabilize the family, the family may need therapy so that the child may become free to abandon the sick role. Family therapy is useful to help parents regroup as a couple and remove the child's symptoms as they focus on their relationship. In addition, the healthy part of the child should be supported to help him relinquish the sick role. Developmentally appropriate activities can increase the child's sense of mastery and self-esteem. But implementation of such activities may require prescription by the pediatrician and enforce mobilization by the staff. A nutritional rehabilitation program may be necessary for the anorectic child or the failure-to-thrive child; a physical rehabilitation program may be a necessary component for the child with the "clenched first syndrome." Psychotropic medication may be employed depending on the specific psychiatric disorder or the specific symptom for which relief is sought.

> A 16-year-old girl, hospitalized because of the recent onset of disabling headaches, was referred for psychiatric consultation after an extensive organic work-up that yielded no pathologic findings. The patient's mother had frequently criticized the physicians and nurses for inadequate attention to her daughter's pain. The staff reported that the girl's symptom was situation-dependent—the pain seemed to worsen when the mother was present, and it was not mentioned when she was with her friends. The patient, who appeared several years older than her actual age, did not seem ill. She was the youngest of six children; her parents had been divorced for 7 years. She lived with her mother who had been housebound with back pain since the divorce. When asked, "If there were one person you could punch in the nose, who would that be?," the girl complained of an intense headache and asked to leave the room. The consultant pointed out to her that repressed feelings can be communicated through pain, and that she learn other ways of expressing her feelings. It became apparent that the pain was a family mode of communication, and that the girl could easily develop a lifelong pain syndrome. She agreed to outpatient psychiatric follow-up.

These ambiguous cases put a great deal of pressure on the consultant and the consultant should feel no shame in seeking support and/or advice from fellow consultants.

Suicide gestures

Suicide is the third leading cause of death among males and the fourth leading cause of death among females aged from 15 to 24 years.[20] (See chapter 14.) Furthermore, suicide attempts among adolescents are on a sharp increase. Although the incidence of completed suicide among children aged 6 to 12 years may be relatively low, suicidal threats and attempts by children in this age group are not uncommon.[21] We recommend almost without exception that all children who have made a suicide gesture be admitted for pediatric (or occasional psychiatric) hospitalization. A brief hospitalization gives the staff sufficient time to complete a thorough evaluation and arrange disposition. Specific suggestions for the assessment of the suicidal child:

1. Gather all the details of the suicide attempt.
2. Pursue the child's understanding of death.
3. Pursue with the child what he expects would happen after the death. Who would attend the funeral? How would the family react? Get as good a history as possible of when the suicidal feelings started and whether there was a clear precipitant to the event (the less impulsive and the more planned, the worse the prognosis).
6. Explore why the attempt was not successful and whether the child or adolescent experiences any remorse about the event.
7. Have a family interview.

The assessment of a suicidal child or adolescent should address the risk of the attempt, the wish to be rescued, whether a plan was present to kill oneself, feelings of hopelessness, helplessness and despair, psychosis, syntonic drug or alcohol abuse, previous suicide attempts, identification with someone who has committed suicide, the intensity of the anger or depression, the presence of support systems, vulnerability to impending losses, and ability to use help. Family issues that should be assessed include a family history of depression, whether a family is "modeling" suicide, interpersonal tension, and real or imagined rejection of the suicidal child by the parents. The consultant is initially asked to decide the appropriate ward management for the suicidal child—whether the child needs one-to-one staffing, four-point restraints, sedation, or none or some or all of the above. The consultant then needs to determine, often within 24 to 48 hours, whether the child or adolescent can be managed as an outpatient living at home, needs psychiatric hospitalization, or requires a more temporary shelter, pending further evaluation of the family. The Department of Nursing often puts pressure on the consultant to make a rapid decision about disposition. Nursing departments are often forced to provide the funding for one-to-one staffing which may not be adequately allocated in their budget. Communication with nursing administration around this issue is often critical in order to avoid nursing resentment toward the patient or unduly hasty decision by the psychiatric consultant. Although some of these suicidal patients may be severely depressed and require antidepressant medication, such intervention is usually not indicated in the first 24 to 48 hours when the thorough assessment is ongoing. Criteria for psychiatric hospitalization include serious risk of death through suicide, little wish to be rescued, psychosis, identification with someone who has committed suicide, syntonic drug or alcohol abuse, intense feelings of hopelessness and helplessness, intense anger or severe depression, lack of support systems, history of inability to use help, and vulnerability to further losses.

Familial grief

The families referred for consultation are often overwhelmed in response to the death of their children, and require careful assessment and observation. The assessment should include how families have responded to traumatic events in the past, whether they are chronically grieving, whether there is a history of psychiatric problems, whether there exists a current family member with depressive disorder, and what marital supports are available. Occasionally a family member will require psychiatric hospitalization or a mild sedative. However, most frequently family members are responsive to phone or personal interview follow-up.

Behavior problems

Some children are referred for consultation for the management of specific behavioral symptoms. Their symptoms may include excessive activity, agitation, verbal or physical threats to staff and other children, seizurelike episodes, and temper tantrums. A careful assessment, including medical, developmental, and social history from the child and family, a neurologic examination, nursing observations, and school reports, is needed. When attention deficit disorder with hyperactivity is diagnosed, the child may respond quite dramatically to the prescription of stimulants or an antidepressant. In a chronically impulse-disordered adolescent, the use of a sedative such as thioridazine at a low dose may be helpful. Occasionally an underlying psychosis may be discerned and the appropriate antipsychotic agent should be instituted. At times a neuropsychiatric disorder, such as partial complex seizures, are noted and anticonvulsants instituted. There are ward issues around such patients. Staff and patients may feel unsafe and need to be reassured. There may be disagreements between staff members concerning the management of a given child and the child may be acting out this disagreement. A team meeting with various staff may reduce the extent of this symptomatology. Sometimes these children cannot be managed on a pediatric ward and require placement in a setting that has the necessary staffing for the management of emotionally disturbed children.

Problems specific to the preschool child

Referrals specific to preschool children are requested for the child with failure to thrive, developmental delays, or suspected or confirmed sexual and/or physical abuse. Evaluation of the child's physical, intellectual, and emotional involvement, themes in play, and interaction with family, staff, and consultant form the foundation of the assessment. The use of dolls may be helpful in such an evaluation to understand the child's concern about abuse or aggression. The consultant may also note the child to be hypervigilant and to have great difficulty trusting anyone. It is important with such children to assess attachment behavior. Does the child have a special attachment to a parent or does the child attach the same to all providers? It is equally important to assess the parent.

Fraiberg[22] has proposed a specific intervention for the infant: the form of mother-infant therapy. In mother-infant therapy the mother and infant are seen together. The mother-infant intervention involves not only the mother's description of her feelings but the active demonstration of these feelings in relation to her infant. With the parent, the consultant addresses past and present feelings of hate and how the infant contributes to these feelings. Interactional issues in the mother-infant sphere are clarified. In addition, education regarding child development is provided. Treatment intervention may also include the filing of a statement of concern for the child's welfare to the state welfare board, and a request for investigation of the family; a request of the court that the child be placed outside the family; specific treatment for a psychiatric condition of the parents; a nutritional rehabilitation program (for the child with failure to thrive); child-play therapy; or a child-stimulation program including physical therapy, occupational therapy, and speech therapy.

The pediatric intensive care unit

Children 12 years old and under define the world in terms of a familiar, controllable environment. The PICU bears no resemblance to home or school and denies the patient any sense of control over his surroundings. Children, like the elderly, often react to intensive care hospitalization with confusion, withdrawal, or anxiety. The use of familiar toys, blankets, photos, and accessories may be helpful in such reactions.

The conscious child is usually solemn and preoccupied with his physical condition. He experiences adjustment problems related to control, protection, and pain.[8] The child wants to know, "Where am I?", and "What is happening to me?" He requires direct explanations and careful prediction of what is going to take place to feel some sense of control. The child wants to know, "Who is here to protect and care for me?" The child needs to know that someone caring and familiar is close by. The child's coping strategies usually include dependence on the parenting figure, and thus open parental visiting and vigil are encouraged. The child is also in acute fear of pain. Adequate local anesthesia or IV anesthesia should be used for painful procedures. Sedation may also be indicated. The consultant can minimize the child's pain through awareness, acknowledgment, and explanation. While examining the child in as short a time as possible, the intensive care physician may handle a child or talk about him without sensitivity to his actual or potential disorder. An example might include the clinician applying pressure to the arm of a child receiving IV fluids, unaware of an impending phlebitis.

Psychiatric consultation in the PICU setting has several features: urgency, constant availability, minimal privacy, considerable noise and distraction, and pressure to make major changes immediately.[8] Reasons for referral to the psychiatrist in a PICU include depression, suicide attempts, postoperative nightmares, psychosis, delirium, and developmental assessment. In a psychotic or delirious child the differential diagnosis includes hypoxia, hypoglycemia, meningitis, and drug ingestion. Postoperative nightmares are common in the intensive care setting. Often the comfort of a familiar figure is all that is needed. However, for some the nightmares are chronically accompanied by agitation. For these children the nightmares often involve misconceptions of what their surgery involved and, occasionally, uncontrolled pain is a hidden factor.

An "ICU syndrome" has been noted in children—primarily younger children aged 18 months to 6 years. The syndrome refers to a transient psychotic state and delirium, characterized by depression, confusion, disorientation, hallucinations, and/or paranoid delusions. Some children become withdrawn, do not speak, and are passive. Others are hostile and agitated. Contributing factors include sleep and sensory deprivation, inappropriate parental reactions, and overstimulation. The syndrome is generally alleviated by increased parental contact, familiar toys, and reduced lighting and decreased noise to facilitate sleep. The child may need to be relocated to a less noisy or less frightening area, with increased parental visitation, and a more active play program. In rare circumstances the administration of haloperidol may be helpful.

Staff Liaison in the PICU.   Liaison activities include the understanding of medical, nursing, and social staff so that they are better able to communicate and tolerate the stress that is part of an intense caring for ill children.[4] Increasing the staff's capacity to bear anxiety and to be in empathic contact with suffering children and families can be accomplished through group work and individual case review.

> A 6-year-old child with chronic renal failure was hospitalized in the PICU after renal transplant rejection. He had had two previous transplant rejections and was well known to the PICU staff. He was extremely short for his age and had crippling bone disease secondary to his renal insufficiency. On the unit he had several cardiac arrests and was resuscitated. The nursing staff and house staff were of the opinion that the child should not be resuscitated, despite the wishes of the attending physician that all care be instituted for this child. The PICU staff are accustomed to intensive care treatment and response and not to the managment of chronic disease. Several group meetings with the nursing and house staffs served to educate them about the course of such illness—including what is known and also what is not known. These sessions also focused on the feelings that the patient engendered in the staff. Gradually the staff developed a more objective perspective, became more united in their planning, and were able to understand some of the emotional sources of staff conflict.

Physicians are often psychologically unavailable to nurses and can be condescending. Nurses sometimes feel that they are not given adequate respect. Young house staff can feel inadequate and frightened by the technical and psychological demands of caring for ill children. They are tired and feel constantly judged. At times they feel the nurses are not working with them. It is common for the rage associated with feelings of helplessness in the care of sick children to be projected onto the child, family, staff, or spouse. Such feelings can adversely influence the quality of care given and affect the staff's interest in their work. Weekly groups for nursing and house staff[23] and multidisciplinary rounds with intensive case review are necessary to provide opportunities for sharing information, identifying and acknowledging feelings, tolerating painful affects, and supporting one another.

Child psychiatry consultation liaison work is a tremendous challenge requiring a special character structure. The consultant can be defeated by the child, the family, the referring physician and/or the ward staff. The consultant needs to be available, accessible, flexible, and articulate. Assessment techniques vary with the developmental style of the child and treatment interventions may include individual psychotherapy, family therapy, pharmacotherapy, behavioral management and/or staff meetings. Liaison activities are central to the development of a child psychiatry consultation service and improve the care of hospitalized children.

REFERENCES

1. Schowalter JE: Hospital consultation as therapy, in Noshpitz JE (ed): *Basic Handbook of Child Psychiatry*. Vol 3, 1979 pp 365–375.
2. Mutter AZ, Schliefer MH: The role of psychological and social factors in the onset of somatic illness in children. *Psychsom Med* 1966; 28:333–343.
3. Stocking M, Rothney W, Grosser G, et al: Psychopathology in the pediatric hospital: implications for the pediatrician. *Am J Public Health* 1972; 62:551–556.
4. Jellinek MS, Herzog DB, Selter LF: A psychiatric consultation service for hospitalized children. *Psychosomatics* 1981; 22:29–33.
5. Anders TF, Niehans M: Promoting the alliance between pediatrics and child psychiatry. *Psychiatr Clin North Am* 1982; 5:241–258.
6. Rosenn D, Loeb L, Jura M: Differentiation of organic from non-organic failure to thrive syndrome in infancy. *Pediatrics* 1980; 66:689–704.
7. Minuchin S: The use of an ecological framework in the treatment of a child, in Anthony J, Koupernik C (eds): *The Child in His Family*. New York, John Wiley & Sons, Inc, 1970.
8. Herzog DB: Psychiatrist in the pediatric intensive care setting, in Manschreck TC, Murray GB (eds): *Psychiatric Medicine Update*. New York, Elsevier Biomedical Press, 1984, pp 133–142.
9. American Psychiatric Association: *Diagnostic and Statistical Manual of Mental Disorders*, ed 3 [DSM-III]. Washington, American Psychiatric Association, 1980.
10. Kashani JG, Barbero GJ, Bolander FD: Depression in hospitalized pediatric patients. *J Am Acad Child Psychiatry* 1981; 20:123–134.
11. Herzog DB, Rathbun JM: Childhood depression: developmental considerations. *Am J Dis Child* 1982; 136:115–120.
12. Puig-Antich J: Affective disorders in childhood. *Psychiatr Clin North Am* 1980; 3:403–424.
13. Puig-Antich J, Novacenico H, Davies M, et al: Growth hormone secretion in prepubertal children with major depression. *Arch Gen Psychiatry* 1984; 41:455–460.
14. Petti TA, Law W: Imipramine treatment of depressed children: a double-blind pilot study. *J Clin Psychopharmacol* 1982; 2:107–110.
15. Kashani JH, Shekim WO, Reid JC: Amitriptyline in children with major depressive disorder: a double-blind crossover pilot study. *J Am Acad Child Psychiatry* 1984; 23:348–351.
16. Biederman J, Jellinek MS: Psychopharmacology in children. *NEJM* 1984; 310:948–972.
17. Preskorn SH, Weller EB, Weller RA: Depression in children: relationship between plasma imipramine levels and response. *J Clin Psychiatry* 1982; 43:450–453.
18. Gittleman-Klein R: Diagnosis and drug treatment of childhood disorders, in Klein DF, Gittleman R, Quitkin F, et al (eds): *Diagnosis and Drug Treatment of Psychiatric Disorders: Adults and Children*, ed 2. Baltimore, Williams & Wilkins Co, 1980, pp 590–775.
19. Herzog DB, Harper G: Unexplained disability. *Glin Pediatr* 1981; 20:761–768

20. Eisenberg L: Adolescent suicide: on taking arms against a sea of troubles. *Pediatrics* 1980; 66:315–320.
21. Pfeiffer CB, Zuckerman S, Plutchik R, et al: Suicidal behavior in normal school children: a comparison with child psychiatric inpatients. *J Am Acad Child Psychiatry* 1984; 23:416–423.
22. Fraiberg S: *Clinical Studies in Infant Mental Health*. New York, Basic Books, Inc, 1980.
23. Beardslee WR, DeMaso DR: Staff groups in a pediatric hospital: content and coping. *Am J Orthopsychiatry* 1982; 52:712–718.

26

Psychotropic Drug Prescribing

JERROLD G. BERNSTEIN

Since the appearance of the first edition of this handbook, several useful new therapeutic agents have been introduced into the practice of psychopharmacology. We have gained new information that further supports biological factors in the etiology of psychiatric disorders and we have learned more about the optimal use of psychotropic medications in patients. As with any advance in medicine, unwanted effects have also occurred. Increasing concerns have surfaced about the possible long-term adverse effects of psychotropic medications, particularly with respect to tardive dyskinesia resulting from long-term neuroleptic treatment.[1] Although it is unlikely that anyone can distill our current and expanding knowledge of psychopharmacology into one chapter, I have attempted to present practical considerations regarding the administration of a wide variety of medications in the treatment of psychiatric disorders. Since medication prescribing rests fundamentally upon a knowledge of the pharmacology of those mediations which are being prescribed, I have attempted, at times in overly simplified form, to present basic information regarding the pharmacologic mechanisms of the various psychotropic medications. Since drug interactions are discussed in chapter 27, I will not discuss in detail these issues in this chapter. I will, however, attempt to focus on specific issues related to the prescribing of these medications in the setting of the general hospital. The discussion presented here will address itself to important psychotropic drugs within various therapeutic categories according to the system of classification presented in Table 26-1.

ANTIANXIETY DRUGS

Anxiety is a common complaint among patients hospitalized for nonpsychiatric indications. The most common form of anxiety seen in the general hospital setting may be termed "anticipatory anxiety." This form of anxiety may be spoken of as "nervousness," resulting from fears about a possible adverse diagnosis or fears associated with scheduled

Table 26-1. Classification of Psychotropic Drugs

Antianxiety Drugs	Antipsychotic Drugs	Antidepressant Drugs	Mood-Stabilizing Drugs
Benzodiazepines Short half-life 　Alprazolam (Xanax) 　Lorazepam (Ativan) 　Oxazepam (Serax) 　Triazolam (Halcion) Long half-life 　Chlorazepate (Tranxene) 　Chlordiazepoxide hydrochloride (Librium) 　Diazepam (Valium) 　Halazepam (Paxipam) 　Prazepam (Centrax) Propanediol Carbamate 　Meprobamate (Equanil) Barbiturates 　Amobarbital (Amytal) 　Phenobarbital (Luminal) Antihistamine 　Hydroxyzine (Vistaril)	Phenothiazines Aliphatic 　Chlorpromazine (Thorazine) Piperidine 　Thioridazine (Mellaril) 　Mesoridazine (Serentil) Piperazine 　Trifluoperazine hydrochloride (Stelazine) 　Fluphenazine hydrochloride (Prolixin) 　Perphenazine (Trilafon) Thioxanthenes Aliphatic 　Chlorprothixene (Taractan) Piperazine 　Thiothixene (Navane) Butyrophenone 　Haloperidol (Haldol) Dihydroindolone 　Molindone hydrochloride (Moban) Dibenzoxazepine 　Loxapine succinate (Loxitane)	Tricyclics Tertiary Amine 　Amitriptyline hydrochloride (Elavil) 　Imipramine hydrochloride (Tofranil) 　Doxepin hydrochloride (Sinequan) Secondary Amine 　Desipramine hydrochloride (Norpramin) 　Nortriptyline hydrochloride (Pamelor) 　Protriptyline hydrochloride (Vivactil) Dibenzoxazepine 　Amoxapine (Asendin) Tetracyclic 　Maprotiline (Ludiomil) Phenylpiperazine 　Trazodone hydrochloride (Desyrel) Monoamine Oxidase Inhibitors 　Isocarboxazid (Marplan) 　Phenelzine sulfate (Nardil) 　Tranylcypromine sulfate (Parnate) 　Pargyline hydrochloride (Eutonyl)	Lithium carbonate (Eskalith) Carbamazepine (Tegretol)

diagnostic or therapeutic procedures. Anticipatory anxiety is, in a sense, a normal form of anxiety which occurs quite rationally in response to unpleasant or stressful experiences. Minor degrees of anticipatory anxiety may best be managed, nonpharmacologically, with simple reassurance and support. More extensive degrees of anxiety may make the patient extremely uncomfortable as he proceeds through his diagnostic and therapeutic hospitalization. Furthermore, severe anxiety in a hospital setting may give rise to insomnia and have a deleterious effect on the patient's ability to maintain the strength to proceed with ongoing medical treatment. Although minor degrees of insomnia may not justify pharmacologic intervention, persistent inability to sleep may require the administration of medication in order to keep the patient comfortable. The watchword of medicating the patient who is experiencing normal anxiety and insomnia in the general hospital setting is: Be conservative; prescribe the lowest dose of medication for the shortest period of time.[1]

Some individuals suffer from severe chronic anxiety which may be associated with insomnia as well as a variety of unpleasant physiologic symptoms including rapid heart rate, sweating, and diarrhea. Patients with chronic anxiety who are hospitalized for medical treatment are likely to experience increased levels of anxiety and insomnia and will require the administration of medication to deal with these unpleasant symptoms. Specific anxiety disorders include phobic anxiety wherein patients experience extreme anxiety often in association with irrational fears, and panic anxiety, wherein there are acute, discrete episodes of severe anxiety and panic, apparently unrelated to external events. Patients who experience phobic anxiety or panic attacks may suffer from either independent of the other or, not uncommonly, from both of them simultaneously.[2] These forms of anxiety are not necessarily associated with insomnia though insomnia occurs in some phobic patients. Some patients with panic attacks awaken with these episodes from a deep sleep. These latter two anxiety disorders generally require pharmacologic treatment and may benefit from benzodiazepines such as alprazolam or from treatment with tricyclic antidepressants or monoamine oxidase inhibitors (MAOIs). Phobic disorders and panic attacks may be so incapacitating to individuals that they are prevented from working, attending school, or, indeed, leaving their own home. Although patients with anticipatory anxiety generally are best treated with intermittent administration of benzodiazepines, those individuals who are incapacitated by severe chronic anxiety generally require long-term continuous administration of medication as do patients that suffer from phobic disorders and panic attacks.[2]

Most antianxiety drugs are CNS depressants that exert a dose-related action ranging from a mild, calming effect to drowsiness and sedation with the induction of sleep when higher doses are administered. Alcohol has been used since ancient times as a sedative. More recent additions to the armamentarium have included bromides, barbiturates, meprobamate, and the now more widely used benzodiazepines. All of these drugs share in common one significant unwanted effect, namely, the potential of producing addiction. Patients receiving any of these CNS depressant drugs, over a prolonged period of time, will become tolerant to their action, requiring greater and greater dosage to be administered.[1] When these medications are suddenly discontinued, patients may experience a withdrawal syndrome with the possible occurrence of seizures and delirium following addiction to barbiturates, benzodiazepines, or any CNS depressant drug. Since patients with chronic anxiety are likely to take these medications over prolonged periods of time, they are particularly vulnerable to developing drug dependency.

Many middle-aged and older individuals who are admitted to hospitals for treatment of a variety of medical disorders do not provide adequate historical information to allow the physician to make a judgment of possible drug dependency. It is of great importance to talk carefully with all patients admitted to general hospitals in order to determine the possibility that they may have been taking a variety of antianxiety, sedative, or hypnotic drugs on a regular basis. Failure to get this information may expose the patient to the unwanted risk of a withdrawal syndrome during a medical hospitalization.

Patients who have become dependent on sedative drugs may require a pentobarbital tolerance test to clarify the extent of their addiction and a subsequent period of gradual drug withdrawal generally employing phenobarbital.[1] Although the addiction potential of alcohol and barbiturates is well appreciated by physicians, it is important to emphasize that meprobamate and the various benzodiazepines also have significant addiction potential. In the general hospital setting, it is important to be aware that the drowsiness and sedation produced by antianxiety drugs may be additive to the drowsiness and sedation produced by a variety of nonpsychotropic drugs discussed in chapter 27.

The sedating effect of antihistamines, such as hydroxyzine and diphenhydramine hydrochloride, may make these compounds useful, nonaddicting sedatives which may decrease anxiety or help to produce sleep in a patient for whom one does not wish to prescribe chloral hydrate, barbiturates, or benzodiazepines. It must be remembered, however, that most antihistamines also possess some anticholinergic activity and may therefore give rise to increased heart rate, and if large doses are employed, particularly in the elderly, confusional states may occur. On the positive side, the antihistamines have no potential for inducing drug dependency or addiction, and do not produce extrapyramidal effects or tardive dyskinesia following long-term use.

In the past, neuroleptic or antipsychotic drugs, particularly the more strongly sedating agents such as chlorpromazine and thioridazine have been recommended in the treatment of chronic anxiety. Occasionally, high-potency neuroleptics such as trifluoperazine hydrochloride have also been recommended in the treatment of severe chronic anxiety. In view of continuing concerns about the possible occurrence of tardive dyskinesia in patients receiving neuroleptic medications over a prolonged period of time, it is generally preferable to avoid the use of such drugs in the management of chronic anxiety in nonpsychotic patients. In rare instances, wherein a series of medications has been tried extensively without benefit, cautious use of neuroleptics in the treatment of severe anxiety over short periods of time may be appropriate.[1] Indeed, patients suffering from extreme degrees of agitation following cardiac surgery may benefit from the temporary oral or parenteral administration of haloperidol.[3] Although the antipsychotic drugs will be discussed in more detail below, it is important to note here that they should be used only infrequently and for very short periods of time in the management of severe anxiety in nonpsychotic patients.

Although the use of barbiturates in the treatment of anxiety and insomnia has largely been supplanted by the benzodiazepines, occasionally short-acting barbiturates such as pentobarbital may be useful for brief periods of administration in the treatment of insomnia in hospitalized patients. Furthermore, some anxious individuals achieve a beneficial effect with relatively low doses of barbiturates such as phenobarbital, amobarbital, and butabarbital sodium. Among barbiturates, phenobarbital has a relatively long duration of action with a half-life approximating 24 hours.[4] Phenobarbital produces less tolerance and less likelihood of dependence than shorter-acting barbiturates. Unfortunately, phenobarbital can induce the number of hepatic microsomal enzymes, and may therefore enhance the speed of metabolism of a variety of coadministered drugs, including tricyclic antidepressants and warfarin-type anticoagulants.[4] Chloral hydrate is frequently a useful hypnotic which may be used to induce sleep at a dose of 1 g nightly at bedtime in hospitalized patients. Elderly patients are likely to be more sensitive to the sedative action of chloral hydrate and may require a lower dose.[5] Furthermore, chloral hydrate displaces warfarin-type anticoagulants from plasma protein–binding sites and may therefore increase prothrombin time in anticoagulated patients. Chloral hydrate should not be administered in patients receiving these anticoagulants.

The most pronounced disturbing symptoms of anxiety are often those of excessive sympathetic nervous system activity, including persistent sinus tachycardia, excessive sweating, tremors, urinary urgency, and diarrhea or abdominal cramping. Many of these physiologic symptoms of anxiety respond favorably to the β-adrenergic blocker, propranolol hydrochloride. Propranolol is widely used in the treatment of cardiac arrhythmias, angina pectoris, and hypertension. Although the use of propranolol is not approved in the United States for the treatment of anxiety, it has been extensively used experimentally here and abroad and has been shown to be specifically beneficial in alleviating many of the physiologic symptoms of anxiety, thereby reducing the patient's perception of this dysphoric state. Propranolol has no addicting potential, which is, of course, an advantage for any agent that may be used over a prolonged period of time in a given patient. Propranolol is contraindicated for patients with a history of bronchial asthma, and may produce or worsen congestive heart failure in susceptible individuals.[4] If propranolol is used for anxiety, the patient should be carefully examined by an internist, and it is preferable that he be followed simultaneously by an internist and psychiatrist because of the potential unwanted medical complications of this drug. Nevertheless, some patients who have failed to respond to a variety of medications have achieved satisfactory control of their anxiety through judicious use of propranolol.[1,6] In the treatment of anxiety, propranolol hydrochloride is generally effective in a dosage range of 10 to 20 mg taken three to four times daily. Propranolol is also of interest to the psychiatrist because of its usefulness in the treatment of neuroleptic-induced akathisia, essential tremor, and the tremor induced in some patients by lithium carbonate therapy.[1,7] The effective dosage of propranolol hydrochloride for control of akathisia, essential tremor, and lithium-induced tremor is generally 10, 20, or 40 mg three to four times daily.

Propranolol is not a sedative and does not depress the CNS. It may, however, produce or worsen depression when large doses are employed and may also occasionally produce confusion and clouding of consciousness. β-Adrenergic blockers such as metoprolol and atenolol do not cross the blood-brain barrier as readily as propranolol and may be useful in blunting some of the peripheral autonomic symptoms of anxiety, though these drugs have not been extensively studied in anxiety disorders.[1,4]

Benzodiazepines are the most widely prescribed drugs in the treatment of anxiety and insomnia. Various compounds in this group differ from

Table 26-2. Half-Lives and Dosage Ranges of Common Benzodiazepines

Drug	Half-life (h)	Dosage Range (mg/d)	Indication
Alprazolam (Xanax)	12–19	0.125–6.0	Anxiety, Panic
Chlordiazepoxide (Librium)	12–48	5–200	Anxiety
Diazepam (Valium)	20–90	2–40	Anxiety
Flurazepam (Dalmane)	24–100	15–30	Insomnia
Lorazepam (Ativan)	10–20	1–10	Anxiety
Oxazepam (Serax)	8–21	10–90	Anxiety
Temazepam (Restoril)	12–24	15–30	Insomnia
Triazolam (Halcion)	1.7–3.0	0.125–0.5	Insomnia

each other in terms of their duration of action, half-life, and dosage, as demonstrated in Table 26-2. As noted in the table, some of these compounds are primarily indicated for the treatment of insomnia while others are primarily indicated for anxiety. In general, drugs in this group can be used interchangeably for either anxiety or insomnia.[4] The half-lives shown in Table 27-2 represent published figures for the various compounds and are generally based upon single-dose administration. With continued administration of any benzodiazepine, including those which are shorter acting, the half-life tends to become prolonged beyond the figures quoted. Drugs with longer half-lives exert a more cumulative effect with prolonged administration than do those with shorter half-lives. Excessive drowsiness and sedation are the most common side effects of benzodiazepines, the action of which is increased when taken in conjunction with alcohol or other CNS depressant drugs.[1,4]

The anxiolytic action of benzodiazepines appears to be related to their interaction with specific neuronal benzodiazepine receptors. Indeed, there is some correlation between receptor binding affinity and anxiolytic potency.[8] γ-Aminobutyric acid (GABA) is a naturally occurring inhibitory neurotransmitter which appears to increase the affinity of benzodiazepines for the receptor site. Benzodiazepines increase the frequency with which anion channels open in response to GABA. This, in turn, is associated with hyperpolarization of the postsynaptic neuron, decreasing the frequency of neuronal firing.[8] The actions of benzodiazepines appear to be closely related to GABA effects on anion channels. Quite conceivably, some of the basic mechanisms of anxiety within the CNS may relate to the inhibitory neurotransmitter GABA.[8] In all likelihood, other neurotransmitter systems, including norepinephrine and substance P may likewise be involved in anxiety disorders. Since the benzodiazepines produce a variety of effects including anxiolysis, muscle relaxation, and anticonvulsant action, it is likely that several subtypes of benzodiazepine receptors exist.[8]

In prescribing benzodiazepines for anxiety or insomnia, it is generally preferable to use those drugs with shorter half-lives since they are less likely to produce excessive sedation as a result of continued accumulation through repetitive administration. In the treatment of anticipatory anxiety requiring pharmacologic intervention, the administration of the smallest dose of a shorter-acting compound such as alprazolam, lorazepam, or oxazepam is preferable to the use of longer-acting drugs such as diazepam.[1] In anticipatory anxiety or anxiety that occurs in response to life events, these medications may be administered intermittently and, generally, infrequently. The use of shorter-acting benzodiazepines administered one or two times daily is preferred to more frequent administration.

Proper education of the patient regarding the necessity to minimize the dose of medication taken may allow for a satisfactory therapeutic response with minimum risk of drug dependency since the latter is more likely to occur when larger doses are taken more frequently and for longer periods of time. Patients with simple anxiety disorders should be encouraged to utilize their medication intermittently and not to continue taking the benzodiazepine in the absence of symptoms. Likewise, patients with intermittent insomnia should be encouraged to utilize the medication only when needed rather than on a regular nightly basis.[5] The practice of routinely prescribing hypnotics at bedtime to hospitalized patients should be discouraged in favor of a program of prescribing which takes into account the patient's specific need for pharmacologic intervention.[15] Oxazepam or temazepam at doses of 15 to 30 mg at bedtime may be equally satisfactory to induce sleep. Either of these compounds may be far preferable to diazepam or flurazepam hydrochloride, both of which have significantly longer half-lives and a greater likelihood of cumulative effects. Triazolam, which has the shortest half-life of any marketed benzodiazepam, may, in many respects, be the ideal hypnotic. Since sedatives are generally more effective in inducing sleep than they are in keeping patients asleep for a long period of time, the rapid onset of action and short half-life of triazolam may be advantageous. Furthermore, the short half-life significantly reduces the risk of continuing daytime sedation following a bedtime dose.[5]

Phobic disorders and panic attacks are frequently responsive to treatment with benzodiazepines, particularly alprazolam which has been extensively studied in this form of anxiety.[2,9] Unlike anticipatory anxiety and stress-induced anxiety, which are often responsive to low doses of benzodiazepines administered intermittently, patients who suffer from phobic disorders and panic attacks generally require larger doses of benzodiazepines administered on a continuous basis. Controlled clinical trials of alprazolam documents the superior efficacy of this compound as compared to either placebo or other potentially active drugs.[2,9] Patients who have phobic disorders, particularly agorophobia and those who have discrete panic attacks are often responsive to continuous administration of alprazolam, generally in the dosage range of 3 to 6 mg/d. When initiating treatment for such individuals, the dosage needs to be started relatively low, perhaps 0.25 mg three times daily with progressive dosage increase until an optimally effective and tolerated dose is achieved. If patients are started on excessively high doses or if the dosage is titrated upward too rapidly, excessive sedation is likely to occur prior to achieving the desired antiphobic or antipanic effect.[2] Once an effective dosage has been reached, generally patients continue to be responsive without further increase.

It is of utmost clinical importance in treating phobic disorders and panic anxiety to gradually titrate the dosage downward rather than abruptly discontinue alprazolam since continuing administration of this medication may be associated with drug dependence and the occurrence of a withdrawal syndrome following abrupt discontinuation.[1,2] Many patients who are not responsive to alprazolam will experience more satisfactory control of their phobic disorder or panic attacks when they are treated with a tricyclic compound such as imipramine hydrochloride or an MAOI such as phenelzine sulfate.[2] It is important when converting the therapeutic regimen from alprazolam to one of the latter compounds to titrate the dosage gradually downward rather than abruptly discontinuing the alprazolam as the new medication is begun.

When prescribing any sedative, it is important for the physician to be aware of the potential additive interaction between the antianxiety drug and a variety of nonpsychotropic medications which may produce drowsiness.[1] These interactions are discussed in more detail in chapter 27. The physician must also be aware that elderly patients, patients with organic brain dysfunction, and patients with impaired hepatic or renal function will be more sensitive to the action of any benzodiazepine or other sedative compound and will thus require significantly lower doses of such medications.

ANTIPSYCHOTIC DRUGS

Antipsychotic drugs, or neuroleptics, are used in the treatment of acute psychotic symptoms associated with schizophrenia, mania, and psychotic depression. These drugs are also employed in the prophylaxis of recurrent psychotic symptoms in schizophrenic patients. They may also be useful in the treatment of acute psychotic symptoms that occur in association with organic brain dysfunction. Psychotic manifestations that may occur as a result of drug intoxication are generally not treated with antipsychotic medications, although these drugs are occasionally employed for brief intervals in controlling the psychotic agitation that may be induced by adverse reactions to drugs or by intentional drug intoxication such as that produced by phencyclidine hydrochloride (angel dust.)

When encountering an acutely psychotic patient in the general hospital setting, the physician must first attempt to make a diagnosis. If the psychotic symptoms are the result of chemical intoxication, such as that produced by anticholinergic drugs, avoidance of neuroleptics may be the most appropriate first step in the assessment and treatment of the patient. Indeed, anticholinergic deliria may present a diagnostic puzzle which can be clarified by the cautious, slow intravenous (IV) administration of 1 mg of physostigmine diluted in a total volume of 10 mL of normal saline.[1] The physician encountering an acutely psychotic patient in the general hospital with a negative past psychiatric history must investigate the possibility that the patient's psychotic symptoms are related to his medical problem or are secondary to therapy.

Patients experiencing their first acute psychotic episode during the course of a medical hospitalization may also be suffering from a drug withdrawal syndrome associated with the abrupt discontinuation of alcohol, barbiturates, benzodiazepines, or other sedative drugs. Such patients may require the administration of benzodiazepines or a pentobarbital tolerance test to assess their dependency upon sedatives. The administration of chlorpromazine to a patient withdrawing from alchohol or sedatives may provoke hypotension and convulsions, thus significantly worsening an already difficult clinical situation. Patients who experience hallucinations during the course of withdrawal from alcohol or other sedatives may benefit from the administration of small doses of haloperidol in conjunction with oxazepam, other benzodiazepines, or phenobarbital. Although haloperidol should not be relied upon as the sole agent during sedative withdrawal, its ability to lower seizure threshold is significantly less than that of chlorpromazine and its potential for producing hypotension is minimal.

Antipsychotic drugs have a specific ability to control hallucinations, delusions, and disordered thinking associated with psychotic illnesses. They vary considerably in their clinical potency which closely parallels their affinity for binding with dopamine receptor sites in the brain.[10,11]

Increasing evidence suggests that schizophrenic disorders have a genetic predisposition which gives rise to a biochemical disturbance wherein there is increased central dopaminergic activity.[1,12] The ability of antipsychotic drugs to block dopamine receptor sites appears to explain their antipsychotic action.[11] Table 26-3 presents the characteristics of some of the more commonly used antipsychotic drugs. The neuroleptic agents are listed in order from highest to lowest potency. As can be seen from the table, their clinical potency closely parallels their affinity for dopamine receptor sites as measured by inhibition of haloperidol binding. The table also demonstrates their relative affinity for cholinergic receptor sites.[14] In addition to the potency differences of the various antipsychotic drugs, these compounds also differ one from the other in terms of their likelihood of producing a variety of unwanted effects, including anticholinergic side effects, extrapyramidal effects, sedation, and hypotension. Furthermore, among antipsychotic drugs, chlorpromazine has the greatest ability to lower seizure threshold and therefore provoke convulsions, while thioridazine and haloperidol are much less likely to effect convulsive threshold and provoke seizures. Patients with convulsive disorders should generally not receive chlorpromazine.

The anticholinergic action of antipsychotic drugs is responsible for blurred vision, dry mouth, constipation, urinary retention, and tachycardia, which may accompany their administration. Patients with gastrointestinal (GI) disorders may be particularly sensitive to the anticholinergic action of these drugs, particularly if they are simultaneously receiving other medications with anticholinergic activity. Men with prostatic enlargement are apt to experience urinary retention when they receive strongly anticholinergic compounds. Patients with cardiovascular disease may be adversely effected by strongly anticholinergic agents such as chlorpromazine or thioridazine which may increase heart rate, thereby decreasing time for ventricular filling and thus producing a decrease in cardiac output. High-potency antipsychotic drugs such as haloperidol, fluphenazine hydrochloride, thiothixene, and trifluoperazine produce less anticholinergic side effects than do the low-potency agents such as chlorpromazine and thioridazine.[1,14] On the other hand, the low-potency antipsychotic agents produce less acute extrapyramidal or parkinsonian effects than do the high-potency agents. The high-potency neuroleptic medications tend to produce significantly less sedation and hypotension than do the low potency antipsychotic drugs.[1] In the general hospital setting, where patients are likely to be simultaneously suffering from complicated medical disorders, haloperidol is generally the antipsychotic agent of choice from the standpoint

Table 26-3. Characteristics of Commonly Used Antipsychotic Drugs

Clinical Potency of Antipsychotic Action from Most to Least Potent* (Chemical Class)	Inhibition of (^3H) Haloperidol Binding, K_1 (nmol)[13]	Relative Affinity for Muscarinic (Cholinergic) Receptor[14]	Anticholinergic Effects Clinically Observed	Parkinsonian Effects Clinically Observed	Sedation Clinically Observed	Hypotension Clinically Observed
Haloperidol (Haldol) [butyrophenone]	1.5±0.14	0.21	+	+++++	++	+
Fluphenazine hydrochloride (Prolixin) [piperazine-phenothiazine]	1.2±0.12	0.83	++	+++++	++	++
Thiothixene (Navane) [piperazine-thioxanthene]	1.4±0.11	0.78	++	++++	++	++
Trifluoperazine hydrochloride (Stelazine) [piperazine-phenothiazine]	2.1±0.34		++	++++	+	++
Perphenazine (Trilafon) [piperazine-phenothiazine]		0.91	++	++++	+++	+++
Molindone hydrochloride (Moban) [dihydroindolone]			+++	+++	+	++
Loxapine succinate (Loxitane) [dibenzoxazepine]			+++	+++	+++	++
Chlorpromazine (Thorazine) [aliphatic-phenothiazine]	10.3±0.2	10.0	++++	++	+++++	++++
Thioridazine (Mellaril) [piperidine-phenothiazine]	14.0±0.2	66.7	+++++	+	++++	+++++

* Drugs are listed in order of clinical potency, from most potent to least potent in their action against psychotic symptoms, based upon the author's clinical experience and review of a wide range of published data. Likelihood of producing various side effects is likewise based upon the author's observations of patients and a review of published information from numerous sources.

of its high potency and relatively minor side effects with the exception of its propensity for producing acute extrapyramidal reactions. Generally, dosage adjustment or the coadministration of an appropriate antiparkinsonian medication will provide adequate control of these unwanted extrapyramidal effects.

Treatment of schizophrenia with antipsychotic drugs can be divided into three phases. The initial phase of treatment is aimed at providing behavioral control and reducing agitation, fear, anxiety, disturbed thinking, hallucinations, and delusions. If one conceptualizes acute psychosis as a disorder involving excessive action of dopamine or related neurotransmitters, one may think of treatment in the acute phase as being aimed at producing dopaminergic receptor blockade. Achievement of this pharmacologic effect with neuroleptic medication parallels the initial phase of clinical improvement. The term "pharmacolysis" seems applicable to describe the acute phase of drug treatment of psychosis. A rapid antipsychotic effect may best be achieved by administration of adequate doses of specific antipsychotic medications, either by the oral or intramuscular (IM) route.[1,15]

The next phase of antipsychotic chemotherapy involves stabilization of the patient with gradual reduction of antipsychotic dosage in order to achieve the best possible control of symptoms with the lowest effective dose of medication, thereby reducing the risk of drug side effects. The third phase is the maintenance phase involving the long-term continuous administration of the lowest possible dose of medication in order to prevent recurrence of the psychotic illness.

In the schizophrenic patient, these three phases of treatment are generally best accomplished by starting and continuing treatment with a single antipsychotic drug provided that the patient is able to tolerate this medication without incapacitating side effects. If side effects do develop, it may be necessary to add an antiparkinsonian medication or change to a different antipsychotic drug.[1,16] In general, the administration of haloperidol or another high-potency antipsychotic agent such as trifluoperazine or thiothixene is preferable to the use of low-potency antipsychotic drugs in the acutely psychotic schizophrenic patient. Although low-potency antipsychotic agents, such as chlorpromazine and thioridazine which possess considerable sedative action, may be useful and tolerated by acutely psychotic patients, the likelihood of these drugs producing excessive sedation, anticholinergic action, and hypotension makes them less desirable than the high-potency antipsychotic agents.

The psychiatric consultant in caring for an acutely manic patient on a medical or surgical ward should initiate treatment with a high-potency antipsychotic compound in conjunction with lithium carbonate in order to achieve behavioral control.[1] Although lithium carbonate is highly effective in reducing manic symptoms, it tends to act rather slowly requiring 1 to 2 weeks for a beneficial effect to be observed.[17] Haloperidol is more rapid in its onset of action, and is likely to produce significant behavioral control of the acutely manic patient within one to three days.[17] Haloperidol is more effective in normalizing the acutely manic patient than is chlorpromazine, although the latter may achieve significant sedation with a less pronounced improvement in the manic quality of behavior.[17] In acute mania, the initial starting dose of haloperidol should be 5 mg orally or IM. However, patients with manic psychosis often require larger doses of haloperidol or other antipsychotic agents than do schizophrenic patients. It is not uncommon for acute manic patients to require 40 to 80 mg of haloperidol/d in the early phase of treatment. With symptomatic improvement on a combined halo-peridol–lithium carbonate regimen, the dose of the antipsychotic medication may be gradually decreased and subsequently discontinued as the patient stabilizes on a maintenance regimen of lithium carbonate.[1] Although concerns have been raised in the literature about a possible specific toxic syndrome associated with the simultaneous administration of lithium and haloperidol, evidence suggests that this syndrome does not exist. In a series of 425 patients receiving a combined lithium-haloperidol regimen, none developed this specific syndrome.[18]

Treatment of the psychotically depressed patient is usually best initiated by the administration of a high-potency antipsychotic medication alone, followed by the addition of an appropriate tricyclic or MAOI antidepressant.[1,19] Once initial recovery is noted in the patient with psychotic depression, treatment may often be continued with the antidepressant drug alone following gradual discontinuation of the antipsychotic agent. In some patients with severe depression with psychotic features, a more prolonged course of antipsychotic medication must be administered along with the appropriate antidepressant. Some patients with recurrent severe psychotic depressive disorders are optimally benefitted by a regimen of antidepressant medication in conjunction with lithium carbonate once the initial psychotic phase of the illness begins to remit in response to antipsychotic chemotherapy.[19]

Molindone hydrochloride and loxapine succinate are chemically distinct from each other and from other antipsychotic agents. Loxapine is chemically a dibenzoxazepine, which is structurally similar to amoxapine, one of the newer antidepressant drugs.[20] Molindone is an indole derivative, structurally similar to the neurotransmitter serotonin.

Both of these compounds can be considered intermediate-potency antipsychotic agents, being less potent than the piperazine phenothiazines and more potent that chlorpromazine. Molindone exerts the least sedative action of all currently marketed antipsychotic agents.[21] This compound also has an ability to decrease appetite and may, in fact, allow patients to lose weight while taking it, in contradistinction to most other antipsychotic drugs which tend to promote weight gain. On some occasions, molindone has been noted to promote seizurelike activity and may therefore not be desirable in the treatment of patients with convulsive disorders. Loxapine, which can be administered either by the oral or IM route, may possess some antidepressant activity and may be particularly useful in the treatment of borderline patients. These compounds, being neither phenothiazines nor butyrophenones, may be of value in the treatment of patients who have developed allergic reactions to other neuroleptic medications.

In prescribing antipsychotic drugs for elderly patients and for those with organic brain dysfunction, high-potency drugs such as haloperidol are preferable because of their more specific antipsychotic action and their lesser likelihood of producing anticholinergic and hypotensive side effects. In such patients, it is reasonable to start at very low doses (eg, haloperidol 0.25 to 1.0 mg every four to 12 hours) and titrate the dosage gradually as clinically necessary and tolerated.

Patients receiving antipsychotic drugs may develop withdrawal dyskinesia if the dosage is abruptly reduced or discontinued. Clinically, withdrawal dyskinesia generally begins with abnormal oral or facial movements which resemble tardive dyskinesia. Tardive dyskinesia, which appears in approximately 15% to 20% of patients receiving chronic neuroleptic treatment is the major long-term risk of antipsychotic drug therapy. Contrary to earlier thinking, tardive dyskinesia may disappear spontaneously several months after neuroleptics are discontinued, and a variety of pharmacologic interventions have been successfully employed with a resultant diminution or disappearance of dyskinetic movements.

Neuroleptic Malignant Syndrome

Neuroleptic malignant syndrome (NMS) is a rare complication of antipsychotic drug therapy which physiologically and mechanistically resembles malignant hyperthermia of anesthesia. This syndrome can occur at any point in antipsychotic drug therapy with either high-potency or low-potency neuroleptics. It is most likely to occur during an acute phase of psychotic illness, in the course of treatment with multiple neuroleptic drugs simultaneously, or following multiple changes from one neuroleptic to another.[1] Neuroleptic malignant syndrome is characterized by the following findings: stiffness with catatonia, hyperthermia (100.5° F to 106° F), autonomic dysfunction with either hypotension or hypertension, bradycardia or tachycardia, siallorhea, sweating, dyspnea, and dysphagia. Patients with NMS tend to become seriously ill as a result of dehydration, electrolyte imbalance, aspiration pneumonia, pulmonary emboli, and secondary infectious complications.[22] Patients developing this syndrome should have neuroleptic medications immediately discontinued and be given IV fluid replacement along with careful monitoring of physiologic functions and fluid and electrolyte balance.

Physical therapy for help with ambulation, and antiembolism stockings are useful adjuncts to treatment. It is preferable when encountering a patient with NMS to avoid the administration of all medications, certainly neuroleptic medications and those drugs with pronounced autonomic effects. Cautious use of low doses of benztropine mesylate may be useful in the treatment of stiffness and siallorhea, but may present an added risk in terms of further complicating an already disturbed autonomic balance. Bromocriptine, a dopamine agonist, and dantrolene, an antispasticity drug, have both been used with considerable success individually and combined in the treatment of NMS, and should be considered for any patient who is seriously ill with this syndrome.[21,22]

ANTIDEPRESSANT DRUGS

Depressive disorders vary considerably in severity, ranging from mild depressions provoked by losses or other life crises to more severe, incapacitating depressions which may occur spontaneously in the absence of traumatic life events. Some individuals will experience a single episode of depression in their lifetime, provoked by difficulties in their personal lives or the occurrence of a serious medical illness. On the other hand, many individuals, unfortunately, suffer from recurrent episodes of depression which may begin as early as the teenage years or as late as the eighth decade of life. Severe depressive disorders are more apt to occur in individuals who have a family history of affective illness. There is significant evidence for a genetic predisposition to major affective disorders, both the unipolar and bipolar types.[23] Patients who are severely depressed often develop anorexia and lose considerable weight. Depressed patients frequently have a disturbance of their sleep pattern and tend to awaken during the night or in the early morning hours. At either time they are unable to fall back to sleep. Although anorexia and insomnia are most commonly found in depressed patients, depression sometimes can cause an increase in appetite and hypersomnia.

Depressed patients feel sad and hopeless and generally lose interest in their usual work and leisure time activities. The inability to achieve pleasure from normally pleasurable activities is the hallmark of depression. Decreased sexual interest and decreased frequency of sexual activity are common in depression. The energy level is almost always low and there is a sense of fatigue and the feeling of being physically slowed down. Some depressed patients experience psychotic thinking and become preoccupied with thoughts of guilt and self-reproach. Concentration and memory are often impaired and indecisiveness is common in depression, as are thoughts of death and ideas of suicide.

The psychiatric consultant in the general hospital setting will encounter all degrees of depression among patients who are hospitalized for medical illnesses. Many of those patients who do not have prior histories of affective illness can be helped by psychotherapeutic intervention, while those who have reactive depressions that are persistent and incapacitating may require pharmacologic treatment. Patients with severe depressions, particularly when associated with appetite and sleep disturbances and with somatic symptoms, will most likely require pharmacologic intervention in conjunction with whatever psychotherapy is provided.

Extensive clinical and scientific investigation has provided strong support for a biological or biochemical basis for the major depressive disorders. Patients who experience severe or recurrent depressive illnesses appear to have a biochemically based illness related to deficiencies of neurotransmission within the brain.[24] The neurotransmitters that have been most often associated with depressive illness include norepinephrine, and serotonin.[24] The medications that are helpful in the treatment of depression exert their beneficial effect by increasing the availability or activity of these neurotransmitters within brain synapses.[24,25] In the early days of antidepressant chemotherapy, it was generally held that only severe endogenous depressions should be treated pharmacologically and that minor depressions or reactive depressions should be treated psychotherapeutically without medication. Current thinking strongly supports the use of pharmacologic treatment in any depressive disorder which has been present and incapacitating over a period of several weeks. There is increasing evidence that individuals who suffer from persistent reactive depressions can benefit significantly by pharmacologic treatment and can be restored to a more functional and rewarding life more rapidly by this approach than by a long course of psychotherapy.[1] There is no reason to avoid medication in a depressed patient who is being treated psychotherapeutically and there is no reason to avoid psychotherapy in a depressed patient who is receiving medical management.

Prior to the availability of our currently used effective antidepressant drugs, the amphetamines were commonly employed in the treatment of depression. Drugs of this group, including dextroamphetamine and methylphenidate hydrochloride, have an ability to stimulate norepinephrine neurotransmission within the brain.[2] These compounds are capable of increasing energy, and improving the mood. Unfortunately, patients tend to become tolerant to these drugs and may experience only a short-lived antidepressant effect.[1,2] Nevertheless, amphetamines, including the related compound methylphenidate, are sometimes useful in the treatment of depression in individuals who do not tolerate tricyclic- or MAOI-type antidepressant drugs.[1] In general, the preferred pharmacologic treatments of depression consist of a series of tricyclic antidepressants, the MAOIs, and several newer compounds which are chemically distinct from the tricyclic antidepressants, but which appear to exert their therapeutic effect by similar mechanisms.

As can be seen in Table 26-4, the currently marketed tricyclic antidepressants, including two nontricyclic antidepressants, differ from one another in their relative effects in inhibiting norepinephrine and serotonin reuptake mechanisms. These drugs also differ in terms of their relative likelihood of producing sedation and anticholinergic side effects as can be seen in the table. Inhibition of neuronal reuptake mechanisms for serotonin and norepinephrine increase the availability and activity of these neurotransmitters within the brain.[3,4] Although various mechanisms of action have been proposed for these antidepressant drugs, current evidence suggests that their ability to alleviate depressive symptoms is based upon a correction of the deficient neurotransmitter function present in the patient. The MAOIs, by decreasing the metabolic degradation of norepinephrine and serotonin, will likewise increase the availability of these neurotransmitters within the brain and thus, presumably, help to correct the symptoms of depressive illness. Amephetamines, which increase norepinephrine neurotransmission and fenfluramine hydrochloride, which increase central serotonergic activity, likewise possess antidepressant activity.[4] Preliminary research suggests that the administration of L-tryptophan or L-tyrosine, amino acid precursors of serotonin and norepinephrine respectively, may also exert an antidepressant effect, presumably as a result of increased

Table 26-4. Pharmacologic Profiles of Tricyclic and Tetracyclic Antidepressants

	Anticholinergic Effect	Sedative Effect	Reuptake Antagonism	
			Norepinephrine	Serotonin
Tricyclic				
Tertiary Amines				
Amitriptyline hydrochloride (Elavil)	+++++	+++++	+	++++
Imipramine hydrochloride (Tofranil)	++++	+++	++	+++
Trimipramine (Surmontil)	++++	++++	Uncertain*	
Doxepin hydrochloride (Sinequan)	++	++++	Uncertain*	
Tricyclic				
Secondary Amines				
Desipramine hydrochloride (Norpramin)	+	+	+++++	0
Protriptyline hydrochloride (Vivactil)	+++	+	Uncertain*†	
Nortriptyline hydrochloride (Aventyl)	+++	++	+++	++
Tricyclic				
Dibenzoxazepine				
Amoxapine (Asendin)	++	++	++++	+
Tetracyclic	++	++++	+++++	0
Maprotiline (Ludiomil)				
Triazolopyridine				
Derivative				
Trazodone hydrochloride (Desyrel)	++	+++++	0	+++++

* Tertiary amine structure suggests greater effect on serotonin reuptake than norepinephrine reuptake.
† Secondary amine structure suggests greater effect on norepinephine reuptake than serotonin reuptake.

Relative anticholinergic and sedative potencies of the various antidepressant drugs are based upon a composite of multiple published clinical studies of each drug as well as the clinical observations of the author.

Relative effects of the various antidepressant drugs on nerve reuptake of norepinephrine and serotonin are based in each case upon published laboratory and clinical investigations. Referencs providing documentation for these data are:

Brogden RN, Heel RC, Speight TM, et al: Trazodone: A review of its pharmacological properties and therapeutic use in depression and anxiety. *Drugs* 1981; 21:401–429.

Greenblatt EN, Lippa AS, Osterberg AC: The neuropharmacological action of amoxapine.

Arch Int Pharmacodyn Ther 1978; 233:107–135.
Hollister LE: Tricyclic antidepressants (part I). *N Engl J Med* 1978; 299:1106–1109.
Maas JW: Biogenic amines and depression. *Arch Gen Psychiatry* 1975; 32:1357–1361.
Maitre L, Waldmeier PC, Greengrass PM, et al: Maprotiline—Its position as an antidepressant in the light of recent neuropharmacological and neurobiological findings. *J Int Med Res* 1975 (suppl 2): 3:2–15.
Snyder SH, Yamamura HI: Antidepressants and the muscarinic cholinergic receptor. *Arch Gen Psychiatry* 1977; 34:236–239.

synthesis of these neurotransmitters within the brain. According to some research studies, measurement of urinary 3-methoxy-4-hydroxy-phenylglycol (MHPG) may have some predictive value in determining whether a given depressed patient will be more likely to respond to a serotonin-active drug such as amitriptyline hydrochloride or a norepine-phrine-active drug such as desipramine hydrochloride.[25] Unfortunately, more recent investigations indicate that measurement of urinary neuro-transmitter metabolites has thus far only very limited ability to predict antidepressant drug responsiveness.[26] Therefore the choice of a parti-cular antidepressant drug relies more on clinical decision-making and the administration of a therapeutic trial of antidepressants.

Antidepressant drugs differ considerably in their side effect profiles. As can be seen in Table 26-4, amitriptyline, trimipramine, doxepin hydro-chloride, maprotiline, and trazodone hydrochloride are likely to produce a greater sedative effect and therefore may be particularly desirable for a depressed patient who has difficulty sleeping. In these situations, the administration of the total daily dose at bedtime may avoid the coadministration of sedatives or hypnotics in order to induce sleep. Desipramine, protriptyline hydrochloride, nortriptyline hydrochloride, and amoxapine are significantly less sedating than the previously mentioned drugs and may be particularly useful in the withdrawn, depressed patient who tends to sleep excessively. These latter medica-tions may be administered in divided doses throughout the day, or may be administered as a single bedtime dose.

The anticholinergic action of tricyclic antidepressants is particu-larly troublesome since this pharmacologic mechanism may give rise to dry mouth, blurred vision, constipation, urinary retention, and tachy-cardia. In addition to these peripheral manifestations of cholinergic blockade, the stronger anticholinergic antidepressants are likely to produce CNS effects of impairment of memory and concentration, speech blockage, confusional states, and delirium.[27,28] Elderly patients and patients with organic brain syndromes are particularly vulnerable to anticholinergic side effects.

Among commonly used antidepressants, desipramine appears to have the least anticholinergic activity followed by amoxapine, maprotiline, trazodone, and doxepin. According to some studies, doxepin exerts a moderate degree of anticholinergic activity, although in clinical practice, most patients do not complain of such side effects. Strongly anticholinergic antidepressants may also decrease sweating and impair temperature regulation, particularly in the elderly, or in patients exposed to very warm climates or working conditions. As discussed in more detail in chapter 27, more strongly anticholinergic tricyclics such as amitriptyline should generally be avoided in patients with unstable cardiac conditions. In general, antidepressant drugs should be avoided immediately following acute myocardial infarction. In prescribing antidepressant drugs for patients with cardiovascular disease the dosage should be started at a lower than normal level and titrated up more slowly than conventional regimens suggest. Furthermore, the continuing administration of divided doses, as opposed to a single bedtime dose, is advantageous in the elderly or in patients with cardiovascular disease.[1]

Among antidepressant drugs, amoxapine is unique in that it has a rapid onset of action, often producing a response within the first week of therapy.[1,29] The side effects of amoxapine, from the standpoint of sedation and anticholinergic action, are relatively mild, making the drug generally well tolerated. Amoxapine is also unique in that it possesses some neuroleptic or dopamine blocking activity which may give rise to occasional occurrences of extrapyramidal side effects.[30] Because of its dopamine-blocking activity, amoxapine has been suspected of being a potential risk in the production of tardive dyskinesia following long-term therapy. However, having used the drug in a large series of patients, I have encountered akathisia on only one occasion and have not seen more severe extrapyramidal side effects or tardive dyskinesia.

Trazodone, another of the second-generation antidepressants, has the unique characteristic of decreasing appetite in many patients which may be an advantage in individuals who gain weight on other antidepressants. Despite its relatively low anticholinergic activity, trazodone may produce impaired or slow thinking in some individuals which appears to be related to this anticholinergic mechanism. A few instances of drug-induced delirium have also been reported with trazodone.[31] From the standpoint of efficacy, although trazodone is a primary inhibitor of serotonin reuptake, generally this drug appears less effective than amitriptyline. Another of the second-generation antidepressants is maprotiline, which, although effective against depression, appears to reduce seizure threshold and may provoke convulsions in patients with convulsive disorders or in those individuals who take large doses therapeutically or who overdose on the drug.[32] Maprotiline should generally be avoided in patients who have convulsive disorders.

Nomifensine maleate (Merital) a structurally unique antidepressant, inhibits both norepinephrine and dopamine reuptake mechanisms. This drug has minimal sedative and low anticholinergic potency and may produce an activating antidepressant effect with less stimulation of appetite.[33] Some patients receiving this drug have developed fever and hemolytic anemia, therefore, it has been withdrawn from the American market.[33]

Bupropion hydrochloride (Wellbatrin), another antidepressant which is neither a tricyclic nor an MAOI, exerts its therapeutic action by an as yet unknown mechanism. This drug appears not to inhibit norepinephrine or serotonin reuptake although it has some inhibitory action on dopamine reuptake mechanisms.[34] Preliminary studies suggest low sedative and anticholinergic potency and minimal effect on appetite, weight gain, and cardiovascular parameters.[34] It has been associated with a high incidence of seizures and therefore withdrawn from the American market

Patients who suffer from psychotic depressive disorders, particularly in the presence of delusional thinking, hallucinations, and agitation, generally should be started on a low to moderate dose of a high-potency antipsychotic agent such as trifluoperazine or haloperidol. As the psychotic symptoms begin to improve, by the end of the first week of treatment, a tricyclic antidepressant may then be added to the neuroleptic medication.[1] Psychotically depressed patients, who have pharmacotherapy initiated with antidepressants in the absence of antipsychotic drugs, may experience increased psychotic symptoms and agitation. Use of fixed-dose combinations of amitriptyline and perphenazine is to be discouraged since adequate dosage adjustment of the antidepressant is often associated with excessive doses of the neuroleptic. Furthermore, as the psychotic features of the depression improve, it is generally preferable to reduce the dose of antipsychotic medication to a minimum while continuing the patient on a full dose of an antidepressant, which cannot be adequately accomplished with a fixed-dose combination. Likewise, patients who have nonpsychotic depressive disorders should not be treated with fixed-dose combinations of amitriptyline and perphenazine since, in most instances, the administration of a neuroleptic is not necessary in nonpsychotically depressed patients.

Some patients who have severe depressive disorders, in the absence of psychotic features may, however, benefit from temporary use of low doses of high-potency neuroleptics such as trifluoperazine or haloperidol in conjunction with their antidepressant regimen. Neuroleptics are capable of increasing serum concentrations of tricyclic antidepressants and may also be beneficial in reducing agitation and anxiety which may accompany even nonpsychotic depressive disorders. Most such patients, following a brief course of combined antidepressant and neuropleptic medication, may have the neuroleptic discontinued. However, some individuals continue to benefit from low doses of neuroleptics (2 to 6 mg/d) along with a continuing antidepressant drug regimen. Patients whose depression is refractory to treatment with conventional tricyclics or MAOIs may benefit from the addition of either a low dose of a high-potency neuroleptic to the antidepressant regimen or from the addition of lithium carbonate or tri-iodothyronine (25 μg/d). Although the mechanism of the facilitation of antidepressant response by either lithium carbonate or tri-iodothyronine is not clearly understood, numerous studies document the action of this combination therapy.[35,36]

Most sophisticated clinical laboratories are capable of measuring serum tricyclic antidepressant concentrations. The measurement of tricyclic antidepressant blood levels is not a necessary part of routine antidepressant drug therapy.[1] It is a useful technique in patients who fail to respond to therapeutic doses of antidepressant drugs. In such patients a tricyclic blood level will determine the adequacy of their serum concentration. Patients who have repetitive side effects with a variety of tricyclic antidepressants can benefit from tricyclic serum levels because these may reveal excessive serum concentrations at ordinary therapeutic dosages.[1] In the elderly tricyclic serum measurement is useful since the antidepressant drug dose generally needs to be about 50% of that required in younger persons to achieve comparable therapeutic serum concentrations.[37] Tricyclic blood levels are also of some value in documenting compliance.

In treating any patient with a tricyclic antidepressant, it is important to achieve an adequate dosage level to provide satisfactory clinical improvement. It is also important not to discontinue the antidepressant abruptly since this may be associated with a rapid recurrence of depressive symptoms or, in some cases, with the occurrence of manic symptoms.[1] Once an adequate course of antidepressant drug therapy has been administered, a gradual tapering of the dose of the drug over a period of 4 to 12 weeks is preferable to a swift cessation of therapy. Patients who have had persistent or recurrent depression generally require a longer course of antidepressant drug therapy than patients whose depression has been of shorter duration or less severe proportions.[1] Patients who have had a recent onset of depression and who have responded promptly to antidepressant medication may well achieve the desired therapeutic result with a 3- to 4-month course of antidepressant drug therapy. Longer sieges of depression may require 12 months of treatment or continuous maintenance for an indefinite period of time.[1]

One major advantage of the MAOI antidepressants as compared with the tricyclic antidepressants is their virtual lack of any anticholinergic effect. This accounts for the infrequent occurrence of blurred vision, dry mouth, and constipation in MAOI-treated patients. The MAOI antidepressants appear less likely to provoke cardiac arrhythmias than tricyclic drugs. Although the risk of hypertensive reactions to MAOIs is the most widely known potential side effect of these drugs, its occurrence is quite rare in the presence of reasonable care with respect to dietary and medication intake. The commonest side effect seen with MAOI antidepressants is postural hypotension.[1] Among these drugs, phenelzine is somewhat more likely to produce postural hypotension than isocarboxazid, which, in turn, is somewhat more likely to produce postural hypotension than tranylcypromine sulfate.[1] The postural hypotensive response to MAOI antidepressants is most likely due to decreased sympathetic outflow to small arterioles.[4] The hypotensive action of this group of drugs has been utilized to therapeutic advantage by one member of the group, pargyline hydrochloride, which is useful in patients who have hypertension and depression. Another side effect not infrequently seen with the MAOI antidepressants is difficulty falling asleep and a tendency to nighttime awakenings. Tranylcypromine, an MAOI antidepressant with an amphetaminelike structure, is somewhat more stimulating than other drugs of this groups, and more likely to produce sleep disturbances.

When prescribing MAOI antidepressants, they should be given in divided doses throughout the day. By so doing one may minimize the severity of hypotensive reactions to these drugs. Patients who experience a favorable therapeutic response but who are troubled by symptoms of postural hypotension (lightheadedness, dizziness, and headache) may experience somewhat less hypotension if they receive simultaneously a daily dose of 25 µg of tri-iodothyronine or 100 to 150 µg of thyroxine.[1] In addition, these thyroid hormones appear to enhance the antidepressant response to MAOI compounds as they do when used with tricyclic antidepressants.[38] Another frequently effective technique in minimizing postural hypotension associated with MAOI antidepressants is to recommend that patients increase their daily salt intake by more heavily salting their food. Salt tablets in divided doses totalling 4 to 6 daily can also be employed. In my clinical experience, the use of supplemental salt in this fashion has not been associated with any untoward effects and has allowed many patients who could otherwise not tolerate MAOI antidepressants to take them with a good outcome. Some clinicians recommend fludrocortisone acetate to counteract the hypotensive effects of MAOI antidepressants.[2] In my experience, the administration of supplemental salt is equally effective, safer, and less costly.

The *Physicians' Desk Reference* is cautious in its recommendations regarding MAOI antidepressants, suggesting their use only in those depressed patients who fail to respond to other antidepressant drugs. Certainly, one indication for the use of these agents is with patients unresponsive to other antidepressants. On the other hand, those individuals who have previously had difficulty tolerating the side effects of tricyclic drugs should be treated initially with MAOI antidepressants, rather than forcing a retrial of tricyclics. Although some investigators have suggested that patients with severe depression and associated vegetative signs are good candidates for MAOI treatment, many such individuals do indeed respond favorably to these drugs.[1,39] There is evidence that patients with atypical depressions with hypochondriasis and obsessive-compulsive features may be particularly responsive to MAOI antidepressants as compared to tricyclic drugs.[40,41]

In addition to the usefulness of these compounds in the treatment of depressive disorders, they are highly effective in nondepressed individuals with obsessive-compulsive disorders, and in patients with agoraphobia.[3,41] Although tricyclic antidepressants and alprazolam may be of some use in agoraphobia and in panic disorders, there is strong evidence that MAOI antidepressants are significantly more effective than these other compounds both in phobic disorders and in patients with recurrent panic anxiety.[1] Patients who abuse alcohol may achieve a favorable response in terms of anxiety and depression with MAOI drugs. Alcoholics present a particular risk in terms of potentially dangerous interactions with these drugs, and should receive them only under conditions of careful monitoring. In view of the potentially dangerous food and drug interactions of the MAOI antidepressants, they should generally be avoided in patients who are highly suicidal or who have a history of multiple prior suicide attempts. Because of their potentially energizing and stimulating effects, they might, theoretically, increase the risk of self-destructive behavior in some patients, and if this is a concern their use must be carefully weighed against alternative treatment.[1]

Any patient for whom MAOI antidepressants are prescribed must be carefully instructed orally and in written form regarding the dietary and medication restrictions. Tyramine-rich foods, particularly fermented cheeses, and red wine, especially Chianti, must be scrupulously avoided. Some food and beverage products which may, if taken in large quantity, present a risk of a hypertensive reaction, must be avoided at the initial phase of therapy, and then introduced only cautiously and in small quantities once the patient has stabilized on MAOI therapy.[1] Although not mentioned in any of the generally published lists of dietary restrictions, monosodium glutamate (MSG) should probably be avoided in MAOI-treated patients. Taken in moderate to large quantity, MSG may produce a variety of autonomic effects and it has, in my experience, been associated with sweating, dizziness, and headache in some MAOI-treated patients.[1] Soy sauce may also produce similar effects and should likewise be minimized in the diet of patients receiving MAOI drugs.

Patients being treated with this group of antidepressant drugs must be even more cautious about drug interactions than food interactions. Specifically, appetite suppressants and stimulants, including amphetamines and phenylpropanolamine hydrochloride must be avoided because they may provoke severe hypertensive reactions. Similar risks exist with the majority of prescription and over-the-counter cough syrups, cold remedies, nasal decongestants, and nose drops. Cocaine use is exceedingly dangerous in patients receiving MAOI antidepressants since hypertensive reactions and acute psychotic episodes may result from the combination of these drugs. Meperidine hydrochloride is exceedingly dangerous in MAOI-treated patients since it may produce severe agitation, tachycardia, hyperpyrexia, hypertension, convulsions, and a potentially fatal result.[1] Figure 26-1 presents an outline of important food and drug restrictions to be followed by patients receiving MAOI antidepressants. A printed list such as this should be provided to all patients receiving these medications.

Surgical anesthesia may be dangerous in patients receiving MAOI antidepressants if the anesthesiologist is unaware of the patient's therapeutic regimen. For this reason, it is useful to suggest that patients receiving these medications carry a wallet card describing their medication or wear a Medic Alert bracelet. Since monoamine oxidase levels generally return to normal five days following discontinuation of these medications, routine surgery can generally be done approximately 1 week thereafter. Most anesthesiologists prefer to wait 2 weeks for an elective procedure. In the case of emergency surgery, as long as the anesthesiologist is aware of the presence of MAOI therapy, anesthesia can be cautiously and safely administered provided sympathomimetic drugs and meperidine are avoided. When patients on MAOIs are to

Patients taking monoamine oxidase inhibitor (MAOI) antidepressants must not consume the following foods:
1. Fermented cheeses (eg, cheddar or other strong cheeses)
2. Pickled herring, sardines, and anchovies
3. Chicken livers
4. Canned or processed meats (eg, Spam)
5. Pods of broad beans
6. Canned figs
7. Yeast extract (eg, Marmite, and brewer's yeast tablets
8. Red wine and beer

The following drugs must be avoided while receiving MAOI antidepressants:
1. Amphetamines
2. Cocaine
3. Stimulants
4. Appetite suppressants
5. Nose drops and nasal decongestants
6. Cold remedies containing decongestants
7. Cough syrups containing decongestants
8. Asthma medications
9. Dental or other local anesthetics containing epinephrine
10. Meperidine hydrochloride (Demerol)

Patients taking MAOI antidepressants should either drink decaffeinated coffee or decaffeinated cola drinks, or limit their intake to a total of two cups or glasses of caffeine-containing beverage per day. Patients on these medications should not eat more than 2 oz of chocolate candy per day. Chocolate-flavored cookies, cake, and ice cream may be consumed while on MAOI antidepressants. Alcoholic beverages should be avoided while taking MAOI antidepressants. However, one may occasionally have a single cocktail or 2 or 3 oz of white wine. While being treated with MAOI antidepressants, one should not eat more than 2 oz of sour cream, yogurt, cottage cheese, American cheese, or mild Swiss cheese per day. All other cheese products or food products whose manufacturing process involves fermentation should be avoided in the diet. Soy sauce and monosodium glutamate (MSG) should be avoided or used only in minimal amounts.

Figure 26-1. Dietary and medication restrictions for patients taking monoamine oxidase inhibitors.

receive local anesthesia for dental or other procedures, they should receive a drug which does not contain epinephrine.

In prescribing MAOI therapy for depression, phenelzine is generally preferable in the presence of moderate to severe anxiety since it has a greater sedating effect and perhaps more prominent antianxiety effect than tranylcypromine.[1] For most patients, the usual therapeutic dose of phenelzine hydrochloride is 60 mg/d administered in three or four divided doses. Generally, this medication should be started at a dose of 15 mg twice daily and gradually titrated upward as tolerated and as necessary to achieve the therapeutic response. Some patients will require doses up to 90 mg daily and others will be responsive to doses as small as 15 to 30 mg daily. In some individuals, once the therapeutic response has been achieved, if there is an intolerable degree of postural hypotension, the dose may be gradually titrated downward. Isocarboxazid is chemically similar to phenelzine, and appears to be comparably effective as an antidepressant when given in divided doses totaling 30 to 40 mg/d.

Tranylcypromine appears to have a more rapid onset of action than the two previously mentioned MAOIs, often producing some initial therapeutic response after three or four days in comparison with the usual period of 1 to 2 weeks with other MAOI antidepressants. Tranylcypromine also differs from the other drugs in that it exerts a more stimulating effect and may be particularly useful in withdrawn anergic depressed patients. Patients who tend to sleep excessively during the daytime may be particularly benefitted by tranylcypromine. The usual daily antidepressant dosage ranges between 30 and 60 mg given in three or four divided doses.[1] The antianxiety effect of tranylcypromine is generally less than that seen with phenelzine, and some patients receiving tranylcypromine feel excessively stimulated or experience increased anxiety and sleep disturbances. Tranylcypromine is somewhat less likely than phenelzine to produce significant postural hypotension. Sexual dysfunction occasionally occurs during the course of MAOI therapy. Any of these compounds may diminish sexual interest and drive. Likewise, they may decrease erectile ability in men and delay or inhibit ejaculation.[42] This group of antidepressants may also impair sexual sensitivity, stimulation, and achievement of orgasm in women.[43] Some persons experience less sexual dysfunction with tranylcypromine or isocarboxazid than with phenelzine.[1]

In the early years of antidepressant drug therapy, it was generally accepted that tricyclic and MAOI antidepressants should not be administered simultaneously. Since the mid-1970s, numerous well-conducted clinical investigations have been done utilizing combined regimens of these drugs.[44] Initially, several reports provided documentation that patients receiving amitriptyline could have phenelzine cautiously added to their regimen, with both drugs given in full therapeutic dosage without any higher incidence of adverse effects than was encountered by the patient receiving a full dose of either antidepressant alone.[44] Subsequent studies have provided documentation for the safety of combining either phenelzine or tranylcypromine with a variety of tricyclic and second-generation heterocyclic antidepressant drugs.[45–47] In none of the published controlled clinical investigations was there a significantly higher incidence of adverse effects with the combined regimen than with either drug administered singly. The early studies of combined regimens suggested amitriptyline as the safer tricyclic to use because of its greater serotonin reuptake activity and less activity on norepinephrine reuptake mechanisms.[44] Subsequently, numerous antidepressants, including those preferentially acting upon serotonin and those preferentially acting on norepinephrine, have been combined with MAOI antidepressants.[1] Documentation for the safety of the combined regimens is quite solid.

With respect to the question of efficacy, there is as yet no evidence based on controlled studies that combined regimens are more effective than single-agent therapy. In my clinical experience, I have frequently found that the combination tricyclic-MAOI regimen appeared more effective in alleviating severe depressive illness than did any one of a series of antidepressants administered singly to the same individual. I have not observed any increased incidence of adverse effects.

Many times patients who are not responding to a particular antidepressant drug will need to have their regimen changed, sometimes from an MAOI to a tricyclic, and at other times in the opposite direction. Based upon experience with combined regimens, it no longer seems necessary to withdraw all drug therapy for a period of time prior to instituting the new antidepressant treatment. Too many patients suffer such increased morbidity from their depression that hospitalization is needed in order to withdraw medication for a period of time. With careful patient monitoring, including frequent visits with blood pressure and pulse measurements, patients can be changed from one type of antidepressant to another with gradual dosage increase of the new medication while having their previous medication slowly withdrawn without undue risk.[1]

There is no undue risk in combining lithium carbonate with MAOI antidepressants. The addition of lithium may enhance the antidepressant activity of MAOIs just as it does with tricyclic antidepressants.[1] In the event that there is a clinical need to administer neuroleptic medication to patients being treated with MAOI antidepressants, only high-potency neuroleptics such as haloperidol or trifluoperazine should be used. Chlorpromazine, mesoridazine, and thioridazine should be avoided in any patient receiving an MAOI antidepressant since these low-potency, strongly hypotensive, neuroleptic medications will undoubtedly provoke significant hypotensive reactions.[1]

The MAOI antidepressants not infrequently increase the amplitude of deep tendon reflexes. Not uncommonly, patients receiving these medications may also exhibit clonus, either sustained or unsustained.

Neither of these changes in the neurologic examination appear to have pathologic significance and they are not indicative of a hypertensive crisis or an impending crisis.[1] Patients receiving these drugs may also experience muscular irritability and periodic "jumping" movements of the extremities, particularly when lying still in bed.[1] These jumping movements may or may not be associated with "electric shock sensations."[2] Monoamine oxidase inhibitor therapy may be associated with vitamin B_6 (pyridoxine) deficiency and it is often useful to administer pyridoxine in a dose of 100 to 400 mg daily. The administration of this vitamin may minimize the jumping movements and muscular irritability.[2]

MOOD-STABILIZING DRUGS: LITHIUM CARBONATE AND CARBAMAZEPINE

Unlike other psychotropic drugs which are complex organic molecules, lithium carbonate is a simple compound which may be classified chemically as a salt. Following observations of the sedative potential of lithium compounds used for nonpsychiatric medications, Cade first demonstrated the efficacy of lithium salts in controlling agitated, psychotic states in ten manic patients. In the intervening years, since Cade's dramatic discovery, a vast number of studies have been conducted to explore the psychotropic effects and therapeutic potential of lithium carbonate, the most commonly used lithium salt. The clinical actions of lithium are quite variable under different circumstances. Indeed, it seems paradoxical that the same substance can both calm agitated, manic patients and alleviate depression. It is for this reason that the term "mood-stabilizing drug" seems to be the most appropriate description for its actions. This term implies the ability of lithium to stabilize or normalize mood, whether the starting point be a "high" (mania) or a "low" depression. The term mood-stabilizing drug also implies the ability of lithium carbonate to act prophylactically in preventing recurrent episodes of both mania and depression.

In recent years, carbamazepine, initially employed in the 1960s in the treatment of trigeminal neuralgia and convulsive disorders, has been found to have a lithiumlike effect. Carbamazepine has demonstrated usefulness in controlling agitated manic states as well as in the prophylaxis of recurrent mania in patients who are either intolerant to or unresponsive to lithium salts. Because of its newly found therapeutic action, carbamazepine is included here under mood-stabilizing drugs in spite of the fact that this therapeutic use has not yet been approved by the Food and Drug Administration.

Although the mechanism of action of lithium is uncertain, this alkalai metallic element can substitute for sodium, potassium, or both, and can alter the functions of potassium, calcium, magnesium, and phosphate ions.[48] Lithium flow involves an active transport mechanism rather than passive diffusion across the cell membrane.[48] This ion also appears to enhance blood-brain barrier (BBB) permeability, to stimulate sodium entry into cells, to reduce choline uptake, and to increase CSF amino acid concentrations.[48,49] Lithium can also activate sodium-potassium-magnesium adenosine triphophatase (ATPase) in biological membranes and can interact with anionic membrane phospholipids, particularly in nervous tissue.[50]

Chronic lithium administration can block presynaptic and postsynaptic dopamine receptor supersensitivity induced either by nigrostriatal lesions or by drugs which block dopamine receptors or decrease the availability of dopamine at the receptor sites.[50] These findings may explain lithium's ability to prevent recurrences of mania.

Lithium has a number of effects involving norepinephrine. It may increase the turnover of norepinephrine in the brain, increase norepinephrine neuronal uptake, and inhibit stimulus-induced norepinephrine release.[48] Lithium increases urinary excretion of the norepinephrine metabolites vanillylmandelic acid (VMA), normetanephrine, and MHPG, and increases MHPG in CSF during the initial phase of lithium administration.[52] Lithium also appears capable of preventing supersensitivity, not only of dopamine receptor sites, but also of α- and β-adenergic receptors.[48] Since it has been suggested that a reduction in synaptic norepinephrine in the brain may be associated with depression, the reduction in β-adenergic supersensitivity noted with lithium partially explains its antidepressant effect.

Lithium also interacts with serotonin in a variety of ways. It increases brain concentrations of tryptophan, the precursor of serotonin, stimulates serotonin synthesis, and increases 5-hydroxyindolacetic acid (5-HIAA) in CSF. Lithium appears to stimulate serotonin uptake in human platelets and either has no effect or inhibits serotonin turnover within the brain. It has been suggested that chronic lithium administration may reduce serotonin receptors within the brain.[48].

Lithium administration chronically enhances acetylcholine synthesis and release, and increases acetylcholine and choline content in the brain. Since cholinergic stimulation may have an antimanic effect, the increase in brain acetylcholine activity may partially explain its antimanic action.[48] Interference with norepinephrine and dopamine release mechanisms, turnover, and receptor site sensitivity may also be important in the antimanic action of lithium. It is conceivable that the biphasic actions of lithium in both depression and mania may be related to changes in receptor site conformation within brain tissue.

The primary indications for lithium carbonate therapy, and the only two approved by the FDA, are its use in the treatment of acute mania and its long-term administration in the prophylaxis of recurrent mania.[1] Lithium has, however, been used therapeutically for a wide range of psychiatric disorders. Although lithium has been suggested by some to be beneficial as a single agent in the treatment of depression, its value as an antidepressant in severely depressed patients appears limited in most clinical circumstances. As mentioned earlier, however, many patients who have had partial responses to tricyclic or MAOI antidepressants may experience considerable enhancement of a therapeutic response when lithium is added to the antidepressant drug regimen.[53] Lithium has some value when used alone in the prophylaxis of recurrent depression, particularly in bipolar patients. However, its prophylactic use in depression is somewhat less efficacious than its prophylactic value in mania.[48] Approximately one third of patients receiving lithium for the prophylaxis of recurrent depression will need intermittent courses of antidepressant medication in conjunction with lithium in order to properly manage depressive episodes which may occur in spite of continuous lithium therapy.[1]

Patients with schizoaffective illness may benefit acutely as well as during the course of maintenance therapy with a combined regimen of lithium carbonate in full therapeutic dosage along with low doses of high-potency neuroleptics such as haloperidol or trifluoperazine.[54,55] Clinical studies indicate greater efficacy of combined regimens in schizoaffective illness than that observed when either therapeutic agent is administered singly. Atypical affective disorders, including affective episodes in borderline patients and in those individuals with emotionally unstable character disorders (EUCD), may benefit significantly from lithium carbonate therapy.[56] Lithium has also been found to be of value in patients with impulse disorders and in those exhibiting episodic violence.[57] Its use has been suggested and, at times, found useful in women with premenstral syndrome, particularly when associated with cyclic depressions.[1] The use of lithium in schizophrenia is controversial.

The generally accepted range of serum lithium concentrations is 0.6 to 1.2 mEq/L. Patients in the acute phase of manic psychosis are generally best treated with lithium doses which achieve serum concentrations at the upper end of this therapeutic range.[48] Most patients maintained on lithium carbonate do well at serum lithium concentrations between 0.6 and 0.8 mEq/L. Some patients who experience side effects with lithium, particularly tremor and GI disturbances, feel better and achieve an adequate therapeutic response with serum lithium concentrations in the range of 0.5 to 0.6 mEq/L.[1] According to some studies, the lithium efficacy has been demonstrated in a number of patients with bipolar affective illness at serum concentrations between 0.3 and 0.6 mEq/L.[58] In patients with bonafide affective illness who appear to respond favorably to lithium but cannot tolerate conventional therapeutic doses, the clinician should try maintenance at a lower blood level. There is a good possibility that this will be efficacious while minimizing lithium side effects. It is wise to use the same lithium preparation (brand) in each patient since minor variations in formulation, tablet compression density, and inert ingredients may effect the bioavailability thereby alter serum lithium concentration.[1] The use of a standard brand lithium product does not add significantly to the cost.

There has been concern about the possible renal toxicity of lithium. Although many patients taking lithium experience polyuria or polydipsia, which may be associated with excessive thirst, lithium is generally not nephrotoxic when cautiously used in patients with normal renal function.[48] There have been no reported instances of severe azotemia or renal failure produced by lithium as the sole offending agent.[59] Although the last decade has seen a number of reports in the literature indicating microscopic changes in glomeruli and renal tubules on kidney biopsy specimens of lithium-treated patients, the pathologic significance of these abnormalities does not appear to be great.[48] Nevertheless, lithium should be reserved for those patients who have a psychiatric disorder likely to benefit from this medication. Its continuing use in a given patient should be predicated on evidence of a therapeutic response. The majority of patients with abnormal kidney biopsies while on lithium have either had multiple episodes of lithium intoxication or have had long-standing severe polyuria and polydipsia.[59] Patients with persistent severe polyuria need to be assessed in order to decide the appropriateness of either continuing lithium therapy or using another drug such as carbamazepine.[1] During the course of lithium therapy, renal concentrating ability decreases and measurements of urine osmolality following a 12-hour fast are likely to reveal decreased osmolality.[1] Generally, following a brief lithium holiday renal concentrating ability returns toward normal. In patients who have renal disease or who develop severe polyuria or recurrent lithium intoxication, consultation with a nephrologist may be obtained.

The use of lithium, whether therapeutic or prophylactic, must follow certain guidelines in order to facilitate effective and safe treatment with this potent and valuable drug. Prior to the administration of lithium carbonate, certain baseline laboratory studies should be performed. A baseline ECG is important since therapeutic doses of lithium may be associated with minor ECG changes, particularly in the ST segment and T wave.[1,48] If ECG changes occur during lithium treatment, the baseline ECG is useful to document their relationship to lithium rather than to coronary disease. Since lithium intoxication can be associated with abnormalities of cardiac conduction and rhythm, the pretreatment ECG is of further value in the long-term management of the patient.[1] Lithium carbonate treatment may be associated with goiter or decreased thyroid hormone production or release. For this reason, pretreatment levels of T_4 (thyroxine), T_3 (tri-iodothyronine) and TSH (thyroid-stimulating hormone) should be obtained.[1,60]

These may be of value in helping to clarify a potential thyroid abnormality which may occur in the future during lithium treatment.[1,48] It is of utmost importance to obtain serum creatinine or BUN measurements, or both, prior to starting lithium treatment. Abnormalities in these tests imply renal functional impairment that may give rise to excessive lithium concentrations in the presence of the usual therapeutic doses of lithium.[1,48] In patients with cardiac, respiratory, or renal disease or in patients receiving diuretics, it is important to measure serum electrolytes prior to instituting lithium treatment.[1,48]

Lithium is removed from the body almost entirely by renal excretion. The half-life of lithium in normal healthy adults is generally about 18 hours, while in elderly or infirm individuals the lithium half-life may double.[48] Sodium and lithium are reabsorbed competitively by the proximal tubules of the kidney.[48] Sodium is further absorbed in the distal tubules although lithium is not. Salt restriction will increase lithium retention and may lead to toxic serum concentrations. Diuretic drugs, which act at the distal tubules, will facilitate the excretion of sodium but not of lithium; therefore diuretics tend to facilitate lithium retention and may lead to lithium toxicity.[48] With the exception of salt restriction and diuretic drugs other dietary changes or medications have little effect on the therapeutic or toxic actions of lithium carbonate.

In order to make lithium treatment as safe as possible, it is preferable to start with relatively low doses.[1] In healthy individuals with normal renal function lithium carbonate may be prescribed in doses of 300 mg three or four times daily. In elderly patients or in those with renal disease, lower doses should be employed. These patients may be safely treated with lithium if low enough doses are selected and blood levels are adequately monitored. It is important in instituting lithium treatment to advise patients not to take the drug on an empty stomach. If lithium is taken at mealtimes or with small snacks, the likelihood of gastric irritation, nausea, and epigastric distress will be minimized.[1] Lithium is absorbed rapidly from the stomach over a period of three to six hours following each dose. Because serum lithium concentrations tend to peak within a short time after ingestion, it is important to measure serum lithium concentrations at a stable interval following drug administration. For practical purposes, it is advisable to measure serum lithium concentrations approximately eight to 12 hours after the previous dose of lithium.

It is often helpful to note in the patient's record the time interval between the last dose of lithium and the time of blood drawing in order to clarify laboratory results that appear to be inappropriate. During the initial phases of treatment with lithium in the acutely manic or depressed patient, serum determination should be done once or twice weekly. Once the patient demonstrates the ability to tolerate lithium, blood levels should be taken at weekly intervals for a month, then every 2 weeks during the second month of treatment. After that, lithium levels may be measured every 3 to 4 weeks. After several months of treatment with a relatively stable serum lithium concentration, the patient can safely be followed with determinations taken every 6 to 8 weeks.[1] Although some clinicians favor infrequent serum lithium measurements during long-term management, it is preferable to allow intervals of no less than 2 or 3 months for serum monitoring over years of treatment with this drug. Aside from the advantage of spotting an abnormal lithium level or perhaps an abnormal behavior pattern, the regular measurement of lithium levels is beneficial subjectively because it helps the patient's understanding of the importance of medication use and follow-up to continued well-being.

Most patients in the initial phase of treatment with lithium experience relatively few side effects. Unlike other psychotropic drugs, lithium does not produce autonomic nervous system side effects or measurable sedation except in the manic or hypomanic patient. The occasional patient's complaint of appetite loss or epigastric distress will usually abate rapidly either spontaneously or by rearranging lithium dosages to coincide with meals.[1] These GI symptoms may also appear in patients as early signs of lithium toxicity, and this problem must be explored by measuring lithium blood levels if the symptoms persist.[48]

Some patients experience dryness of mouth or a metallic taste when starting lithum treatment; often these symptoms disappear, but in some cases they persist throughout treatment and the patient learns to tolerate or ignore them. Muscle tremors are often seen at the outset of lithium treatment, but they generally disappear within the first week or two. Persistent tremors of the hands and fingers in association with lithium treatment may be helped by reducing the dose of lithium or by changing the pattern of administration so that peak lithium levels reached following each dose are minimized by giving multiple smaller doses.[1] In some patients, persistent tremor may require treatment with propranolol, as mentioned earlier in this chapter. The association of tremor with ataxia, muscle weakness, or muscle hyperirritability may be a sign of lithium intoxication and should be investigated by measuring the serum lithium concentration. A variety of neurologic symptoms, including vertigo, slurred speech, incontinence, and seizures, may be associated with lithium toxicity and should be evaluated and treated promptly by discontinuing lithium and administering an adequate volume of fluid.[48] Additional medical aspects of lithium are discussed in detail in chapter 28.

The daily maintenance dose of lithium carbonate varies among individual patients. The required dosage of lithium does not necessarily vary directly with body size. Some elderly individuals may be maintained adequately with satisfactory blood levels of the drug by administering 300 to 450 mg of lithium daily. On the other hand, some patients require daily maintenance doses of 1800 mg or more. Both the therapeutic and maintenance dosages of lithium should be guided by clinical observation of the patient along with measurements of serum lithium concentration. Patients taking lithium should be encouraged to phone their physician in the event of the development of any intercurrent illness that may increase the likelihood of lithium intoxication. Patients taking lithium should also be encouraged to discontinue their medication for a day or two in the event of the development of fever, nausea, vomiting, or diarrhea.[1] The development of these symptoms in a previously asymptomatic individual should signal the need for obtaining lithium blood level measurements. Indeed, any change in behavior or symptoms in a patient being maintained on lithium should be investigated by measuring the serum lithium concentration and observing the patient clinically.[1]

Carbamazepine (Tegretol) is an iminodibenzyl compound structurally similar to the tricyclic antidepressant drugs.[4] It has been used extensively as an anticonvulsant, particularly for temporal and limbic seizure activity in patients with temporal lobe epilepsy.[1,4] According to research which has suggested a "kindling" model for affective disorders, carbamazepine was initially tried as a potential antimanic drug.[61] In open studies as well as in well-controlled double-blind investigations, carbamazepine has demonstrated efficacy in the treatment of acute manic episodes.[61] Subsequent research has indicated that carbamazepine may be a useful antimanic drug in patients who do not respond satisfactorily to lithium carbonate or who do not tolerate lithium.[62] In some investigations, carbamazepine has been used alone in the treatment of mania, while in other studies it has been used in conjunction with lithium carbonate in patients demonstrating limited lithium responsiveness.[63] Increasing numbers of clinical investigations have documented the efficacy of carbamazepine alone and in combination with lithium in the treatment of acute manic psychosis. Additional studies have documented the efficacy of carbamazepine in the prophylaxis against recurrent mania.[64] It has also been used in conjunction with neuroleptic medications in the treatment of agitated psychotic states other than mania.[65] Because of its structural similarity to the tricyclic antidepressants, it has been suggested that carbamazepine may exert antidepressant activity or may be useful in the prophylaxis of recurrent depressions.[1,64] Though its efficacy against depressive illness seems less dramatic than its antimanic action, carbamazepine does appear to have a useful role when used along with antidepressant drugs or when used in the maintenance treatment of patients subject to recurrent depressive episodes.

The mechanism of action of carbamazepine in affective illness is not clearly known although its pharmacology is complex and interesting. Carbamazepine does not block dopamine receptor sites, unlike neuroleptic drugs, and therefore it does not appear to have the potential for producing extrapyramidal reactions or tardive dyskinesia.[62] Carbamazepine blocks reuptake of norepinephrine and inhibits stimulation-induced release of norepinephrine at synaptic sites.[64] Carbamazepine appears to decrease GABA turnover in animals whereas GABA levels in CSF are unchanged in affectively ill patients treated with this drug.[64] Carbamazepine decreases CSF concentrations of somatostatin and may also interact pharmacologically with other nonmonoamine neurotransmitters, including peptides.[64]

The ability of carbamazepine to produce hypotensive or anticholinergic side effects is minimal. Some patients experience slight dizziness or headache and many patients experience stomach upset or nausea when starting treatment with this drug.[4] If the dosage of carbamazepine is started low and titrated upward gradually, GI disturbances are minimize.[1] Likewise drowsiness, which can occur in response to carbamazepine, occurs to a lesser extent when the drug is administered in small doses with gradual dosage titration or when the majority of the daily dose is administered at bedtime.[1] Indeed, bedtime administration of carbamazepine may actually have a useful sleep-inducing or sleep-prolonging effect.[1] The most serious side effect of carbamazepine is the possible production of leukopenia, or, more rarely, agranulocytosis or aplastic anemia.[4] Leukopenia is infrequent and may, to some extent, be dose-related.[1,61] More serious hematologic side effects are rare and are generally reversible if the diagnosis is established early and the drug is discontinued.[61] It is important to do white blood cell and differential counts prior to instituting carbamazepine therapy, preferably at weekly intervals during the first month or two of treatment and, then with gradually decreasing frequency.[1,61] Patients who are on carbamazepine for long-term maintenance should generally have white cell and differential counts done every 1 to 3 months during the course of treatment.[1,64] The appearance of leukopenia during the course of carbamazepine therapy should lead to discontinuation of the medication and reassessment of the patient prior to reinstituting therapy with this drug.[1]

In view of the fact that carbamazepine has not been approved by the FDA for the treatment of affective disorders, this issue must be fully discussed with the patient and, preferably, a family member prior to instituting treatment. It is also advisable to document in the medical record that other therapeutic options have been offered and to list the specific reasons for using carbamazepine in the present clinical situation.

The dosage of carbamazepine generally used in the treatment and prophylaxis of mania ranges between 400 and 1200 mg/d given in divided doses. It is preferable to start most patients at daily doses of approximately 400 mg and titrate dosage as clinically dictated by the patient's response. When used in the treatment of seizure disorders, the ordinary therapeutic blood level of carbamazepine is in the range of 8 to 12 μg/mL.[1] The therapeutic blood level of carbamazepine in the treatment and prophylaxis of affective illness has not been well established and though it is useful to periodically measure blood levels, one cannot safely assume that a particular blood level implies the likelihood of a favorable response and the absence of side effects.[62] Indeed, some of the patients studied with carbamazepine therapy at the National Institute of Mental Health have required higher dosages and higher blood levels than those described above. As mentioned elsewhere in this volume, carbamazepine may impair renal excretion of lithium and may effect intestinal absorption of this ion leading to increased serum lithium concentrations when combined lithium-carbamazepine therapy is used. Patients receiving these drugs in combination should have periodic careful blood level determinations of both drugs. Although carbamazepine and neuroleptics have been safely used in combination with an enhanced therapeutic effect in agitated psychotic states, a potential neurotoxic side effect has been reported with this combined regimen.[66]

REFERENCES

1. Bernstein JG: Handbook of Drug Therapy in Psychiatry. Boston, John Wright–PSG Inc, 1983.
2. Sheehan DV: The treatment of panic and phobic disorders, in Bernstein JG (ed): Clinical Psychopharmacology, (ed 2). Boston, John Wright–PSG Inc, 1984, pp 93–109.
3. Sos J, Cassem NH: Intravenous use of haloperidol for acute delirium in intensive care unit settings, in Speidel H, Rodwald G (eds): Psychic and Neurological Dysfunctions after Open Heart Surgery. Stuttgart, Georg Thieme Verlag, 1980, pp 196–199.
4. Gilman AG, Goodman LS, Gilman A (eds): Goodman and Gilman's The Pharmacological Basis of Therapeutics, (ed 6). New York, MacMillan Publishing Co, 1980.
5. Hartmann E: Insomnia: diagnosis and treatment, in Bernstein JG (ed): Clinical Psychopharmacology, (ed 2). Boston, John Wright–PSG Inc, 1984, pp 177–188.
6. Shehi M, Patterson WM: Treatment of panic attacks with alprazolam and propranolol. Am J Psychiatry 1984; 141:900–901.
7. Lipinski JF, Zubenko GS, Cohen BM, et al: Propranolol in the treatment of neuroleptic-induced akathisia. Am J Psychiatry 1984; 141:412–415.
8. Ticku MK: Benzodiazepine-GABA-receptor-ionophore complex: current concepts. Neuropharmacology 1983; 22:1459–1470.
9. Sheehan DV, Coleman JH, Greenblatt DJ, et al: Some biological correlates of panic attacks and agoraphobia and their response to a new treatment. J Clin Psychopharmacol 1985; 4:66–75.
10. Snyder SH: Dopamine receptors, neuroleptics and schizophrenia. Am J Psychiatry 1981; 138:460–464.
11. Snyder SH: Receptors, neurotransmitters, and drug responses. N Engl J Med 1979; 300:465–472.
12. Kety SS: Mental illness in the biological and adoptive relatives of schizophrenic adoptees: findings relevant to genetic and environmental factors in etiology. Am J Psychiatry 1983; 140:720–727.
13. Creese O, Burt DR, Snyder SH: Dopamine receptor binding predicts clinical and pharmacologic potencies of antischizophrenic drugs. Science 1976; 192:481–483.
14. Snyder S, Greenberg D, Yamamura HI: Antischizophrenic drugs and brain cholinergic receptors. Arch Gen Psychiatry 1974; 31:58–61.
15. Donlon PT, Hopkin J, Tupin JP: Overview: Efficacy and safety of the rapid neuroleptization method with injectable haloperidol. Am J Psychiatry 1979; 136:273–278.
16. Keepers GA, Clappison VJ, Casey DE: Initial anticholinergic prophylaxis for

neuroleptic-induced extrapyramidal syndromes. *Arch Gen Psychiatry* 1983; 40:1113–1117.

17. Shopsin B, Gershon S, Thompson H, et al: Psychoactive drugs in mania. *Arch Gen Psychiatry* 1975; 32:34–42.

18. Baastrup PC, Hollnagel P, Sorenson R, et al: Adverse reactions in treatment with lithium carbonate and haloperidol. *JAMA* 1976; 236:2645–2646.

19. Price LH, Conwell Y, Nelson JC: Lithium augmentation of combined neuroleptic-tricyclic treatment of delusional depression. *Am J Psychiatry* 1983; 140:318–322.

20. Zisook S, Click MA Jr: Evaluations of loxapine succinate in the ambulatory treatment of acute schizophrenic episodes. *Int Pharmacopsychiatry* 1980; 15:365–378.

21. Binder R, Click I, Rice M: A comparative study of parenteral molindone and haloperidol in the acutely psychotic patient. *J Clin Psychiatry* 1981; 42:203–206.

22. Caroff SN: The neuroleptic malignant syndrome. *J Clin Psychiatry* 1980; 41:79–83.

23. Weissman MM, Kidd KK, Prusoff BA: Variability in rates of affective disorders in relatives of depressed and normal probands. *Arch Gen Psychiatry* 1982; 39:1397–1403.

24. Bernstein JG: Neurotransmitters and receptors in pharmacopsychiatry, in Bernstein JG (ed): *Clinical Psychopharmacology*, (ed 2). Boston, John Wright–PSG Inc, 1984; 59–76.

25. Maas JW: Biogenic amines and depression. *Arch Gen Psychiatry* 1975; 32:1357–1361.

26. Muscettola G, Potter WZ, Pickar D, et al: Urinary 3-methoxy-4-hydroxy-phenylglycol and major affective disorders. *Arch Gen Psychiatry* 1984; 41: 337–342.

27. Schatzberg AF, Cole JO, Blumer DP: Speech blockage: a tricyclic side effect. *Am J Psychiatry* 1978; 135:600–601.

28. Livingston RL, Zucker DK, Isenberg K, et al: Tricyclic antidepressants and delirium. *J Clin Psychiatry* 1983; 44:173–176.

29. Hekimian LJ, Friedhoff AJ, Deever E: A comparison of the onset of action and therapeutic efficacy of amoxapine and amitriptyline. *J Clin Psychiatry* 1978; 39:633–637.

30. Cohen BM, Harris PQ, Altesman RI, et al: Amoxapine, neuroleptic as well as antidepressant? *Am J Psychiatry* 1982; 139:1165–1167.

31. Damlouji NF, Ferguson JM: Trazodone-induced delirium in bulimic patients. *Am J Psychiatry* 1984; 141:434–435.

32. Schwartz L, Swaminathan S: Maprotiline hydrochloride and convulsions—a case report. *Am J Psychiatry* 1982; 139:244–245.

33. Rickels K (ed): Nomifensine: the preclinical and clinical profile of a second generation antidepressant. *J Clin Psychiatry* 1984; 45(No. 4, section 2):1–105.

34. Zung WWK, Walker JI, Stern WC (eds): New directions in the treatment of depression: bupropion. *J Clin Psychiatry* 1983; 44(No. 5, section 2):1–211.

35. Stern SI, Mendels J: Drug combinations in the treatment of refractory depression: a review. *J Clin Psychiatry* 1981; 42:368–373.

36. Schatzberg AF: Evaluation and treatment of the refractory depressed patient, in Bernstein JG (ed): *Clinical Psychopharmacology*, (ed 2). Boston, John

Wright–PSG Inc, 1984, pp 77–92.

37. Nies A, Robinson D, Friedman MJ, et al: Relationship between age and tricyclic antidepressant plasma levels. *Am J Psychiatry* 1977; 134:790–793.

38. Goodwin FK, Prange AJ, Post RM, et al: Potentiation of antidepressant effects by L-triiodothyronine in tricyclic non-responders. *Am J Psychiatry* 1982; 139:34–38.

39. Tyrer P: Towards rational therapy with monoamine oxidase inhibitors. *Br J Psychiatry* 1976; 128:354–360.

40. Kayser A, Robinson DS, Nies A, et al: Response to phenelzine among depressed patients with features of hysteroid dysphoria. *Am J Psychiatry* 1985; 142:486–488.

41. Sheehan DV, Ballenger J, Jacobson G: Treatment of endogenous anxiety with phobia, hysterical and hypochondriacal symptoms. *Arch Gen Psychiatry* 1980; 37:51–59.

42. Rapp MS: Two cases of ejaculatory impairment related to phenelzine. *Am J Psychiatry* 1979; 136:1200–1201.

43. Barton JL: Orgasmic inhibition by phenelzine. *Am J Psychiatry* 1979; 136:1616–1617.

44. Ravaris CL, Robinson DS, Ives JO, et al: Phenelzine and amitriptyline in the treatment of depression. *Am J Psychiatry* 1980: 137:1075–1080.

45. White K, Pistole T, Boyd JL: Combined monoamine oxidase inhibitor tricyclic antidepressant treatment: a pilot study. *Am J Psychiatry* 1980; 137:1422–1425.

46. White K, Simpson, G: Combined MAOI–tricyclic antidepressant treatment—a reevaluation. *J Clin Psychopharmacol* 1981; 1:264–282.

47. Riise IS, Holm P: Concomitant isocarboxazid/mianserin treatment. *J Affective Disord* 1984; 6:175–179.

48. Ortiz A, Dabbagh M, Gershon S: Lithium: clinical use, toxicology and mode of action, in Bernstein JG (ed): *Clinical Psychopharmacology*, (ed 2). Boston, John Wright–PSG Inc, 1984, pp 111–144.

49. Preskorn SH, Irwin GH, Simpson S, et al: Medical therapies for mood disorders alter the blood-brain barrier. *Science* 1981; 213:469–471.

50. Hauser H, Shipley GG: Crystalization of phosphatidylserine bilayers induced by lithium. *J Biochem* 1981; 256:1377–1380.

51. Pert A, Rosenblatt JE, Sivit C, et al: Long-term treatment prevents the development of dopamine receptor supersensitivity. *Science* 1978; 201:171–173.

52. Schildkraut JJ: Pharmacology—the effects of lithium on biogenic amines, in Gershon S, Shopsin B (eds): *Lithium: Its Role in Psychiatric Research and Treatment*. New York, Plenum Press, 1973, pp 51–73.

53. DeMontigny C, Grunberg F, Mayer A, et al: Lithium induces rapid relief of depression in tricyclic antidepressant nonresponders. *Br J Psychiatry* 1981; 138:252–256.

54. Biederman J, Lerner Y, Belmaker RH: Combination of lithium carbonate and haloperidol in schizoaffective disorder. *Arch Gen Psychiatry* 1979; 36:327–333.

55. Delva NJ, Letemendia FJJ: Lithium treatment in schizophrenia and schizoaffective disorders. *Br J Psychiatry* 1982; 141:387–400.

56. Rifkin A, Quitkin F, Carillo C: Lithium carbonate in emotionally unstable

character disorder. *Arch Gen Psychiatry* 1973; 27:519–523.

57. Sheard MH, Marini JL, Bridges CI, et al: The effect of lithium on impulsive aggressive behavior in man. *Am J Psychiatry* 1976, 133:1409–1413.

58. Coppen A, Abou-Saleh M, Millen P, et al: Decreasing lithium dosage reduces morbidity and side effects during prophylaxis. *J Affective Disord* 1983; 5:353–362.

59. Lippmann S: Is lithium bad for the kidneys? *J Clin Psychiatry* 1982; 43:220–224.

60. Cooper TB, Simpson GM: Effects of lithium on thyroid function. *Am J Psychiatry* 1969; 125:1132–1135.

61. Ballenger JC, Post RM: Carbamazepine in manic depressive illness: a new treatment. *Am J Psychiatry* 1980; 137:782–790.

62. Post RM, Uhde TW, Putnam FW, et al: Kindling and carbamazepine in affective illness. *J Nerv Ment Dis* 1982; 170:717–731.

63. Nolen WA: Carbamazepine: a possible adjunct or alternative to lithium in bipolar disorder. *Acta Psychiatr Scand* 1983; 67:218–225.

64. Post RM: Use of the anticonvulsant carbamazepine in primary and secondary affective illness: clinical and theoretical implications. *Psychol Med* 1982; 12:701–704.

65. Klein E, Bental E, Lerer B, et al: Carbamazepine and haloperidol v placebo and haloperidol in excited psychosis. *Arch Gen Psychiatry* 1984; 41:165–170.

66. Kanter GL, Yerevanian BI, Ciccone JR: Case report of a possible interaction between neuroleptics and carbamazepine. *Am J Psychiatry* 1984; 141:1101–1102.

27

Drug Interactions

JERROLD G. BERNSTEIN

Advances in the practice of medicine have in part have due to the availability of new medications, which has, in turn, given rise to a problem of ever-increasing complexity, that of drug interactions. Since many psychotropic medications may produce adverse pharmacologic effects and since medications used to treat nonpsychiatric illness may yield behavioral complications, the consulting psychiatrist must be familiar with a wide variety of unwanted drug reactions.[1] Furthermore, the psychiatrist in the general hospital setting must be alert to potential interactions between the medications which he prescribes and those prescribed by other physicians simultaneously. This chapter will focus on those interactions between therapeutic agents which are likely to be seen in the course of psychiatric consultation as well as adverse reactions to individual psychotropic and nonpsychotropic medications. Patients not infrequently first come to psychiatric attention as the result of behavioral or cognitive changes that are drug-induced. The psychiatrist who prescribes medications must be equally conversant with their favorable and their unfavorable actions. This chapter will stress the pharmacologic basis of drug interactions and adverse drug effects in the clinical setting.

MECHANISMS OF DRUG-DRUG INTERACTIONS

The three general mechanisms of drug-drug interactions include the pharmacokinetic, pharmacologic, and idiosyncratic interactions.[2]

Pharmacokinetic Interactions

Pharmacokinetic interactions include those interactions involving drug absorption wherein one drug may enhance or impair gastrointestinal (GI) absorption of another. For example, drugs that reduce GI motility may slow the transit time of another drug, thus allowing it to be present in the GI tract for a longer period of time, thereby enhancing systemic absorption of the second drug. Drugs may speed GI motility to

538

the extent that there is decreased absorption of another therapeutic agent. Furthermore, the coadministration of cholestyramine resin or of a gel antacid, along with a phenothiazine may result in formation of an insoluble complex which is not absorbed through the GI tract, thereby decreasing the therapeutic effect of the administered psychotropic medication.[3]

Another pharmacokinetic interaction involves the binding of a drug to plasma proteins with the resultant availability of a lower concentration of free drug. If another drug is administered which displaces the first drug from plasma protein–binding sites, the concentration and pharmacologic action of the first drug, now freed from the binding sites, is increased. A common example of this is the displacement of warfarin from plasma protein–binding sites by the coadministration of chloral hydrate.[3] In addition to protein binding, lipid solubility and binding are extremely important in that all psychotropic medications, with the exception of lithium carbonate, are quite freely lipid-soluble. As the fat to lean body mass ratio increases in the elderly patient, increased plasma concentration are encountered with a variety of lipid-soluble psychotropic medications.[4]

Interactions at the site of biotransformation are another form of pharmacokinetic drug interactions. For example, barbiturates induce a variety of hepatic microsomal enzymes, thus enhancing the rate of metabolic degradation of many drugs, including the anticonvulsant phenytoin. On the other hand, inhibition of drug-metabolizing enzymes by one drug may increase plasma concentration and pharmacologic action of another drug. The monoamine oxidase inhibitors (MAOIs) not only diminish the activity of this enzyme, thereby enhancing the effects of a variety of sympathomimetic amines, but also have the ability to impair metabolic degradation of unrelated drugs, including sedatives and narcotics, thereby increasing the pharmacologic effects of a given dose of one of these compounds.[3,4]

Finally, pharmacokinetic drug interactions at the site of drug elimination may enhance or impair the pharmacologic action of a variety of medicinal substances. Alkalinization of the urine by the administration of sodium bicarbonate, for instance, may hasten the excretion of long-acting barbiturates such as phenobarbital; this interaction may thus be useful in the treatment of phenobarbital overdoses. However, the same interaction may prevent the desired pharmacologic effect of a carefully chosen phenobarbital dose in a patient with a seizure disorder.[3] Acidification of the urine by ascorbic acid or ammonium chloride increases the rate of excretion of amphetamines and phencyclidine hydrochloride (PCP). Thus the administration of acidifying agents may be an important therapeutic technique in the treatment of PCP or amphetamine intoxication.

Pharmacologic Interactions

Pharmacologic interactions occur when two simultaneously administered drugs act similarly on the same receptor site or antagonize the action of each other at the receptor site. At times, a desired and therapeutic effect can be achieved by administering two drugs that act similarly at the same receptor site. Two drugs acting at the same receptor site in a similar fashion may, however, produce an unwanted additive drug interaction as in the case of a patient developing an anticholinergic delirium when receiving a combination of neuroleptic, tricyclic antidepressant, and antiparkinsonian medication. Two drugs, each with important and desired therapeutic effects, may antagonize the action of each other, thus preventing a desired therapeutic response. The classical example of this kind of drug interaction occurs when a hypertensive patient on a regimen of guanethidine receives amitriptyline hydrochloride or another tricyclic antidepressant and thereby loses the antihypertensive effect of guanethidine. All tricyclic antidepressants block nerve reuptake mechanisms which are necessary to achieve the antihypertensive action of guanethidine, clonidine hydrochloride, and related drugs.

Idiosyncratic Reactions

Another form of drug-drug interaction is the idiosyncratic phenomenon wherein we do not understand the mechanism of interaction leading to either a diminished therapeutic response of one or the other drug or the occurrence of a toxic or adverse effect of one drug when administered in the presence of another. One form of idiosyncratic reaction involves allergic reactions to drugs, wherein the patient has presumably been sensitized by the prior administration of a similar medication to the extent that a classical immunologically mediated reaction occurs.[2,4] Although in the idiosyncratic category, allergic reactions are, by definition, largely unpredictable, it should be borne in mind that familiarity with chemical structural similarities between various therapeutic agents may allow the clinician to avoid allergic reactions to a specific pharmacologic agent when the patient has previously experienced an allergic reaction to a chemically related substance.[4] As we obtain greater understanding of the mechanism of action and adverse effects of a variety of medications, we will encounter fewer and fewer idiosyncratic drug interactions. As we understand mechanisms better, we may be able to avoid combined therapeutic application of substances which have previously been demonstrated to interact with each other in an adverse fashion.

Having reviewed some mechanisms of common drug interactions, we will now focus on specific interactions between various psychotropic drugs and medications administered for nonpsychiatric illness. The role of coexisting medical and neurologic disorders in the occurrence of adverse drug reactions as well as the psychiatric complications of nonpsychotropic medications will also be discussed. Since so many adverse drug reactions have been recorded in the literature and are indeed being discovered almost on a daily basis, it is impossible to discuss all known drug interactions or adverse effects. Those reactions which are discussed have been well documented in published literature and are common enough that the average sophisticated clinician should be prepared to recognize them.

SEDATIVES

A wide variety of chemical compounds including barbiturates, benzodiazepines, antihistamines, meprobamate, methaqualone, glutethimide, ethchlorvynol, chloral hydrate, and ethanol are used to treat anxiety and insomnia. Sedatives are also known as minor tranquilizers or antianxiety drugs.

All sedatives, with the exception of antihistamines, have the capability of producing a dose-related CNS depressant effect. Administration of excessive doses of these compounds or their use in combination with each other or with other centrally acting drugs, may give rise to profound CNS depression and respiratory depression. Certainly, patients suffering from chronic obstructive pulmonary disease may be excessively sensitive to respiratory depression induced by these drugs and may suffer prolonged respiratory embarrassment. These drugs, with the exception of the antihistamines, are capable of inducing tolerance, physical dependence, and addiction when administered over a prolonged period of time. Patients suddenly withdrawn from any of these drugs following the appearance of an addictive syndrome, may suffer a withdrawal reaction marked by seizures, delirium, high fever, and even death. Patients who have become dependent on any of the sedative drugs require careful gradual detoxification under medical supervision. Although benzodiazepines have relatively minor anticholinergic action, confusional states and prolonged sedation resulting from their use may be reversed by the cautious intravenous (IV) administration of physostigmine.[5] A toxic delirium has been reported when ethchlorvynol is used in combination with tricyclic antidepressants, presumably related to the enhancement of anticholinergic action of the latter drug by the former.[6]

Barbiturates, particularly phenobarbital, are potent enzyme inducers and may enhance metabolic degradation of a variety of drugs including phenytoin and anticoagulants, reducing the therapeutic effects of the latter compounds.[3]

Benzodiazepines, which were initially believed to be relatively free of drug interactions, have been found to interact with a variety of therapeutic agents. Cimetidine inhibits benzodiazepine metabolism, producing increased and prolonged effects, particularly of longer-acting benzodiazepines such as chlordiazepoxide hydrochloride and diazepam.[7] Likewise, disulfiram, which decreases benzodiazepine metabolism, may enhance and prolong the pharmacologic action of these compounds.[8] When diazepam is administered along with neuromuscular blocking drugs such as gallamine triethiodide or succinylcholine chloride, prolonged neuromuscular blockade and paralysis result.[9]

Chloral hydrate, which displaces a variety of drugs from plasma protein–binding sites may, by this mechanism, enhance the anticoagulant effects of warfarin and related compounds, and may also interact with the diuretic furosemide to produce diaphoresis and a hypertensive reaction.[10]

Hydroxyzine, a sedating antihistamine without CNS depressant or addictive effect, has been reported to interact with phenothiazines, particularly thioridazine, tricyclic antidepressants, and lithium to increase the risk of cardiac arrhythmias.[11] Table 27-1 presents an outline of some of the more commonly encountered drug interactions involving sedatives.

ANTIPSYCHOTIC DRUGS

Antipsychotic or neuroleptic drugs include five chemically distinct groups of therapeutic agents: the phenothiazines, thioxanthenes, butyrophenone, dihydroindolone, and dibenzoxazepine. These drugs alleviate hallucinations, delusions, disordered thinking, and other major manifestations of psychotic illness, as a result of their ability to block dopamine receptors within the brain. The various antipsychotic drugs differ from one another in their potency and selectivity with respect to dopamine receptor blockade. They also differ from one another in respect to their side effects. Chlorpromazine, mesoridazine, and thioridazine are most sedating whereas haloperidol, loxapine succinate, molindone hydrochloride, and the piperazine phenothiazines such as trifluoperazine

Table 27-1. Drug Interactions: Sedatives

Drug	Interacts with	Effect	Mechanism
Barbiturates	Phenytoin	Decreased phenytoin effect	Enzyme induction
Barbiturates	Anticoagulants (warfarin, dicumarol)	Decreased anticoagulant effect	Enzyme induction
Barbiturates Methaqualone Chloral hydrate Glutethimide	Tricyclic antidepressants	Decreased antidepressant effect	Decreased tricyclic antidepressant serum concentration
Benzodiazepines (except oxazepam, lorazepam, alprazolam)	Cimetidine	Increased benzodiazepine effect	Decreased benzodiazepine metabolism
Benzodiazepines	Disulfiram	Increased benzodiazepine effect	Decreased benzodiazepine metabolism
Benzodiazepines	Antacids	Decreased benzodiazepine effect	Impaired GI absorption
Chloral hydrate	Anticoagulants (warfarin, dicumarol)	Increased warfarin effect	Trichloroacetic acid displaces warfarin from plasma protein
Chloral hydrate	Furosemide	Diaphoresis, hot flashes, hypertension	Uncertain
Diazepam	Gallamine triethiodide Succinylcholine chloride	Prolonged neuromuscular blockade	Uncertain
Ethanol	CNS depressants	CNS depression	Additive effect
Ethchlorvynol	Tricyclic antidepressants	Delirium	Uncertain
Hydroxyzine	Phenothiazines Tricyclic antidepressants Lithium carbonate	Cardiac toxicity	Increased effect on cardiac repolarization
Phenytoin	Anticoagulants	Phenytoin toxicity	Decreased phenytoin metabolism

hydrochloride are much less sedating. If a highly sedating antipsychotic agent is used in combination with a barbiturate or benzodiazepine, the patient may experience excessive somnolence and an additive drug interaction. He may become difficult to arouse or may experience respiratory depression, particularly if there is underlying chronic obstructive pulmonary disease or if the patient is elderly.[4,6]

Chlorpromazine, mesoridiazine, and thioridazine are potent α-adrenergic blocking agents and may thereby produce considerable hypotension. If these drugs are combined with coronary, cerebral, or peripheral vasodilators or with antihypertensive drugs, more profound degrees of hypotension may be encountered.[1,4] Likewise, the combination of the previously mentioned phenothiazines with an MAOI antidepressant can produce profound hypotension which may be difficult and indeed dangerous to reverse since the MAOI may increase the risk of any pressor agent administered and the phenothiazine will reduce the response when a pressor agent is administered.[4,6] Hypotension resulting from these drug interactions is best treated by keeping the patient in a recumbent position and providing IV fluid replacement through a large catheter with careful patient monitoring to avoid congestive heart failure which may result from too vigorous fluid replacement. If pressor agents must be administered, phenylephrine hydrochloride is the safest to employ, but it must be used cautiously because of the need to balance reduced sensitivity to the drug as a result of phenothiazines versus the increased sensitivity to the drug resulting from monoamine oxidase inhibition. Epinephrine should be avoided because it may, as a result of its β-adrenergic stimulant effect, induce further hypotension. The use of indirect acting agents, such as metaraminol bitartrate, which release catecholamines from the adrenal medulla, may be associated with unwanted hypertensive and arrhythmic effects.[12]

Haloperidol has the least α-adrenergic blocking effect, and is least likely among antipsychotic drugs to induce hypotension. The likelihood of an additive interaction with vasodilators or antihypertensive drugs is less with haloperidol than with the previously mentioned phenothiazines. Haloperidol and the piperazine phenothiazines such as trifluoperazine are safer if used in conjunction with MAOIs than are the previously mentioned lower-potency more hypotensive neuroleptics. When used alone, haloperidol is much less likely than other neuroleptics to induce unwanted hypotensive effects. When phenothiazines are used in combination with a variety of anesthetics such as halothane, enflurane, and isoflurane, there is considerable likelihood of a profound hypotensive reaction; therefore, this drug combination should be avoided.[13] It should be kept in mind that phenothiazines may produce an additive drug interaction with succinylcholine resulting in prolonged neuromuscular blockade in association with anesthesia employing this muscle relaxant.[14]

Numerous drugs prescribed by psychiatrists exert a pronounced anticholinergic effect. Indeed, most antiparkinsonian medications exert their therapeutic action as a result of cholinergic blockade. Tricyclic, tetracyclic, and related antidepressants produce pronounced anticholinergic action. Among antipsychotic drugs, thioridazine and mesoridazine are most likely to produce pronounced cholinergic blockade. Chlorpromazine is also strongly anticholinergic while the piperazine phenothiazines including trifluoperazine and the butyrophenone compound haloperidol exert much less anticholinergic action. Clinicians are generally aware that anticholinergic drugs produce blurred vision, dry mouth, tachycardia, constipation, and urinary retention. It is all too easy to forget that anticholinergic agents may also have a central effect including the production of stuttering speech and impaired memory and concentration.[4] Since patients receiving neuroleptic drugs frequently are also receiving antiparkinsonian medication, and, not uncommonly, tricyclic antidepressants as well, there is a strong likelihood of the patient experiencing excessive cholinergic blockade as a result of his psychotropic drug regimen.

Patients receiving neuroleptic drugs in combination with tricyclic antidepressants should generally not be given an antiparkinsonian medication. The latter will generally be unnecessary for controlling extrapyramidal side effects and will certainly add to the potential for an adverse central or peripheral anticholinergic syndrome. Clinicians must realize that patients often take nonprescription medications in addition to those which have been prescribed. Many over-the-counter cold remedies, tranquilizers, and sleeping medications contain potent anticholinergic agents and antihistamines. It is not inconceivable that a patient may therefore be taking at any given time three to five separate medications with anticholinergic activity, thus heightening the risk of an anticholinergic delirium or of peripheral manifestations of cholinergic blockade including tachycardia and dysrrhythmias. Similar toxic anticholinergic syndromes are commonly seen in patients who have taken an overdose of a variety of prescribed and over-the-counter medications. Physostigmine is a cholinesterase inhibitor which may be used as a diagnostic test to assess anticholinergic toxicity.

Neuroleptic drugs, by virtue of their ability to block depamine receptor sites, commonly induce a variety of extrapyramidal effects including stiffness, tremors, increased salivation, and a parkinsonian gait with small steps and reduced accessory movements. The high-potency antipsychotic agents such as piperazine, phenothiazines, and haloperidol are more likely to produce acute extrapyramidal effects than are the lower-potency agents such as chlorpromazine and thioridazine. The simultaneous administration of a variety of antiparkinsonian medications including trihexyphenidyl hydrochloride and benztropine mesylate is useful to reduce or obliterate these unwanted extrapyramidal effects of antipsychotic medications. Patients who have spontaneously occurring Parkinson's disease are likely to have the symptoms of their movement disorder worsened by the administration of neuroleptic drugs, although such medications may be essential if the patient has developed a psychotic illness. In a patient with Parkinson's disease, it may be worthwhile to initiate antipsychotic drug treatment with a lower-potency agent such as chlorpromazine or thioridazine rather than a higher-potency dopamine blocker.

Patients receiving levodopa for Parkinson's disease will, in all likelihood, have the beneficial effect of that medication rather quickly reversed if neuroleptic medication is prescribed.[9] Despite its beneficial effects, levodopa itself may produce psychotic symptoms. In a parkinsonian patient who requires antipsychotic chemotherapy, it may be best to utilize anticholinergic antiparkinsonian medications alone or in combination with amantadine hydrochloride to control symptoms of the movement disorder rather than continue the administration of levodopa in conjunction with antipsychotic chemotherapy. A levodopa-treated parkinsonian patient who develops psychotic symptoms may best be treated by terminating levodopa therapy, and observing for evidence of behavioral improvement before aggressively instituting antipsychotic chemotherapy unless the situation is clinically urgent. In such patients, temporary administration of amobarbital sodium or a short-acting benzodiazepine such as oxazepam, may control agitation while awaiting clearance of a potential toxic levodopa reaction.

Although it is fairly well known that tricyclic antidepressants may inhibit the antihypertensive effects of guanethidine, clonidine, and related drugs, it is important to realize that chlorpromazine itself, a neuroleptic, has some ability to block nerve reuptake mechanisms and may therefore antagonize the therapeutic action of these antihypertensive medications.[9] Another type of interaction involving neuroleptics and antihypertensives is the occurrence of a transient dementia in patients receiving haloperidol in combination with methyldopa.[15,16] This interaction appears to result from the ability of the antipsychotic drug to block dopamine receptor sites and the antihypertensive drug to reduce neurotransmitter synthesis.[16] The ability of methyldopa to reduce central as well as peripheral neurotransmitter synthesis appears to explain the ability of this drug to induce severe depression when administered as the sole therapeutic agent for hypertension.[13] This finding is certainly reminiscent of reports nearly 30 years ago that reserpine administered for the treatment of hypertension could induce profound depression and suicidal behavior.[17]

Since phenothiazines may exert prominent α-adenergic blockade, their administration in conjunction with epinephrine may result in a reversal of the pressor action of epinephrine with the occurrence of a hypotensive reaction due to unopposed β-adenergic stimulation induced by epinephrine.[4,12] Tricyclic antidepressants have long been associated with disturbances of cardiac rhythm.[18] Likewise, some phenothiazines, most notably thioridazine and chlorpromazine, have been associated with the occurrence of cardiac arrhythmias. An important and potentially dangerous drug interaction may occur when thioridazine is administered simultaneously with quinidine, resulting in depressed myocardial function and dysrrhythmias, presumably due to the fact that both drugs exert similar electrophysiologic effects on the myocardium.[14] It is likely that other antiarrhythmics and other phenothiazines may interact in a similar fashion based upon our knowledge of their electrophysiologic effects. Significant ECG effects and interactions with cardiac drugs have not been reported for haloperidol even though the latter drug has been used in a number of studies in rather high dosage in patients following acute myocardial infarction or open heart surgery.[4]

In addition to the interesting variety of drug-drug interactions that have been observed with phenothiazines, it is important to note that their administration concomitantly with antacids, cholestyramine, or activated charcoal may decrease their GI absorption and pharmacologic effects.[6] Likewise, cigarette smoking has been reported to decrease the antipsychotic action of chlorpromazine, possibly related to increased chlorpromazine metabolism.[14] The common practice of mixing liquid preparations of various phenothiazines with various beverages such as fruit juices to increase palatability presents considerable risk since many juices and other beverages when mixed with liquid phenothiazines result in the formation of an insoluble precipitant whose GI absorption appears to be poor, resulting in the possibility of therapeutically inadequate serum drug concentrations.[6] Liquid preparations of haloperidol are compatible with beverages, do not form insoluble precipitates, and are readily absorbed from the GI tract.

Neuroleptics, especially chlorpromazine, lower seizure threshold and increase the risk of convulsions occurring in patients with seizure disorders.[4] Likewise, when these drugs are taken in overdoses, they may provoke seizures. Thioridazine and haloperidol are least likely to provoke seizures in normal persons and in those with underlying convulsive disorders. Chlorpromazine should generally be avoided in patients who have convulsive disorders. Patients receiving any neuroleptic drug in combination with an anticonvulsant should have periodic monitoring of the latter to be certain that pharmacotherapy is adequate and thereby reduce the risk of seizures. Table 27-2 demonstrates important antipsychotic drug interactions.

TRICYCLIC ANTIDEPRESSANTS

Although various mechanisms of action have been proposed for tricyclic, tetracyclic, and chemically unrelated antidepressants such as trazodone hydrochloride, the most widely accepted mechanism of action involves the ability of these drugs to inhibit nerve reuptake of either norepinephrine or serotonin or both. Many depressed patients respond differentially to drugs affecting one or the other of these transmitters. In addition to their differential effect on reuptake mechanisms, these antidepressants differ from one another in their propensity to produce various side effects commonly associated with this group of therapeutic agents. The tricyclic drugs, amitriptyline hydrochloride and doxepin hydrochloride; the tetracyclic antidepressant, maprotiline; and the triazolo compound, trazodone, are the most sedating of currently prescribed antidepressants and, likewise, are more likely to produce an additive interaction with other sedatives including barbiturates, benzodiazepines, and neuroleptics, producing excessive drowsiness and sedation.

Tricyclic antidepressants and the previously mentioned structurally unique antidepressant drugs all possess considerable anticholinergic action. Amitriptyline, imipramine hydrochloride, and trimipramine are relatively more anticholinergic than doxepin, amoxapine, maprotiline, trazodone, and desipramine hydrochloride.[4] As mentioned previously, the anticholinergic actions of one type of medication are clearly additive with the cholinergic receptor blocking actions of other agents, be they neuroleptic, antiparkinsonian, or antisecretory drugs. The central and peripheral manifestations of cholinergic blockade have been described in the previous section on antipsychotic drugs. Physostigmine is a useful diagnostic test to assess anticholinergic toxicity due to antidepressant drugs. The clinician is strongly advised that in prescribing medication for the elderly patient or the patient who must receive other anticholinergic

Table 27-2. Drug Interactions: Antipsychotics

Drug	Interacts with	Effect	Mechanism
Antipsychotic drugs	Levodopa	Decreased levodopa effect	Dopamine blockade
Chlorpromazine	Guanethidine Clonidine	Decreased antihypertensive effect	Chlorpromazine inhibits uptake mechanisms
Chlorpromazine	Cigarette smoking	Decreased antipsychotic effect	Increased chlorpromazine metabolism
Haloperidol	Methyldopa	Dementia	Dopamine blockade and decreased catecholamine synthesis
Phenothiazines (especially chlorpromazine, thioridazine mesoridazine)	Antihypertensive drugs and coronary vasodilators	Hypotension	Peripheral vasodilation
Phenothiazines	Epinephrine	Hypotension, vasodilation	α-Adrenergic blockade and β-adrenergic stimulation
Phenothiazines	Monoamine oxidase inhibitors	Hypotension	α-Adrenergic blockade and direct vasodilation
Phenothiazines	Anesthetics: enflurane, isoflurane, halothane	Hypotension	Potentiation of vasodilation, myocardial depression
Phenothiazines	Opiates Sedatives Hypnotics Barbiturates Benzodiazepines Antihistamines	Prolonged somnolence, respiratory depression	Additive CNS depression and hypotension
Phenothiazines	Succinylcholine chloride	Prolonged neuromuscular blockade	Phenothiazines decrease levels of cholinesterase
Phenothiazines	Antacids, tea, coffee, milk, fruit juice, cholestyramine resin	Decreased phenothiazine effect	Impaired GI absorption
Thioridazine	Quinidine	Cardiac arrhythmias, myocardial depression	Additive myocardial and electrophysiologic effects

agents, those drugs having the least anticholinergic potency are safest.

Since tricyclic antidepressant drugs inhibit nerve reuptake of biogenic amines centrally as well as peripherally, they may increase myocardial norepinephrine; this in conjunction with their anticholinergic action, and their quinidinelike effect, may give rise to cardiac arrhythmias.[4,18] Arrhythmias can be characterized by the presence of atrial or ventricular premature beats and in some cases, the latter may be multifocal or give rise to short runs of ventricular tachycardia.[19] The arrythmogenic effect of tricyclic antidepressants is more likely to occur in those individuals with underlying coronary or valvular heart disease, and particularly in patients who have had a recent myocardial infarction.[1,19] Patients who have had occasional extrasystoles may experience an increased frequency of these abnormal beats during the course of tricyclic antidepressant drug therapy. Patients receiving antidepressants in conjunction with sympathominetic amines such as isoproterenol or ephedrine for asthma, or stimulants such as amphetamines, are more likely to experience cardiac arrhythmias.[4,18] Likewise, the elderly are more apt to experience the dysrrhythmic effect of tricyclic antidepressants.

In contradistinction to these tricyclic effects, the ability of these drugs to exert a quinidinelike membrane-stabilizing action may actually suppress atrial or ventricular premature beats.[19] Furthermore, this membrane-stabilizing effect of tricyclic antidepressants may be additive with a similar mechanism produced by a variety of antiarrhythmic drugs including quinidine, procainamide hydrochloride, and disopyramide. This additive interaction may not only suppress cardiac disrrhythmias, but may also give rise to depressed myocardial contractility and congestive heart failure.[18,19] Indeed, even when administered alone in conventional therapeutic dosage, tricyclic antidepressants may depress the myocardium with the resultant worsening of previously existing congestive heart failure or the appearance of heart failure de novo.[18] Tricyclic antidepressants and some neuroleptics, particularly thioridazine and chlorpromazine, may produce a variety of ECG changes including ST segment depression, and decreased voltage, inverted, or biphasic T waves.[1,20] Conduction disturbances may also occasionally occur in patients receiving tricyclic antidepressants or thioridazine.[19,20]

Although tricyclic antidepressants do not produce α-adrenergic blockade, they commonly induce postural hypotension, most likely due to their ability to relax vascular smooth muscle, resulting in peripheral vasodilation.[4,18,19] This hypotensive effect of tricyclic antidepressants may be additive with a variety of vasodilator and antihypertensive medications, giving rise to uncomfortable or occasionally even dangerous hypotensive reactions.[4] Although hypertensive reactions have been the adverse effect most commonly attributed to the interaction of tricyclic with MAOI antidepressants, the risk of enhanced hypotension occurring with this combined regimen is probably greater than the risk of a hypertensive reaction.[4,6]

When tricyclic antidepressants are administered to patients receiving guanethidine, clonidine, bethanidine sulfate, or debrisoquin sulfate, the antihypertensive actions of these drugs are inhibited giving rise to an elevation in blood pressure.[3,4] The mechanism of this interaction is well known and is due to the ability of tricyclic drugs to inhibit nerve reuptake, not only of norepinephrine and serotonin, but also of the previously mentioned antihypertensive drugs.[4,12] It has been reported previously that doxepin does not antagonize the antihypertensive action of these drugs. There is, however, clear pharmacologic evidence to support the statement that doxepin will indeed antagonize those antihypertensive drugs whose mechanism of action requires their active uptake into nerve endings.[4]

One useful drug-drug interaction involving tricyclic antidepressants and phenothiazines is the ability of phenothiazines to slow the metabolism of tricyclic antidepressants, thereby boosting the beneficial therapeutic effects of the latter.[21] Indeed, some depressed patients who do not respond to tricyclic antidepressants when administered alone achieve a favorable response when these drugs are administered in combination with relatively low doses of phenothiazines.[4]

Anticonvulsant drugs, including phenytoin and phenobarbital, may increase the rate of tricyclic antidepressant metabolism, thereby decreasing the antidepressant effect.[9] As in the case of chlorpromazine and other phenothiazines, the tricyclic antidepressants lower the seizure threshold and may provoke seizures when used in ordinary therapeutic dosage in patients with convulsive disorders. Convulsions are a common manifestation of antidepressant drug overdose. One of the newer antidepressants, a tetracyclic drug, maprotiline, appears to have a somewhat greater ability to lower seizure threshold and provoke seizures than some of the older conventional tricyclic antidepressants. Another potential drug interaction is the ability of stimulants, including amphetamines and methylphenidate hydrochloride, to inhibit metabolism of tricyclic antidepressants, thereby increasing both tricyclic serum concentration and therapeutic response.[4,15] Table 27-3 delineates some of the common drug-drug interactions involving tricyclic antidepressants.

MONOAMINE OXIDASE INHIBITOR ANTIDEPRESSANTS

Monoamine oxidase inhibitors produce their antidepressant action as the result of increasing brain concentrations of monoamine neurotrans-

Table 27-3. Drug Interactions: Tricyclic Antidepressants

Drug	Interacts with	Effect	Mechanism
Tricyclic antidepressants (TCA)	Direct-acting sympathomimetics (epinephrine, norepinephrine)	Hypertension, arrhythmias	Inhibition of neuronal uptake mechanisms
TCA	Stimulants: amphetamines, methylphenidate hydrochloride	Increased antidepressant effect	Inhibition of TCA metabolism; increased brain levels of stimulants
TCA	Stimulants, including cocaine	Agitation, psychosis	Same mechanisms
TCA	Anticonvulsants	Decreased effect of TCA	Increased TCA metabolism
TCA	Anticonvulsants	Seizures	TCAs lower seizure threshold
TCA	CNS depressants: alcohol, anesthetics, barbiturates, benzodiazepines	Increased CNS depression, hypotension	Additive CNS depressive effects and adrenergic blockade and direct vasodilation
TCA	Alcohol Barbiturates Chloral hydrate Lithium carbonate	Decreased TCA effect	Lowered TCA serum concentration, enhanced TCA metabolism

TCA	Diazepam Antipsychotics Antiparkinsonian drugs Antisecretory drugs	Increased TCA effect, confusion, delirium, tachycardia urinary retention, ileus	Decreased TCA metabolism, anticholinergic toxicity
TCA	Phenothiazines	Enhanced effects of both drugs	Decrease metabolism of each other
TCA	Antihypertensives: guanethidine, clonidine hydrochloride, bethanidine sulfate, debrisoquin sulfate	TCA block antihypertensive effects; hypertension may occur	TCA inhibit nerve uptake of these antihypertensive drugs
TCA	Antiarrhythmic drugs: quinidine, procainamide hydrochloride, disopyramide, lidocaine, propranolol hydrochloride, etc	Myocardial depression, decreased contractility, dysrrhythmias	Additive quinidinelike effects on myocardium and conduction system
TCA	Monoamine oxidase inhibitors (MAOI)	Increased TCA effect, increase or decrease blood pressure	Monoamine oxidase inhibition with reuptake blockade

mitter substances by blocking monoamine oxidase (MAO)–catalyzed metabolic degradation of these substances.[4] Since both reuptake mechanisms and metabolic inactivation of neurotransmitters may increase their availability and activity within the brain, these two antidepressant mechanisms are theoretically complementary. Since the beginning of antidepressant drug therapy, however, most people have considered the potential toxic effects of combined antidepressant therapy to be too dangerous to recommend it as a viable treatment approach. However, newer research strongly suggests that MAOIs, alone or in combination with tricyclic drugs, may be far safer than previously thought.[22,23] It is theoretically possible that combined therapy could provoke a higher incidence of hypertensive reactions. Based upon controlled studies and clinical observation, this drug combination does not appear to be associated with a high risk of hypertensive crises.[23] The most commonly encountered unwanted effect of MAOI antidepressants is the production of postural hypotension, which may, in fact, be enhanced in some patients receiving tricyclics in combination with MAOIs. The guideline, however, in cases where combined therapy regimens are utilized is that patients be carefully monitored before and during treatment, and it is preferable that the patient previously receive both types of antidepressant singly so that the adverse effects of the individual drug may be seen before the patient is exposed to combination therapy.

Tranylcypromine sulfate is a nonhydrazine, while phenelzine sulfate and isocarboxazid are both hydrazine compounds. The hydrazine structure may be potentially hepatoxic, though the incidence of reported liver damage with these drugs is exceedingly low. Tranylcypromine structurally resembles the amphetamines and may produce some direct stimulant action in addition to the pharmacologic effects resulting from enzyme inhibition. Although hypertensive reactions to tranylcypromine in the absence of food or drug interactions have been suggested, there is no convincing evidence that they do in fact occur. On the other hand, it is conceivable that a patient who has been treated with phenelzine and subsequently abruptly started on tranylcypromine may experience a hypertensive reaction. Therefore in changing treatment from one MAOI to tranylcypromine, a five-day drug-free interval is advised; when changing from tranylcypromine to another MAOI a drug-free interval is not required.

The most widely known drug interaction in psychiatry is the hypertensive reaction which may occur when tyramine-rich foods or beverages are consumed by a patient being treated with an MAOI. In reality, hypertensive reactions to tyramine-rich foods are quite uncommon among MAOI-treated patients.[4] Those hypertensive reactions which do occur are more frequently associated with the consumption of prescription or over-the-counter medications containing stimulants or vaso-constrictor decongestants. Nevertheless, patients being treated with MAOI antidepressants should be clearly warned, both orally and in writing, to avoid consuming significant quantities of the following foods and beverages:

1. Fermented cheeses, specifically cheddar and other strong cheeses
2. Pickled herring, sardines, and anchovies
3. Chicken livers
4. Canned or processed meats
5. Pods of broad beans
6. Canned figs
7. Yeast extract
8. Wine and beer

Patients being treated with MAOIs should generally limit their daily intake of caffeine-containing beverages, including coffee, tea, and cola drinks to two or three cups or glasses per day. If an individual tends to consume large quantities of these beverages, they should be advised to drink decaffeinated products. White wine is generally less likely to contain significant quantities of tyramine than is red wine, Chianti being particularly high in its tyramine content. Many beers are also rich in tyramine. Fermented liquors generally do not contain significant quantities of tyramine, but, since MAOIs tend to potentiate alcohol, the effects of these beverages may be enhanced by drug therapy. A single cocktail or 3 oz of white wine can be safely consumed. Small quantities, not exceeding 2 oz per day of sour cream, yogurt, cottage cheese, American cheese, mild Swiss cheese, or chocolate may be consumed during the course of MAOI therapy, generally without ill effect.

Patients receiving MAOI antidepressants should be told specifically to avoid the use of nose drops, cold remedies, nasal decongestants, cough syrups, diet pills, and any other prescription or over-the-counter remedy which may contain vasoconstrictor or stimulant-type drugs. The current epidemic of cocaine abuse indicates the necessity to specifically warn patients against the use of cocaine while taking an MAOI. The author has seen two patients who have experienced this unfortunate drug interaction which was manifested clinically by moderate hypertension and a pronounced but relatively transient acute psychosis. One of the patients experienced this reaction on several occasions despite strong warnings to avoid cocaine use. Patients suffering from bronchial asthma who may be medicated with ephedrine, epinephrine, or other broncho-dilators have a rather high risk of experiencing a drug-drug interaction during the course of MAOI antidepressant therapy. Therefore, generally, asthmatic patients should not receive this form of antidepressant treat-ment unless their asthma can be adequately controlled by the inter-mittent use of steroid inhalers such as beclomethasone dipropionate.

Patients who develop hypertensive reactions as a result of the com-bination of vasoactive substances with MAOI antidepressants frequently respond adequately to mild sedation administered in a quiet, darkened room. More severe hypertensive reactions generally are best treated by the intravenous (IV) administration of phentolamine (Regitine) in a dose of 5 mg. Propranolol hydrochloride, a β-adrenergic blocking agent administered slowly IV alone or in combination with the α-adrenergic blocking drug phentolamine, may also be useful in the presence of a severe hypertensive crisis.

Pargyline hydrochloride (Eutonyl), an MAOI, has been used for a number of years as an antihypertensive drug. This compound also exerts an antidepressant effect and may be very useful in the treatment of depressed hypertensive patients. There are a number of potential drug interactions between MAOIs and antihypertensive medications. Guanethidine when initially administered causes the release of nore-pinephrine from nerve endings.[12] An MAOI-treated patient who is started on guanethidine may experience a hypertensive reaction; therefore these drugs are incompatible.[12] Hydralazine hydrochloride is likely to produce more pronounced tachycardia and quite possibly an elevation in blood pressure in an MAOI-treated patient.[9] Methyldopa can also theoretically provoke a hypertensive reaction in a patient receiving MAOI antidepressants.

The most common unwanted effect of MAOI antidepressants is a decrease in blood pressure, most prominent with postural change from a reclining or sitting position to a standing position.[4] Any vasodilator is likely to enhance the hypotensive reaction.[4,6] Phenothiazines, particu-larly low-potency agents such as chlorpromazine and thioridazine, are particularly likely to provoke significant hypotensive reactions when given to patients receiving MAOIs. If a neuroleptic is necessary in conjunction with this form of antidepressant drug therapy, piperazine phenothiazines such as trifluoperazine or the butyrophenone halo-peridol, are clearly the safest drugs with the least likelihood of producing a hypotensive reaction. Levodopa, a common antiparkinsonian medi-cation, may provoke pronounced CNS stimulation and hypertension in conjunction with MAOIs.[6,12] A similar reaction may occur with the respiratory center stimulant doxapram hydrochloride.[6]

Central nervous system depressants including alcohol, barbiturates, benxodiazepines, chloral hydrate, and opiates are generally potentiated in the presence of therapy so that excessive sedation and CNS depression results.[4,6]

The narcotic analgesic, meperidine hydrochloride, when administered to an MAOI-treated patient, may provoke a serious and fatal adverse reaction.[6,13] The MAOI-merperidine reaction is characterized by agitation, restlessness, headache, rigidity, and hyperpyrexia. It may be associated with profound hypotension or dramatic hypertension, convulsions may occur, the patient may become comatose and, indeed, deaths have been reported from this syndrome.[13] The administration of meperidine to MAOI-treated patients is absolutely contraindicated.

Although emergency surgery under general anesthesia can be safely accomplished during the course of MAOI therapy, it is generally preferable to delay elective surgical procedures for 1 to 2 weeks after discontinuing these drugs. In addition to the risk of a drug interaction involving the administration of pressor agents to an MAOI-treated patient during the course of surgery, several drug interactions involving anesthetics have been reported. Halothane and enflurane have both been observed to produce muscle stiffness and hyperpyrexia in MAOI-treated patients.[13] Succinylcholine and related muscle relaxants may have their paralytic effect enhanced and prolonged as the result of MAO inhibition.[13] Furthermore, as stated previously, barbiturates, including those used for general anesthesia may be potentiated by this form of antidepressant drug therapy.[13] Table 27-4 delineates the spectrum of drug interactions involving MAOIs.

LITHIUM CARBONATE

Lithium carbonate, a salt of the alkalai metal lithium, is the simplest chemical substance used in psychiatric treatment. This drug has been repeatedly demonstrated to exert a therapeutic and prophylactic effect in manic illness, and has frequently been demonstrated to be of value in the treatment and prophylaxis of depression as well as a variety of other psychiatric syndromes.[4] In spite of its simplicity from a chemical standpoint, the physiologic actions of this ion are quite complex, and the mechanism of its therapeutic action is not yet well understood.[24]

Lithium is not metabolized by the body, but is filtered, reabsorbed, and excreted by the kidneys. The pharmacokinetics of lithium are intimately tied to the physiology of sodium, chloride, potassium, and fluid balance. Sodium depletion resulting from a salt-restricted diet or the administration of diuretics will enhance lithium retention, thereby increasing the serum concentration of this ion and the potential risk of lithium

Table 27-4. Drug Interactions: Monoamine Oxidase Inhibitor Antidepressants

Drug	Interacts with	Effect	Mechanism
Monoamine oxidase inhibitors (MAOIs)	Tricyclic antidepressants (TCA)	Increased TCA effect; increased or decreased BP	MAO inhibition; blocks reuptake
MAOI	Other MAOIs	Hypertension, hyperpyrexia	Sympathomimetic effect of tranylcypromine sulfate in presence of other MAOIs
MAOI	Phenothiazines	Hypotension	Vasodilation and α-adrenergic blockade
MAOI	Anesthetics: halothane, enflurane	Muscle stiffness, hyperpyrexia	Impaired drug metabolism, increased catecholamines
MAOI	Meperidine hydrochloride	Agitation, restlessness, hypotension, hypertension, headache, rigidity, hyperpyrexia, convulsions, coma, death	Elevation of brain serotonin levels by MAOI and impaired hepatic metabolism of narcotics due to enzyme inhibition by MAOI
MAOI	Benzodiazepines	Enhanced effect of benzodiazepines	?Enzyme inhibition
MAOI	Alcohol Barbiturates Chloral hydrate Opiates	CNS depression	?Enzyme inhibition
MAOI	Spinal anesthesia	Hypotension	Potentiated vasodilation
MAOI	Doxapram hydrochloride	CNS stimulation, agitation, hypertension	Catecholamine release

MAOI	Levodopa	CNS stimulation, hypertension	Increased catecholamine synthesis
MAOI	Sympathomimetics: amphetamines, cocaine, dopamine, ephedrine, epinephrine, metaraminol bitartrate, norepinephrine, phenylpropanolamine hydrochloride, phenylephrine hydrochloride, tyramine, etc	Hypertensive crisis, CNS stimulation, agitation, acute psychotic reaction	Impaired metabolism of endogenous catecholamines, and exogenous sympathomimetic compounds
MAOI	Tyramine-rich foods: beer, wine, cheese, fermented meat and fish products, yeast derivatives, broad beans	Hypertensive crisis	Impaired GI degradation of tyramine and endogenous catecholamines
MAOI	Succinylcholine chloride, suxamethonium chloride, d-tubocurarine chloride	Prolonged muscle relaxation, muscle paralysis	MAOI decreases plasma concentration of pseudocholinesterase

toxicity. Hypokalemia, which may occur during the course of diuretic therapy, enhances the toxic potential of the lithium ion.[24] When lithium was first used in psychiatry, diuretics were thought to be contraindicated in conjunction with lithium therapy. The accumulation of considerable clinical experience with the therapeutic use of lithium indicates that it may be safely administered in conjunction with diuretic therapy provided serum lithium concentration as well as serum electrolytes, particularly potassium, are monitored at regular intervals.[4,24] Patients receiving stable diuretic regimens for hypertension or congestive heart failure whose serum potassium concentration remains normal can generally tolerate lithium therapy without ill effects or undue risk. Medically ill patients, particularly those receiving vigorous diuretic regimens for acute congestive heart failure or other serious conditions, may require temporary discontinuance of lithium. The occurrence of hypokalemia during the course of diuretic therapy may necessitate temporary discontinuance or dosage reduction if lithium is being simultaneously administered. Hypokalemia not only enhances the toxicity of lithium, but also significantly increases the risk of digitalis intoxication.[24] Digitalis preparations such as digoxin may be used safely in conjunction with lithium provided that normal electrolyte balance is maintained and hypokalemia does not ensue. In the absence of excessive serum lithium concentration, lithium is not likely to produce cardiac arrhythmias or conduction disturbances. However, the presence of toxic serum concentrations of lithium may provoke atrial or ventricular premature beats and intraventricular conduction abnormalities.[25,26] Hypokalemia and digitalis toxicity likewise present the risk of cardiac dysrrhythmias and may enhance the arrhythmogenic potential of lithium even when the latter is maintained at therapeutic serum concentration.[19,26]

Lithium interferes with iodine trapping by the thyroid gland and the formation of thyroid hormones.[24] In the course of lithium therapy, patients may develop goiter with normal thyroid hormone levels or may experience hypothyroidism in the absence of clinically observable thyroid gland enlargement. In such cases, lithium carbonate therapy may be continued along with properly monitored thyroid hormone replacement.[26] It is useful to palpate the thyroid gland and obtain laboratory studies including tri-iodothyronine (T_3), thyroxine (T_4), and thyroid-stimulating hormone (TSH) prior to instituting lithium carbonate therapy.[4] These measurements may subsequently be repeated every year or two during the course of treatment. Lithium has been reported to decrease glucose tolerance in some patients, although its ability to induce diabetes is doubtful.[6,26] There have been reports of the combined administration of phenothiazines with lithium potentially increasing the risk of hyperglycemia.[6] Not uncommonly, patients receiving lithium carbonate have elevated WBC counts, in the range of 14,000 to 16,000/mL or occasionally higher. There is no known significant adverse effect of lithium on the hematopoietic system and the occurrence of leukcocytosis does not suggest a need to modify the regimen.[24]

About a decade ago, a specific toxic syndrome was reported to occur when patients were treated simultaneously with lithium carbonate and haloperidol.[27] Subsequently, similar syndromes marked by the presence of an abnormal EEG, confusion, impaired cognition and mentation, and a variety of autonomic symptoms was reported when lithium was used in conjunction with a variety of other neuroleptics including thioridazine and fluphenazine hydrochloride.[28] A review of 425 patients treated with the combination of haloperidol and lithium failed to confirm even one case of the previously described toxic syndrome.[29] In the experience of this author, such a syndrome does not exist. However, patients receiving neuroleptic drugs may develop the neuroleptic malignant syndrome (NMS) which bears considerable resemblance to the previous reports of specific toxic syndromes involving combined therapy with neuroleptics and lithium. Likewise, many of these syndromes described findings not inconsistent with lithium intoxication and, in the case of the initial reports involving haloperidol, the patients' serum lithium concentrations were all well above the generally accepted therapeutic range of 0.6 to 1.2 mEq/L.[77] Since lithium is most commonly used in conjunction with neuroleptic drugs in the treatment of acute manic psychosis, it would be inappropriate to delete this form of combination drug treatment from our therapeutic armamentarium.[24,26]

Numerous drugs when combined with lithium are capable of increasing the serum concentration of the latter ion. Tetracycline administered to lithium-treated patients increases serum lithium concentration and may provoke lithium intoxication either as a result of increased lithium absorption from the GI tract or impaired lithium renal excretion.[30] A variety of nonsteroidal anti-inflammatory drugs, including phenylbutazone, indomethacin, and piroxicam have been reported to increase serum lithium concentration and provoke lithium intoxication, apparently as a result of their ability to increase renal tubular reabsorption of the lithium ion.[31,32]

Carbamazepine, through a mechanism which is at this point unclear, may enhance the therapeutic effect of lithium, and has also been reported on occasion to increase serum lithium concentration with the possibility of producing lithium toxicity.[33,34] There is a case report of a lithium-treated patient who experienced increased serum lithium concentrations during the course of marijuana smoking, the putative mechanism being that marijuana slowed GI motility, thereby increasing lithium absorption.[35] The combination of methyldopa with lithium has been reported to be associated with lithium toxicity; though the mechanism is uncertain, this interaction may depend more on neurotransmitter activity of the two drugs rather than on changes in drug absorption or excretion patterns.[36]

Prolonged muscle paralysis has been reported in lithium-treated patients who have received succinylcholine, pancuronium bromide, or decamethonium bromide as muscle relaxants during the course of surgical anesthesia.[13,33] The mechanism of interaction between lithium and these muscle relaxants appears to be a synergistic effect at the neuromuscular junction.[13] Hydroxyzine has been reported to interact with lithium producing disturbances in cardiac conduction, presumably as a result of an increased effect of lithium on cardiac repolarization mechanisms.[11] Table 27-5 gives the drug interactions involving lithium carbonate.

PSYCHIATRIC COMPLICATIONS OF NONPSYCHOTROPIC MEDICATIONS

Many nonpsychotropic medications prescribed in the general hospital setting produce unwanted cognitive or behavioral side effects. The presence of psychiatric illness, organic brain dysfunction, or impaired renal or hepatic function may predispose a particular patient to these unwanted drug effects. The remainder of this chapter will briefly outline some of the psychiatric complications of medications. When an adverse behavioral effect is suspected, the situation can generally be clarified by temporarily withdrawing the suspected agent and, where necessary or feasible, substituting a less toxic alternative therapy.

Cardiovascular Drugs

Digitalis, one of the oldest drugs in current use, may produce a variety of side effects including visual distortions, disturbed color perception, and flickering lights. In addition, depression, hallucinations, and delirium have occasionally been reported with digitalis, generally with excessive blood levels of the drug.[1]

Antiarrhythmics. Numerous drugs used in the treatment of cardiac arrhythmias may produce psychiatric symptoms. Delirium, confusion, and hallucinations have all been reported with quinidine. These effects may occur with excessive doses of the drug but are also known to occur

Table 27-5. Drug Interactions: Lithium Carbonate

Drug	Interacts with	Effect	Mechanism
Lithium	Marijuana	Increased lithium concentration	Increased lithium absorption
Lithium	Tetracyclines	Lithium intoxication	Enhanced lithium absorption; impaired lithium excretion
Lithium	Muscle relaxants: succinylcholine chloride, pancuronium bromide, decamethonium bromide	Prolonged muscle paralysis	Synergism at neuromuscular junction
Lithium	Carbamazapine	Enhanced lithium effect	?Synergistic effect
		Possible lithium toxicity	Uncertain
Lithium	Methyldopa	Lithium toxicity	Uncertain
Lithium	Phenylbutazone Indomethacin Piroxicam	Lithium toxicity	Increased tubular reabsorption of lithium
Lithium	Hydroxyzine	Cardiac conduction disturbance	Increased effect of lithium on cardiac repolarization
Lithium	Phenothiazines Neuroleptics	May enhance neurologic toxicity of each other, hyperglycemia	Additive effect— central dopamine blockade; ? effect on catecholamine turnover rate
Lithium	Thiazide diuretics	Increased lithium concentration	Increased Na and K execretion and lithium reabsorption

in some individuals who are sensitive to quinidine when ordinary dosages are employed.[1] A high index of suspicion must be maintained with respect to possible psychiatric side effects of drugs. An elderly woman with dementia who was taking quinidine over a number of years experienced a dramatic improvement in mental status when quinidine was discontinued.[37]

Procainamide may also produce depression, giddiness, and psychotic symptoms, including hallucinations, in susceptible individuals.[38] Disorientation, confusion, and hallucinations have been noted in patients receiving lidocaine IV for the treatment of cardiac arrhythmias.[1] Psychotic reactions have been reported in patients receiving disopyramide, an antiarrhythmic drug which possesses considerable anticholinergic effect as does quinidine.[39]

Propranolol and a variety of other β-adrenergic blocking drugs are used for the treatment of cardiac arrhythmias, angina pectoris, hypertension, and an ever-increasing series of clinical conditions. Of the β-adrenergic antagonists, propranolol is the compound most often associated with unwanted cognitive and behavioral effects. Vivid dreams and nightmares occasionally occur with propranolol therapy. Hallucinations and toxic psychosis may occur in some patients receiving propranolol. These effects tend to occur more often in the elderly although age is not an inviolable barrier to their occurrence.[4] These toxic behavioral effects are not dose-dependent and may take place in some individuals receiving doses as low as 20 to 40 mg/d of propranolol hydrochloride. Depression appears to be distinct from the toxic psychoses which may occur with propranolol administration and is more likely to be seen when daily dosage is 120 mg or greater. Some of the newer β-adrenergic antagonists have limited ability to cross the blood-brain barrier when ordinary therapeutic doses are utilized, and are therefore less likely to cause psychiatric side effects. Patients who have experienced cognitive or behavioral complications with propranolol will often tolerate atenolol or metoprolol without these unwanted effects.

Antihypertensives.   Reserpine, the earliest effective antihypertensive drug, has played a major part in our understanding of the role of neurotransmitters in psychiatric illness. Reserpine depletes stores of norepinephrine and serotonin in various tissues, including the brain, and can induce severe depressive states and may provoke suicidal behavior. The depressogenic effect of reserpine appears more likely to occur in patients with prior affective illnesses. However, even patients with no prior history of depression may become severely depressed while receiving this drug. Depression is more likely to occur when larger doses of reserpine are administered; however, depression may occur with daily doses as low as 0.1 to 0.25 mg.

Methyldopa may produce drowsiness, impaired concentration, hallucinations, and paranoid ideation.[40] The commonest psychiatric effect of methyldopa, however, is the production of depression which may be severe enough to necessitate specific antidepressant drug therapy.[40] Although, more likely to occur in patients with prior depressive histories, depression may occur in association with methyldopa in patients with completely negative psychiatric histories. The occurrence of depression in a patient who is being treated with reserpine or methyldopa dictates that the antihypertensive therapy be changed to a less depressogenic drug as the first step in treating the depressive illness.

Clonidine may produce drowsiness, anxiety, hallucinations, and depression, although the latter is far less common than with reserpine or methyldopa.[1] Guanethidine rarely may also produce depression.[1] Since both clonidine and guanethidine inhibit nerve uptake of tricyclic antidepressants, these antihypertensive compounds must be discontinued prior to the administration of antidepressant drugs. Depression is a rare side effect of hydralazine and prazosin hydrochloride, but the presence of depression in a patient who is receiving one of these drugs should at least raise the possibility of modifying the antihypertensive regimen.[1] Sodium nitroprusside, used in the treatment of hypertensive crises, has been reported to potentially produce a toxic psychosis.[1] Depletion of intracellular potassium by diuretics may induce weakness; even minor degrees of hypokalemia may produce symptoms suggestive of depression. Therefore the occurrence of depressive symptoms in a patient who is receiving diuretics indicates the necessity of measuring serum potassium and, quite possibly, providing oral potassium supplementation.

In males, erectile or ejaculatory dysfunction may occur with a variety of drugs including clonidine, guanethidine, methyldopa, reserpine, and β-adrenergic blocking drugs.[1]

Respiratory Drugs

Bronchodilators, including ephedrine, albuterol, isoproterenol, metaproterenol sulfate, and terbutaline sulfate possess sympathomimetic actions and may produce palpitations, tremor, and nervousness. A toxic psychosis resembling amphetamine psychosis may occur with ephedrine, especially when larger doses are employed.[41] Psychotic symptoms have also been reported with albuterol.[42] Central nervous system stimulation, agitation, and anxiety may be produced by aminophylline and theophylline.[1] Aminophylline may play an etiologic role in the toxic psychosis which occasionally accompanies respiratory failure.[43]

Gastrointestinal Drugs

A wide variety of compounds have been utilized to decrease GI secretion and motility. These compounds exert their effect largely by virtue of their anticholinergic action. The nature of anticholinergic deliria and related complications has been discussed previously in this chapter. One of the most widely prescribed drugs in the treatment of GI disorders is cimetidine, to which has been attributed a number of psychiatric side effects.

Cimetidine is a competitive antagonist of histamine H_2 receptors; it inhibits histamine-stimulated gastric acid secretion, and also blocks gastrin and acetylcholine.[44] Delirium is the most widely reported behavioral complication of cimetidine, occurring in 25 of the 35 cases described in the literature. Toxic behavioral effects of this compound tend to occur more often in older patients who are seriously ill, particularly those with renal or hepatic impairment. As expected, these patients generally achieve higher blood levels with conventional doses of this compound. When deliria occur, they most often become noticeable within the first 24 to 48 hours of treatment, and they tend to clear within 24 hours after discontinuation of cimetidine.[45] Although toxic deliria, hallucinations,[46] and confusion are more apt to occur in the acutely ill hospitalized patient, some individuals receiving maintenance cimetidine outside of the hospital setting will experience an apparent drug-associated depression.[47]

Anticonvulsant Drugs

Phenytoin, a widely used anticonvulsant, may produce inappropriateness of affect, confusion, drowsiness, and occasionally hallucinations.[48,49] Carbamazepine, which may be useful in the treatment of mania, can facilitate the therapeutic effect of lithium and, at times, may increase serum lithium levels and provoke lithium intoxication with associated obtundation or confusion.[4] Carbamazepine possesses some anticholinergic action and has been reportedly associated with delirium in a patient who was simultaneously receiving neuroleptics.[50] Carbamazepine, even in therapeutic doses, may produce excessive sedation and ataxia. Clonazepam, a benzodiazepine with anticonvulsant properties, is capable of producing CNS depression and a state of intoxication not dissimilar to that seen with other benzodiazepines.[4]

Hormones

Adrenal corticosteroids may yield a variety of psychiatric symptoms, whether produced endogenously as in the case of Cushing's syndrome or administered therapeutically as anti-inflammatory drugs. Endogenous Cushing's syndrome is more often associated with depression than with mania, although either may occur.[51] Hypercortisolism resulting from the therapeutic administration of steroids may have either manic or depressive features, though steroid-induced mania is more common than steroid-induced depression. Affective symptoms may occur when steroid dosage is stable, though these symptoms are more likely to be noted as the steroid dosage is being increased or decreased.[51] Suicide may occur in association with endogenous or exogenous hypercortisolism. Steroids may also produce confusion, paranoia, and hallucinations in the absence of clear manic or depressive symptomatology.[1]

There are no clear data on the role of prior psychiatric illness in increasing the vulnerability to steroid-induced mood changes. A positive history for affective illness may increase the risk of behavioral complications of steroids, though such a substratum is not required for the occurrence of these symptoms.[4] Lithium has a clear beneficial role in the treatment of steroid-induced mania, regardless of the prior history of affective illness.[4] Neuroleptics are often necessary in the initial treatment of steroid-induced mania and antidepressants are often necessary and helpful in the treatment of steroid-induced depression.[4]

Thyroid hormones (thyroxine and tri-iodothyronine) may facilitate the antidepressant action of tricyclics and MAOIs.[4] Thyroid hormones can produce agitation and anxiety, particularly when larger doses are administered. Acute psychotic reactions resembling either mania or schizophrenia may occur in response to administration of thyroid hormones, even in the absence of other drugs or a prior history of psychiatric illness.[1,52] Thyroid hormone administration can occasionally produce emotional lability and crying episodes.[52]

Oral contraceptives have long been known to produce depression. One epidemiologic study reported a 7% incidence of depressive symptoms in patients taking oral contraceptives.[53] Progesterone is the birth control component linked to depressive symptoms, and the risk of depression may be minimized by administering those preparations which contain minimal amounts of this hormone. A significant proportion of patients developing depression while taking oral contraceptives will need treatment with an antidepressant, though initially the birth control pill should be discontinued and the patient observed for a period of time. Estrogenic hormones, the other component of birth control pills, may improve the patient's sense of well-being and may exert a mild antidepressant effect.

Analgesic and Anti-Inflammatory Drugs

Propoxyphene is a nonnarcotic analgesic that is structurally similar to methadone and capable of inducing addiction indistinguishable from a true narcotic addiction. Propoxyphene may cloud consciousness and produce psychotic reactions including hallucinations.[4,12] Addiction to propoxyphene requires careful detoxification, often including the administration of methadone. Pentazocine is a potent analgesic, which although technically not a narcotic exerts narcotic agonist and antagonist effects.[54] This compound may provoke a withdrawal syndrome when administered to patients addicted to narcotics that is similar to that seen when naloxone hydrochloride is administered to such patients. Pentazocine itself is an addicting substance when administered orally or intramuscularly over a prolonged period of time.[54] This drug is also capable of producing hallucinations. Furthermore, when patients addicted to pentazocine are suddenly withdrawn they may develop a withdrawal syndrome identical to that seen with opiate drugs, except that pentazocine withdrawal often includes the appearance of hallucinations.[54] Patients addicted to this drug generally require detoxification under medical supervision, most commonly utilizing gradually decreasing doses of methadone.[55]

Indomethacin, an anti-inflammatory drug, is most often employed in the treatment of inflammatory arthritis and bursitis. Confusional states occasionally occur as the result of indomethacin treatment. Depression may be produced or worsened by indomethacin; it has also been associated with suicidal ideation and suicide attempts.[12] Less frequently, indomethacin treatment may be associated with acute psychotic reactions including auditory or visual hallucinations.[4,12] Behavioral toxicity of indomethacin may be severe enough to require discontinuation of the medication as well as specific pharmacologic treatment of the depressive or psychotic reaction.

Antibacterial Drugs

Isoniazid (INH) is an antituberculous drug which inhibits both monoamine and diamine oxidase enzymes. Isoniazid may produce memory impairment, confusion, euphoria, and acute psychotic reactions.[4] Psychoses induced by this drug generally require that it be discontinued and that appropriate antipsychotic agents be administered.

Although seizures have frequently been reported with high-dose penicillin administration, this compound has generally not been associated with behavioral toxicity. Cephaloridine has infrequently been implicated in the occurrence of hallucinations.[56] Rifampin, an antibiotic used in the treatment of gram-negative infections and tuberculosis, has been reported to produce impaired concentration and confusional states.[56] Two other antituberculous drugs, ethionamide and cycloserine, have been reported to produce depression and confusional states.[56] Cyclo-

serine has been implicated in the production of toxic psychoses as well.[56]
Dapsone, used in the treatment of leprosy, may produce nervousness and
acute psychotic reactions.[56]

REFERENCES

1. Jefferson JW, Marshall JR: *Neuropsychiatric Features of Medical Disorders.*
New York, Plenum Medical Book Co, 1981.
2. Burrows GD, Norman TR: Psychotherapeutic drugs: Important adverse
reaction and interactions. *Drugs* 1980; 20:485–493.
3. Ragheb M: Drug interactions in psychiatric practice. *Int Pharmacopsychiatry* 1981; 16:92–118.
4. Bernstein JG: *Handbook of Drug Therapy in Psychiatry.* Boston, John
Wright–PSG Inc, 1983.
5. Avant GR, Speeg KV, Freeman FR, et al: Physostigmine reversal of diazepam-
induced hypnosis. *Ann Intern Med* 1979; 91:53–55.
6. Gaultieri CT, Powell SF: Psychoactive drug interactions. *J Clin Psychiatry*
1978; 39:720–729.
7. Ruffalo RL, Thompson JF: Effect of cimetidine on the clearance of benzodiazepines. *N Engl J Med* 1980; 303:753–754.
8. Shader RI, Greenblatt, DJ: Clinical implications of benzodiazepine pharmacokinetics. *Am J Psychiatry* 1977; 134:652–656.
9. Hansten PD: *Drug Interactions,* ed 4. Philadelphia, Lea & Febiger, 1979.
10. Malach M, Berman N: Furosemide and chloral hydrate. *JAMA* 1975;
232:638–639.
11. Hollister LE: Hydroxyzine hydrochloride: Possible adverse cardiac interactions. *Psychopharmacol Commun* 1975; 1:61–65.
12. Gilman AG, Goodman LS, Gilman A (eds): *Goodman and Gilman's The
Pharmacological Basis of Therapeutics,* ed 6. New York, Macmillan Publishing Co, 1980.
13. Demuth GW, Ackerman SH: Methyldopa and depression: A clinical study
and review of the literature. *Am J Psychiatry* 1983; 140:534–538.
14. Janowsky EC, Risch C, Janowsky DS: Effects of anesthesia on patients taking
psychotropic drugs. *J Clin Psychopharmacology* 1981; 1:14–20.
15. Thornton WE, Pray BJ: Combination drug therapy in psychopharmacology. *J
Clin Pharmacol* 1975; 15:511–517.
16. Thornton WE: Dementia induced by methyldopa with haloperidol. *N Engl J
Med* 1976; 294:1222–1223.
17. Qvetsch RM, Achot RWP, Litin EM, et al: Depressive reactions in hypertensive patients. *Circulation* 1959; 19:366–375.
18. Jefferson JW: A review of the cardiovascular effects and toxicity of tricyclic
antidepressants. *Psychosom Med* 1975; 37:160–179.
19. Risch SC, Groom GP, Janowsky DS: Interfaces of psychopharmacology and
cardiology, pt 1. *J Clin Psychiatry* 1981; 42:23–34.
20. Risch SC, Groom GP, Janowsky DS: Interfaces of psychopharmacology and
cardiology, pt 2, *J Clin Psychiatry* 1981; 42:47–59.
21. Overo KF, Gram LF, Hansen V: Interaction of perphenazine with the kinetics
of nortriptyline. *Acta Pharmacol Toxicol* 1977; 40:97–105.
22. Ravaris CL, Robinson DS, Ives JO, et al: Phenelzine and amitriptyline in

the treatment of depression. *Arch Gen Psychiatry* 1980; 37:1075–1080.

23. Ranzani J, White KL, White J, et al: The safety and efficacy of combined amitriptyline and tranylcypromine antidepressant treatment: A controlled trial. *Arch Gen Psychiatry* 1983; 40:657–661.

24. Ortiz A, Dabbagh M, Gershon S: Lithium: Clinical use, toxicology and mode of action, in Bernstein JG (ed): *Clinical Psychopharmacology*, ed 2. Boston, John Wright–PSG Inc, 1984.

25. Shon M: Electrocardiographic changes during treatment with lithium and with drugs of the imipramine type. *Acta Psychiatr Scand Suppl* 1963; 169:258–259.

26. Jefferson JW, Greist JH, Ackerman DL: *Lithium Encyclopedia for Clinical Practice*. Washington, DC, American Psychiatric Press Inc, 1983.

27. Cohen WJ, Cohen NH: Lithium carbonate, haloperidol, and irreversible brain damage. *JAMA* 1974; 230:1283–1287.

28. Spring GH: Neurotoxicity with combined use of lithium and thioridazine. *J Clin Psychiatry* 1979: 40:135–138.

29. Baastrug PC, Hollnagel P, Sorenson R, et al: Adverse reactions in treatment with lithium carbonate and haloperidol. *JAMA* 1976; 236:2645–2646.

30. McGennis AJ: Lithium-tetracycline: Toxic interaction. *Br Med J* 1978; 1:1183.

31. Reimann IW, Diener U, Frolich JC: Indomethacin but not aspirin increases plasma lithium ion levels. *Arch Gen Psychiatry* 1983; 40:283–286.

32. Kerry R, Owen G, Michaelson S: Possible toxic interaction between lithium and piroxicam. *Lancet* 1983; 1:418–419.

33. Jefferson JW, Greist JH, Baudhuin M: Lithium: Interactions with other drugs. *J Clin Psychopharmacology* 1981; 1:124–134.

34. Nolen WA: Carbamazepine: A possible adjunct or alternative to lithium in biopolar disorders. *Acta Psychiatr Scand* 1983; 67:218–225.

35. Ratey JJ, Ciraulo DA, Shader RI: Lithium and marijuana. *J Clin Psychopharmacology* 1981; 1:32–33.

36. O'Regan JB: Adverse interactions of lithium carbonate and methyldopa. *Can Med Assoc J* 1976; 115:385.

37. Gilbert GJ: Quinidine dementia. *JAMA* 1977; 237:2093–2094.

38. McCrum ID, Guidry JR: Procainamide-induced psychosis. *JAMA* 1978; 240:1265–1266.

39. Falk RH, Nisbet PA, Gray TJ: Mental distress in patient on disopyramide. *Lancet* 1977; 1:858–859.

40. Whitlock FA, Evans LEJ: Drugs and depression. *Drugs* 1978; 15:53–71.

41. Roxanas MG, Spalding J: Ephedrine abuse psychosis. *Med J* 1974; 80:411.

42. Gluckman L: Ventolin psychosis. *NZ Med J* 1974; 80:411.

43. Faden A: Encephalopathy following treatment of chronic pulmonary failure. *Neurology* 1976; 26:337–339.

44. Weddington WW, Muelling AE, Moosha HH: Adverse neuropsychiatric reactions to cimetidine. *Psychosomatics* 1982; 23:49–53.

45. Strauss A: Cimetidine and delirium: Assessment and mangement. *Psychosomatics* 1982; 23:57–62.

46. Adler LE, Sadja L, Wilets G: Cimetidine toxicity manifested as paranoia and hallucinations. *Am J Psychiatry* 1980; 137:1112–1113.

47. Jefferson JW: Central nervous system toxicity of cimetidine: A case of depres-

sion. *Am J Psychiatry* 1979; 136:346.
48. Franks RD, Richter AJ: Schizophrenia-like psychosis associated with anticonvulsant toxicity. *Am J Psychiatry* 1979; 136:973–974.
49. Tollefson G: Psychiatric implications of anticonvulsant drugs. *J Clin Psychiatry* 1980; 41:296–302.
50. Kanter GL, Yerevanian BI, Ciccone JR: Case report of a possible interaction between neuroleptics and carbamazepine. *Am J Psychiatry* 1984; 141:1101–1102.
51. Fawcett JA, Bunney WE: Pituitary adrenal function and depression. *Arch Gen Psychiatry* 1967; 16:517–535.
52. MacCrimmon DJ, Wallace JE, Goldberg W, et al: Emotional disturbance and cognitive deficits in hyperthyroidism. *Psychosom Med* 1979; 41:331–340.
53. Malek-Ahmadi P, Behrmann PJ: Depressive syndrome induced by oral contraceptives. *Dis Nerv System* 1976; 37:406–408.
54. Brogden RN, Speight TM, Avery GS: Pentazocine: A review of the pharmacologic properties, therapeutic efficacy, and dependence liability. *Drugs* 1973; 5:6–9.
55. Swanson DW, Weddige RL, Morse RM: Hospitalized pentazocine abusers. *Mayo Clin Proc* 1973; 48:85–93.
56. Snavely SR, Hodges GR: The neurotoxicity of antibacterial agents. *Ann Intern Med* 1984; 101:92–104.

28

The Psychiatric Nurse Clinical Specialist in Liaison Psychiatry

SUZANNE O'CONNOR and CAROLYN B. BILODEAU

Meeting the emotional, psychological, and spiritual needs of patients has long been acknowledged as an integral part of comprehensive nursing care. Nursing's challenge is not only to assess each patient's physical status, but also to identify these emotional, psychological, and spiritual needs. In addition, nursing is responsible for planning, implementing, and evaluating appropriate therapeutic interactions and interventions.

The psychiatric nurse clinical specialist (PCS) plays a major role in assisting staff to apply and integrate the specialized skills of psychiatric–mental health nursing into the general hospital setting.

The purpose of this chapter is to describe the scope of the PCS's role as it is currently practiced, with specific emphasis on the unique contribution which the clinical specialist makes to consultation psychiatry.

WHAT ARE THE RESPONSIBILITIES OF PSYCHIATRIC NURSE CLINICAL SPECIALISTS?

Several authors describe the role of the PCS as a comprehensive role of consultant, change agent, educator, and liaison to patients, families, and staff.[1–5] Others focus on the clinical specialist as primarily a consultant to staff, guiding their interventions with specific "problem" patients by following through with staff to outline and modify appropriate plans of care.[6–10] Robinson describes the goals of nursing specialists as "providing consultation to staff and strengthening their skills to provide more psychotherapeutic intervention to the patients."[11]

Psychiatric nurse clinical specialists are expert practitioners in psychiatric–mental health nursing with experience in medical-surgical nursing and committed to upholding the highest standards of nursing. They have master's degrees in psychiatric–mental health nursing and are trained to be sensitive observers who can conceptualize their observations within a theoretical framework. A synthesis of theoretical models in psychiatry, nursing, systems and consultation theory, crisis intervention, and adult learning create the theoretical model for practice.[10] They have working knowledge of the institution's organizational structure, operational policies and practices, and directional goals.

DEVELOPMENT OF NURSE CLINICIAN ROLE AT MASSACHUSETTS GENERAL HOSPITAL

The position of nurse clinician (currently referred to as clinical specialist) at Massachusetts General Hospital (MGH) was an outgrowth of a 9-month experiment begun in 1965 by the Department of Nursing.[12] Through the cooperation of the psychiatric and medical head nurses and nursing administration, a plan was devised whereby one experienced staff nurse at a time was rotated from the psychiatric unit to a medical unit to serve as consultant. The psychiatric head nurse provided daily supervision to the nurse consultant.

Evaluation of the experiment identified the following effects:

1. As communication improved, the nursing staff on the medical unit developed increased awareness of patients' and staff's needs, greater skill in meeting these needs, and heightened job satisfaction.

2. Those who served as consultants became increasingly cognizant of the stresses and demands inherent in a medical setting and skillful in providing support and offering concrete suggestions for nursing intervention.

3. Those serving as consultants to the medical unit also recognized their need for more formal preparation for this role.

Based on these results, a full-time psychiatric nurse clinician position was created in 1966. The role of the nurse clinician involved collaborating with the head nurse and other health disciplines in identifying the emotional needs of patients and in designing an integrated patient care plan. The nurse was employed in a staff position under the direction of the medical nursing supervisor and worked with patients, families, and staff members on six medical units.

Creating and introducing a new and unfamiliar position within the Department of Nursing was not without its difficulties. Members of the health care team needed to learn how the psychiatric nurse clinician would function and what she would accomplish. Some members of the medical staff wondered how she could function without upsetting, antagonizing, or frightening patients. Some nursing staff members thought the clinician would take over the "talking" aspect of their work, would notice they were not competent in interpersonal relationships, and would become aware of their "negative" reactions to patients. Others were envious of her relative freedom and autonomy and her lack of direct patient assignment. At times, the clinician herself felt isolated and uncertain in developing this new role. She had no explicit administrative authority but had to gain authority indirectly from nursing staff through her competence, her ability to establish rapport, and her genuine concern for the problems of patients, families, and staff.

Despite these initial reactions, the position became accepted and integrated into the health care delivery system. Gradually, additional psychiatric nurse clinician positions were created throughout the hospital.

THE HOSPITAL SETTING

There are some aspects of the hospital setting that affect patient and family responses. Massachusetts General Hospital is a major medical teaching hospital located in a busy metropolitan area (Boston). It is viewed by many as a hospital for the acutely ill where one goes for the latest in diagnostic, medical, and surgical treatment. Due to the severity of their illnesses, some patients require extensive surgery, radical treatment, and long-term hospitalization. Both patients and families may expect miracles from the referred physician, who is often one of the experts in the specialty. The patient's and family's preconceived image of physician and nursing staff may lead to interpersonal frustration, mistrust, and conflicts if the patient's condition does not improve.

Many environmental factors of a large teaching hospital may compound anxiety over illness. Often, patients are uprooted from their community and family supports and travel long distances for this hospitalization. Their isolation, displacement, and fears of urban life add to their adjustment problems. The costs of telephone calls to significant others and the cost of lodging and meals for relatives who accompany the patient add to the financial burden the patient has to bear.

Within the hospital setting, the patient and family may be confronted with unfamiliar equipment, procedures, and environment as well as meeting a host of strangers. The hospital's focus on education implies the patient may be confronted with a large number of students from a variety of disciplines. The need for research and the use of relatively new and unfamiliar drugs and treatments may enhance a patient's suspiciousness and his feeling like a guinea pig. Also, multiple transfers to and from specialized units requiring continual adjustment often occur. The patients and families are not only frightened for themselves, but also are made aware of the myriad of catastrophic events, including death, occurring to other patients.

Each of the stress situations mentioned above heightens the patients' and families' anxiety and increases the need for support.

CURRENT STATUS OF PSYCHIATRIC NURSE CLINICAL SPECIALISTS AT MGH

In 1966, MGH hired its first psychiatric nurse clinical specialist (formerly referred to as a nurse clinician) and throughout the years has remained committed to providing the services of the PCS to the hospital population. Currently, there are seven part-time and five full-time PCS's. Each is assigned to a specific nursing service (eg, neurological, pediatric, medical, surgical, etc) so that the entire hospital is covered.

The PCS reports directly to the chairman of psychiatric nursing, who is responsible to the director of nursing. In addition to being administratively responsible, the chairman also provides supervision to each specialist.

The PCS is in a staff position rather than a line position. Without supervisory and administrative responsibility for the consultee, the PCS is in an optimal position to be trusted and utilized by all levels of nursing.

ROLE IMPLEMENTATION

Administrative support, demonstrated by encouragement and sanction of the role through support for the PCS's ideas and projects, recognition of PCS expertise, and active defense when the PCS is under fire, has been identified as vital to PCS success and satisfaction.[10]

The 12 psychiatric nurse clinical specialists at MGH were surveyed by O'Connor and Berry to determine what positions in the organizational structure could be identified as having the greatest impact on their own success as clinical specialists (unpublished data, 1983). This survey revealed that the top three positions in order of importance were (1) the head nurse, (2) the nursing chairman of the assigned service, and (3) the nursing supervisor. The acceptance by these three specialists of the specialist as a person with whom they can establish rapport along with their commitment to the role, led to easier access to the staff nurses.

This survey identified regularly scheduled meetings as a most useful way to establish alliances with leadership. These meetings served as a forum for gaining information about a unit's needs; for dispelling fears, biases, and stereotypes about psychiatric clinical specialists; and for imparting information about what the specialist feels are the limits and contributions of the role.

When the gatekeepers have allowed the clinical specialist access to staff, it is essential for the clinical specialists to maintain visibility and provide rapid availability when consulted, in order to solidify the consultative alliance. The responsibility for initiating and maintaining this collaborative relationship lies with the PCS.

The survey suggested entry strategies to help the PCS become visible to staff:

Having coffee with staff to share one's sociability

Attending change-of-shift report

Attending and giving didactic teaching sessions

Summarizing the role for hospital-wide and unit orientees

Interviewing patients and families with a staff member present and then collaborating on a care plan

Documenting every contact with the referred patient

Offering realistic, concise, and practical suggestions for all nursing shifts

A useful question the clinical specialist may ask herself is, "What does this nurse need in order to let me in?" For example, while discussing with the head nurse the possibility of establishing psychosocial nursing groups, the clinical specialist may identify the head nurse's need to be in control. The specialist might then suggest they colead the group sessions.

Knowing that for some nurses asking for help implies inadequacy, the PCS remains nonjudgmental when her assistance is requested. She also acknowledges those perceptive observations the staff has made, the appropriateness of the referral, and the complexity of the situation. The PCS does not cross-examine staff or imply blame by questions such as, "Why did you do that?" but rather, "That's interesting; can you tell me more?" Until the relationship is secure, the clinical specialist gives help at the level at which it is requested, rather than confronting the nurse with the purpose of the request.

The recommendations by the PCS should reflect her understanding of the demands and pressures felt by the nursing staff over a 24-hour period. She must be aware of the staff's capabilities and be able to translate her psychiatric knowledge into practical suggestions that can be readily utilized by the staff.

The staff's anxiety about caring for a patient often serves as a catalyst for consulting with the PCS. However, their stereotypes of psychiatric personnel as weird, able to read your mind, and unaware of the stressors in medical-surgical nursing, can inhibit the collaborative relationship. The consultant needs to dispel these myths through the use of humor, a professionally appropriate appearance, avoidance of psychiatric jargon, acknowledging the stresses on the staff, and clarification of the scope and limitations of the PCS role.

Some nurses may wonder whether the PCS reports every observation of staff functioning and interaction to nursing administration. To foster trust and rapport with staff, the PCS respects confidentiality and assures staff she is not a hotline to administration. What is discussed with administrative personnel encompasses overall themes and generalized observations.[13]

Ongoing alliances with staff require continual evaluation and feedback if the relationships are to grow. The PCS needs to be cautious to avoid the following:

> Losing objectivity as her relationship with consultees becomes more familiar and comfortable
>
> Interpreting the consultee's behavior or feelings unless this is necessary for case management
>
> Increasing dependence on the PCS which may lessen the consultee's confidence in problem solving
>
> Meeting the PCS's own needs to decrease isolation by socializing with staff members

The PCS's proven clinical competence, which can be maintained by supervision and a supportive peer group, can be the most sustaining factor in successful consultation.[14] The overall success of the consultative alliance depends on the mutual responsibility and commitment that the consultant and consultee make to work together. Clarifying mutual expectations and being receptive to feedback can help keep the relationship vital.

While there are many facets of the role, the remainder of this chapter will discuss direct and indirect consultation with patients, families, nursing staff, and administrative personnel. The specific ways in which each PCS functions vary with her style, experience, skills, and the setting and specialty in which each works. Although there are unique features in the practice of each PCS at MGH, the common goal is to improve the quality of patient care. The following is not meant to describe exclusively the functioning of one clinical specialist but rather to present a composite picture.

PSYCHIATRIC NURSE CLINICAL SPECIALISTS IN THEIR WORK WITH INDIVIDUAL PATIENTS

The PCS becomes involved with an individual patient by either a referral or by case finding. A request may come from (1) a nurse, (2) a physician, (3) another member of the health term, or (4) the family.

1. A nurse

    Head nurse: One of our patients has presented a confusing picture to all involved. Four months ago his physician diagnosed liver metastases from colon cancer treated 2 years previously. His current admission was for uncontrollable abdominal pain which has decreased with a stronger narcotic. When discharge was imminent he complained of increased pain and refused to eat. I wonder if you could assess what fears he might have about leaving here and if these fears could be contributing to his symptoms?

    Nurse caring for patient: She drives everyone away from her. The minute I mention I'm going to change her dressing, she dictates exactly the way she wants it done and what not to do and talks to all of us as if we're stupid. She'll be here for weeks with this deep infected wound and we need to find a way to help her trust us more and have confidence that we know what we're doing.

    Supervisor: A patient was just admitted for surgery tomorrow. Staff suspect that he is a heavy drinker. Would you look into this and see if we need to call in a psychiatry consult preop?

2. A physician

    Internist: I've been working for years with this remarkable woman with progressive vascular disease. She is very depressed because her vascular disease hasn't responded to medications this time. I'm sure an amputation of her leg will be required. I wonder if you'd see her to assess if she's ready to hear about surgery now?

    Psychiatrist: I've been seeing Mr A. to gradually withdraw his narcotics. He has recently become a management problem on the unit and has taken a manipulative, passive-aggressive stance with staff. I thought if you could see him and observe his behavior and the staff's responses to it, you could offer additional support and management ideas to the staff.

3. Another member of the health team

    Respiratory clinician: I'm trying to wean Mr R. from his respirator because all agree he has the lung capacity to breathe without the machine. He's terrified of weaning and demands that staff be with him constantly. Your help in identifying ways we can get him to believe he can be weaned safely would be useful to us.

    Ostomy clinician: Mrs S. has refused to look at her colostomy for 2 weeks. When I try to teach her, she defers to her sister who has agreed to take full responsibility for care of the colostomy. We believe the patient needs to learn the care also since we can't fully rely on the sister who lives a half-hour away. What am I missing that would help her be more comfortable with and accepting of her colostomy?

4. The family

    My husband was recently told his cancer has spread to his liver. I've never seen him so depressed and he won't even talk to me anymore. I'm scared he's going to do something to himself.

After receiving the referral, the PCS discusses the referral further with the consultee. The PCS then involves the charge nurse and/or the primary nurse and reviews the patient's record and care plan to gather additional data. Strain and Grossman emphasize the importance of also evaluating the request for consultation to determine the hidden agenda as well as to evaluate the impact of family, culture, physician, and milieu on the patient.[15] Lewis and Levy coined the phrase "diagnosing the total consultation" to describe the process the PCS uses to decide to become involved either indirectly or directly with the patient.[10]

Indirect Intervention

In working primarily with the staff, the PCS serves as a resource to the patient's primary nurse and/or the nurse consultee. The PCS may interpret the nurse's observations and commend her accomplishments in observing and meeting the patient's psychological needs.

Staff often question, "What can I do with all I have observed?" The PCS assists by helping identify further areas that need exploration, interpreting possible meanings of behavior, summarizing the themes or collective ideas that staff express, and adding objectivity to often highly emotional issues. As the data are collected, the PCS focuses on diagnosing the problem(s) and offering realistic interventions that staff feel capable of implementing.

Working directly with staff improves their psychosocial assessment, interviewing, and problem-solving skills along with their professional self-esteem and work satisfaction. The use of this indirect approach to consultation is founded in the staff nurse's experience with similar issues, perceptiveness, and, most significantly, willingness to work with the patient and PCS.

> Mr C., a 37-year-old single lawyer, appeared to recover satisfactorily following a lobectomy for cancer. On the morning of discharge, Mr C. reported blood in his stool. A gastrointestinal work-up revealed numerous tumors. Both Mr C. and his mother became increasingly agitated and demanding. Mr C.'s primary nurse asked the PCS for "help" during this crisis.

The PCS, knowing that the primary nurse had successfully related to other distressed patients in the past and had wanted to become even more comfortable with and supportive to such patients, decided to work directly with the primary nurse. The PCS met daily with the primary nurse to process the events of the past 24 hours. Specifically they discussed what new information was given to the patient, how he responded to this and past information, and what his expressed and implied needs were. The clinical specialist helped the staff nurse identify behavior patterns and coping styles and discussed appropriate staff interventions. These informal meetings with the clinical specialist gave the primary nurse the opportunity to verbalize her feelings and concerns and to identify and set priorities on issues raised. The primary nurse then found it easier to be more objective and motivated to deal directly with the patient and his mother's emotional crisis. The PCS focused on the trust which had developed rapidly between the patient, his mother, and the nurse and pointed out how the nurse had become a significant resource.

Following an exploratory laparotomy, Mr C.'s physician informed him that his prognosis was very poor but that everything possible would be done to stabilize him so that he could return home. Mr C. was devastated and gradually talked about many unresolved issues that plagued him, the most troubling being his ambivalent relationship with his mother. The staff helped him share with his mother his past regrets and resentments which had limited his expression of love. Their relationship flourished despite his deteriorating physical condition.

The clinical specialist recognized the emotional drain that this situation created for staff and acknowledged their efforts and willingness to provide optimal emotional care. The PCS listened as staff members explored the impact on them of this young man's impending death and worked through personal grief issues which had interfered with their listening to him. The PCS focused on the positive feedback shared by the patient, family, and physician about the significant impact of staff on the patient's ability to cope with his eventual death.

Direct Intervention

The most prevalent reason for direct intervention by the PCS is to evaluate a patient's adjustment to illness. Other indications include providing support to a patient, assessing factors that may have contributed to the staff nurse feeling overwhelmed or inexperienced, and gaining insight into the nurses' experiences in caring for this patient.

The clinical specialist encourages the primary nurse and/or consultee to be present, when appropriate, during the interview with the patient to assist in the following ways:

Help the patient feel less anxious

Foster the patient's relationship with the nurse and not solely with the PCS

Provide an opportunity for the PCS to serve as a role model in communication to help the consultee improve interviewing skills, sensitivity, and perceptiveness

Assist the nurse to take responsibility needed for nursing care
Facilitate a realistic and mutual assessment of the interview.

Perceptive "diagnosis of the total consultation" using the nursing process leads the clinical specialist to make a nursing diagnosis* based on the observations and information obtained. The specialist documents the observations in the patient's chart and offers pertinent suggestions for patient management and recommendations for other referrals such as chaplain, psychiatrist, or social worker. The primary nurse generally incorporates these ideas into the patient's care plan. In addition, the PCS will contact the patient's physician directly if the observations warrant the physician's immediate attention, for example, if the patient appears actively suicidal.

The clinical specialist routinely follows the patient's progress with the primary nurse. On the basis of the initial interview as well as the ongoing information received, the PCS determines whether and how many subsequent visits to the patient are necessary. Some patients require continued support throughout their hospitalization and into the immediate discharge period. The following is an example of the clinical specialist's direct intervention:

> Mr G., a 41-year-old accountant, married, with two young children, was diagnosed with myasthenia gravis 10 years ago. His adjustment was fostered by his obsessive-compulsive personality style which helped him adhere strictly to his medication regimen and keep his illness under control until 2 years ago. His myasthenia became less responsive to medication and his total body weakness led to four emergency admissions necessitating a respirator and intensive care. During the first emergency admission, the PCS was asked to lessen his panic reaction to his near-death episode. Diagnosing the total consultation and assessing the extreme anxiety of patient and staff, the PCS decided to see the patient directly.

Following the initial interview with Mr G. and his wife, the clinical specialist made the nursing diagnoses of (1) severe anxiety due to fear of dying by suffocation, (2) depression due to loss of hope for maintaining his independence and role as father and husband, and (3) anger due to a loss of control of his chronic illness and dependence on a respirator. She planned further daily visits with patient and wife.

---

* "Nursing diagnoses, or clinical diagnoses made by professional nurses, describe actual or potential health problems which nurses, by virtue of their education or experience, are capable and licensed to treat."[16]

Her relationship with Mr and Mrs G., fostered by respect, perserverence, and willingness to work at enhancing communication, developed rapidly during the crisis. Mr G. became more direct with his anger and despair. During periods of intense emotional distress, Mr G. spoke rapidly and inarticulately. When lip reading became too difficult, Mr G. resorted to writing, pantomime, or pointing to a word chart to convey his message. The PCS emphasized the expertise and number of intensive care unit (ICU) staff and their high degree of interest in him, which enhanced his cooperation with them.

Because Mrs G. reported that her husband coped best when he understood intellectually what was happening and felt in control, the clinical specialist encouraged physicians and nurses to involve Mr G. more directly in their plans and to be aware of his need for information. What helped reduce his anxiety most was a key physician's sharing daily progress reports and hopeful comments about the time-limited symptoms and future reversal of respiratory distress.

The PCS held numerous conferences with nursing staff to discuss the needs of Mr and Mrs G., possible ways to meet these needs, and reactions and feelings of staff in response to the couple. As Mr G. improved, the clinical specialist and staff from the ICU met with the neurologic floor nurses to share what they had learned about Mr G. and assist in the transition to a new unit. The transfer went well and Mr G. was discharged a month later.

The clinical specialist followed Mr G. and his family during his three remaining emergency admissions for respiratory distress. Her consistent relationship and commitment to follow them closely and intervene with new staff to anticipate Mr and Mrs G.'s needs and fears made their crises manageable.

During his last admission, his team of medical specialists concluded that his diminished respiratory function and total body sepsis were no longer treatable. His primary neurologist of 10 years had great difficulty accepting the conclusions of the team and continued to treat him aggressively in the ICU for several days.

Mr G. communicated to the PCS that he knew he was dying and shared his fears and needs. Two unresolved issues emerged: "How can I tell my trusted doctor and friend that I want to be allowed to die more peacefully?" and "What can I say to my wife to help her and the children accept this?" Knowing how perceptive Mr G. was and how he needed control, the PCS asked, "What can I do to be most useful to you?" He readily responded that he wanted the clinical specialist to prepare his physician for his need to talk openly about the reality of his dying and thoughts about the aggressiveness of his treatments. The PCS spoke with the physician about Mr G.'s general thoughts and his high respect and appreciation for this physician's commitment to Mr G.'s care.

The physician then expressed some of his grief and guilt over needing to modify his aggressive treatments. He was ready to hear what Mr G. needed to say and, after their talk, discontinued all unnecessary diagnostic and painful procedures, increased Mr G's comfort, and transferred him to the neurologic floor where he could spend more time with his family and the staff he knew well.

Mr G.'s second request was for the clinical specialist to be with him as he talked to his wife. She did so and was there when Mr G. told his wife that his time was limited and how grateful he was for the years they had spent loving each other. In the most moving exchange, he expressed his grief, anger, fears, and regrets about leaving her and the children. Then, in his usual style, he addressed what he hoped for and wanted for his children. Later, Mr G. expressed appreciation to the clinical specialist for being the catalyst in helping his wife and him to face his dying as a couple.

PATIENT AND FAMILY GROUP INTERVENTION

In addition to working with individual patients, the PCS utilizes the group meeting for both hospitalized and recently discharged patients. Clinical specialists have led support groups for patients and families who are coping with burns, cardiac conditions, paralysis, amputations, dermatologic problems, cancer, and acquired autoimmune deficiency syndrome (AIDS).

One PCS led group meetings for hospitalized vascular patients with new or impending amputations. Since the number of available and appropriate patients varied, the meetings were scheduled as needed. The purpose of these meetings was to provide patients the opportunity to share reactions to body image changes, guilt over smoking, concerns over their ability to function independently and become rehabilitated, and reactions to illness and hospitalization. Group discussions anticipated the difficulties that might be encountered after discharge. Ideas about coping with stress were exchanged and support was readily provided by the group. Although some patients were embarrassed and reluctant to attend the meetings initially, they responded positively to encouragement from staff and PCS. Most group members felt that the group discussions had helped them feel normal in their grieving, more prepared to face posthospitalization challenges, and hopeful about a successful adjustment. Staff nurses who attended as observers learned about their patients' specific needs and concerns and used this information to make more individualized discharge plans.[17]

Another example of patients helping patients is the use of peer counseling. The medical team serves as a catalyst in initiating this technique by introducing a patient who has successfully coped with an illness to a patient recently disabled with the same problem. The veteran patient can become a credible role model through the sharing of feelings, experiences, and practical suggestions with the newly disabled patient.[18]

PSYCHIATRIC NURSE CLINICAL SPECIALISTS AND FAMILY MEMBERS

The nursing staff is concerned not only with the patient's emotional needs but also with the effects of the illness on family members. The PCS may meet with family directly to offer support during a specific crisis such as death, elicit their help when a patient is resistant to nursing care or when the goals of staff differ from those of the patient and/or family, and evaluate their responses and facilitate their adjustment to the patient's illness and nursing intervention.

The clinical specialists share their observations with nursing staff and help them integrate the family into the total care of the patient. They may also recommend a referral to other members of the health care team for additional support.

Weekly family groups have been led by the PCS for families of oncology, neurology, cardiology, and ICU patients. These groups provide a forum for sharing concerns, asking questions, and giving and receiving support. The tremendous supportive value of these groups led to the initiation of a group for families and friends of AIDS patients, which was postponed due to low attendance.[17]

In the above summary of Mr G., the PCS was also closely involved with Mrs G., meeting with her as often as needed. (A social worker met weekly with Mrs G. and her two children to best facilitate their communication about Mr G's poor prognosis.) The clinical specialist helped Mrs G. devise ways to communicate with her respirator-dependent husband, to set limits on Mr G.'s regression and overdependence on her, and to work through her guilt over taking care of her own needs by occasionally not visiting daily. Mrs G. also learned from the clinical specialist how to relate more effectively with key members of the nursing staff in negotiating change and gathering accurate information. According to Mrs G., the PCS helped give her the strength to listen to Mr G.'s urgent need to talk honestly and, as a result, they were able to work through many unresolved issues before he died.

PSYCHIATRIC NURSE CLINICAL SPECIALISTS AND
NURSING STAFF

While discussion thus far has been focused on the role of psychiatric clinical specialists in patient and family situations, the predominance of their time and effort is directed toward staff. The specialists' ultimate goal is that of working themselves out of a job. While in reality there is an ongoing need for the position, having this goal helps the clinical specialists set priorities. They assist staff members in developing their expertise and autonomy in evaluating coping mechanisms, assessing the impact of emotions on illness and recovery, and planning appropriate intervention. The staff's active involvement often provides them with optimal learning. The PCS steps into a situation only when it cannot be handled equally well by a member of the nursing staff. They are concerned with promulgating their role as a resource to nurses rather than as independent practitioners.

The group method of consultation has been a cost-effective and timesaving vehicle in helping the psychiatric nurse clinical specialists achieve their goals with staff members. They meet weekly at a scheduled time with nursing staff on each of their units. The meetings are usually nonstructured and focus on solving problems raised by the staff to improve care or resolve staff conflicts. The degree of rapport and trust among themselves and with the PCS affects the extent to which the group feels comfortable in exploring and sharing feelings and working toward a resolution of the problem raised. Ideally, the meetings offer the individual staff member insight, support, and recognition from colleagues and foster group creativity and cohesiveness.

The meetings are not group therapy, and only the issues that have relevance to the work setting are appropriate for discussion. Feelings about staff members can only be discussed if both parties are present. The specialists recognize that the more internal conflict is present, the less energy is available for external goal activity. Energy that could be channeled into improving patient care is spent on interpersonal struggles.[19]

In addition to scheduled weekly meetings, the staff may request a meeting to deal with an immediate crisis, such as a combative patient or a patient who is dying. On an individual basis, staff members consult the PCS not only to discuss patients but also to raise issues of personal concern or to request assistance in initiating counseling services for themselves. The clinical specialist serves only as a referral source, not as a therapist to staff.

Many staff nurses and managers attend the numerous workshops taught by the PCS on the integration of psychological aspects into patient care, such as contracting, management of the difficult patient, death and dying, ethics, stress management, pain, interpersonal relationships, alcoholism, and human sexuality. Several PCS's have videotaped interviews with patients to enhance further the nursing staff's awareness of the emotional needs of patients. Through this technique, the PCS serves as a role model for nursing practitioners and makes a lasting contribution to nursing education.

ADMINISTRATIVE CONSULTATION

Providing clinical expertise to nursing administrators by integrating psychological principles with systems theory and adhering to the guidelines of consultation theory can be a useful contribution to the nursing department by the PCS. Over the years, administrative consultation has become increasingly utilized by head nurses, supervisors, and chairmen of nursing services as administrators contend with more financial pressures, higher activity, and lowered census and staff shortage.

Typical requests for help may involve the administrator's dilemma in handling problem staff members, low morale due to budget cuts, staff turnover, and communication problems with other disciplines. Specific requests for consultation include how to counsel a staff nurse to accept a role in a less acute setting when the nurse is neither comfortable nor meeting the standards of the ICU. Another administrator may request advice on how she can approach staff who are repeatedly late or sick. Head nurses often ask for help in understanding intrastaff personality conflicts and how to keep morale up. When major changes in roles or implementing care are anticipated, the PCS may be consulted as to how to pave the way for the change to ensure positive support from staff.

In the following example, a supervisor talks with the PCS about the difficulty she has with a head nurse who uses considerable overtime to fill vacancies in staffing.

> *Supervisor:* She [head nurse] allows staff to make last-minute changes in the time plan, leaving the unit with below-minimum staffing. Then she asks someone to work overtime—she's already over budget —or she asks me to float staff from another area of the hospital.
> *PCS:* What have you done about her behavior in past situations?
> *Supervisor:* For 6 months I've been on her for the exact issue! [Very angrily gives a lengthy history with full details.]
> *PCS:* [Carefully avoids agreeing such as by nodding, siding with her, or becoming embroiled in her anger. Attempts to look for perceptions

and assumptions.] What do you think the head nurse might be doing?
Supervisor: [Expounds on the complexity of the problem.]
PCS: What are your feelings about this?
Supervisor: [Expounds.]
PCS: [Matter-of-factly and objectively summarizes what she thinks she heard the supervisor say and asks her to validate its accuracy. When there is mutual agreement on what has been stated, problem solving can begin.] What do you think needs to be done about the problem?
Supervisor: [Offers possible solutions.]
PCS: [Helps the supervisor weigh the benefits and disadvantages of each solution. When the supervisor chooses a solution(s), the PCS offers suggestions for implementation.]

Throughout the discussion, the PCS aims to unravel the complexity of the problem by increasing the supervisor's sensitivity to the head nurse's perspective and her insight into the possible viewpoints the head nurse may have. The PCS actively listens for recurrent themes, such as control, and highlights these for the supervisor's reflection. The PCS tries to elicit the supervisor's thoughts on approaches to the problem and offers suggestions that may be useful. The supervisor and PCS mutually weigh the merits of both sides of the issue. The supervisor is then free to decide to accept or reject the ideas of the PCS. Administrative consultation involves issues that are usually highly charged and profoundly impact an individual or a group. The administrator may look at the PCS for partisan leanings, especially in interpersonal conflicts that may lead to poor evaluations or termination of staff. It is essential for the PCS to maintain a neutral position regarding administrative decisions.[20] Occasionally, the PCS's listening and nodding may be misconstrued as agreement with the administrator's views. To maintain neutrality, the PCS may need to say to the administrator, "I'm neither agreeing nor disagreeing but this is what I have heard you say. . . ." The PCS must help the administrator to articulate and evaluate her observations and plan of action so that the PCS is not identified with the administrator's decision. Maintaining neutrality can be difficult for the PCS for reasons that may relate to the human tendency over time to develop biases and alliances. To avoid this the PCS must seek supervision and peer support meetings with psychiatric colleagues.

FRUSTRATIONS AND SATISFACTIONS

Initially, the PCS faces many frustrations in her work. Among these are setting priorities, time constraints, isolation, lack of feedback, and coping with resistant staff. To best persevere, the PCS must actively seek a peer support system to provide objectivity, a close working relationship, and an exchange of ideas within the group. The awareness of the need for a peer group is as essential to the success of PCS functioning as is education, experience, and supervision.[10] Weekly peer group meetings at MGH have been vital to reduce isolation and offer support, and to keep the individual specialist positive and creative in the role. Some members meet monthly with other hospital psychiatric nurse specialists; this adds to their improved functioning. Supervision is also an invaluable source of objectivity, feedback, professional autonomy, and esteem. It is essential that hospital administration demonstrate its encouragement and sanction of the PCS. This can be achieved by administrators permitting the PCS freedom to introduce new ideas and recognizing the contribution of the PCS to quality patient care.[21,22]

The Department of Psychiatry's weekly seminars have helped to enhance the PCS's knowledge of consultation psychiatry. The collaborative working relationship with the members of consultation psychiatry enables the nurse specialist to receive informal consultation as needed.

A survey by O'Connor and Berry of the twelve PCS's at MGH revealed that ten specialists believed that the greatest initial challenge in the role was to develop trust and rapport with all consultees and make accurate patient assessments and pertinent interventions (unpublished data, 1983). In the role of PCS most were initially stymied by the vast amount of knowledge necessary to understand the effect of illness on patients' psychological and physical well-being. In addition to knowledge concerning the effects of illness, it is essential for the PCS to propose interventions appropriate for each unit and patient situation. Many specialists felt that their greatest reward was to motivate staff to independently assess and intervene in patient management. The PCS indicated professional satisfaction from contributing to improved staff morale and interstaff communication on the various units.

UNIQUE CONTRIBUTIONS

The PCS makes a distinct contribution to the field of consultation psychiatry. The psychiatrist represents the resource in psychopathology, psychosomatic medicine, pharmacology, and differential diagnosis. Psychiatric clinical specialists are primarily concerned with contributing to the ongoing nursing assessment of patients' psychological needs, treatments, nursing care, and methods of coping with illness. Unlike psychiatrists they do not prescribe medication, order treatments, or make recommendations for medical management. Because they are nurses, other nurses can directly request the specialist's intervention for themselves or their patients. Familiarity with the demands placed on the nursing staff throughout a 24-hour period enables the PCS to be sensitive and realistic in making recommendations. At times patient referrals may be more appropriate for a psychiatrist; however, the patient, family, or physician may resist this idea. The PCS can intervene and often pave the way for acceptance of a psychiatrist.

The social worker represents the resource in family dynamics as well as social and family-related aspects of illness. The psychiatrist, psychiatric clinical specialist, and the social worker can be joint resources in psychodynamics, psychotherapy, and crisis intervention. In collegial relationships with psychiatry and social service, the PCS can bring to the team a knowledge of nursing and sensitivity to the difficulties inherent in nursing care. The PCS can assist other disciplines to be realistic and practical in their consultative suggestions to nurses. An interdisciplinary approach to the delivery of care requires each discipline to understand and respect the other's unique base of operation, contributing to quality patient care.[10]

The changes in health care brought on by rising health care costs has led to greater competition among hospitals. Hospitals and community agencies need to attract more consumers to use and recommend their services to best maintain their census. One of the best sources of marketing quality care can be nurses, since they spend a large amount of time working directly with patients and families. They are on the front lines to uphold the standards of care and the philosophy of the hospital. Individualizing each person's care and involving the patient in the planning and the control of his treatment is a key factor in satisfying patients.

The financial crisis in health care has necessitated more efficient delivery of health care through prevention and early detection of problems and through rapid formulation of treatment and discharge plans. Staff nurses are challenged to prepare patients physically and emotionally to adjust to the fears and losses of surgery, body image changes, prognosis, and treatments. The patient's usual regression needs to be minimized so that patients and families can prepare for self-care and discharge. How to maintain a good relationship with patients and families, while urging them to take responsibility sooner than they feel is comfortable is a question staff nurses frequently ask the PCS. The stress is intense on all disciplines directly involved with patients and families as well as on the administration to maintain employee morale during stringent budget cuts. All psychiatric liaison resources are in a pivotal position to assist the many patients and families that have entrusted their care to the hospital.

REFERENCES

1. Zahourek R, Tower M: The psychiatric nurse as therapist, liaison and consultant. *Perspect Psychiatr Care* 1971; 9:64–71.
2. Weinstein L, et al: Organizing approaches to psychiatric nurse consultation. *Perspect Psychiatr Care* 1979; 17:66–71.
3. Goldstein S: Psychiatry clinical specialist in the general hospital. *Nurs Adm* 1979; 9:34–37.
4. Grace M: The psychiatric nurse specialist and medical surgical patients. *Am J Nurs* 1974; 74:481–483.
5. Herz F: The psychiatric clinical specialist in the general hospital: a view. *Supervisor Nurse* 1971; 2:75–81.
6. Marcus J: Nursing consultation: a clinical speciality. *J Psychiatr Nurs* 1976;
7. Caplan G: *The Theory and Practice of Mental Health Consultation.* New York, Basic Books, 1970.
8. Cohen R: Providing emotional support for the seriously ill. *RN* 1974; 37:62–70.
9. Colbert L: The psychiatric nurse clinical specialist works with the nursing service. *J Psychiatr Nurs* 1971; 9:21–22.
10. Lewis A, Levy J: *Psychiatric Nursing: The Theory and Clinical Practice,* Reston, Va, Reston Publishing Co, 1982.
11. Robinson L: *Liaison Nursing.* Philadelphia, FA Davis Co, 1974.
12. Bilodeau C: The nurse clinician. *Q Rec MGH Nurs Alumni Assoc* 1971; 61:5–8.
13. Barbiasz J, et al: Establishing the psychiatric liaison nurse role: collaboration with the nurse administrator. *J Nurs Adm* 1982; 12:9–14.
14. Shields J (ed): *Peer Consultation in a Group Context: A Guide for Professional Nurses.* New York, Springer-Verlag, 1985.
15. Strain J, Grossman S: *Psychological Care of the Medically Ill: A Primer in Liaison Psychiatry,* New York, Appleton-Crofts, 1975.
16. Gordon M: Nursing diagnosis and the diagnostic process. *Am J Nurs* 1976; 76:1299–1304.
17. Pearlmutter D, et al: Models of family and centered care in one acute care institution. *Nurs Clin North Am* 1984; 19:173–187.
18. Guggenheim F, O'Hara S: Peer counseling in a general hospital. *Am J Psychiatry* 1976; 133:1197–1199.
19. Deloughery G, et al: *Consultation and Community Organization in Community Mental Health Nursing.* Baltimore, Williams & Wilkins Co, 1971.
20. Pearlmutter D: The role and functions of a psychiatric clinical nurse specialist in a general hospital, in *Advances in Psychiatric Mental Health Nursing,* 1982, vol 1, lesson 9.
21. Shaefer J: The satisfied clinical: administrative support makes the difference. *J Nurs Adm* 1973; 3:17–20.
22. Culman M: Role strain experienced by the nurse clinician, *thesis.* Case Western Reserve University, Cleveland, 1971.

29

Legal Aspects of Consultation

JAMES E. GROVES and JAMES M. VACCARINO

The law protects the physician who acts as a good doctor but poor lawyer more than one who acts as a good lawyer but poor doctor. Consultants—whether lawyers or psychiatrists—to physician-consultees have as the first and major task that of convincing consultees that their safest haven within the law is good faith, common sense, and the highest standard of care for the patient. Physicians suddenly confronted with legal problems tend to see the law and lawyers as adversarial to good patient care. They become constricted, defensive, and convoluted in their logic; they panic and become arrogant.

Such situations are not uncommon. During his first week as a consultant to our medical and surgical services, a psychiatric resident was asked by five different physicians seven questions of a medicolegal nature:

1. Is commitment to a mental hospital a possible disposition for this demented old man?
2. What do I do with this patient who wants to sign out against advice but won't sign the AMA form?
3. What is the liability of a house officer who forgets to note in the chart that the patient is leaving the emergency ward against advice?
4. What *is* "brain death" anyway?
5. Is this woman competent to manage her own funds?
6. What is the service's liability for actions by a resident who treats a patient in that patient's home?
7. (From a female physician) Do I have to transfer this man to a male's care just because he doesn't happen to like women doctors?

Such questions portend matters of some delicacy, and consultants not only must be familiar with relevant legal concepts but also must use this knowledge to diminish consultees' anxiety and enhance their effective functioning. When consultation requests have legal overtones, psychiatric consultants have to expand their purview. Consultees are seeking help in combating anxiety and gloom arising not only from lack of knowledge of a medical specialty not their own but also because

591

of unfamiliarity with facts entirely outside medicine—and to these facts of law they attach fearful, sinister import.

Since statutes vary from state to state and change from year to year, the following pages represent an attempt to articulate durable principles applicable to the psychiatric consultation rather than to analyze specific fine points of law.

PHYSICIANS' RIGHTS AND OBLIGATIONS

1. *Negligence, malpractice,* and *liability* are terms that are often misunderstood by physician-consultees. What they mean and what they imply are simply a physician's responsibility to the patient for failure to adhere to the accepted standard of medical practice that resulted in a compensable injury. The accepted standard of care is not inflexible or unreasonable, but a deviation from it must be justified in court by the use of testimony of unbiased observers or experts.

2. *Confidentiality* between patients and physicians is usually demanded and protected by statue and custom. Exceptions occur when keeping such confidences could reasonably be expected to endanger the life of the patient or other persons. In a California case* this concept was affirmed when it was held: "The Court recognizes the public interest in supporting effective treatment of mental illness and in protecting the rights of patients to privacy. But this interest must be weighed against the public interest in safety from violent assault." An exception to the obligation for confidentiality may occur in the case of physicians being sued by patients when the confidences are needed by the physicians for their own defense.

3. *"Good Samaritan" laws* exist in most states. They are an attempt to ensure that no liability will ensue to practitioners who volunteer their expertise at the scene of an accident. Although it is of some comfort to physicians to have such safeguards, it is, in most cases, an untested concept and quite possibly unnecessary since there exist other common law principles that afford similar protection.

4. *Refusal to treat patients,* in hospital or out, is a right that most physicians are unaware that they possess. This right obtains when no agreement to treat, implied or expressed, has been consummated. For example, maintaining a walk-in clinic or emergency room can be construed as an implicit agreement to treat. If no "contract" such as this exists, then physicians cannot be legally compelled to consider a patient's case. In a situation in which a prospective patient discusses his

---

* *Tarasoff v the Regents of the University of California,* December 1974.

or her history with a physician, it may be difficult to assert that no relationship has been established, particularly if the patient is under the impression that such exists. Physicians must clarify at the outset that they may or may not accept a case. Clearly this situation does not embody the emergent or even urgent medical problem. When the physician elects not to treat an individual, the physician should make every effort to provide an alternative course to avoid claims of abandonment, which is similar to negligence. The optimal care of the patient is the first consideration. Whenever a physician desires to dismiss a patient from treatment or to transfer the patient to another physician, the transferring physician must ensure a continuity of care by specific arrangement with the physician who is going to treat the individual. Also the physician should enter in the medical record the course pursued and the reasons and indications for such a transfer of care. In the event no physician-patient relationship has been created, referral of such a patient to a health-care facility such as a walk-in clinic demonstrates concern for the patient without necessarily creating an obligation to treat.

Knowing about the doctor's right *not* to treat is important for consultants because, often, the knowledge that a physician can cease the care of a particular patient allows enough "give" in a confrontation so that the physician's anxiety diminishes and negotiation can begin.

5. *The dying patient and the care of the hopelessly ill* are receiving such attention in the media that consultants may expect high-voltage requests for help from physicians who find themselves in situations in which the question of patients' competence to understand the nature of their acts is raised. Primarily, it should be remembered that although patients can request that no heroic efforts be employed to preserve them in the case of hopeless prognosis, this is clearly distinct from requests for active intervention to precipitate death, hence euthanasia, which is absolutely illegal. In the former case, such requests are, in their proper perspective, helpful to physicians in making their decisions with regard to future treatment modalities. Consulting psychiatrists in such circumstances should be concerned with determining whether requests against heroic efforts stem from depression or pain and whether or not patients are capable of understanding the nature of their acts and therefore capable of understanding the nature of their requests. In the instance of minor children who suffer terminal conditions, in the absence of any overriding legal requirements in any jurisdiction, competent parents should likewise be able to make such decisions against extraordinary efforts. Finally, the psychiatrist should do what he

or she can to ensure the comfort of the patient, such as seeing that treatment of clinical depression and alleviation of tractable pain are not overlooked in the anxiety that surrounds the dying patient (see chapter 17). Developing and documenting written guidelines for the management of these difficult situations can be very helpful in assuring rational constancy in approach. Appendixes I and II are offered as examples of such documents.

THE CIVIL RIGHTS OF PATIENTS

Much needed and long-awaited measures for the protection of the civil rights of mentally ill and medical patients are sometimes poorly comprehended by physicians, who may view these protections as intrusions into their domain of clinical judgment and as instruments that hamstring them in their attempts to provide optimal clinical care. In some states bills have been passed explicitly spelling out patients' "bill of rights" (see appendix III). One such is appended at the end of the chapter. Food and drug laws, new and experimental treatments and procedures, commitment and restraint laws—all recently modified— enlarge the area of anxiety for physicians who previously had to concern themselves with only consent, competency, and refusal of treatment against medical advice.

1. *New drugs, treatments, and procedures* should not be used without informed consent by patients or next of kin where indicated and proper authorization from hospital and governmental agencies. Even a commonly used drug may not be administered for an uncommon or not officially recognized indication without approval by the Food and Drug Administration and hospital committees on ethics and experimentation.

2. *Commitment and physical restraint* are areas generally poorly understood by patients and physicians alike. In most states psychiatrists can restrain patients to examine them against their wills, provided the examination takes place immediately. In some states, psychiatrists are empowered to commit patients to a mental hospital for evaluation without themselves having examined those patients. This power, however, is best left unused except by the courts. Usually, if a physician restrains a patient and then decides that the patient is not committable, the physician is not liable to civil or criminal action, provided the physician had reasonable cause to restrain in the first place and acted in good faith. In a general hospital, if a medical or surgical patient is psychiatrically committable but requires medical or surgical treatment, the wisest course is to enact commitment procedures and request the mental health facility to accept the patient but allow him or her to

remain in the general hospital for care. This commitment action must later be reassessed when the clinical status of the patient changes.

One of the most common questions for psychiatric consultants concerns delirious, demented, or psychotic patients who are being treated on a medical or surgical ward. Patients with such conditions as delirium tremens, postoperative psychosis, senile dementia, and acute or chronic psychotic illnesses with a concurrent medical illness are often frightened, confused, disoriented, and assaultive; they tend to lash out at staff, try to leave their beds or the ward, and create general havoc. Frequently the psychiatric consultant is called after patients have been restrained, not only because management recommendations are sought, but also because the staff wishes the consultant to lend sanction to the physical restraint of these patients.

The nursing care, psychotropic medications, and physical management of psychotic patients are covered in chapter 11. The legal aspects of restraint of patients on a medical or surgical ward are the concern here. In situations in which patients are incapable of understanding the nature of their acts, are in need of hospitalization, and yet are not committable under any relevant statute, it is defensible as in the best interest of patients to protect their own personal integrity by customary and acceptable methods, including restraint. In these cases the consent of the patients' next of kin should be sought as well. The justification for restraint, including history and formal mental status examination, should be clearly documented in the medical record, along with psychiatric differential diagnosis, treatment, and management recommendations.

While restraining patients may open a physician to charges of "battery" (the unpermitted, unprivileged touching of another person) or of "false imprisonment," not restraining may lead to charges of negligence (failure to follow accepted standards of practice). Although exposure to an action for battery is possible, if the action of restraint was reasonable under the circumstances and the medical record reflects such justifications, the chances for successful litigation against a physician are remote. Alternatively, a failure to restrain where such is indicated carries a greater risk of loss, both to patients who injure themselves (or others) and to the physician who is sued for negligence.

3. *The right of a patient to refuse a specific form of treatment or procedure* is ancient and has generally been well understood by physicians (eg, the right of Jehovah's Witnesses to refuse blood transfusion while retaining the right to other medical treatments). But this right is not absolute (eg, the lack of a right by Jehovah's Witnesses to refuse

transfusion of a minor child). In medical emergencies that appear to endanger the patient or in acute situations that threaten the safety of staff and other patients, the physician who acts in good faith while administering a treatment or procedure is generally not liable. In the case of chronic medical conditions, ongoing situations, and "heroic" measures to sustain life, the balance shifts back and the competent patient may legally refuse.

4. *Leaving treatment against medical advice* is the prerogative of any competent, nonconsenting patient. If patients are able to understand the nature of their acts and are unimpaired in judgment beyond those stresses commonly imposed by the hospital situation, they can leave against advice (provided they are able to understand and judge such advice) whether or not they sign an instrument acknowledging that they are leaving against advice. The consultant frequently arrives to find a patient detained on a ward by the security police not because he or she wishes to leave against advice but because the patient refuses to sign a form acknowledging that. If patients appear competent and nonconsenting, they may be asked for their signature, but they must be released even if they will not give it. Patients who are not competent and for whom it would be dangerous to leave should, of course, be restrained.

The threat to sign out against medical advice is generally more a psychological problem than a legal one (see chapter 14). If there is time for the consultant to work with the patient, the consultant often finds that there has been some interruption of communication between physician and patient; if this can be healed, the patient will often be dissuaded from leaving. If the patient leaves, major tasks for the consultant are to mollify the staff so that the patient may return later if necessary and to reassure the patient that return is permitted. This provision of some "give" in a confrontation is sometimes effective in aborting a threat to leave against advice.

CONSENT AND COMPETENCY—UNDERSTANDING AND JUDGMENT

Considerations of commitment and restraint lead logically into issues of consent and competency, of understanding and judgment. Patients may be competent and not give consent; they may be incompetent but try to give consent; they may be incompetent and not give consent; or they may be competent and give consent. But the crux of the matter is that there can be no consent unless there is first competency.

There is one instance, however, in which neither consent nor competency should be considered. That is the case of dire and obvious medical emergencies. If patients are brought to the hospital or encountered outside it with life-threatening medical emergencies and physicians, in the pressure of time, act with their best judgment and in good faith, they should not fear civil or criminal action. In an obvious medical emergency a physician must act without studying the legal aspects unless a next of kin to the patient is there and actively staying the physician's hand. Even in such an instance, physicians who act in good faith and with good clinical judgment are not very likely to suffer more than some inconvenience after the fact. Nonetheless, once the emergency is over, it is wise for the physician to chart immediately in the medical record or office notes what occurred and why the physician acted as he or she did.

Now, to return to consent and competency, there can be no consent unless there is first competency. Competency is usually *specific* and defined in relation to a specified act—to make a will, stand trial, consent to or refuse a proposed treatment, and the like. Being competent to perform one act does not mean that one is necessarily competent to perform another. Hence the components necessary for each act must be specific. About the question of competency to stand trial, for example, most statutes are comparatively clear—individuals must be able to understand the charges against them and must be able to participate in their own defense. Patients may be competent in some situations but not in others. Competency in medical matters, such as diagnostic procedures, medical, and surgical treatment, and leaving the hospital against advice must be judged by the patient's assessment of that particular situation. Nor should it be forgotten that even a patient already deemed by a court incompetent to manage his or her own funds, to make a will, or to enact a contract (such as marriage) can still be quite competent to refuse an operation judged lifesaving by the physicians. Hence the first response to the question "Is this patient competent?" should be "Competent for *what?*" When this is specified, eg, competent to refuse amputation of a gangrenous foot, the judgment hinges on the patient's understanding of three things: the illness (that something is wrong and, to some degree, how wrong), the treatment (what is proposed and why it is relevant to what is wrong), and the consequences of the decision. So notions like "live or die," "take away the pain," and "find out why you can't keep food down," become the concrete points which guide the dialogue between consultant and patient.

Concreteness, dogged persistence, and the thoroughness to satisfy oneself what the patient's true grasp of the situation is will usually produce data for a reasonable psychiatric judgment. The consultant must

Table 29-1. Factors in Selection of Competency Tests

	Risk-Benefit Ratio of Treatment	
Patient's Decision	Favorable	Unfavorable or Questionable
Consent	Low test of competency (cell A)	High test of competency (cell D)
Refusal	High test of competency (cell B)	Low test of competency (cell C)

Reproduced with permission from Roth LH, Meisel A, Lidz CW: Tests of competency to consent to treatment. *Am J Psychiatry* 1977; 134:279–284.

begin with a thorough grasp of the risk-benefit ratio of what is proposed. In fact, the strictness of the competency test should be varied as this ratio changes. Table 29-1 illustrates this relationship. The more favorable to the patient the risk-benefit is, the less one would require for consent and more for refusal to be competent. For the patient advised to undergo incision and drainage of an obvious wound abscess, acceptance hardly deserves a vigorous cross-examination. Refusal, on the other hand, could not be taken so lightly, and the more serious the abscess, the more intense the examination of competency would have to be. If the risk-benefit ratio were unfavorable to the patient, eg, proposed intrathecal cytarabine hydrochloride as a possible treatment for disabling multifocal leukoencephalopathy, refusal would not have to be challenged as meticulously as consent.

Unfortunately, patients who are incompetent for psychiatric reasons can seem competent to observers other than the consultant. The subtleties have to be spelled out. Distended, vomiting, and complaining of abdominal pain, a patient was found to be obstructed and diagnosed as having a gangrenous bowel. Surgery was recommended, but she refused. Fully oriented and intelligent, she stated she realized that failure to undergo laparotomy and excision of dead bowel was most likely to mean she would die. Psychiatric examination revealed that she was suffering from severe major depression and past psychiatric records revealed that a month before the onset of her abdominal symptoms she had stated that she devoutly wished she were dead. Detailing this information the consultant stated that her refusal could not be taken at face value. Her family was summoned and guardianship procedures begun.

Incompetence may be temporary, as when mental alertness fluctuates. Disruption occurs when a patient changes a decision with these fluctuations. An agreement with both the patient and family can be made when the patient is competent, so that care can flow as smoothly as possible. Sometimes the cause of incompetence is treatable. Occasionally a patient will refuse a procedure because of intense pain—and may even prefer death just to terminate the pain. Narcotics sufficient to relieve the pain would in this case be required before an adequate competency examination can be made. When depression is a factor, as in the case mentioned above, psychostimulants, which act within one or two days, may restore the patient's perspective so that the decision to refuse or accept can be competently made. Consulting notes in the chart, as well as other statements, must clarify that the wish to be dead is a *symptom* of the psychiatric disorder, just as fever is a symptom/sign of infection. Delirium and agitation are frequent factors in treatment decisions. A neuroleptic is the treatment of choice when no specific cause of the confusional state can be found. Failure to administer such an agent would be as remiss as refusing to correct hypoglycemia. Even in a state like Massachusetts, where the courts seem to classify neuroleptics in a separate category, their use is justifiable in an emergency. Psychological suffering (depression, paranoia, confusion, psychosis) may be even more unpleasant to a patient than the type dignified by the term "physical," and they are fully biological realities. Consultants may have to point these facts out repeatedly. Even psychotic patients have clear reasons for refusing a treatment—but it may be that voices are telling them not to be treated, that they do not deserve to get well, that the surgeon is a designated spy planted by the telephone company, and other reasons which, if only known, make it clear why competency must be questioned.

It is not the physician's task to answer questions about financial competency, testamentary capacity, competency to enact contracts, and the like. If such questions arise in the consultation, the psychiatrist's only task is to inform the consultee so that such decisions may be properly left to the courts or to the patient's legal representative. Similarly, the physician may not pronounce a patient "incompetent" in the legal sense; this pronouncement requires a formal court proceeding. A physician may not opine on issues of a patient's general legal competency unless asked to do so by the courts. Consent depends on the patient's ability to make an understanding, informed judgment on the particular question at hand. Patients who are uninformed because of communication difficulties, such as a foreign language, deafness, or aphasia, and patients who are ignorant of important aspects of their care cannot technically give consent, whether or not they are competent.

Since unconsented treatments or procedures are in most states considered battery and are more frequently considered negligence, and since consent hinges on understanding, it is at his or her own peril that a physician goes through with a procedure or treatment on a passive, confused, or fearfully mute patient who seems compliant or willing. The ancient maxim *Qui tacet consentire videtur* ("silence gives assent") will not protect physicians and is not defensible. Physicians must obtain informed consent from competent patients or from their next of kin if the patients are incapable of granting it.

Most states accept the psychiatric definitions of understanding and judgment, but these should be documented in the chart or office notes of the physician in the form of a mental status examination. Impairments of intellect, memory, attention, and consciousness flaw understanding; impairments in reality testing, sense of reality, impulse control, and formal logic flaw judgment. The presence or absence of any and all of these flaws should be noted in the formal, recorded mental status examination and their bearing on the context of an illness, procedure, or treatment should likewise be elaborated.

There are important exceptions to these guidelines for seeking and obtaining informed consent. The instance of the medical emergency has been mentioned. Another is the case of an emergent medical situation coupled with a psychiatric condition that would make the patient committable—such as the suicidal patient who refuses treatment as a means to a suicidal end.

The issue of obtaining informed consent is complicated in the case of minors. First of all, the age of minority varies from state to state. Second, the rights and consentability of minors vary from state to state and from medical condition to medical condition. Massachusetts, for instance, permits minors to give consent for treatment of drug addiction irrespective of parental authority. Third, the reason for denial of consent by a parent may protect the physician's actions—such as lifesaving measures prohibited by the parents on religious grounds. Finally, there is the notion of the "emancipated minor," a minor who is free from parental control and dominance. Generally, informed consent by an emancipated minor, carefully documented in the record, protects the physician's action from criticism by the parent or guardian of that minor.

The decision-tree for seeking and obtaining informed consent is summarized in Figure 29-1. The Massachusetts General Hospital's policy statement and consent form is appended to this chapter (appendix IV).

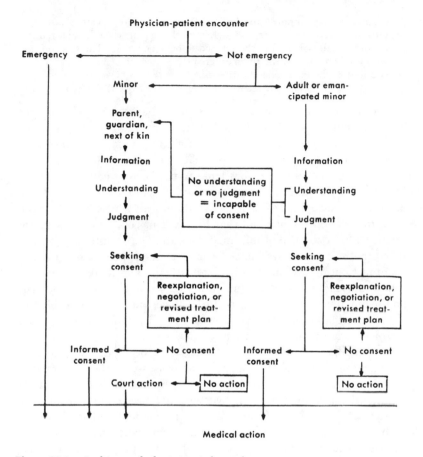

Figure 29-1. Seeking and obtaining informed consent.

THEORY VERSUS PRACTICE: LAW AND MEDICINE

This is a hypothetical case example on which most physicians would agree among themselves and most lawyers would agree among themselves—but one group would not agree with the other.

> Mrs R. was a 30-year-old woman without previous psychiatric history who suffered acute onset of abdominal pain. In the emergency ward she showed signs and symptoms of an acute abdomen that was clinically diagnosed as gangrenous bowel. She rapidly became comatose as signs of shock developed and she was rushed to the operating room for

exploratory laparotomy. Just before the induction of anesthesia she returned to consciousness, jumped from the operating table, and ran down the hall, saying that she refused to be operated on. The surgeon, who was scrubbing at the time, ordered the patient to be brought back, strapped to the table, and anesthetized. Gangrenous bowel was found, resected, and the patient recovered uneventfully from the surgery.

Under the law the surgeon's actions might have constituted battery. The patient may well have been incompetent and certainly was not consenting, but she was not examined for competency and no consent was sought from her next of kin. Fortunately the patient was happy with the result, as was her family, but had she not been or had she died, the outcome for the surgeon could have been serious indeed. Had this surgeon been sued, his best defense would probably have been that this was a medical emergency and that he acted in good faith to save the patient's life in absence of informed consent. The plaintiff might have argued that the patient was able to run from the operating room and so was in fact not in imminent danger of death and that there was time for seeking consent. And so the arguments might have gone, back and forth, and the outcome is anyone's guess. Juries in general would probably find for the surgeon, but not always. The best rule is, if at all possible, seek informed consent from the patient or next of kin.

We would like to conclude this chapter as we began it, saying that the best friend under the law that a physician possesses is the best standard of clinical care of the patient. But from the hypothetical case it may be seen that there is sometimes—and we wish to stress, rarely—an apparent conflict between optimal clinical care of the patient and the law.

What we wish to stress is that such apparent contradictions are rare, that they occur under the pressures of time and anxiety, and that anticipation, communication, compromise, and common sense often are effective in reconciling such differences. When anticipation, communication, compromise, and common sense are lacking in an apparent contradiction between the law and good clinical care, it is the job of the consultant to try to provide them.

Dr B. was a brilliant surgical resident. She called for a psychiatric consultant for Mr J. one night because the patient had refused to allow her to examine him, saying that he didn't like women. She was strongly reluctant to place him in the care of a male physician on another team, but was concerned about what might happen if his clinical condition worsened. Mr J. was a 50-year-old hemophiliac who had been hospitalized with a large inguinal hernia with question of incarcerated bowel. The psychiatric consultant found him to be a healthy-looking man who was frightened, demanding, and angry but not psychotic or suicidal. He was rational and had intact formal judgment. He told the consultant that he had "a grudge" against women because "they are carriers of hemophilia but can't get it themselves." He blamed his mother for giving him the disease and he bitterly complained that she had made him miserable throughout his childhood. "And now this dame comes along and wants to poke around in me. No dice." The consultant discovered on talking with the patient that what the patient feared was the rectal examination, which was used periodically to make sure that he had not begun to bleed into his bowel. The consultant then got a supply of rubber gloves, lubricant, and guaiac papers and taught the patient how to do his own test for occult blood. He informed the patient that he considered him not insane and not incompetent, but that the hospital was not obligated to provide a male physician in such a nonemergency situation. He told the patient, in short, that he might have to choose between the female surgeon and no physician at all. And he told the surgeon about the fear of the rectal examination and that the patient was able to do his own monitoring for occult bleeding. He also told her that she was not obligated to transfer the patient nor liable if she did not. But he did ask her to "compromise" with the patient. The surgeon and the patient agreed on an interim solution for the night: the physician could examine him if she believed he needed it, but he could do his own rectal examination.

In this instance the physician and the patient backed away from a confrontation. Enough "give" was placed in the system so that they could compromise. The consultation involved the patient's consent, which he would not at first give and then later did in a somewhat qualified way. It involved his competence to make judgments on the basis of his understanding of his clinical condition. It involved the physician's liability in the case, by which she had at first felt trapped. If the patient had begun to hemorrhage or decompensate emotionally (or both) during the night, the consultation might have come to involve a decision on restraint. If a solution had not been worked out, the situation might have come to a threat to leave against medical advice, which would have necessitated another assessment of the patient's clinical status against his ability to understand and make judgments. A changing clinical course might have altered the physician's liability in the face of a possible change in the patient's competence to consent.

Whatever might have happened, it still would have come down to an informed judgment on the part of the consultant set against the backdrop of the changing fact-patterns of the case—a weighing of the clinical course against the mental status of the patient against the physician's rights and responsibilities against probable outcome and, finally, against what was humanly workable. The consultant's ability to see what was humanly workable helped to resolve the apparent conflict between law and medicine. As Alfred North Whitehead remarked, "Reason is the horse we ride after we have decided which direction we want to go."

CONCLUSION

The psychiatric consultant to the physician having a medicolegal problem should, in addition to the usual consultation, take the following steps:

1. Know the clinical facts of the consultation.
2. Know or find out the salient facts of law concerning the consultation.
3. Know the nature of any apparent conflict between clinical care and the law.
4. Know the hospital attorney; share information and attempt to develop a multidisciplinary team approach to patient care.
5. Try to gain some time for resolution; for example, attempt to push back deadlines for procedures, treatment, leaving the hospital against advice, and the like.
6. Know the personalities of the physician and the patient.
7. Know the next of kin to the patient, their understanding, fears, biases, personalities, and the probabilities of informed consent from them.
8. Act as go-between, diminishing anxiety and communication gaps among physician, patient, family, and try to find areas for compromise and agreement.
9. Search out covert disagreements and hidden fears in the physician and patient; try to find commonsense measures that would remedy these and search for "loopholes" and areas in which conflicts can be mended or avoided.
10. Provide detailed documentation in the patient's medical record or chart of the patient's understanding, judgment, consentability, and clinical and psychiatric status, as well as the course pursued.
11. Use such consultations to teach physicians that they have little to fear from the law and to teach patients that they have little to fear from their physicians.

Appendix I

GUIDELINES FOR DETERMINATION OF BRAIN DEATH
Memorandum from the General Director, Massachusetts
General Hospital, May 15, 1984.

I. Preface

The medical and legal communities have indicated the "locally accepted guidelines" are to be used for the diagnosis of brain death. The following are proposed guidelines which may be helpful in determining brain death. These guidelines do not replace the physician's judgment in individual cases, since brain death is a clinical diagnosis. These are not intended to encourage the use of resources in order to establish the diagnosis of brain death nor do they indicate the physician's role once the diagnosis has been made. They may, however, be referred to as reasonable, current and generally acceptable criteria.

II. Technical Criteria

With the exception of II.B.2 (Ancillary Testing) all of the following criteria should be met.

A. Clinical

1. Cerebral unresponsiveness: The patient should be deeply comatose with no evidence of withdrawal or posturing to painful stimuli. Spinal level movements such as the flexor toe response or isolated triple flexion do not preclude the diagnosis of brain death.

2. Brainstem unresponsiveness:

   a. Apnea test: The proper determination of severe medullary damage requires an apnea test.

   The patient should be removed from the respirator and CO_2 allowed to accumulate while the thorax is observed and palpated carefully for spontaneous respiration. At the end of a period of time estimated to bring the arterial PCO_2 to above 50 torr, (a PCO_2 rise of approximately 2.5 torr/min can be expected in most patients), a blood gas sample is drawn and the patient is reconnected to the ventilator. If arterial PCO_2 at the end of the test exceeds 50 torr and pH is below 7.35, apnea has been adequately demonstrated.

   During this test vital functions are supported by the use of diffusion oxygenation. This may be accomplished by preoxygenation for five minutes with 100% O_2 and the use of a tracheal cannula supplying 8–12 L/min O_2 through the tracheal tube (not a T-piece). An acceptable change in pulse or blood pressure or the appearance of cyanosis requires termination of apnea testing.

      b. Absence of other brain functions:

         (1) Pupils—The pupils should be 4 mm in diameter or larger and unreactive to bright diffuse light. They should not be oval in shape since this demonstrates residual midbrain function.

         (2) Eye Movements—There should be no spontaneous eye movement. Oculovestibular testing with 30 mL ice water irrigation of each ear separately should produce no eye movement. The patient's head should be elevated 30 degrees during testing and the external auditory canals cleared.

         (3) Other—There should be no corneal external facial movement, or bulbar function such as gagging or coughing with tracheal stimulation.

         (4) Spinal reflexes—The presence of deep tendon or other spinal mediated reflexes does not preclude the diagnosis of brain death; decerebrate or decorticate posturing, however, does.

  B. Laboratory Testing

    1. Electroencephalogram: An EEG recording of at least 30 minutes duration should show no electrocerebral activity; ie, the absence of nonartifactual activity greater than 2 μV in amplitude with electrode impedances between 100 and 3000 Ω and interelectrode distances at least 10 cm. There should be no change with auditory, visual, or painful stimulation. ECG artifact should be visible. There is no need for the patient to be normothermic and recordings with core body temperature above 90 degrees are acceptable. A recording showing no EEG activity should be read by a staff member prior to the determination of brain death and appear in the record.

    2. Ancillary testing: Radionuclide or contrast angiographic demonstration of absent cerebral blood flow are not necessary but can be used in special cases (see below). Evoked potentials may be helpful in the diagnosis of brain death but are not diagnostic alone.

III. Period of Observation and Underlying Illness

A period of observation of at least 24 hours without clinical neurologic change is recommended and necessary if brain hypoxemia-ischemia have occurred. Toxicologic screening for central nervous system depressant drugs is recommended in all cases where such toxins may play a role. If the cause of coma is known with certainty and drug-metabolic causes have been excluded, then in extraordinary circumstances a period of observation of six hours with no change in clinical state is adequate.

IV. Special Cases

  A. Children and neonates: The above criteria in general form can be applied to children and neonates under the following conditions and with the following exceptions:

    1. A diagnosis that the brain has ceased functioning is precluded if there is a phenobarbital level greater than 10 μg/mL, a pentobarbital level of greater than 2 μg/mL, a thiopental level of 5 μg/mL, and a valproate level of 40 μg/mL.

    2. Brain blood flow techology is not yet sufficiently well-established or understood to justify its use in determining that the brain of a child/infant has ceased functioning.

3. Twenty-four (24) hours must elapse between that time when the guideline criteria have been met and the determination of death is made.
4. Either [Chief of Pediatrics] or [Chief of Pediatric Neurology] is to be consulted in all such instances.
5. Documentation that death has occurred is to be entered in the patient's record by the patient's physician or his/her designee; it must include a record of those examinations (and the time they were performed) which led to the determination that the brain had ceased functioning and that, therefore, the patient was dead.

B. The previous therapeutic use of high dose barbiturates for raised intracranial pressure or seizures does not preclude the diagnosis of brain death if serum levels at the time of examination are very low, ie, less than 1 mg/mL. Brain blood flow examination may be useful in circumstances where barbiturates are present.

C. Inability to examine the brainstem: When circumstances do not permit the examination of the eyes or pupillary reaction and eye movements, the diagnosis of brain death may generally be made by demonstrating EEG inactivity and apnea. In questionable cases cerebral blood flow studies are recommended.

D. Hypothermia and hypotension: Except when extreme, below 90 degrees, hypothermia does not produce the clinical or EEG phenomena associated with brain death. The diagnosis of brain death should not be made if the systolic blood pressure is below 90 torr.

V. Consultation and Recording

If the patient is under the care of a nonneurologic physician, then a staff neurologist or neurosurgeon should concur in the diagnosis of brain death. A note to the effect that the patient is declared dead and the explicit criteria used for this determination should be written, dated, and signed in the patient's chart. Physicians associated with the transplantation team or a potential organ recipient should not be involved in the determination of brain death.

Appendix II

POLICY ON "DNR" ORDERS
Approved by the General Executive Committee,
Massachusetts General Hospital, April, 1980

To indicate "Do Not Resuscitate":

A. A physician wishing to implement a DNR order must ensure that a written order is entered and signed either (1) by the patient's Attending Physician or (2) in the name of such Physician by his designee—who must be a member of the Professional Staff to whom the Attending Physician delegates the authority to so act.

B. DNR orders must be written in the Patient's Medical Record and in the Doctors' Order Book. The note in the Patient's Record should include:
   1. The patient's physical condition warranting the order
   2. The patient's mental competence and the basis of such determination
   3. A record of discussions held with the patient, his Immediate Family, or Guardian regarding the prognosis and the Order
   4. Pertinent Court orders, if there are any, relating to the Patient.

C. DNR orders must be renewed in writing at 48-hour intervals. Unless so extended, a DNR order shall automatically expire 48 hours after the entry.

Appendix III

PATIENTS' BILL OF RIGHTS

Massachusetts Acts of 1979, Chapter 214
Approved May 23, 1979

AN ACT PROVIDING CERTAIN RIGHTS TO PATIENTS AND RESIDENTS IN HOSPITALS, CLINICS AND CERTAIN OTHER FACILITIES.

Be it enacted by the Senate and House of Representatives in General Court assembled, and by the authority of the same, as follows:
Chapter 111 of the General Laws is hereby amended by inserting after section 70D the following section:—

Section 70E. As used in this section, "Facility" shall mean any hospital, institution for the care of unwed mothers, clinic, infirmary maintained in a town, convalescent or nursing home, rest home, or charitable home for the aged, licensed and subject to licensing by the department; any state hospital operated by the department; any "Facility" as defined in section three of chapter one hundred and eleven B; any private, county or municipal facility, department or ward which is licensed or subject to licensing by the department of mental health pursuant to section twenty-nine of chapter nineteen; any "Facility" as defined in section thirty-eight of chapter one hundred and twenty-three; the Soldiers' Home in Holyoke, and the Soldiers' Home in Massachusetts.

The rights established under this section shall apply to every patient or resident in said facility. Every patient or resident shall receive written notice of the rights established herein upon admittance into such facility, except that if the patient is a member of a health maintenance organization and the facility is owned by or controlled by such organization, such notice shall be provided at the time of enrollment in such organizations, and also upon admittance to said facility. In addition, such rights shall be conspicuously posted in said facility.

Every such patient or resident of said facility shall have, in addition to any other rights provided by law, the right to freedom of choice in his selection of a facility, or a physician or health service mode, except in the case of emergency medical treatment or as otherwise provided for by contract, or except in the case of a

---

Reproduced from Curran WJ: Massachusetts patients' bill of rights: cabbages, kings, sausages and laws. *N Engl J Med* 1979; 301:1433–5. See also similar statements by the American Hospital Association (840 North Lake Shore Drive, Chicago, Ill 60611) and the American College of Physicians (*Ann Intern Med* 1984; 101:129–37, 263–274).

patient or resident of a facility named in section fourteen A of chapter nineteen; provided, however, that the physician, facility, or health service mode is able to accommodate the patient exercising such right of choice.

Every such patient or resident of said facility in which billing for service is applicable to such patient or resident, upon reasonable request, shall receive from a person designated by the facility an itemized bill reflecting laboratory charges, pharmaceutical charges, and third party credits and shall be allowed to examine an explanation of said bill regardless of the source of payment. This information shall also be made available to the patient's attending physician.

Every patient or resident of a facility shall have the right:

(a) upon request, to obtain from the facility in charge of his care the name and specialty, if any, of the physician or other person responsible for his care or the coordination of his care;

(b) to confidentiality of all records and communications to the extent provided by law;

(c) to have all reasonable requests responded to promptly and adequately within the capacity of the facility;

(d) upon request, to obtain an explanation as to the relationship, if any, of the facility to any other health care facility or educational institution insofar as said relationship relates to his care or treatment;

(e) to obtain from a person designated by the facility a copy of any rules or regulations of the facility which apply to his conduct as a patient or resident;

(f) upon request, to receive from a person designated by the facility any information which the facility has available relative to financial assistance and free health care;

(g) upon request, to inspect his medical records and to receive a copy thereof in accordance with section seventy, and the fee for said copy shall be determined by the rate of copying expenses;

(h) to refuse to be examined, observed, or treated by students or any other facility staff without jeopardizing access to psychiatric, psychological, or other medical care and attention;

(i) to refuse to serve as a research subject and to refuse any care or examination when the primary purpose is educational or informational rather than therapeutic;

(j) to privacy during medical treatment or other rendering of care within the capacity of the facility;

(k) to prompt life saving treatment in an emergency without discrimination on account of economic status or source of payment and without delaying treatment for purposes of prior discussion of the source of payment unless such delay can be imposed without material risk to his health, and this right shall also extend to those persons not already patients or residents of a facility if said facility has a certified emergency care unit;

(l) to informed consent to the extent provided by law; and

(m) upon request to receive a copy of the bill or other statement of charges submitted to any third party by the facility for the care of the patient or resident.

Every patient or resident of a facility shall be provided by the physician in the facility the right:

(a) to informed consent to the extent provided by law;

(b) to privacy during medical treatment or other rendering of care within the capacity of the facility;

(c) to refuse to be examined, observed, or treated by students or any other facility staff without jeopardizing access to psychiatric, psychological or other medical care and attention;

(d) to refuse to serve as a research subject, and to refuse any care or examination when the primary purpose is educational or informational rather than therapeutic;

(e) to prompt life saving treatment in an emergency without discrimination on account of economic status or source of payment and without delaying treatment for purposes of prior discussion of source of payment unless such delay can be imposed without material risk to his health;

(f) upon request, to obtain an explanation as to the relationship, if any, of the physician to any other health care facility or educational institutions insofar as said relationship relates to his care or treatment, and such explanation shall include said physician's ownership or financial interest, if any, in the facility or other health care facilities insofar as said ownership relates to the care or treatment of said patient or resident;

(g) upon request to receive an itemized bill, including third party reimbursements paid toward said bill, regardless of the sources of payment; and

(h) in the case of a patient suffering from any form of breast cancer, to complete information on all alternative treatments which are medically viable.

Any person whose rights under this section are violated may bring, in addition to any other action allowed by law or regulation, a civil action under sections sixty B to sixty E, inclusive, of chapter two hundred and thirty-one.

No provision of this section relating to confidentiality of records shall be construed to prevent any third party reimburser from inspecting and copying, in the ordinary course of determining eligibility for or entitlement to benefits, any and all records relating to diagnosis, treatment, or other services provided to any person, including a minor or incompetent, for which coverage, benefit or reimbursement is claimed, so long as the policy or certificate under which the claim is made provides that such access to such records is permitted. No provision of this section relating to confidentiality of records shall be construed to prevent access to any such records in connection with any peer review or utilization review procedures applied and implemented in good faith.

No provision herein shall apply to any institution operated or listed and certified by The First Church of Christ, Scientist, in Boston, or patients whose religious beliefs limit the forms and qualities of treatment to which they may submit.

No provision herein shall be construed as limiting any other right or remedies previously existing at law.

Appendix IV

STATEMENT OF POLICY ON INFORMED CONSENT
Massachusetts General Hospital, July 23, 1984

COMMUNICATION AND CONSENT

A physician performing a medical or surgical procedure on a patient must obtain the patient's informed consent to that procedure. This is essential to good medical practice. It is also required by law.

Informed consent involves a process of effective communication in which the physician must provide enough information for the patient to make an informed judgement on the proposed treatment. Specifically, the physician must disclose in a reasonable manner all significant medical information that (a) the physician possesses or reasonably should possess as a physician with appropriate knowledge and technical skill practicing in that specialty, and (b) is material to an intelligent decision by the patient. This information should include:

1. The nature of the patient's condition
2. The proposed treatment and possible alternatives (including no treatment)
3. The benefits of the proposed treatment and alternatives
4. The nature and probability of risks of the proposed treatment and alternatives
5. The inability of the physician to predict results and the irreversibility of the procedure when that is the case.

The information which must be provided will vary according to the patient's intelligence, experience, age, and other similar factors. Information the physician reasonably believes is already known to the patient (eg, the risk of infection associated with any surgical procedure) need not be specifically disclosed.

DOCUMENTATION

Under Hospital policy, the physician must document, on the approved Hospital form, consent for all therapeutic and diagnostic procedures where disclosure of significant medical information, including major risks involved, would assist a patient in making an intelligent decision whether to undergo the proposed procedure. Such procedures include but are not limited to:

a. All procedures performed under general or local anesthesia, including paracentesis, thoracocentesis, and arthrocentesis
b. All biopsies and excisions (including bone marrow)
c. Cardiac catheterizations and angiography

   d. All endoscopies, excluding sigmoidoscopy and proctoscopy without biopsy
   e. Invasive diagnostic and therapeutic radiologic procedures
   f. Extracorporeal and peritoneal dialysis
   g. Radiation therapy
   h. Invasive cancer chemotherapy
   i. Electroconvulsive therapy
   j. Administration of general or regional anesthesia
   k. Insertion of centrally placed venous lines.

It is anticipated that, in the future, each medical and surgical service or department will prepare and update annually a supplemental list of all procedures performed by that service or department for which informed consent must be *documented* on the Hospital form. These lists will be kept on file in the service or department and in the Office of the General Director.

No procedure on the above list or on the supplemental list of the services and departments may be performed, except in an emergency when the patient's well-being would otherwise seriously be endangered, unless the physician has obtained the patient's informed consent, documented that consent on the Hospital form, obtained the patient's signature, and entered the form in the patient's record.

Although the best practice is for the person performing the procedure to obtain and document the informed consent, another licensed physician who is also a member of the physician group responsible for caring for the patient may obtain the consent and complete and file the form, indicating on the form the name of the physician for whom consent has been obtained. (On resident services, the chief resident would generally be the appropriate person to do so.) If a surrogate obtains the informed consent, the physician with ultimate responsibility is urged to countersign the form. The form may be completed in a physician's office but, if so, must nevertheless be placed in the hospital record, in approximate chronological order, prior to the preparation of the patient for the procedure.

If the patient is unable to sign the form, the physician should so document with an appropriate note in the medical record. A family member or close friend may sign on the patient's behalf to the extent permitted by Hospital policy and good medical practice.

Where a different form is required by law or other Hospital policy (eg, research subjects), consent must be documented on that form. If documentation on a form is not required, it is nevertheless highly desirable to write a note in the chart indicating that consent has been obtained.

IMPLEMENTATION

As a matter of Hospital policy, a patient shall not be given preprocedural medication or transported to an operating room unless consent to the procedure has been obtained and a consent form has been entered by the physician in the record. In case of difficulty, nurses or other involved personnel are requested to contact the physician and, if the difficulty is not quickly resolved, the Administrator on-call. In any case involving use of an Operating Room, the Administrator on-call will contact the Director of the Operating Rooms.

The General Executive Committee of the Professional Staff (GEC) has created a Committee on Informed Consent to oversee compliance with this policy and issue further guidelines as indicated. Members of this committee are available to meet with each service or department to communicate this policy and to instruct staff on the need for communication and documentation.

The Utilization Review Committee will institute procedures for screening records to insure that informed consent has been documented in the manner provided by this policy and will regularly bring compliance data for individual departments and services to the GEC.

MASSACHUSETTS GENERAL HOSPITAL

PROCEDURE CONSENT FORM

Patient Identification Stamp

DATE:

PATIENT:

UNIT NO:

PROCEDURE:

I have explained to the patient the nature of his/her condition, the nature of the procedure, and the benefits to be reasonably expected compared with alternative approaches.

I have discussed the likelihood of major risks or complications of this procedure including (if applicable) but not limited to loss of limb function, brain damage, paralysis, hemorrhage, infection, drug reactions, blood clots and loss of life. I have also indicated that with any procedure there is always the possibility of an unexpected complication.

Additional comments (if any):

All questions were answered and the patient consents to the procedure.

_____M.D.

Dr._____has explained the above to me and I consent to the procedure.

Signature _____

If signature cannot be obtained, indicate reason in comments section above.

SUGGESTED READINGS

Albert HD, Kornfeld DS: The threat to sign out against medical advice. *Ann Intern Med* 1973; 79:888–891.

American College of Physicians: Ethics manual. Part I: History of medical ethics, the physician and the patient, the physician's relationship to other physicians, the physician and society. Part II: Research, other ethical issues, recommended readings. *Ann Intern Med* 1984; 101:129–137, 263–274.

Applebaum PS: The Supreme Court looks at psychiatry. *Am J Psychiatry* 1984; 141:827–835.

Bedell SE, Delbanco TL: Choices about cardiopulmonary resuscitation in the hospital. *N Engl J Med* 1984; 310:1089–1093.

Beresford HR: Legal issues relating to electroconvulsive therapy. *Arch Gen Psychiatry* 1971; 25:100–102.

Bok S: Personal directions for care at the end of life. *N Engl J Med* 1976; 295:367–369.

Bosk CL: Occupational rituals in patient management. *N Engl J Med* 1980; 303:71–76.

Butler Hospital Symposium: Human rights, the law, and psychiatry. *Bull Am Acad Psychiatry Law* 2:1974.

Clinical Care Committee of the Massachusetts General Hospital: Optimum care for hopelessly ill patients. *N Engl J Med* 1976; 295:362–364.

Consents to medical or surgical procedures, in *Hospital Law Manual Attorney's Volume.* Health Law Center, Aspen Systems Corporation, February, 1973. (See especially section 4–9, Mental Incompetents, and section 6, Refusal of Consent.)

Curran WJ: Malpractice by psychiatrists in a private hospital. *Am J Public Health* 1970; 60:1528–1529.

Curran WJ: Legal psychiatry in Massachusetts: another step forward. *N Engl J Med* 1971; 284:713–714.

Curran WJ: Insanity defense in the District of Columbia: end of an era. *N Engl J Med* 1972; 287:702–703.

Curran WJ: The first mechanical heart transplant: informed consent and experimentation. *N Engl J Med* 1974; 291:1015–1016.

Curran WJ: Confidentiality and the prediction of dangerousness in psychiatry. *N Engl J Med* 1975; 293:285–286.

Curran WJ: Malpractice claims: new data and new trends. *N Engl J Med* 1979; 300:26–27.

Curran WJ: Massachusetts patients' bill of rights: cabbages, kings, sausages and laws. *N Engl J Med* 1979; 301:1433–1435.

Curran WJ: Retaliatory actions in malpractice: doctors against lawyers and patients. *N Engl J Med* 1981; 304:211–212.

Curran WJ: Court involvement in right-to-die cases: judicial inquiry in New York. *N Engl J Med* 1981; 305:75–76.

Curran WJ: Breaking off the physician-patient relationship: another legal hazard. *N Engl J Med* 1982; 307:1058–1060.

Curran WJ, Shapiro ED: *Law, Medicine and Forensic Science,* ed 3. Boston, Little, Brown & Co, 1982.

Daedalus: Ethical aspects of experimentation with human subjects. *J Am Acad*

Arts Sci Spring 1969; also *Proc Am Acad Arts Sci* 1969; 98:(2).

Dawidoff DJ: *The Malpractice of Psychiatrists.* Springfield, Ill, Charles C Thomas Publisher, 1973.

Fried C: Terminating life support: out of the closet! *N Engl J Med* 1976; 295:309–391.

Gutheil TG, Applebaum PS: *Clinical Handbook of Psychiatry and the Law.* New York, McGraw-Hill Book Co, 1982.

Gutheil TG, Bursztajn H: Clinicians' guidelines for assessing and presenting subtle forms of patient incompetence in legal settings. *Am J Psychiatry* 1986; 143:1020–1023.

Gutheil TG, Bursztajn H, Brodsky A: Malpractice prevention through the sharing of uncertainty: Informed consent and the therapeutic alliance. *N Engl J Med* 1984; 311:49–50.

Guttmacher MS: *The Role of Psychiatry in Law.* Springfield, Ill, Charles C Thomas Publisher, 1968.

Hamilton J: Malpractice from the private practice and institutional psychiatric viewpoints. *Md State Med J* 1970; 19:69–74.

Hoch PH, Zubin J: *Psychiatry and the Law.* New York, Grune & Stratton, Inc, 1955.

Imbus SH, Zawacki BE: Autonomy for burned patients when survival is unprecedented. *N. Engl J Med* 1977; 297:308–311.

Jackson DL, Youngner S: Patient autonomy and "death with dignity." *N Engl J Med* 1979; 301:404–408.

Joost RH, McGarry AL: Massachusetts mental health code: promise and performance. *Am Bar Assoc J* 1974; 60:95–98.

Katz J, Goldstein J, Dershowitz AM: *Psychoanalysis, Psychiatry, and Law.* London, Collier-Macmillan Ltd, 1967.

Lidz CW, Meisel A, Osterweis M, et al: Barriers to informed consent. *Ann Intern Med* 1983; 99:539–543.

Lo B: The death of Clarence Herbert: withdrawing care is not murder. *Ann Intern Med* 1984; 101:248–251.

McNeil BJ, Pauker, SG, Sox HC, et al: On the elicitation of preferences for alternative therapies. *N Engl J Med* 1982; 306:1259–1262.

Miles SH, Cranford R, Schultz AL: The do-not-resuscitate order in a teaching hospital. Ann Intern Med 1982; 96:660–664.

Moore M: Some myths about "mental illness." *Arch Gen Psychiatry* 1975; 32:1483–1497.

Paris JJ: The New York Court of Appeals rules on the rights of incompetent dying patients. *N Engl J Med* 1981; 304:1424–1425.

The principles of medical ethics with annotations especially applicable to psychiatry: official actions. *Am J Psychiatry* 1973; 130:1058–1064.

Quill TE: Partnerships in patient care: a contractual approach. *Ann Intern Med* 1983; 98:228–234.

Rabkin MT, Gillerman G, Rice NR: Orders not to resuscitate. *N Engl J Med* 1976; 295:364–366.

Rothblatt HB, Leroy DH: Avoiding psychiatric malpractice. *Cal West Law Rev* 1973; 9:260–273.

Saxe DB: Psychiatric treatment and malpractice. *Med Leg J* 1969; 37:187–196.

Schwartz VE: Civil liability for causing suicide: a synthesis of law and psychiatry.

Vanderbilt Law Rev 1971; 24:217–255.

Slawson F: Patient-litigant exception. *Arch Gen Psychiatry* 1969; 21:347–352.

Slawson F: Psychiatric malpractice: a regional incidence study. *Am J Psychiatry* 1970; 126:136–139.

Steinbrook R, Lo B: Decision making for incompetent patients by designated proxy. *N Engl J Med* 1984; 310:1598–1601.

Stone A: The right to treatment. *Am J Psychiatry* 1975; 132:1125–1135.

Wanzer SH, Adelstein SJ, Cranford RE, et al: The physician's responsibility toward hopelessly ill patients. *N Engl J Med* 1984; 310: 955–959.

30

Treatment Decisions in Irreversible Illness

NED H. CASSEM

Urs Peter Haemmerli, Chief of Medicine at the Triemly City Hospital in Zurich, a man of stature and impeccable credentials, was arrested at his home in Zurich on January 15, 1975, accused of murdering by starvation an unspecified number of unnamed elderly patients at his hospital. The accusation was brought by a journalist who had interviewed Haemmerli and was told that patients in irreversible coma were maintained on saline and water alone.[1] Providers of critical care have been under increasing fire from public and private sectors because of the technology we possess to provide advanced life support. Professionals in intensive care settings are in a no-win situation. Occasionally, when they try to limit treatment as Haemmerli did, they are accused of murder. More often, when using the technology in an effort to restore health, they are accused of prolonging dying, being sadistic, or misusing technology for inhumane ends. In short, we are damned if we use our skill and damned if we do not.[2]

When patients are losing their struggle against their disease, both neglect and excessive treatment are hazards. Just as neglecting to give patients treatment that would benefit them is unthinkable, use of every available technology to counter organ failure cannot always be sanctioned, even on the starkest medical grounds. A patient semicomatose from glioblastoma and in failure from cardiomyopathy is not a candidate for cardiac transplant. Nor would any physician be willing to prolong the resuscitation of the advanced cancer patient (even if it were possible) until brain death had occurred. Choices have to be made and some judgments can be difficult. This chapter will discuss certain ethical principles which can guide decisions to stop or continue treatment, a procedure for decision making, and specific situations that commonly vex patients, families, and physicians. The decisions include medical, ethical, legal, emotional, and spiritual issues. Consultation with a psychiatrist will be necessary in a number of these situations.

A MINI-COURSE IN MEDICAL ETHICS

Ethics is a philosophical discipline of which medical ethics is but one part. For the practical purpose of considering treatment decisions in patients with irreversible illness, three basic principles are extracted for discussion.

First Principle

The first principle of all ethics can be stated in the tautologic form, "Good must be done and evil avoided." Each branch or subdivision of ethics then specifies the specific good and specific evil unique to it. In medical ethics, the first principle is traditionally divided into two parts. The first of the two principles specifies the evil to be avoided, namely *primum non nocere*, "first do no harm." The good to be done by the physician is stated in a twofold manner: the doctor must restore health and must relieve suffering. As Slater pointed out, problems of treatment limitation arise when these two aspects of moral good conflict: For some patients the more we do to restore their health, the more suffering we cause them.[3] When a young woman with breast cancer metastatic to liver and lungs and negative estrogen-binding receptor protein presents herself for treatment, almost anything done to attack a malignancy has a 90% chance or better of making her feel worse, without any therapeutic impact on the cancer.

By definition, the patients discussed in this chapter are beyond restoration of health, if such is construed as "cure." As the disease worsens, the treatment goal shifts toward avoidance of undue procedures, preoccupation with side effects, and attention to comfort. Nevertheless, portrayal of this shift does insufficient justice to the spirit of aggressive optimism that should pervade a treatment program. A good model, fully in keeping with this first principle of medical ethics, would be: "Palliate everything, exacerbate nothing." Appropriately aggressive in tone, it addresses that necessary eagerness to maximize the patient's health, while including judicious caution for minimizing suffering.[4]

Second Principle

The second principle stresses the primacy of the patient's will in the decision-making process and is sometimes stated, "Let the will of the patient, not the health of the patient, be the supreme law." Based on the patient's legal right to privacy, this principle affirms the patient's right to refuse any treatment. In other words, from the point of view of a contract, the first principle guarantees that the physician recommends a decision that is medically best for the patient, whereas the second principle guarantees that the patient is free to accept or reject it. (In a sense these two poles represent the ethics of the 1950s and 1960s—the best for the patient—and the ethics of the 1970s—the autonomy of the patient.) The patient's right to receive treatment or to demand a specific treatment are separate, distinct issues.

However, five factors may impair the patient's ability to choose competently.

1. Pain and other physical symptoms may be so intense that the patient would rather die than consider any procedure. Prolonged, severe discomfort can distort a person's ability to make rational decisions, sometimes leading the patient to reject helpful measures or to grasp at useless ones. Immediate relief of such suffering should be sought. Afterward, a better determination can be made of whether the patient genuinely desires to refuse treatment.

2. Treatable depression may make it impossible to take a patient's treatment refusal at face value. For example, a rather healthy patient with recurrent colon cancer was found with acute fever, cough, increased sputum production, and clinical signs of pneumonia. He had been severely depressed for a month and had expressly stated on several occasions that he wished he were dead and wanted to die. He refused transfer to the emergency ward and when asked whether he understood that this could result in a fatal outcome he replied that he not only understood it but wanted to die. The problem in accepting his judgment is that he wanted to die before he ever got the pneumonia, so that this refusal of treatment seems possibly more related to his prior depression than to his pneumonia. Aggressive treatment of depression is part of appropriate palliation.

3. An emergency may arise in which the patient cannot express an opinion, when the physician must act in accord with the patient's best interests as the physician sees them.

4. The patient may become incompetent by reason of delirium, dementia, coma, or some mixture of all three. In such a case the dialogue about treatment choices is then ordinarily conducted with the patient's next of kin, whose obligation is to judge what the patient (not they) would want done. If the delirium is treatable, psychiatric consultation could be extremely helpful as it could in paragraph 3.

5. Some patients may accept or refuse lifesaving treatment based on coercion by another party. A family may want the patient to hang on longer than the patient does or undergo suffering the patient does not want to endure, or they may wish the patient to give up quickly so that

they themselves may be spared suffering, come into an inheritance earlier, not squander family resources on treatment, etc.

The Dialogue

Dialogue with a competent patient can be viewed as a discussion of the risk-benefit ratio of a specific treatment course. The physician's responsibility is to spell out the nature of the treatment, the probable benefits to the patient, and the cost (including suffering). The patient's responsibility is to state whether he will take these risks in exchange for that benefit. Moreover, the patient almost always expects the physician to express his best clinical judgment about the balance of good and bad and to offer a recommendation for or against the option. For a patient whose recurrent bladder cancer was becoming progressively symptomatic, the question of further surgery may arise. The physician might say, "At this point, it is worth raising the question about another exenteration procedure. The second procedure was an ordeal for you. It was painful, and we had a good deal of trouble controlling the infection and hemorrhage. After those 5 weeks in the hospital, in spite of a pulmonary embolus, you managed to get back on your feet and got around reasonably well for 3 months. A third procedure surely guarantees even more trouble with pain, infection, hemorrhage, and other complications. If you do recover from it, I would not expect you to remain well for 3 months. I am reluctant to recommend the procedure."

After further dialogue about these realities, one patient might reply, "On no account would I go through that again," whereas another might say, "Even if there is a remote chance for a bit more decent quality time, I'd like to take it." There are no fortune tellers in medicine, only fallible clinicians, and second opinions are welcome. However, patients appreciate being able to count on the physician's honest judgment to protect them from foolish and costly risks.

Third Principle

Stopping a treatment is ethically no different from never starting it. Granted, discontinuing a mechanical ventilator for a comatose patient is much more difficult psychologically than never starting it, but ethically and legally, the two acts are equivalent. Let us suppose that 2 months after achieving an excellent remission from a lymphoma, a 25-year-old man is brought to the emergency ward comatose and without spontaneous respiration. Initial examination does not reveal a cause for his deterioration, or, if the cause is known (eg, hemorrhage), whether it can be reversed. Does one intubate him? If, at that point, God appeared and announced that the patient had developed extensive infiltrating brainstem involvement that left him beyond treatment, the physicians would thank Him, dispense with the intubation and resuscitation, and pronounce the patient dead when asystole came. Lacking this diagnostic and prognostic gift, however, they intubate and sustain him in the intensive care unit (ICU). Two weeks later, they have come to the same diagnostic conclusion about the patient, who has remained in coma, his breathing sustained by the ventilator.

Now, however, should a physician point out that the ventilator is no longer necessary, an accuser is likely to emerge, announcing that discontinuation of the ventilator is tantamount to homicide, since the patient will die when it is disconnected. But what justified the initial use of the ventilator was the possibility of the patient's coma being reversible. It is this that continues to justify use of the ventilator. Once it is clear that the coma is not reversible, the ventilator is no longer necessary. In this patient, moreover, it cannot be justified and should be discontinued. Emotionality clouds and prevents effective use of this principle. Any medical treatment is justified by the benefit it brings to the patient. When it is begun and later found to provide no such benefit, it ceases to be necessary.

A PROCESS FOR MAKING TREATMENT CHOICES

No universal criterion or formula exists whereby a specific choice can be made. At times, medical expertise clearly dictates the options. For instance, in evaluating a gastrointestinal (GI) bleeder, it may be quite clear that definitive means for treating the hemorrhage have been exhausted or have no possibility of working, as in considering a third gastric or esophageal reconstruction for a patient whose second procedure made such a conclusion unmistakable. Many decisions seem much less clear.

Judging reversibility. Whether, in fact, the illness can be reversed, or how far it can be reversed is the first and most basic question. Will an individual recover from coma? Will further surgery or chemotherapy result in some improvement or only more suffering? These are not ethical but clinical questions best answered by persons with the most advanced knowledge and best clinical judgment. In our experience the first and more urgent question raised by patients and families is focused on the severity of the illness. Some of the ethical literature seems to assume that this question has already been answered. In fact, the problem is actually worsened by discussion of "hopelessly" or "irreversibly" ill patients, because the label assumes the outcome is already known. In most cases, the confidence with which the label "irreversible" can be applied depends entirely on the clinical judgment of the primary physician along with the best available consultations. No committee is equipped to give this expertise (unless explicitly chosen and designated as a prognosis committee). This concern about reversibility—or how helpful any treatment can be—is best shared by the physician with the patient and family. It is a mutual concern.

Introducing the dialogue. How can one tell a patient that treatment limitation is appropriate for discussion and yet not rob him or her of hope? Honesty requires the admission that it may be impossible. The physician needs some way of introducing a discussion of carefully chosen options. The earlier in the course of treatment this occurs, the more comfortably it is likely to proceed. There is no need to start the discussion with direct focus on the incurability of the disease. To the young woman mentioned above who was found to have stage IV breast cancer, the physician might say: "Since we will have to be making decisions about the treatments that are best for you, let me describe a philosophy for choosing. First, no matter how complex the technology of the treatment, if it's sure to help, it will always be available to you. At the same time, many of our treatments for cancer are dangerous and harmful. I refuse to use treatments just because they are there. If a treatment were proposed for you, for example, which I thought would only hurt and not help you, I would tell you that I am against using it and why."

The point of this opening is to reassure the patient that her doctor intends to protect her from inappropriate treatments. It is not a small favor. Moreover, this introduction is brief, and should be followed by silence in order to allow the patient to respond. If given the opportunity, the patient will often specify goals and preferred methods for making judgments about treatments. Some patients will even spell out their wishes about resuscitation, life prolongation, respirators, and the like. By contrast, the physician who tries to deliver an uninterrupted didactic lecture is likely not only to fail, but also to get himself into unnecessary trouble, usually due to the patient's misinterpretations of something in the lecture. The opening statement, then, states or restates the concern about doing no harm to the patient, and is made deliberately brief to give the patient the opportunity for self-disclosure. An additional element in the dialogue might be an invitation to the patient to share responsibility for the choice: "Whenever we start one of these potentially harmful treatments, I need to know that you have some idea of what you're getting into and that you agree to it."

Detailed reviews of history.   No matter how well prepared, some patients or families will still be horrified when the physician introduces the notion that treatment limitation may be necessary. Reminding them at that point in detail what the patient has been through can be powerful and helpful. An elderly woman with small cell carcinoma metastatic to brain, responsive only to pain, had suffered a series of episodes of aspiration pneumonia. Someone has suggested use of a gastrostomy tube, but it had not been placed. After another episode of pneumonia, more extensive than the last, the patient was hospitalized for intravenous (IV) antibiotic therapy at her family's insistence. After ten days, she was still spiking fevers.

When the physician expressed his plan for switching the patient to oral antibiotics and returning her home to die, the family was initially horrified and thought this was "practicing euthanasia," by which they meant neglectful homicide. The doctor then reviewed her course: diagnosis, lobectomy, radiation, 6 good months, discovery of brain metastases with slow but relentless deterioration, inadequate gag reflexes, and increasingly frequent pneumonias not prevented by placement of a nasogastric tube. To prevent aspiration, she already required round-the-clock suctioning, a procedure manifestly uncomfortable to the patient. After explaining that the nasogastric tube failed to prevent aspiration because of the nearly constant aspiration of oropharyngeal secretions, the physician then spelled out what might be required to stop the aspiration definitively: surgical placement of a gastrostomy tube, tracheostomy, and perhaps surgical closure of the vocal cords and upper trachea. The family began by thinking the therapeutic intervention relatively simple: How could anyone refuse this patient antibiotics? The itemization of details and consequence of the treatment and especially hearing the context of the entire illness erased their doubts about its appropriateness. "We'd never want to put her through that, doctor."

Thinking ahead.   Forethought is important to ensure appropriate treatment when the unexpected happens. Suppose, in desperation, a patient with advanced cancer asked for a trial of a phase I drug and was placed on it. After 1 week, he feels neither better nor worse. What should be done if he has a sudden cardiac arrest? The physician who prescribed the drug, fearing it may have caused the arrest, may automatically assume the patient should be resuscitated. Such an assumption is erroneous and would be motivated primarily by guilt. The decision to resuscitate depends, as argued above, on the chances of the treatment being sufficiently successful to satisfy the patient. If the phase I drug caused ventricular tachycardia which could be reversed by administration of lidocaine or countershock, the doctor might reasonably try these without questioning their appropriateness. If an asystolic arrest, however, appeared to be the result of the natural disease process, it would be much more difficult to justify initiation of cardiopulmonary resuscitation (CPR). The decision may not be easy, but guilt feelings about the use of a potentially dangerous agent, to which the patient agreed, are extraneous. The situation is similar to that of choosing high-risk surgery over a lingering illness. Even if death occurs, it was a risk that the patient chose to take and, in fact, one he preferred over living as he was prior to surgery.

Change. There is no guarantee that having made a decision the patient will not change his or her mind about CPR or about the general amount of suffering that is an acceptable price to pay for a little more time or for the chance of "getting back to baseline" briefly. If the woman with stage IV breast cancer chose to forego any treatment, discussion could proceed as follows: "Of course, our goal will be to keep you functioning as well as possible at all times and to avoid hospitalization unless necessary. You should call us and discuss any new symptoms or problems. If you develop something serious like a pneumonia, it might be more comfortable for you to be in the hospital; it certainly is always available to you. [Pause. She replies she'd like to avoid hospitalization at all costs.] I'll remember that and support it, although you can change your mind at any time. By the way, if something totally unexpected happens—say, if you faint, your family is likely to zip you right in here anyway." Whether the patient approves of her family doing this or not, this is an excellent opportunity to remind her that the family cannot be realistically excluded from these choices. Decisions will be much more harmonious, and usually more easily made when family members are included from the start.

Consensus. No "right" decision may be available. Choices must be made and some consensus has to be reached with the realization that surprises are in store. For example, as a patient's respiratory distress worsens progressively, a choice must be made between giving more morphine for comfort and resorting to additional diagnostic tests or brief aggressive therapy. If the choice were made to give morphine and the patient slowly improved, was it the "wrong" choice? Choices are made frequently and the results usually help to clarify subsequent choices. But choices have to be made. Nor does agreement by all guarantee a pleasant outcome: Death is inevitable and despite all efforts to prevent it, suffering is common.

For practical reasons physicians should be cautious about defining "quality of life" for the patient, since an outcome repulsive to one may be acceptable to another. Mental anguish is subjective. Some religious persons "offer up" their sufferings as part of their commitment to a transcendent plan or accept it as part of their relationship to God. The physician's philosophical or religious reasoning may be of no interest to the family—in fact, it may be viewed as hostile if it differs from theirs, especially at times of life-and-death crises. Keeping things basic, the physician is better off saying something like, "Look, my expertise is in the nature of body organs, how they go wrong, what has to be done to make them work better, and what dangers accompany drugs and other treatments we can use to help." When the parents of a retarded child with terminal cancer already have a highly developed sense of their child's right to the best medical care, efforts to restrict treatment on the basis of retardation would be not only unethical but unkind. Pointing out, however, that the child's inability to understand the purpose of a treatment could increase his suffering is both necessary and helpful in a discussion of treatment limitation.

COMMITTEE CONSULTATION ABOUT TREATMENT DECISIONS

In late 1973 at Massachusetts General Hospital (MGH) a subcommittee of the Critical Care Committee was formed to study the treatment of irreversibly ill patients. The initial task of the subcommittee, named the Optimum Care Committee, was to compile data. Shortly thereafter the committee became official and functioned on a regular basis in the hospital.[5]

The number on the committee was deliberately kept at a minimum: a psychiatrist as chairman, an oncologist, a general surgeon, the nursing supervisor of all the ICUs, the hospital lawyer, and a patient, a woman who had undergone a shoulder disarticulation for a rare and highly malignant bone tumor. The psychiatrist (the author) is a Jesuit priest with formal training in ethics, the nursing supervisor was a religious sister, and the patient was a physical therapist at another hospital. Three members of the committee were women, three were men; five members were white, one was black. Representation of varying disciplines was limited to one member from medicine and one from surgery. More important in the selection of the physician members was that they be widely respected by the members of their own specialty and that they be known for their ability to get along with practically everybody. Whenever committees are involved, primary physicians may feel criticized. Individuals who are least threatening in this way are therefore most valuable because a wide basis for trust has already been established.

The committee has undergone some change. The patient member decided after 2 years that the reasons for inclusion of a layman on the committee were insufficient to justify her continuing and there was no reason for such a presence other than window dressing. The oncologist died and was replaced by a cardiologist with a JD degree. Another nursing supervisor has replaced the first member. The hospital lawyer was replaced and then was advised by chief counsel of the hospital to withdraw from the committee because of conflict of interest.

The committee gives a consultation, and, like any consultant, serves in an advisory capacity only to physicians, in situations where a decision about continuing or stopping life-support therapy exists. The request must come from the responsible physician, although on occasion pressure can be brought to bear on this individual by an ICU director or head nurse. The responsible physician may reject the committee's recommendations, although this is rare.

When a consultation is called, the chairman notifies two of the remaining three committee members—the internist for a medical patient and the surgeon for a surgical patient. The two physicians go to the patient's floor, read the chart, and talk to whomever they need to talk to to learn about the case. The nurse member interviews the nursing staff on the floor to find out what they know about the patient, the family, the dilemma, and whether there are any staff nurses who would be opposed to limitation of treatment on the given patient. When some consensus is reached the committee chairman writes a formal note in the patient's chart.

Committee consultation is rare when compared with all the treatment limitation decisions made in the hospital. Physicians and families together are usually able to make these difficult decisions. When consultation is requested, the problem discovered often requires psychiatric consultation. Some of these are listed below.

OBSTACLES TO REACHING CONSENSUS ABOUT TREATMENT LIMITS

Family conflict. Most common of all obstacles is the setting in which physicians and most family agree that the patient, typically incompetent, should not undergo CPR or further aggressive medical treatments aimed at restoring an irreversible illness. One family member, however, disagrees. If the problem is difficult enough to reach a committee consultation, either individual or family pathology or both is usually serious. Most commonly the objecting family member is hostile toward the patient. Typical is the son who lives on the opposite coast, has not had any regular contact with the patient for one to two decades, and materializes at the end of life to criticize all those involved in the patient's treatment. Although some of these persons have relatively stable personality disorders, others are severely disturbed. Psychiatric evaluation may be helpful if the family member will accept it, which is not common.

It is not uncommon for a mother to go to irrational lengths to protect a child (no matter the child's age), although extraordinary resistance may be an effort to see whether or not the physicians really believe that the illness is hopeless. Most of these women had no intention of encouraging harmful treatments, but any uncertainty in the treating physician could be construed as lack of investment in the patient and the treatment limitation recommendation accordingly rejected.

For family conflict a meeting of the family is exceptionally helpful. Usually the pathologic member has been able to function as a quasi-spokesman, but the ability to do this can often be contained if all family members are present.

Physician-nurse conflict caused by consultants. Now increasingly unusual, this problem came to our attention in a few disputed cases where the primary physician wished to proceed with lifesaving treatment and the nursing staff were uniformly opposed. Some of these cases occurred even though the reasons given by the physicians were solid and clearly documented in the chart. It came to light that either the consultants (in the case of private physicians) or an intern (in a case of the chief resident) undermined the confidence of the nurses and the primary medical judgment by making bedside comments such as "What a waste of time" or "This man's EEG is no more active than a grapefruit's." Another junior resident referred to a pending trip of a patient to the operating room as a "warm post[-mortem examination]." The nurses, who were in effect performing 24-hour resuscitation on these very sick patients, were demoralized by these remarks, concluded that their own efforts were meaningless, and questioned the value of therapeutic procedures. Clarification of such issues with physicians and nurses resolves the conflict.

Interdisciplinary conflict. One disputed case brought to light a feeling of conflict between surgeons and anesthesiologists in an ICU. When a surgeon's patient, whose planned gastrostomy generated considerable protest from the ICU physicians, was taken to the operating room for the procedure, he arrived with a systolic blood pressure of 40 mmHg and an arterial pH of 7.09. The surgeons were furious and saw the inadequate ventilation of the patient in transit as the ICU's way of thwarting their own plans to treat the patient, thereby hastening his death. Subsequent discussion revealed that the feelings of mutual mistrust were deeper than the conflict over the care of this one patient. His care had become the occasion for expressing the pre-existing animosity. The two groups were willing to meet jointly so that the conflicts could be minimized in the future.

Patients who don't die "on time." A woman with end-stage cardiac disease, dependent on the intra-aortic balloon pump (IABP), could no longer use this device and it was removed. Death was expected, but she lingered on for several days. On the tenth day there was an outburst among the nursing staff coupled with severe criticisms of the inhumane medical treatment of the woman. When asked what they considered inhumane, they said that the pressor infusion should not be continued. Because they knew, on reflection, that stopping the pressor was followed by pulmonary edema, a terrible way to die, further explanation was sought for their feelings. It turned out that the patient had a rather difficult and contentious personality and remained alert and contentious after the IABP was stopped. The psychological set on the part of both the nursing staff and the patient's family geared them for a short rather than a long vigil. When the time began to drag on, both family and staff found the patient's behavior trying, became more irritable, and blamed "overtreatment" for the problem.

Jackson and Youngner identified other sources complicating treatment decisions in patients: patient ambivalence, major depression, the use of a plea for death with dignity by a patient to identify a hidden problem (it was a plea for attention), a patient who demanded out of fear that treatment be withheld, patient-family conflict, and misconception by some of the ICU staff of a patient's concept of death with dignity.[6]

FURTHER DILEMMAS IN LIMITING TREATMENT

Even when universal consensus about treatment limitations is reached, the choices, though guaranteeing the noble aim of minimizing suffering, remain tinged with tragedy. The patient is going to die. Loss, bereavement, and perhaps feelings of abandonment will follow. Strong feelings about the death of the patient probably account for most or all of the specific difficulties recounted below.

Patient's loss of hope. Hope may be carried by the patient in an exceedingly fragile vessel. Is there a danger that a discussion of limits, "do not resuscitate" (DNR), and the like will shatter that vessel, cause the loss of hope, and produce despair? The strength of patients is commonly underestimated by their families and physicians alike. If the patient has equanimity in the face of terminal illness, it will emerge in early discussions about diagnosis or later ones about appropriate treatment. Sooner or later, the physician will encounter a patient who makes it quite explicit that not only is death frightening but that treatments are the "only hope."

A woman in her mid-50s who, with the help of radiation therapy and combination chemotherapy, had survived with pancreatic carcinoma for 14 months, was hospitalized with bowel obstruction due to recurrence. She was receiving only 5-fluorouracil (5-FU) at the time. Believing chemotherapy was not helping her, her oncologist informed her of his plan to stop it. "What will you give me in its place?" she wanted to know. When he said that he did not intend to replace it with another drug because of the toxicities of other agents, she said "If you are not giving me something for my cancer, I will lose hope." Her oncologist, taken aback, said that her body "needed a rest from chemotherapy for a while," that chemotherapy can also do harm, that the good should not be outweighed by the harm, that 5-FU had not helped over the last 3 months, and that he had pushed it to the point of lowering her white blood cell [WBC] count—the body's way of signaling we had to back off. She countered that she had heard of streptozocin; couldn't he use that? Familiar with the latest drug protocols, he replied that its record was poor, its toxicity significant, and he would not even consider it because he thought it would hurt her. Without treatment, she repeated, she would lose hope. Perplexed, he said that he would return to discuss it further the next day; since her WBC count was marginal, he would hold her 5-FU (as he had in the past).

The next day the oncologist asked the patient if she understood that new, untried drugs could cause her harm without making any impact on her cancer. She understood. Then why would she want such a drug? Again, "If I don't have it I'll lose hope." Mystified, the physician gently asked a crucial question: "Hope *for what*?" The woman was momentarily speechless (this specific question had not occurred to her). "I don't know," she answered, "It certainly is not for cure; I understood from the beginning that this can't be cured. . . . Maybe it is that I want to get home again and back onto the golf course." A new anticancer drug would make that *less* likely, the oncologist told her. The patient replied, "I know that whether or not you give me a drug you will still take care of me, so it isn't that." Although they talked longer, she could not figure out why she had felt so strongly. On the following day she told him that she felt much better and appreciated the prior day's discussion. "My sense of fear is gone; it's still not clear to me, but I've regained the feeling that I'll be all right." Curious, her oncologist asked what she would think if, without informing her, he had given her a placebo and told her it was streptozocin. "Why, that would be a betrayal! I wouldn't approve of that," was her reply. The encouragement to spell out what she meant by hope seemed to have helped this patient considerably.

The problem of nutrition and feeding. Is there a time when food should be forced on the patient? Should it ever be withheld? Almost as simple a given in nature as oxygen, food can likewise present vexing difficulties for those caring for advanced cancer patients. "Starvation? I can't approve of that for anyone!" is an example of the spontaneous emotion generated by the question of withholding food. Reality, however, makes the question unavoidable for certain patients. Some patients' GI tracts become obstructed by extensive metastatic disease, and they cannot eat. In a few cases, a jejunostomy tube may bypass gastric obstruction. Total parenteral nutrition (TPN) is available, but it is an option that many cannot receive at home. Many patients (and physicians) perceive it as "extreme" and do not consider it, especially if they are already being cared for as outpatients. When a patient with intestinal obstruction has been admitted for further diagnosis, placed on TPN, and found to have untreatable extension of disease, then the question of stopping TPN can be a tense one, even when continuation of TPN makes no medical sense.

A discussion with such a patient could begin gently with, "I wanted to discuss with you some reservations I have about TPN and what I see are its disadvantages." Mention each reservation, one at a time, giving the patient adequate opportunity to disclose his thoughts. Examples of topics that could serve sequentially to develop a dialogue include: having to remain hospitalized, lack of freedom of movement, possible aggravation of ascites, complications of the indwelling catheter, and possible (even disproportionate) contribution to tumor growth with consequent worsening of current symptoms. Some patients will quickly reject continuation (or beginning) of TPN. For others, the dialogue will produce the fear, "I will lose hope," as discussed above.

Faced with a nutrition dilemma, the physician returns to the most radical of all questions about treatment: What *good* will it accomplish for the patient? For the advanced cancer patient, *no* procedure or agent can be given unreflective approval. Food is no exception. When illness cannot be reversed and the patient is dying, comfort usually takes precedence. With the conscious patient, the physician may have to argue softly against the benefits of calories. Calories do not necessarily increase comfort. If they do not, what justifies their use? (The principle here remains the "first" one: Every treatment must be justified; only those treatments are justifiable whose benefits outweigh the risks.) The risk of ordering administration of calories is that of increased suffering. The benefits are maintenance of the energy requirements of body organs and single cells. In the patient for whom aggressive treatment is maintaining only marginal aeration or even pain control, will added calories alleviate or worsen the situation? The answer to this question justifies or disqualifies their use. Moreover, a hard-core medical judgment is required by this question. Both the patient and family need this judgment to anchor their own perspective, which seldom if ever allows them to foresee specific medical complications the way the physician does.

Discussions of calories far more commonly arise between doctor and family after the patient has ceased to be competent or even conscious. Some estimate of confidence in the judgment is also owed the family by the physician. Thus, "I have begun to have some (moderate, strong, severe) reservations about the potential effects of feeding here. His pain (breathlessness, potential for further hemorrhage) is relentlessly mounting." When the medical formulation is "I cannot in conscience recommend them," the family benefits from hearing it. By communicating this, the doctor fulfills the medical part of the care contract: to state as specifically as possible the medical judgment of risks and benefits likely to follow initiation or continuation of a medical treatment. Families may naturally say, "We want to save him as long as possible, doctor; even a little life is something precious to cling to." A sympathetic reply would be, "I understand how dear he is to you and only wish I could make him better. Since that is no longer possible, as his physician I must examine every treatment suggested for him in hopes that it will benefit him. I want only the best for him. I am opposed to this treatment because it seems to guarantee him only more suffering."

Hydration.   Often we assume that hydration is essential for comfort, even when caloric intake is not. However, this should not be taken for granted. Dehydration often produces little discomfort, especially among terminally ill patients in whom the cause of inadequate fluid intake is advanced debility and/or altered mental status. Unless the patient is vomiting or the cancer and its treatment directly prevents the passage of liquids into the intestines, the development of dehydration often reflects "poor intake" brought about by general weakness, drowsiness, and so on. Such patients may still experience thirst, but the other sequelae of dehydration—postural hypotension, poor skin turgor, and anorexia (especially in the case of hyponatremic dehydration) or fatigue and mental-status changes—do not commonly produce discomfort.

Thirst and a dry mouth can usually be alleviated by simple mouth care, especially lubrication. Thirst may also be relieved by amounts of water (taken by mouth) that are much smaller than those required to reverse dehydration significantly. Thus, IV rehydration may not be necessary as a comfort measure for many patients, especially those for whom the prolongation of life is not a goal. Its usefulness as a comfort measure is overrated. It will prolong the life of some patients, and may at times be desirable for improving alertness and energy. The patient who is generally well but cannot swallow or retain enough liquids to compensate for current fluid losses will generally benefit from enteral or parenteral fluid administration and, perhaps, nutrition.

Substituted judgment. Substituted judgment is the judgment given by one person for an incompetent person. It is called "substituted" because it is meant to convey what the incompetent person would have wanted in this situation, not what his family or guardian would want. Family members may not understand this. The physician can explain the concept and ask whether the patient ever made any comments on what he would want were he comatose or in the present circumstances: "You or I may want something different for him, but it is his wish we'd really like to know."

No family member wants to think a treatment decision is made because everyone just "gives up" on the patient. Since this is never a legitimate reason, a thoughtful review can emphasize how the doctor and family did not give up. The family may start this dialogue with the question, "How do you really know that he won't get better?" The best answer spells out the flesh-and-blood specifics of treatments, responses, complications, and the turning points that marked the patient's deterioration. For example, one answer could be as follows:

> That's an excellent question, one I've asked myself repeatedly. Remember how 2½ years ago when he was robustly healthy, he had a seizure and we found his astrocytoma? The neurosurgeon removed most of his right frontal lobe, and he then received 6000 rads of radiation therapy to his brain and a course of CCNU [lomustine]. Remember how a year later he still rated himself as "95% effective" and continued to do better than we ever predicted, until last summer, when he just seemed to lose all his pep? It was then the CT [computed tomography] scan showed dilated ventricles, and those lumbar punctures were done to remove spinal fluid, but it didn't help. By September, the neurologists concluded that he had "radiation dementia," and much to all our dismay, he continued to decline. By October, he was incontinent and

deaf and speechless. Even then they told us there was "little to offer" for treatment.

That was 4 months ago, and you have been absolutely heroic about caring for him at home. He had been eating when fed until 3 months ago, when we noticed he had trouble swallowing and developed aspiration pneumonia. That cleared with antibiotics. We put in that feeding tube, but he got pneumonia again last month. Again he cleared with antibiotics. Now he has pneumonia again. That is why we must review the wisdom of what we do to him. But this also reviews for you my perspective and that of the consultants who have seen him; all of us agree he won't get better.

Reviews of illness are particularly important for all individuals involved in the discussion of treatment limitation.

Taking responsibility for decisions to limit treatment is burdensome for all involved, including the physician. Anxiety may cause him to present his opinion in such a way that the family feels that all or undue responsibility has been placed on them. Shortly after a 16-year-old boy was officially pronounced brain dead, the family physician said to the youth's parents: "Well, it's up to you. We can disconnect the respirator now or continue for a little longer." Although the only humane treatment of the dead is provision of dignified passage to burial or cremation, this family interpreted the doctor (who later said that they quoted him incorrectly) as requesting that they "sign the death warrant" for their son. This rather extreme example illustrates how useful it is for the family to hear the physician's explicit opinion. "For my part, I can't in conscience recommend intubating her if she deteriorates further, but I'd want to know if she'd disagree with that," is the sort of statement that aids in the dialogue with a family.

Generally, families are quite sensible about limiting treatment, especially when they are well-informed. Moreover, they tend to be grateful for the care and concern shown them and are rewarding to deal with. Conflict is part of life, however, and can also appear as death approaches. When vehement protest about treatment limitation comes from a family member who has lived for the past several years emotionally (and often geographically) remote from the patient, and the protest is at variance with the wishes of the rest of the family, the behavior is usually pathologic, based on long-standing conflict with the patient. Such a relative may present with disruptive, hostile complaints meant to convey to the world what a devoted son (or brother) he has been, as demonstrated by the extremes he will go to "save" the patient. Even for a psychiatrist, these patients are almost impossible to deal with on an individual basis. A meeting with the entire family will most efficiently clarify the discrepancy in family opinion and make it much more difficult for this remote member to misrepresent family wishes. One might open such a meeting with the following:

> I'm pleased that we could all meet so that we can discuss what course of treatment will ensure the very best for Mrs Jones. It is very helpful that you are here, too, Mr Jones. You would not have come all this distance if you, too, were not very concerned that your mother get the best possible treatment. Now let me review the course of her illness and where we stand. . . .

The request to accelerate death. For some patients and families, death's arrival seems painfully delayed. Even when relatively pain-free, a patient may feel that life is so diminished as to be an imposition rather than a blessing. What can be done for the patient who says, "I want to die now"? A 42-year-old unmarried businessman with recurrent lymphosarcoma had specified to his physician that he preferred comfort measures to further aggressive attempts to slow the progression of his disease. Pleural effusions had been tapped on three occasions to relieve his shortness of breath. A fourth was accepted and performed during an office visit, after which the patient said, "I am quite comfortable at this point. I'd like you to help me die as soon as possible."

His doctor asked whether he had anything specific in mind. Explaining that he tolerated disability and dependency poorly and that he had put all affairs in meticulous order for death, he added that he had assumed physicians had ways to accelerate death in a comfortable and dignified manner. "How would your family view this?" asked his doctor. His parents were dead, and his only sibling, a younger sister, was fully sympathetic—as were his network of friends, a small but devoted group who had impressed the office nurse by their support and availability throughout the patient's illness. The patient was not satisfied that in the future a new pleural effusion or other mediastinal complications might be allowed to progress while he was kept adequately comfortable with morphine, even though the morphine itself might somewhat hasten the moment of death. "Can't you just inject enough morphine to guarantee a rapid death before I ever get to that point?" His physician expressed sympathy for the patient's fears of an uncomfortable or undignified death, then stated her own limits in treatment: that she liberally gave medicine for comfort but would not administer any agent to induce death. Expressing irritation, the patient left but returned to the dialogue in subsequent visits.

The physician noted that the patient refused to bring in his sister or any close friends for discussion of the point, that he denied being suicidal or depressed (nor was he clinically depressed), and that he never took an overdose of his hydromorphone, of which by her calculation he had about 100 tablets. Nor would he consult any other physician, including, in particular, the psychiatrist she recommended. This she suggested after he asked her about a potassium chloride injection, pointing out to him, "I know this is very difficult for you. You have coped superbly—in fact, I have no idea whether I myself could cope half as well were I in your situation. Because it is a matter of continuing to cope, I'd like you to see one of my colleagues, a psychiatrist, who has helped others to get the most out of their coping skills." When he refused, she explored another option. "You probably feel that my treatment limitations are only another burden to bear. Would you like to see another doctor?" "Do you know any doctors who inject potassium chloride for dying patients?" he asked. "No," she replied, "but there are many good oncologists who could review your treatments to see if there is anything I could do better." "I don't want another doctor," he said, confirming his positive attachment to her, which she had felt all along. "The way I look at this as your physician," she said, "is that the illness, like so many things in this world, is bigger than both of us. I am only a physician. Society, wisely, I think, does not license me to kill, even out of motives of mercy. But I have become quite good at minimizing discomforts associated with these illnesses, and I would very much like to remain available to you as each new difficulty presents itself."

The physician in the foregoing example modeled a response when confronted by the request to accelerate death. She stated her own treatment limitations humbly and honestly; explored the meaning of the request in terms of the patient's family, depression, and suicide; suggested psychiatric consultation to decrease emotional distress and increase coping efficiency; was open to another opinion; expressed admiration for the patient's coping ability; and reaffirmed her desire to help, her ability to minimize suffering, and her intention to remain available to the patient (and family) for each difficulty as it would arise. Her soft answers averted his anger at not being able to control her. Her openness helped to explore all the implications of his request. Perhaps most important, her restatement of her commitment to caring for him diminished his fears of abandonment, loss of respect, and ultimate failure to cope with his illness.

DOCUMENTATION

Whenever decisions are made about treatment limitation, the medical record should include an explicit statement of the reasons that led to them, the patient's comprehension of and agreement with them, and the understanding and reactions of other persons significant to the patient, usually the family. The more explicitly this is done, the better the record. Despite contemporary fears of litigation for neglect, malpractice, and homicide, complete honesty is recommended. In the life-and-death struggles with advanced cancer, no therapeutic stone is left unturned to minimize harm and maximize comfort for the patient. Nothing with regard to this goal need be hidden or apologized for. Failure to make orders explicit on the order sheet only jeopardizes care of the patient.

AS DEATH APPROACHES

Treatment team members often hear the question, "What will death be like? How will it come?" Sometimes it is quite possible to forecast the mode of death, as by infection, hemorrhage, or slow lapse into coma. Often behind these questions is the fear that the death will be violent, painful, or humiliating. Since this is usually not the case, it helps to reassure patient and family of this. Cicely Saunders' gentle image of cancer death has been helpful to many: "It is like a candle going out."[7] Management of this phase of illness is described in detail elsewhere in this volume (see chapter 17). Once a decision to limit treatment is made, however, it is important to help the family realize that preparing for a comfortable death is the major task at hand.[8] No further trips to the emergency ward means that we now must cope with the life-threatening process at home. If one stops at the limitation decision itself (eg, no more antibiotics), the family and patient may not have progressed to this next concern: What will they do to cope with the infection? What can they expect? How are they to handle it? Reassurance that the team is as available to them now as it was during the more aggressive treatment phases is essential.

Decisions can change. Death is a natural process, and the course toward it can be punctuated by transient improvement. If a patient recovers spontaneously from aspiration pneumonia without antibiotics, it does not mean the decision to withhold them was "wrong." It was the best possible at the time. Patients and families can be warned ahead of time of these realities. The mature and noble vigil to which health-care professionals commit themselves in the care of their dying patients can be adjusted to these changes with no less equanimity and thoughtfulness than has been shown throughout the illness.

REFERENCES

1. The Haemmerli affair: Is passive euthanasia murder?, editorial. *Science* 1975; 190:1271–1275.

2. Cassem NH: Controversies surrounding the hopelessly ill patient. *Linacre Q* 1975; 42:89–98.
3. Slater E: New horizons in medical ethics. Wanted—a new approach. *Br Med J* 1973; 2:285–286.
4. Cassem EH: Appropriate treatment limits in advanced cancer, in Billings JA (ed): *Outpatient Management of Advanced Cancer.* Philadelphia, JB Lippincott Co, 1985, pp 139–151.
5. Optimum care for hopelessly ill patients: A report of the Critical Care Committee of the Massachusetts General Hospital. *N Engl J Med* 1976; 295:364–366.
6. Jackson DL, Youngner S: Patient autonomy and "death with dignity." *N Engl J Med* 1979; 301:404–408.
7. Saunders C: Care of the dying: The problem of euthanasia. *Nursing Times* 1959; 55(pts 1–6):960–961, 994–995, 1031–1032, 1067–1069, 1091–1092, 1129–1130.
8. Wanzer SH, Adelstein SJ, Cranford RE, et al: The physician's responsibility toward hopelessly ill patients. *N Engl J Med* 1984; 310:955–959.

Index

Obesity, 38
Obsessive–compulsive disorder, 156
Ocular disturbance, 25
Olfactory hallucinations, 22
Ontological denier, 329
Opiate
  barbiturate overdose and, 30
  emergency room patient and,
    434–435
  mixed drug addiction and,
    37–39
  withdrawal and, 34
  see also Narcotic
Oral contraceptive, 567
Organic affective disorder, 228, 248
Organic brain dysfunction
  antipsychotic drugs and, 510
  somatic symptoms of, 129
  suicide and, 273
Organic psychosis, 52
Orientation, 110
Orthostatic hypotension, 239–240
Out–of–body experiences,
  375–376
Outpatient psychotherapy, 5
Overdose, drug
  barbiturate, 29–30
  suicide and, 272
  see also Drug abuse
Over-the-counter medication, 555
Oxazepam, 503
  half–life and dosage range of, 502
  ICU patient and, 364–365
Oxycodone, 441
Oxygenation, cerebral, 425

Pain, 42–68
  burn patient and, 440
  chronic, 54–56
  consultant and, 48–50
  education and, 64–65
  electroconvulsive therapy and, 66
  hypnosis and, 65
  intolerance to, 81–82
  intractable, 413
  measurement of, 47
  medication for, 58–63
  methadone and, 36–37
  nature of, 42–44
  pathologic vs experimental, 44–46

peripheral versus central, 46–47
placebo and, 47–48
postoperative, 74
psychiatric conditions and, 50–54
psychodynamic psychotherapy and,
  65
psychogenic, 141–142
psychosomatic and, 488
schizophrenic patient and, 222
surgery for, 66–67
talking and listening and, 57–58
Palsy, supranuclear, 95–96
Pancreatic carcinoma, 233
Panic disorder, 498, 520
  anxiety and, 156
  benzodiazepines and, 503–504
  medical illness and, 171–172
  somatic symptoms and, 168–170
  surgery and, 77–78
  treatment of, 174–178
Panic mechanism, 157
Paralysis
  external recti and, 25
  spinal cord injury and, see Spinal
    cord injury
Paranoia
  alcoholic and, 17, 24
  amphetamine intoxication and, 38
Parenteral nutrition, 631–632
Paresis, 25
Pargyline hydrochloride, 556
Parkinson's disease
  dementia and, 95–96
  depressions and, 235
  drug interactions and, 546
Paroxysmal pain, 64
Partial seizure
  conversion disorder and, 139
  mental state changes and, 105
Passive-aggressive patient, 292–293
Pathologic anxiety, 154–155
Pathologic dependency, 318–320
  borderline patient and, 199–201
Pathologic pain, 44–46
Patient
  bill of rights for, 609–611
  civil rights of, 594–596
  group intervention and, 583–584
  selection of, for transplantation
    and, 73–74